AF322862

BASIC ISSUES IN PSYCHOPATHOLOGY

Basic Issues in Psychopathology

Edited by
CHARLES G. COSTELLO

THE GUILFORD PRESS
New York London

Library of Congress Cataloging-in-Publication Data

Basic issues in psychopathology / [edited by] Charles G. Costello.
    p. cm.
   Includes bibliographical references and index.
   ISBN 0-89862-139-9
   1. Psychiatry.   I. Costello, Charles G., 1929–
   [DNLM: 1. Psychopathology.   WM 100 B3105]
  RC454.B366   1993
  616.89—dc20
  DNLM/DLC
  for Library of Congress   92-48972
                                      CIP

Contributors

William Avison, PhD, Associate Professor of Sociology, University of Western Ontario, London, Ontario N6A 5C2

Paul Bebbington, FRCPsych, Reader in Social and Epidemiological Psychiatry, MRC Social and Community Psychiatry Unit, Institute of Psychiatry, De Crespigny Park, London, UK SE5 8AF

Richard R. Bootzin, PhD, Professor of Psychology, University of Arizona, Tucson, AZ 85721

Ronald Cobb, BA, doctoral candidate, Department of Psychology, 111-21st Avenue South, Vanderbilt University, Nashville, TN 37420

Charles G. Costello, PhD, Professor of Psychology, University of Calgary, 2500 University Drive, NW, Calgary, Alberta T2N 1N4

Richard A. Depue, PhD, Professor of Human Development, NG21 MVR Hall, Cornell University, Ithaca, NY 14853-7601

Ian H. Gotlib, PhD, Professor of Psychology and Psychiatry, 102 Swift Hall, Northwestern University, Evanston, IL 60208

Lisa Grencavage, BA, doctoral candidate, Department of Psychology, University of Arizona, Tucson, AZ 85721

Richard Harrington, MD, MPhil, MRCPsych, Senior Lecturer in Child and Adolescent Psychiatry, University of Birmingham, Queen Elizabeth Hospital, Mindelsohn Way, Birmingham, UK B15 2QZ

Steven D. Hollon, PhD, Professor of Psychology, 111-21st Avenue South, Vanderbilt University, Nashville, TN 37420

Daniel N. Klein, PhD, Associate Professor of Psychology, State University of New York, Stony Brook, NY 11794-2500

Robin Murray, FRCPsych, Professor of Psychological Medicine, Kings College Hospital and Institute of Psychiatry, De Crespigny Park, London, UK SE5 8AF

Lawrence P. Riso, BA, doctoral candidate, Department of Psychology, State University of New York at Stony Brook, Stony Brook, NY 11794-2500

Varda Shoham, PhD, Associate Professor of Psychology, University of Arizona, Tucson, AZ 85721

Geraldine Strathdee, MRCPsych, Consultant Psychiatrist, Maudsley Hospital, De Crespigny Park, London, UK, SE5 8AF

Graham Thornicroft, MRCPsych, Senior Lecturer, Institute of Psychiatry, De Crespigny Park, London, UK, SE5 8AF

Catherine Walsh, MRCPsych, Research Psychiatrist, Genetics Section, Institute of Psychiatry, De Crespigny Park, London, UK SE5 8AF

David H. Zald, BA, doctoral candidate, Department of Psychology, Elliot Hall, 75 E. River Road, University of Minnesota, Minneapolis, MN 55455

Contents

III. THE COURSES AND CONSEQUENCES OF PSYCHOPATHOLOGY

BASIC ISSUES IN PSYCHOPATHOLOGY

1

Introduction:
Conceptual and Methodological Issues in the Sciences of Psychopathology

CHARLES G. COSTELLO

The title of this introductory chapter refers to the *sciences* of psychopathology rather than the *science* of psychopathology because psychopathology is not one specific form of scientific endeavor. Rather, it is the name given to a scholarly activity that is concerned with the full understanding of behavioral and experiential dysfunctions and that, in attempting to achieve that goal, is in what Healy (1990) has called "the business of providing patterns (frameworks) into which the data of other sciences—biology, psychology, sociology, anthropology, ethology and others—can be fitted" (p. *xiv*). The best psychopathology framework in which to place the data from the contributory sciences remains unknown, and this book will not attempt to argue for any one framework. But it is hoped that the discussions of a number of basic issues with which these sciences have to grapple will be a step toward revealing what the most appropriate framework might be.

Some of the problems specific to each of the contributing sciences are discussed by the authors who have written the chapters of this book. In this introductory chapter I shall discuss some broad conceptual and methodological issues that arise from the subject matter of the sciences of psychopathology and with which all of the contributing sciences have to grapple to some degree. I shall discuss (1) the intricate nature of syndromes, (2) the apparent indistinguishability of some of the phenomena that are currently investigated, (3) the incontrovertible nature of some of the causes of behavioral and experiential disorders that are currently being proposed, and (4) difficulties presented by the interrelationships between the large number of variables that are probably involved in the causes of disorder.

THE INTRICATE NATURE OF SYNDROMES

Most research that is conducted with humans and that seeks the causes of disorders involves the assignment of subjects to diagnostic categories, the core of which is syndromes. This presents the researcher with the following difficult problems.

The Questionable Validity of Psychiatric Diagnoses

It is generally believed that the development of standardized psychiatric interviews (e.g., Present State Examination [PSE], Wing, Cooper, & Sartorius, 1974; Diagnostic Interview Schedule [DIS], Robins, Helzer, Croughan, & Ratcliff, 1981) and diagnostic systems (e.g., ID-CATEGO, Wing et al., 1974; DSM-III-R, American Psychiatric Association, 1987) have resulted in reliable psychiatric diagnoses. In actuality, the evidence for such reliability is questionable because of the methodological weaknesses of most of the studies that have been done. In any case, whatever one's view of the reliability of psychiatric diagnoses, there is general agreement that there is no good evidence for their concurrent, construct, or predictive validity (see Costello, 1992a, 1993b, in press-b, for more detailed reviews of studies of the reliability and validity of psychiatric diagnoses).

The designers of psychiatric interviews and diagnostic systems are constantly trying to improve them when new research data or clinical observations suggest the need for modifications. But this, too, presents a problem because then one cannot confidently relate the findings from studies separated by even quite short periods of time. Although it seems that, in the long run, the progress of science is not a simple function of the accumulation of empirical data (Kuhn, 1970), the comparability of data from studies conducted within short time periods would seem to be necessary.

Inadequate Measurement of Symptoms

Symptoms are the building blocks of syndromes, and syndromes constitute the cores of psychiatric diagnoses. But when one tries to determine if a syndrome is present on the basis of a psychiatric interview, the measurement of each symptom is based on a short answer to a short question or on brief, unsystematized observations. Such patently inadequate measurement casts doubt on their validity, and some data suggest that such doubt is justified. For instance, Mazure, Nelson, and Price (1986) examined the concordance between the ratings of symptoms of depression based on observation and interrogation during a semistructured interview administered to 31 depressed inpatients and the ratings of the corresponding behaviors observed by nurses during a concurrent 3-day period. The four symptom ratings based on observation of behavior during interviews were significantly correlated with the nurses' ratings: lack of responsiveness, $r = .695$; motor retardation, $r = .528$; agitation, $r = .476$; and speech retardation, $r = .471$. But only 5 of the 12 symptom ratings made by the interviewers on the basis of patients' reports were significantly correlated with the nurses' ratings. Four of the seven symptoms, for which the correlations were not significant, were difficulty falling asleep, $r = .100$; early morning awakening, $r = .337$; loss of energy, $r = .275$; and decreased concentration, $r = .148$. These four symptoms are generally considered important in the diagnosis of mood disorders.

Szabadi, Bradshaw, and Besson (1976) have presented data that illustrate the questionable validity of interview assessments of symptoms. They found that, although speech retardation in the form of speech pause time was detectable by objective measures in their depressed patients, it was not observable by trained clinicians. But expecting interviewers to assess speed of speech accurately in addition to all the other characteristics of behavior they are expected to assess is probably asking too much of them. It is also probably asking too much to expect patients to be able to give accurate reports concerning their motor behavior. Lee Robins, who has long labored to develop good psychiatric interviews, has commented in this respect:

> It is not common to have thought about whether one has moved or talked more slowly than normal for a period of two weeks or more. To answer that question one has to decide within the very brief interval that social convention allows between question and response what is normal for oneself, whether there was ever a period different from that normal pattern, and how long that different period lasted. (1989, p. 62)

Research demonstrating the questionable validity of measurements of all of the central symptoms of depression and schizophrenia have been reviewed by the contributors to Costello (1993a, in press-a).

It could be argued that the validity of self-reports of symptoms should not be assessed in terms of how well they predict observable behavior. Lang (1979) has demonstrated that self-reports of fear, behavioral manifestations of fear, and physiological indicators of fear are not highly intercorrelated and has argued that they should be treated as independent manifestations that must be investigated in and for themselves. But if we decide to treat the self-reports of symptoms of disorder as data that are likely to be valuable in and for themselves, irrespective of their correlations with observable behavior, some other way of testing their validity must be found. Furthermore, we will have to remain aware that the self-reports provide only partial information about an individual's problem.

Problems of Misclassification and Confounding

Even when one has good reason to believe that a particular symptom is usually one of the symptoms in a syndrome that forms part of a particular diagnosis, there are problems if one attempts to investigate the symptom in research that uses the diagnosis as the entry point. For instance, Persons (1986) has noted that many researchers whose goal is to test whether a postulated psychological or biological mechanism is responsible for disorders in thinking will test the hypothesis that the mechanism is present in people with a diagnosis of schizophrenia and absent in nonschizophrenics. She has argued that this research strategy is not likely to be successful because (1) not all schizophrenics have thought disorder, and none of the major diagnostic systems requires the presence of thought disorder for a diagnosis of schizophrenia; and (2) even when schizophrenics have thought disorder, they are only episodically so, and their thinking may not be disordered during the testing session. (See Harvey and Neale [1983] for a discussion of this literature.)

Person (1986) has also noted that any difference between schizophrenic and nonschizophrenic groups in the mechanism postulated to be responsible for thought disorder might be a function of (1) schizophrenia, (2) thought disorder, or (3) the joint effects (interaction) of schizophrenia and thought disorder. It may also be a function of some other symptom that frequently occurs along with thought disorder. The problem, of course, arises from the fact that diagnostic classes are polythetic classes, the members of which suffer from different combinations of a set of quite different symptoms that are probably functionally related in quite complex ways.

Difficulties in the Development of Animal Models of Syndromes

The manner in which the intricate and complex nature of syndromes may hinder progress in our understanding of psychopathological disorders also becomes apparent when we consider attempts to develop animal models of syndromes. The learned helplessness model of depression (Seligman, 1975), which, on the face of it, appeared promising, has not yet furthered our understanding of depression, and this may be because researchers have tried to think of the learned helplessness phenomena as constituting a model of some syndrome of depression. But none of the proposed matches between the model and any of the mood disorders has been convincing. On the basis of his extensive review of the literature, Willner (1985) concluded that it was not clear which type of depression learned helplessness models. Overmier and Hellhammer's (1988) review of essentially the same literature led them to the conclusion that learned helplessness is a model of reactive depression. Then again, Healy (1987) concluded that the evidence supported the hypothesis that learned helplessness is a model of endogenous depression.

When one moves away from syndromes and attempts to match the learned helplessness phenomena with specific symptoms of psychopathology, the matches look more promising. For instance, Overmier and Hellhammer's (1988) literature review indicated that uncontrollable shocks reduce the rate of self-stimulation at the nucleus accumbens; they suggest that the experimental procedure that produces learned helplessness might assist in understanding the symptom of anhedonia. Data obtained in research that focuses on how the learned helplessness procedure may affect the brain mechanisms involved in reward also has the advantage that it might help in the understanding of a phenomenon related to a number of psychopathological disorders, for instance, anhedonia in mood disorders and schizophrenic disorders and the reward basis of substance abuse.

INDISTINGUISHABLE CONCEPTS

The problems presented by indistinguishable concepts can be illustrated with George Brown's work on self-esteem. Brown, Andrews, Harris, Adler, and Bridge (1986), in a 12-month follow-up of 303 working-class women in Islington, a district in London, England, found that 150 of the women had a severe life event or chronic difficulty and that some of these women also had low self-esteem. Of the women with a severe life event or chronic difficulty and low self-esteem, 33% developed an onset of depression, as against 13% of the women who did not have low self-esteem. In their further analyses and discussion of the Brown et al. (1986) data in a series of four articles (Brown, Andrews, Bifulco, & Veiel, 1990; Brown, Bifulco, & Andrews, 1990a, 1990b; Brown, Bifulco, Veiel, & Andrews, 1990), Brown and his colleagues noted that the two symptoms of the Present State Examination most directly involving the self, self-depreciation and lack of self-confidence, were highly associated with their measure of low self-esteem. Two further observations suggest that the distinguishability of the concept of "low self-esteem" and the concept of "case depression" is questionable: (1) the definition of a "case depression" required only four symptoms of depression in addition to depressed mood, and (2) the examination of the prevalence of specific symptoms in Brown's Islington sample reported in Chapter 3 of this book indicated that self-depreciation was exhibited by 37% of the womens with depression and lack of confidence by 45%.

The problem of indistinguishable concepts appears in much of the research on the cognitive causes of depression. Researchers test hypotheses derived from cognitive theories such as those of Beck and Seligman, which predict that certain problems in the way people think will cause depression. The way people think is measured by instruments such as the Automatic Thoughts Questionnaire (ATQ) (Hollon & Kendall, 1980), which includes items such as the following: I'm worthless, I can't get started, and My future is bleak. But worthless feelings, lethargy, and pessimism are characteristics of depression itself.

Sullivan and D'Eon (1990), in their study of chronic pain patients, found that a measure of "catastrophizing" was positively correlated with self-reported depression. This is not surprising because the items of the catastrophizing scale are quite obviously depressotypic: I feel my life isn't worth living, I worry all the time about whether it will end, I feel I can't go on, It's terrible and I feel it's never going to get any better, It's awful and I feel that it overwhelms me, and I feel I can't stand it any more. However, further analyses indicated that although catastrophizing was significantly correlated with cognitive items on the depression scale it was not significantly correlated with somatic items after scores on the cognitive items were controlled for. Although, as Haaga (1992) has argued, the conceptual and operational confounding of catastrophizing and depression would be more convincingly demonstrated with multiple measures of these concepts, it is very likely that Sullivan and D'Eon's findings would be replicated.

Other examples of the problem of the indistinguishability of concepts include (1) the higher correlations found between measures of irrational beliefs and measures of distress than between the measures of irrational beliefs themselves (Smith & Allred, 1986; Zurawski & Smith, 1987); (2) the indistinguishability of the concepts of bodily sensations and cognitions in studies of cognitive theories of panic disorder, which has been discussed in Costello (1992b) and Chapter 8 of this book; and (3) the work of Richard Lazarus on the relationships between the frequency of daily hassles and the probability of the occurrence of ill health, including psychopathological disorders (for a recent review see Lazarus, 1990). Dohrenwend, Dohrenwend, Dodson, and Shrout (1984) pointed out that one should not be surprised to find significant associations between reports of hassles and reports of illness because these measures are confounded. Lazarus (1990) has argued that because

stress is always a product of appraisal, then some confounding between
measures of stress and illness is inevitable. It is inevitable because the
independent variable, appraised stress, is bound to contain a subjective sense
of harm, threat or challenge, which in turn overlaps with the dependent
variable of feelings of distress and self-reports of dysfunction. (p. 9)

Lazarus is not enamored of attempts to skirt this confounding by measuring life stress in an objective manner, arguing,

> there is no way to separate person and environment in the appraised person–
> environment relationship without destroying what is meant by psycholog-
> ical stress as conceived in a cognitive–relational theory. Even if totally
> objective input or output measure of stress were possible, it would, perforce,
> mean an abandonment of a cognitive–relational conceptualization and,
> therefore, would describe a totally different phenomenon. We would be
> distorting nature to fit a simpler, mythical metatheory of separable and
> antecedent and consequent variables. (p. 10)

Despite recognizing the likely importance of an individual's appraisal
of stress, one simply cannot accept the confounding of measures in
science. There are two alternatives available to us. We must either develop
new methodologies within the general framework of current scientific
practices (the nature of one these new methodologies as proposed by
Kessler [1987] is described in a later section), or we must embark on quite
different investigative procedures of the kind proposed by writers such as
Gergen (1991).

Another example of the problem of the indistinguishability of concepts can be found in the work of Dworkin (1992), who has demonstrated
that the distinction between affective deficits, supposedly negative symptoms of schizophrenia, and social deficits, supposedly different kinds of
schizophrenic symptoms, is not maintained in current measuring instruments. He pointed out, as an example, that the affective flattening subscale of the Scale for the Assessment of Negative Symptoms (SANS,
Andreasen, 1982) consists of seven symptom ratings (unchanging facial
expression, decreased spontaneous movements, paucity of expressive
gestures, poor eye contact, affective nonresponsiveness, inappropriate
affect, and lack of vocal inflections) that are based on the subject's
behavior during an interview. Dworkin commented: "When the SANS
affective flattening subscale is considered in this context, it becomes clear
that an alternative way of conceptualizing these ratings is that they are
measures of social functioning or social skills" (p. 101).

INCONTROVERTIBLE NATURE OF SOME OF THE
PROPOSED CAUSES OF DISORDER

There are causal concepts that may be distinguishable from concepts of
disorder but measure variables that are so incontrovertibly associated

with the occurrence of the disorder being investigated that the research done with them does not produce findings that are particularly enlightening. For instance, poor self-esteem, even if it can be distinguished from the concept of mood disorder, is such an incontrovertibly depressotypic concept that research on it does not point us in the direction of any genuinely new understanding of the mood disorder.

Incontrovertible concepts tend to get the researcher involved in the kind of reciprocal relationships described by George Brown and his colleagues. Noting their finding that negative interactions in close relationships, particularly with spouse and children, were significantly associated with self-esteem, Brown, Bifulco, Veiel, & Andrews (1990) wrote:

> It is obviously difficult to rule out that devaluing experiences are not the result of low self-esteem itself; and the matter is further complicated by the fact that temperamental or personality characteristics are bound to be involved in some way. Indeed the problem's so recalcitrant that there appears at present to be little hope of satisfactory solution. (p. 225)

Although there are researchers who believe that scientists must begin to investigate such reciprocal processes (e.g., Bandura, 1986; Lazarus, 1990), no generally accepted methodologies for their investigation have been developed. This is due in part to the fact that researchers are often investigating phenomena over which they have no experimental control. Under these circumstances it might be better for researchers to see how far they can get with controvertible concepts that are not as likely to get one involved in bidirectional causal processes and are not as likely to be artificial concepts.

It may be that the concepts that are particularly likely to be so enmeshed are incontrovertible concepts. As I have argued elsewhere (Costello, 1992c), although painstaking research such as that reported by Brown and his colleagues provides us with good descriptions of the sad dance of gloomy dispositions, gloomy events, and gloomy illnesses, we are still left in the dark as to what is at the root of it all. Perhaps researchers will need to look for the causes of disorder in places other than incontrovertible vulnerabilities such as an individual's negative evaluations of the self and incontrovertible stresses such as unpleasant life events, difficulties, and unsupportive spouses. These negative features of an individual's personality and life may simply be further signs of the sick person's misfortune or, at the very most, simply triggers for the release of the proximal cause of the disorder.

Other examples of incontrovertible concepts are negative self-schemas where the emphasis is on the negative content rather than on some hypothesized pathogenic structure of the schema (see review by Kuiper & Olinger, 1986, and Chapter 8 of this book), rigid and inappropriate standards for evaluating self-worth (Kuiper & Olinger, 1989), and hopelessness (Abramson, Metalsky, & Alloy, 1989). Examples of controvertible concepts that have been hypothesized to be among the causes of disorder are poor consolidation of self-schemas (Kuiper & Olinger, 1986), lack of complexity in self-structures (Linville, 1987), and self-focused attention (Ingram, 1990; see also the useful debate in Pyszczynski, Greenberg, Hamilton, & Nix, 1991; and Ingram, 1991)

One of the reasons why researchers prefer to investigate a disorder as it occurs naturally, despite the fact that this approach so often involves incontrovertible concepts, is that such research has greater ecological validity than laboratory research (see Maher, 1991, for a discussion of this issue). But there are times when an emphasis on ecological validity can make it difficult to determine which theory concerning the cause of a phenomenon is the better one. Chow (1987) has discussed this problem and presented an illustrative analogy, which, with slight modifications, goes as follows: Two alternative explanations as to why a road is wet are (1) it has rained and (2) a city crew has washed it. To test the relative validity of the explanations, one may decide to examine streets near the road or examine the leaves on nearby trees. If one is concerned about ecological validity, one may decide to examine the streets because wet streets are likely to be considered ecologically more valid than wet leaves for deciding whether it has rained on the road or a city crew has washed it down. However, both theories can account for wet streets readily, whereas the theory that it has rained is a more likely explanation of the wet leaves. In other words, requiring that the phenomenon investigated be similar to the phenomenon to be explained may diminish the usefulness of the investigation.

COMPLEXITY OF THE MECHANISMS INVOLVED IN THE CAUSES OF DISORDER

Noting their finding that poor self-esteem in combination with negative interactions in close relationships was significantly associated with (1) the occurrence in a 12-month period of severe events arising out of chronic difficulties and severe events that were related to role conflicts and (2) lack of crisis support at the time of occurrence of the severe event, Brown and associates (1990a) wrote: "Psychological and environmental factors relevant for the onset of depression therefore tend to be closely associated and while it would go too far to see the environment and self-esteem as different sides of the same coin it may make little practical sense to worry overmuch about giving one or other causal priority" (p. 242). There is a recognition here that some of the concepts in the best of current research are enmeshed in such a manner that our attempts to compartmentalize them produce artificial concepts.

Reports of the relationships between depression and hypothesized psychosocial causes, such as deficiencies in social supports, unemployment, having a number of small children at home, the occurrence of unpleasant life events, and loss of self-esteem, usually present the findings for each psychosocial variable separately. This would not pose a problem if one could assume that the psychosocial variables are not systematically related to one another. However, a recent supplementary analysis by Champion (1990) of data reported in seven community studies indicated that one of the psychosocial variables that has most consistently been found to be related to depression, that is, lack of intimacy with a spouse, is also significantly correlated with the occurrence of an unpleasant event or the presence of a chronic life difficulty. Such systematic relationships between the postulated causes make it well-nigh impossible in cross-sectional studies to identify the causal mechanisms and even make it extremely difficult to do so in longitudinal studies.

Even if we take into account the intercorrelations between our psychosocial variables in a multivariate analysis of the data, we will probably include only a small proportion of the relevant causal variables, and statisticians have argued that, when we have incomplete control of the variables involved, our estimates of the degree to which one independent variable has an effect on the dependent variable is no more accurate than an estimate of effects excluding control variables entirely (Kessler, 1987). It is sometimes assumed that if one is concerned with the effects of a psychosocial variable that has a discrete time of occurrence such as being fired from a job, and if one can also control for levels of disorder before the psychosocial occurrence, then one can obtain an unbiased estimate of the effects of that psychosocial variable in producing disorder. This is certainly true where initial level of disorder is the only variable that is significantly correlated with the psychosocial variable and the final level of disorder. Even here, as Kessler (1987) has pointed out, one may have the problem of time specification, in other words, the problem of when to measure the initial level of disorder. Kessler gives the following example:

> Imagine a situation where a worker's emotional functioning deteriorated rapidly in an acute episode of major depressive disorder and his supervisor fires him. A prediction equation which assessed baseline levels of emotional functioning several years earlier would totally miss the process of selection into unemployment and would overestimate wildly the impact of unemployment on emotional functioning. (1987, p. 120)

It is not too surprising to find that there is a reciprocal relationship between the putative psychosocial causes of a disorder and the disorder itself. Hammen (1991) in a 1-year longitudinal study found that women with recurrent unipolar depression are exposed to more stress than normal women because of the higher rates of events to which they contributed rather than because of fateful events to which they had not contributed. Obviously, the probability of such reciprocal relationships is even greater in the case of subjectively measured psychosocial variables such as an individual's appraisal of available social support. The adequacy of social support as perceived by an individual may have an effect on the individual's level of disorder, but the level of disorder may also have an effect on the appraisal of social support. Kessler (1983) has described the use of structural equation models to analyze such reciprocal causation. Unfortunately, the procedure requires that one can objectively measure a psychosocial variable that we can assume to have a causal effect on disorder through the intervening influence of the subjective psychosocial variable, and it may not be always evident as to how this is to be done. Kessler provides the following example of a situation where it can be done: If we wish to determine the effects of felt job strain on an individual's emotional condition, we have to take into consideration that the emotional condition probably has a causal effect on the felt job strain. Structural equation models can be applied in this situation because we can obtain objective measures of job strain (e.g., amount of heavy work, the complexity of the work, amount of supervision, etc.). Furthermore, we can safely assume that any causal effects of these job strains on an individual's emotional condition will be mediated by the subjective strain. If the reciprocal causation between the subjective psychosocial variable and the individual's level of emotional functioning is to be teased out, it is also necessary to include in the structural equation objective measures of psychosocial variables that do not have an effect on the objective underpinnings of the subjective psychosocial variable of interest and instead have an effect on that subjective psychosocial variable only through its effects on the level of emotional functioning. In the present example of job strain, one might have objective measures of stress (e.g., serious illness or recent death in the family) that do not have any effect on the objective measures of job strain but have an effect on perceived job strain through their effects on the individual's emotional condition.

But it may be difficult to find suitable objective indicators for some of the most commonly investigated psychosocial variables, such as adequacy of social support and marital intimacy. For instance, we can objectively measure variables such as the extensiveness and density of social networks, but we cannot assume that they are the objective underpinnings of the perceived adequacy of social support, and we cannot assume that any causal effects these objective social support variables have on emotional functioning are mediated by the individual's perception of the adequacy of social support. It may also be difficult to find objective psychosocial variables that have an effect on the subjective psychosocial variable through the effects on the individual's level of emotional functioning but do not have an effect on the objective psychosocial variable. In the present example, even if we had reason to believe that the objectively measured variables of social network extensiveness and density could be considered the underpinnings of the subjective appraisal of social support, one could not safely assume that objectively measured variables such as serious illness and death in the family had no effect on the social network characteristics.

CONCLUSIONS

Progress in the sciences of psychopathology is more likely if researchers (1) avoid the hazards of working with intricate and chameleonic psychiatric diagnoses and focus on specific symptoms of disorder, (2) ensure that the variables they are measuring are distinguishable from one another, (3) test hypotheses that are likely to lead to more information than hypotheses that incorporate incontrovertible correlates of disorder, and (4) pay more than lip service to the problems of disentangling reciprocal causes in human behavior.

REFERENCES

Abramson, L. Y., Metalsky, G. I., & Alloy, L. B. (1989). Hopelessness depression: A theory-based subtype of depression. *Psychological Review, 96,* 358–372.

American Psychiatric Association. (1987). *Diagnostic and statistical manual of mental disorders* (3rd ed., rev.). Washington, DC: Author.

Andreasen, L. N. C. (1982). Negative symptoms in schizophrenia: Definition and reliability. *Archives of General Psychiatry, 39,* 784–788.

Bandura, A. (1986). *Social foundations of thought and action: A social cognitive theory.* Englewood Cliffs, NJ: Prentice-Hall.

Brown, G. W., Andrews, B., Bifulco, A., & Veiel, H. (1990). Self esteem and depression: I. Measurement issues and prediction of onset. *Social Psychiatry and Psychiatric Epidemiology, 25,* 200–209.

Brown, G. W., Andrews, B., Harris, T. O., Adler, Z., & Bridge, L. (1986). Social support, self-esteem and depression. *Psychological Medicine, 16,* 813–831.

Brown, G. W., Bifulco, A., & Andrews, B. (1990a). Self-esteem and depression: III. Aetiological issues. *Social Psychiatry and Psychiatric Epidemiology, 25,* 235–243.

Brown, G. W., Bifulco, A., & Andrews, B. (1990b). Self-esteem and depression: IV. Effect on course and recovery. *Social Psychiatry and Psychiatric Epidemiology, 25,* 244–249.

Brown, G. W., Bifulco, A., Veiel, H. O. F., & Andrews, B. (1990). Self-esteem and depression: II. Social correlates of self-esteem. *Social Psychiatry and Psychiatric Epidemiology, 25,* 225–234.

Champion, L. (1990). The relationship between social vulnerability and the occurrence of severely threatening life events. *Psychological Medicine, 20,* 157–161.

Chow, S. L. (1987). Science, ecological validity and experimentation. *Journal for the Theory of Social Behaviour, 17,* 181–194.

Costello, C. G. (1992a). Research on symptoms versus research on syndromes: Arguments in favour of allocating more research time to the study of symptoms. *British Journal of Psychiatry, 160,* 304–308.

Costello, C. G. (1992b). Problems in recent tests of two cognitive theories of panic. *Behaviour Research and Therapy, 30,* 1–5.

Costello, C. G. (1992c). Conceptual problems in current research on cognitive vulnerability to psychopathology. *Cognitive Therapy and Research, 16,* 379–390.

Costello, C. G. (1993a). *Symptoms of depression.* New York: Wiley.

Costello, C. G. (1993b). Advantages of the symptom approach to depression. In C. G. Costello (Ed.), *Symptoms of depression* (pp. 1–21). New York: Wiley.

Costello, C. G. (in press-a). *Symptoms of schizophrenia.* New York: Wiley.

Costello, C. G. (in press-b). Advantages of the symptom approach to schizophrenia. In C. G. Costello (Ed.), *Symptoms of schizophrenia.* New York: Wiley.

Dohrenwend, B. S., Dohrenwend, B. P., Dodson, M., & Shrout, P. E. (1984). Symptoms, hassles, social supports and life events: The problem of confounded measures. *Journal of Abnormal Psychology, 93,* 222–230.

Dworkin, R. H. (1992). Affective deficits and social deficits in schizophrenia: What's what? *Schizophrenia Bulletin, 18,* 59–64.

Gergen, K. J. (1991). Emerging challenges for theory and psychology. *Theory and Psychology, 1,* 13–35.

Haaga, D. A. F. (1992). Catastrophizing, confounds, and depression: A comment on Sullivan and D'Eon (1990). *Journal of Abnormal Psychology, 101,* 206–207.

Hammen, C. (1991). Generation of stress in the course of unipolar depression. *Journal of Abnormal Psychology, 100,* 555–561.

Harvey, P. D., & Neale, J. M. (1983). The specificity of thought disorder to schizophrenia: Research methods in their historical perspective. In B. Maher (Ed.), *Progress in experimental personality research* (Vol. 12). New York: Academic Press.

Healy, D. (1987). The comparative psychopathology of affective disorders in animals and humans. *Journal of Psychopharmacology, 1,* 193–210.

Healy, D. (1990). *The suspended revolution: Psychiatry and psychotherapy re-examined.* London: Faber and Faber.

Hollon, S., & Kendall, P. (1980). Cognitive self-statements in depression: Development of an automatic thoughts questionnaire. *Cognitive Therapy & Research, 4,* 383–396.

Ingram, R. E. (1990). Depressive cognition: Models, mechanisms, and methods. In R. E. Ingram (Ed.), *Contemporary psychological approaches to depression* (pp. 169–195). New York: Plenum Press.

Ingram, R. E. (1991). Tilting at windmills: A response to Pyszcynski, Greenberg, Hamilton and Nix. *Psychological Bulletin, 110,* 544–550.

Kessler, R. C. (1983). Methodological issues in the study of psychosocial stress. In H. B. Kaplan (Ed.), *Psychosocial stress: Trends in theory and research* (pp. 267–341). New York: Academic Press.

Kessler, R. C. (1987). The interplay of research design strategies and data analysis procedures in evaluating the effects of stress on health. In S. V. Kasl and C. L. Cooper (Eds.), *Stress and health: Issues in research methodology* (pp. 113–140). New York: Wiley.

Kuhn, T. S. (1970). *The structure of scientific revolutions* (2nd ed., Vol. 2, No. 2). *International Encyclopedia of Unified Science.* Chicago: University of Chicago Press.

Kuiper, N. A., & Olinger, L. J. (1986). Dysfunctional attitudes and a self-worth contingency model of depression. In P. C. Kendall (Ed.), *Advances in cognitive–behavioral research and therapy, Vol. 5* (pp. 115–142). New York: Academic Press.

Kuiper, N. A., & Olinger, L. J. (1989). Stress and cognitive vulnerability for depression: A self-worth contingency model. In R. W. J. Neufeld (Ed.), *Advances in the investigation of psychological stress* (pp. 367–391). New York: Wiley.

Lang, P. J. (1979). A bio-informational theory of emotional imagery. *Psychophysiology, 16,* 495–512.

Lazarus, R. S. (1990). Theory-based stress measurement. *Psychological Inquiry, 1,* 3–13.

Linville, P. W. (1987). Self-complexity as a cognitive buffer against stress-related illness and depression. *Journal of Personality and Social Psychology, 52,* 663–676.

Maher, B. A. (1991). Deception, rational man, and other rocks on the road to a personality psychology of real people. In W. M. Grove & D. Cicchetti (Eds.), *Thinking clearly about psychology: Vol. 2. Personality and psychopathology* (pp. 72–88). Minneapolis: University of Minnesota Press.

Mazure, C., Nelson, J. C., & Price, L. H. (1986). Reliability and validity of the symptoms of major depressive illness. *Archives of General Psychiatry, 43,* 451–456.

Overmier, J. B., & Hellhammer, D. H. (1988). The learned helplessness model of human depression. *Animal Models of Psychiatric Disorder, 2,* 177–202.

Persons, J. B. (1986). The advantages of studying psychological phenomena rather than psychiatric diagnoses. *American Psychologist, 41,* 1252–1260.

Pyszczynski, T., Greenberg, J., Hamilton, J., & Nix, G. (1991). On the relationship between self-focused attention and psychological disorder: A critical reappraisal. *Psychological Bulletin, 110,* 538–543.

Robins, L. N. (1989). Diagnostic grammar and assessment: Translating criteria into questions. *Psychological Medicine, 19,* 57–68.

Robins, L. N., Helzer, J. E., Croughan, J., & Ratcliff, K. S. (1981). National Institute of Mental Health Diagnostic Interview Schedule: Its history, characteristics and validity. *Archives of General Psychiatry, 38,* 381–389.

Seligman, M. E. P. (1975). *Helplessness: On depression, development and death.* San Francisco: W. H. Freeman.

Smith, T. W., & Allred, K. D. (1986). Rationality revisited: A reassessment of the empirical support for the rational–emotive model. In P. C. Kendall (Ed.),

Advances in cognitive–behavioral research and therapy, Vol. 5 (pp. 63–87). New York: Academic Press.

Sullivan, M. J. L., & D'Eon, J. L. (1990). Relation between catastrophizing and depression in chronic pain patients. *Journal of Abnormal Psychology, 99,* 260–263.

Szabadi, E., Bradshaw, C. M., & Besson, I. A. O. (1976). Elongation of pause-time in speech: A simple objective measure of motor retardation in depression. *British Journal of Psychiatry, 129,* 592–597.

Willner, P. (1985). *Depression: A psychobiological synthesis.* New York: Wiley.

Wing, J. K., Cooper, J. E., & Sartorius, N. (1974). *The measurements and classification of psychiatric symptoms.* London: Cambridge University Press.

Zurawski, R. M., & Smith, T. W. (1987). Assessing irrational beliefs and emotional distress: Evidence and implications of limited discriminant validity. *Journal of Counseling Psychology, 34,* 224–227.

I

PROBLEMS OF DETECTION, DESCRIPTION, AND DIAGNOSES

2

Psychiatric Disorders: Problems of Boundaries and Comorbidity

DANIEL N. KLEIN

LAWRENCE P. RISO

A classification system can be regarded as a theory, or model, of the underlying structure of a particular domain. The theory's content is contained in a series of assumptions and inferences regarding what constitutes an individual element in the system and how these elements are interrelated (Gould, 1989; Skinner, 1981). Thus, in addition to having implications for the categorization of individual units or cases, the treatment of boundaries and overlap between constituent parts of the system reflects critical hypotheses about the nature and interrelationships of the various classes in the taxonomy (Stein, 1991).

In psychopathology, controversies over the basic boundaries and divisions between disorders have persisted since antiquity (Berrios, 1988; Jackson, 1986). In recent years, there has also been increasing interest in the problem of cooccurrences between disorders, or comorbidity (e.g., Maser & Cloninger, 1990). In this chapter, we outline what we regard as the major conceptual issues related to the boundaries and overlap between psychiatric disorders, and discuss available approaches to studying these problems. We do not attempt to review the extensive literature on the boundaries and comorbidity between specific disorders, although we draw on this literature to illustrate particular conceptual and methodological issues. The problem of the boundaries between psychiatric disorders is addressed first because a discussion of comorbidity presupposes the acceptance of at least several distinct disorders.

BOUNDARIES

Conceptual Issues

The question of boundaries between psychiatric disorders requires an examination of two more fundemental issues in classification. The first is whether disorders are discrete, "natural" classes or artificial categories established by imposing cutoffs at arbitrary points on continua. The second issue concerns whether our interests are better served by categorical or dimensional models of classification. Both of these issues are relevant to understanding the meaning of a boundary and determining its precise location.

Discreteness

Disease constructs tend to be conceptualized as discrete entities.[1] There is, however, no logical reason for this to be the case, and many phenomena that are currently accepted as diseases are continuous with normal functioning (e.g., hypertension). In fact, it is likely that nondiscrete, multifactorial models may be more appropriate for many of the chronic diseases that currently account for most of the morbidity and mortality in modern industrialized societies (Weiner, 1978; Whitbeck, 1977).

Just as there is no generally accepted definition of *mental disorder* (see Gorenstein, 1984; Kendell, 1975; Wakefield, 1992; Widiger & Trull, 1991), there is no clear and unambiguous definition of what is meant by a *type, entity, taxon, nonarbitrary class,* or *discrete category.* In defining *discreteness,* some investigators focus on the distributional features of observable "markers" such as symptomatology. For example, Kendell (1975) defined *discrete entities* by the presence of discontinuity, or a "point of rarity," between the clinical features of a condition and that of its neighbors. Similarly, extending Fleiss and Zubin's (1969) earlier definition, Grove and Tellegen (1987) proposed that *types* be defined as mixtures of multivariate distributions that differ in average location, or population means. In contrast, others have emphasized the form of the underlying etiological process. Thus, Meehl (1977; Meehl & Golden, 1982) argued that discreteness, or *taxonicity,* is indicated by any one of the following conditions: (1) a dichotomous etiological factor that is both necessary and sufficient for a disease syndrome to appear (e.g., the gene for Huntington's disease), (2) a dichotomous etiological agent that is necessary but not sufficient for the disease to be manifested (exposure to the influenza virus), and (3) a threshold effect or step function, which is evident in the relationship between exposure to the causal factor and the probability of exhibiting the syndrome (e.g., ingesting less than the necessary minimum amount of niacin for a sufficient period of time results in pellagra).

Several important problems and distinctions arise in considering the issue of discreteness in psychopathology and in disease more generally. First, discreteness at one level does not necessarily imply discreteness at other levels. A disorder can be discrete with respect to etiology, pathophysiology, or phenomenology, but not at other levels (Cloninger, Reich, & Yokoyama, 1983; Depue & Monroe, 1983). Thus, it is possible for a single set of causal factors to produce qualitatively distinct symptom pictures (phenotypic heterogeneity, or variable expressivity), depending on the severity of the etiological agent, social or environmental circumstances, or other modifying variables (Kendler, Heath, Martin, & Eaves, 1987). For example, Huntington's chorea is transmitted by a single dominant gene, yet can be associated with a wide range of symptom presentations that overlap with a variety of psychiatric disorders (Caine, Hunt, Weingartner, & Ebert, 1978). Similarly, there is evidence suggesting that antisocial personality and somatization disorder result from similar etiological processes that are expressed differently as a function of gender (Cloninger, 1978).

It is also possible for similar clinical presentations to arise from different etiological processes (e.g., mental retardation, dementia). Indeed, it appears likely that most of the major psychiatric disorders are etiologically heterogeneous (Cloninger et al., 1983; Baron, Endicott, & Ott, 1990) and represent "final common pathways" for diverse causal processes (Akiskal & McKinney, 1975).

Given that discreteness may be evident at one level but not another, the question arises as to which level should take precedence in deciding whether a particular disorder is a discrete entity. In medicine, etiology has traditionally been accorded priority, as classifications based on clinical and pathophysiological manifestations have typically been replaced by etiologically based classifications once the latter has been elucidated (Hudson, 1983; Pies, 1979; Weiner, 1978).[2]

Unfortunately, this does not fully address the question, as the concept of etiology is itself problematic. Etiological processes often involve complex causal chains, and it is not always clear which element or process should be regarded as the primary etiological factor (Meehl, 1977; Whitbeck, 1977). Indeed, etiological primacy in medicine has been accorded on a variety of grounds, including the form of the relationship between the causal agent and the disorder (e.g., necessary and/or sufficient conditions; step functions), favoring proximal over remote causes, and giving priority to factors that are more amenable to prevention and/or treatment (Whitbeck, 1977). Thus, whether a disorder is regarded as having a discrete etiology may depend, in part, on which causal factor is accorded etiological primacy.

In addition to identifying the level at which discreteness is sought, it is also important to be specific about which boundaries are to be considered discrete. A psychopathological condition can be discrete with respect to normality, but not other psychiatric disorders. For example, Crow (1990) has hypothesized that the major psychoses lie along a psychotic–affective continuum. However, he has not challenged the assumption that they are qualitatively different from normality. A disorder may also be continuous with normality, but discrete from other psychopathological conditions. For example, Schneider (1958) argued that the difference between normal personality variation and the personality disorders are a matter of degree, rather than kind, but that the personality disorders are qualitatively different from the major symptom disorders. Finally, a psychopathological condition could be discrete with respect to some psychiatric disorders, but not others. For example, many investigators believe that schizophrenia is qualitatively different from normality and most other psychiatric disorders, but is continuous with "spectrum" conditions such as schizotypal personality disorder (Kendler, 1985; Meehl, 1989).

Categorical versus Dimensional Models

Although psychiatric nosologies typically employ a categorical format, many investigators have argued that dimensional models are more appropriate (Achenbach, 1985; Eysenck, Wakefield, & Friedman, 1983; Frances, 1982; Strauss, 1975; Widiger, 1991). This debate is frequently confounded with the issue of discreteness, as proponents of categorical models tend to assume that psychiatric disorders are discrete entities, whereas advocates of dimensional models generally reject the notion of discreteness. However, the question of whether these debates are, in fact, isomorphic depends on existing knowledge of etiology and the level at which discreteness is sought. When etiology is unknown, psychiatric classification is generally based on clinical features. If discreteness is defined in terms of still-to-be-discovered etiological processes, but classification is based on symptomatology, the debates over discreteness and categorical versus dimensional models address different levels. Under these conditions, one might reasonably advocate a categorical approach to classification on the grounds that it is an efficient means of summarizing and communicating information about clinical syndromes without necessarily believing that the disorders will ultimately be shown to be etiologically discrete. This is the position taken by DSM-III-R, which employs a categorical format but states that there "is no assumption that each mental disorder is a discrete entity" (American Psychiatric Association, 1987, p. *xxii*). Then again, it is also reasonable to believe that, although most disorders will ultimately be shown to be discrete, dimensional models are more useful at the stage when little is known about etiology, as arbitrary assumptions about boundaries are not required.

Categorical models have several advantages. First, they simplify communication by using a single term to summarize a large quantity of information. Thus, it is more efficient to give a patient a single diagnosis than to rate them on a number of symptom dimensions.

Second, people often tend to prefer categories to dimensions in everyday speech, even when the construct involved is clearly dimensional in nature. For example, color is a dimensional concept that is associated with the wavelength of visible light. Yet colors are most often referred to as discrete categories (Blashfield, 1990).

Third, a categorical format parallels the form of clinical decision making (Widiger & Trull, 1991). Most clinical decisions are categorical in nature (e.g., prescribe Treatment X versus Treatment Y; continue or discontinue Treatment Z). Hence, if a dimensional system were employed in routine clinical practice, it would frequently be necessary to impose arbitrary cutoffs, converting the system into a categorical format.

Finally, a categorical approach has the potential to provide leverage for discovering rare discrete conditions that might be obscured by a dimensional approach (Meehl, 1979, 1986; Meehl & Golden, 1982). For example, a clinician might notice that a particular cluster of seemingly unrelated symptoms tends to cooccur in a small subgroup of patients. Hypothesizing that this represents an etiologically discrete syndrome, the clinician can then determine whether it is associated with a particular pattern of external correlates, such as course, family history, and treatment response. Indeed, the history of medicine suggests that this is frequently how syndromes are discovered. Within a dimensional system, however, the discovery of such a syndrome would be less likely. Instead, the high scorers on each dimension relevant to the syndrome would be a heterogeneous group that included a very small number of patients with the syndrome and a much larger group of patients without it.

Although the history of medicine indicates that a categorical approach can have great heuristic value, there are no assurances that this track record will apply to psychopathology. Thus, it remains a matter of conjecture how closely the nature and structure of psychopathological disorders will mirror classical medical conditions (Kendell, 1989).

The major strengths of a dimensional approach include the preservation of more information, superior reliability, and greater power in statistical analyses (Eysenck et al., 1983; Frances, 1982; Widiger, 1991). In addition, dimensional systems are less likely to create arbitrary distinctions that result in problematic "border" categories such as schizoaffective disorder and mixed anxiety and depression (Widiger & Trull, 1991). It is curious that in the face of these considerable advantages, no comprehensive dimensional model of psychopathology has been offered for some time. It is likely that part of the problem is the complexity required of any comprehensive dimensional system. It is difficult enough deciding which and how many symptom dimensions to include and how to define them. However, this task rapidly becomes even more complex when one tries to include duration requirements, course factors (e.g., age and type of onset; chronic versus episodic course), and exclusion criteria.

Classification systems can mix categorical and dimensional models. Skinner (1986) has discussed class quantitative and radex models that combine categorical and dimensional features. As an example of the former, Kendell (1969) proposed that patients falling within the broad category of depression be assigned an endogenous–neurotic dimensional score, rather than a traditional subtype diagnosis. It may also be the case that a categorical format is more appropriate for some disorders and a dimensional system more appropriate for others (Gunderson, Links, & Reich, 1991).

Prototype models represent a different form of a mixed categorical–dimensional approach to classification. The prototype approach was developed to account for "fuzzy" boundaries in natural classification (Rosch & Mervis, 1975). Within this framework, category membership is viewed as a matter of degree, rather than something that is present or absent. Members of a particular class vary in their "typicality" as a function of two factors: (1) overlap with the target category, which is generally defined as the number of features of the prototype they exhibit; and (2) dissimilarity from the prototypes of neighboring categories (Cantor & Genero, 1986). Prototype models differ from other mixed models in that the class or disorder is viewed exclusively in categorical terms, rather than including both categorical and dimensional components. It is the individual case, or patient, that is viewed dimensionally, as falling along a continuum of typicality. Although the prototype and dimensional models can both be used to yield dimensional measures of psychopathology, the meaning of the scales are quite different. In the prototype approach, the scale is best interpreted as a measure of diagnostic typicality based on distance from the prototype. In contrast, in the dimensional approach, the scale is a direct attempt to quantify severity of psychopathology.

Discovering and Confirming Boundaries
between Disorders

Over the last two decades, most of the data addressing distinctions between psychiatric disorders derives from the framework proposed by Robins and Guze (1970). This paradigm, which is essentially an application of the process of construct validation (Cronbach & Meehl, 1955) to psychopathology, consists of five phases: clinical description, laboratory studies, delimitation from other disorders, and follow-up and family studies. Following this framework, the validity of a diagnostic category has been supported when its core clinical features are much more common in individuals with, than without, the disorder; the syndrome is stable over time and has a characteristic course and outcome; and the condition has important external correlates such as family history and relevant psychological and biological variables.

This type of data is critical in that it can support a category's construct validity and may also shed light on its etiology and clinical management. In addition, if a diagnosis cannot be validated according to the Robins and Guze framework, it is highly unlikely to reflect a discrete disorder. Regardless of the strength of the evidence, however, this kind of data cannot resolve the issue of whether a disorder represents a distinct class or an arbitrary division along a continuum (Cloninger, 1989; Grove & Andreasen, 1989; Kendell, 1975). For example, one can hypothesize the existence of a discrete syndrome "moderate overweight disorder," which could be identified by the following characteristics: larger waist size than average, as determined by norms for the appropriate sex and age group; avoidance of tight or revealing clothing; negative feelings about one's body image; and a tendency to breath heavily after mild–moderate physical exertion. The diagnosis would be excluded by a diagnosis of obesity. It could be readily demonstrated that these indicators are much more common in individuals with the putative syndrome than in a relevant contrast group. In addition, it is likely that the syndrome would be stable over time, run in families, and be associated with increased morbidity and mortality. Nonetheless, this evidence would not be sufficient to support the hypothesis that "moderate overweight disorder" was a typological condition rather than an arbitrary point along a continuum of weight.

Despite decades (indeed, centuries) of research and debate, none of the currently accepted psychiatric disorders has been conclusively demonstrated to be a discrete entity. The greatest effort in this area has focused on validating Kraepelin's distinction between schizophrenia and the major mood disorders. This work has produced considerable data consistent with the Kraepelinian hypothesis (e.g., Cloninger, Martin, Guze, & Clayton, 1985; Gershon & Reider, 1980). However, these findings are far from conclusive, and sufficient data exist to provide a credible basis for alternative models positing a continuum between schizophrenia and the major mood disorders (Crow, 1990; Gershon et al., 1988; Kendell, 1989; Taylor, 1992).

The data are even less conclusive in other areas of psychopathology. Many investigators have argued that the boundaries between mild–moderate unipolar depression and the anxiety and somatoform disorders are arbitrary and that these conditions should be subsumed under the broader rubric of a "general neurotic syndrome," which is continuous with normal functioning (Andrews, Stewart, Morris-Yates, Holt, &

Henderson, 1990; Sims, 1986; Tyrer, 1989). An even greater number of investigators have challenged the view of personality disorders as discrete entities (e.g., Grove & Tellegen, 1991; Widiger, 1991).

The inability to resolve these fundamental nosological issues is due, in large part, to the difficulty of demonstrating the existence of discrete boundaries between psychiatric disorders. A number of conceptual and statistical approaches have been used in an attempt to address this problem. The two oldest and most frequently used approaches have been (1) examining distributions of scores derived from discriminant analysis for evidence of bimodality and (2) cluster analysis. More recent approaches include mixture analysis, latent class analysis, demonstrating a nonlinear relationship between clinical features and an independent criterion, and finding a "disordinal interaction" between diagnoses and variables from another domain.[3]

In the following section, we provide a brief overview of each of these six approaches. However, before discussing the specific techniques, it is important to recognize that all of these methods, even those using "latent" variables, are limited to addressing the same level as the variables (e.g., clinical features, biological correlates, family history) that are employed in the analysis. Thus, these techniques can be used to test the hypothesis that symptomatology (or variables from another domain) in a given sample is best characterized by two or more clusters, classes, or distributions. However, as discussed previously, the presence or absence of discreteness at the clinical or pathophysiological level does not necessarily correspond to discreteness at the level of etiology. In order to fully resolve the question of discreteness in an etiological sense, it is necessary to have indicators of the underlying causal processes. Because etiology remains unknown for most psychopathological conditions, it is unlikely that any of these techniques, in and of themselves, can produce conclusive results.

This has several implications. First, assuming that discreteness is defined at the level of etiology, the more directly the variables selected by the investigator reflect etiological processes, the greater bearing the results will have on the question of discreteness. In light of this, it is unfortunate that the majority of studies using the approaches discussed later in this chapter have relied exclusively on cross-sectional symptomatology, rather than using variables from other domains that may be more closely related to etiological processes.

Second, this highlights the need for systematic research programs that apply several of these approaches to variables from multiple levels and domains. To the degree that the findings converge across methods and domains, one can have greater confidence in whether particular psychopathological conditions are discrete entities.

Multimodality

The early literature on whether psychiatric disorders were discrete entities focused primarily on the presence or absence of multimodality (particularly bimodality) in the distribution of patients' symptoms (Carney, Roth, & Garside, 1965; Kendell, 1968a; Moran, 1966). The basic premise behind this approach was that, in order to demonstrate a discrete boundary between two disorders, the number of cases exhibiting symptoms of one disorder but not the other (blacks and whites) should be substantially greater than the number of cases with a mixture of symptoms of both disorders (grays). In other words, there should be a point of rarity in the distribution of symptoms between the two disorders.

Typically, studies using this approach begin by selecting patients from two diagnostic categories and assessing a group of variables that are thought to be useful in distinguishing the groups. In most studies, a discriminant function analysis is then conducted to obtain the weighted combination of variables that maximizes the classification of patients into the original diagnostic categories. Each patient is then assigned a canonical coefficient score from the discriminant analysis, and these scores are plotted against the frequency of patients. Finally, the plots are inspected for evidence of bimodality, or a point of rarity.

A number of studies have employed this approach to examine the distinctions between schizophrenia and the mood disorders (Brockington, Kendell, Wainwright, Hillier, & Walker, 1979; Brockington et al., 1991; Kendell & Gourlay, 1970), depressive and anxiety disorders (Roth & Mountjoy, 1982), and psychotic/endogenous and neurotic/reactive depression (Carney et al., 1965; Kendell, 1968a; Kendell & Gourlay, 1970). Unfortunately, bimodality is a poor criterion for determining whether disorders are discrete. A number of factors can obscure bimodality, even when it exists, and a number of factors can create the appearance of bimodality in what is really a unimodal distribution (Everitt, 1981a; Grayson, 1987; Grove & Andreasen, 1989; Murphy, 1964).

At least four factors can obscure bimodality. First, unless the difference between groups is quite large (e.g., greater than two standard deviations on a normally distributed variable), two equimixed groups will yield a unimodal distribution. Second, if one of the two populations of interest is very small, it can easily be obscured within the tail of the larger population. Third, unequal variances between groups can conceal bimodality. Finally, unreliable measures of the criterion groups or symptoms can obscure bimodality (Everitt, 1981a; Grove & Andreasen, 1989; Murphy, 1964). Grove and Andreasen (1989) explored the effects of a number of these factors in a recent Monte Carlo study and found that bimodality was detectable only if two disorders stemmed from very different etiological processes, there was a sharp threshold effect between the underlying etiology and the manifestation of disorder, and the indicators (e.g., symptoms) were both highly reliable and tightly tied to the etiological process.

A related method, bitangentiality, has been proposed as a more powerful alternative to bimodality (Grove & Andreasen, 1989; Harris & Smith, 1949). To demonstrate bitangentiality, there must be two distinct tangents with the same slope on one side of the mode of a unimodal distribution (Grove & Andreasen, 1989). Bitangentiality is more sensitive than bimodality, as it can be demonstrated in the presence of much smaller differences between groups (Harris & Smith, 1949).

There are also at least five factors that can spuriously create the impression of bimodality (Everitt, 1981a; Grove & Andreasen, 1989; Murphy, 1964). First, if the sample is restricted to "pure" forms of the disorders of interest, rather than comprising a representative sample, a point of rarity will be obtained that reflects sampling bias rather than the low prevalence of mixed cases in the real world. Second, bimodality can be artifactually created by referral biases, such as the "institutional taxa" described by Grove (1991; Grove & Andreasen, 1989). For example, if individuals with extreme values on either of two independent, normally distributed traits (e.g., impulsivity and neuroticism) have an increased likelihood of treatment referral, the distribution of patients in clinical samples would provide the misleading impression that impulsive and neurotic patients constituted two distinct classes. Third, observer biases and halo effects can falsely produce the appearance of bimodality (Kendell, 1968b). Fourth, bimodality can be artifactually enhanced or obscured, depending on how histograms are plotted (Grove & Andreasen, 1989; Murphy, 1964). As a result, some studies have employed statistical tests for multimodality (Brockington et al., 1979; Moldin, Gottesman, & Erlenmeyer-Kimling, 1987). However, these procedures are less sensitive than more recent methods, such as mixture analysis (Everitt & Hand, 1981; Fliess, 1972). Finally, Grayson (1987) has demonstrated that dimensional constructs can yield bimodality under certain measurement conditions, such as when all symptoms on a rating scale provide optimal discrimination between groups at a similar level of illness severity.

In light of these difficulties, efforts to demonstrate multimodality in the manner described previously have been largely superseded by mixture analysis, which may have greater power to detect discrete classes. However, it is important to note that all of the other approaches discussed later in this chapter are also susceptible to Type I errors due to sampling, referral, and rater biases and to psychometric artifacts, and to Type II errors due to unreliable measurement (Golden, 1991; Grayson, 1987).

Cluster Analysis

Cluster analysis refers to a variety of statistical techniques that attempt to divide large samples into more homogeneous subgroups, or clusters. Although this approach was introduced into the psychopathology literature more than 50 years ago (Zubin, 1938), cluster analysis was not widely applied to psychiatric disorders until the 1970s, following Sokal and Sneath's (1963; Sneath & Sokal, 1973) classic texts on numerical taxonomy in biological classification. Since then, cluster analysis has been used to derive general typologies for adult (Everitt, Gourlay, & Kendell, 1971) and child (Lessing, Williams, & Gil, 1982) psychopathology and to derive more homogeneous subgroups within the psychotic (Lorr et al., 1963) and mood disorders (Blashfield & Morey, 1979; Grove, Andreasen, Young et al., 1987), parasuicide (Paykel, 1981), alcoholism (Morey & Blashfield, 1981), personality disorders (Morey, 1988), and sexual aggression (Rosenberg & Knight, 1988).

A large number of clustering methods exist. The two most commonly employed classes of techniques are sequential hierarchical agglomerative and partitioning methods (Blashfield & Aldenderfer, 1978; Grove & Andreasen, 1986). Hierarchical agglomerative techniques, such as average linkage and Ward's method, combine small subsets of subjects into progressively larger groups in an attempt to maximize within group similarity. Similarity can be assessed in a variety of ways, including product–moment correlations and various Euclidean distance measures. The investigator must decide at what point to stop the clustering process because hierarchical agglomerative procedures ultimately produce a single large cluster encompassing the entire sample. In contrast, partitioning, or k-means, procedures start with an initial assignment of individuals to a user-specified number of clusters. Subjects are then shifted from cluster to cluster in order to maximize within group similarity (Blashfield & Aldenderfer, 1978; Grove & Andreasen, 1986, 1989; Milligan & Cooper, 1987).

There are a number of unresolved issues in cluster analysis. First, different clustering methods often generate different solutions to the same data (e.g., Everitt et al., 1971; Strauss, Bartko, & Carpenter, 1973). In order to compare the validity of different clustering methods, Monte Carlo studies have been conducted in which a set of clustering algorithms are applied to an artificial data set with a predetermined structure, and the extent to which the various methods "recover" the known structure is determined. These studies indicate that all methods perform best when the data include clearly distinct, homogeneous groups. In addition, most methods are prone to error when the groups exhibit substantial overlap, although different methods perform better, depending on the particular structure of the data set. Overall, Ward's and the convergent *k*-means methods have consistently been among the top performers, hence these appear to be the most robust procedures currently available (Grove & Andreasen, 1986, 1989; Grove & Tellegen, 1987; Hand & Everitt, 1987; Milligan & Cooper, 1987). It is generally recommended that several of the better techniques be applied to the same data and that only solutions that converge across methods be accepted (Blashfield, 1980; Everitt, 1972; Grove & Andreasen, 1986).

Second, there is no clear means of determining how many clusters should be derived from a given analysis. A number of methods for determining the number of clusters in a data set have been proposed, and Monte Carlo studies indicate that they vary considerably in their effectiveness. However, no clear consensus regarding the technique(s) of choice has emerged (Blashfield, 1980; Grove, 1991; Milligan & Cooper, 1987).

A related question is how to determine whether there are any "real" clusters in the data at all. Clustering programs almost invariably generate clusters, even when none exist (e.g., data with a single multivariate normal distribution) (Everitt, 1972; Milligan & Cooper, 1987). Thus, clusters may represent the extremes of a single dimension rather than natural groups (Everitt, 1972). This issue is obviously critical if cluster analysis is to be useful in determining whether a disorder is discrete. In view of the potential for deriving arbitrary clusters, it is generally recommended that clustering solutions should be replicated on a second data set and validated against external variables such as treatment response, outcome, and family history before being accepted (Blashfield, 1980; Everitt, 1972; Kendell, 1975; Milligan & Cooper, 1987; Paykel, 1981). However, although this might support the meaningfulness and utility of a clustering solution, it cannot ensure that clusters are discrete, rather than the extreme ends of a dimension.

An alternative is to develop inferential statistics to test the hypothesis that the data contain two or more real clusters, as opposed to the null hypothesis that the data are drawn from a single population. Unfortunately, work in this area is still at an early stage (Milligan & Cooper, 1987). In a recent simulation study by Grove (1991), only one of four indices proposed in the literature performed even moderately well.

Third, although there are algorithms that can produce overlapping clusters (Sokal, 1974; Milligan & Cooper, 1987), most cluster analytic techniques can only assign subjects to one cluster (Kendell, 1975). This is inconsistent with clinical reality, where patients often exhibit multiple disorders, and failure to take comorbidity into account could obscure "natural" clusters.[4]

A fourth issue concerns the choice of variables to include in the cluster analysis. One of the advantages of cluster analysis, compared with the other methods discussed here, is that a large number of variables can be employed, provided large enough samples are available. Indeed, early numerical taxonomists in biology advocated including as many variables as possible with minimal preselection on theoretical grounds. However, this strength is also associated with significant risks, as an overly inclusive approach to variable selection can lead to the failure to detect important clusters because differences are obscured by irrelevant information (Kendell, 1989). Indeed, Monte Carlo studies indicate that the inclusion of just one "random" variable can greatly reduce the ability of clustering algorithms to recover the known structure of simulated data sets (Milligan & Cooper, 1987).

Finally, the interpretation of the meaning of the clusters obtained is still largely subjective, much like the interpretation of factors in factor analysis. For example, in depression, several cluster analytic studies have yielded clusters with similar labels, but close inspection of their contents indicated minimal overlap (Blashfield & Morey, 1979).

Mixture Analysis

Mixture analysis attempts to estimate the number of populations underlying a given set of continuously distributed data (Everitt & Hand, 1981; Fleiss, 1972; Gibbons et al., 1984; Titterington, Smith, & Makov, 1985). Conceptually, it is an extension of the multimodality approach discussed before. However, as previously noted, multimodality is a very insensitive criterion because mixed populations generally yield unimodal distributions unless they are very widely separated.

Mixture analysis derives from Pearson (1894), who first developed a method for estimating mixtures of two normal distributions. Pearson's method of moments has been largely superseded by maximum likelihood procedures, which were applied to mixture analysis by Day (1969). Most mixture models assume that the admixed populations are normally distributed, although models for other distributions (e.g., exponential models for survival time data) are available (Everitt & Hand, 1981; Titterington et al., 1985).

Mixture analysis is generally applied to continous data (e.g., symptom scales, laboratory values, canonical variate scores from a discriminant function analysis).[5] Multivariate mixture models, which estimate the number of populations underlying the joint distributions of two or more variables, are also available. However, they can be extremely difficult to interpret when three or more variables are employed (Gibbons et al., 1984). Maximum likelihood procedures are used to estimate the number of admixed populations and the mean, standard deviation, and proportion of individuals in each population. The probability of an individual being from each specific population can also be estimated.

Chi-square statistics (e.g., the likelihood ratio chi-square) can be used to determine whether the addition of a second population significantly improves the fit of the model to the data. If a two-population solution provides a better fit, three populations can be tested, and so forth (Everitt & Hand, 1981; Gibbons et al., 1984).

Mixture analysis has been applied to a variety of problems in psychopathology. These have included testing the hypothesis that schizophrenia is a discrete entity (Cloninger et al., 1985), comparing the unitary and binary models of depression (Fleiss, 1972), identifying anhedonic and nonanhedonic subtypes of depression (Fawcett, Clark, Scheftner, & Gibbons, 1983), distinguishing anxiety and somatoform disorders (Sigvardsson, Bohman, von Knorring, & Cloninger, 1986), identifying genetic markers in the relatives of patients with bipolar disorder (Dorus et al., 1983) and schizophrenia (Clementz, Grove, Iacono, & Sweeney, 1992; Iacono, Moreau, Beiser, Fleming, & Lin, 1992), identifying subjects at particularly high risk among the offspring of schizophrenics (Moldin, Rice, Gottesman, & Erlenmeyer-Kimling, 1990), and exploring the latent structure of schizotypy by using psychometric measures in college students (Lenzenweger & Moldin, 1990).

Several issues should be considered in evaluating studies using mixture analysis. First, most mixture models assume that the mixed underlying components are normally distributed and have equal variances. However, it is unclear how robust these procedures are to violations of these assumptions (Grove & Andreasen, 1989).

Second, skewness and kurtosis in the observed data can be incorrectly interpreted as evidence of mixture. Hence, data transformation is often necessary prior to analysis (Gibbons et al., 1984; Grove & Andreasen, 1989).

Third, very large samples are required, particularly when the components are poorly separated and one of the mixing proportions approaches zero (Everitt, 1981b; Everitt & Hand, 1981; Fleiss, 1972; Grove & Tellegen, 1987).

Finally, few Monte Carlo studies, providing an empirical evaluation of the performance of mixture analysis on simulated data, are available (Grove & Tellegen, 1987; Titterington et al., 1985). This is particularly important in light of Everitt and Hand's (1981) suggestion that, given enough components, it will always be possible to find a mixture that fits the data.

Latent Class Analysis

Originally developed by sociologists (Goodman, 1974; Lazarsfeld & Henry, 1968), latent class analysis (LCA) refers to a group of models in which the relationships among categorical observed (or manifest) variables are explained by discrete unobserved (or latent) variables. Thus, LCA differs from mixture analysis, in which the latent variables are also categorical, but the observed variables are continuous.

The basic concept underlying LCA is that of local independence. Assuming that there is a significant relationship among a set of observed variables, it is hypothesized that this association is indirect and can be accounted for by the relationships between the manifest variables and an underlying latent variable (McCutcheon, 1987; Young, 1983; Young & Tanner, 1983). For example, it may be hypothesized that depressive symptoms are intercorrelated because they are all manifestations of major depression. Thus, at a given level of the diagnosis (major depression present or absent), the clinical features of depression would be independent.

LCA begins with a cross-classification table, in which the number of subjects in each possible combination of categories of observed variables is tabulated. The parameters of the hypothesized model are then estimated from the data by using one of several available maximum likelihood procedures (Clogg, 1977; Haberman, 1979). These procedures yield estimates of the number of latent classes and their prevalence in the sample. The probability that an individual in a given latent class will obtain a particular value on an observed variable can also be derived. This provides an index of the relationship between the observed and latent variables, much like factor loadings in a factor analysis, which can be used to interpret the nature of the latent classes. In addition, individuals' latent class assignments can be used as an independent method of classification against which to validate clinical and laboratory diagnoses (Golden, 1982; Grove & Andreasen, 1986; Rindskopf & Rindskopf, 1986). Finally, the goodness-of-fit between the observed frequencies in the cross-tabulation and those predicted by the model is tested by using chi-square procedures (McCutcheon, 1987; Young & Tanner, 1983).

LCA can be used to determine the number of latent classes in a sample and to characterize their features. First, it is determined whether the observed variables (e.g., clinical features) in a set are significantly associated. A lack of association suggests that only a single class is present in the sample. If the basic model of independence can be rejected, then the goodness of fit of a two class model is tested. If that fails to fit the data, a three-class model can be tested, and so forth. The characteristics of the latent classes can then be examined and used to refine clinical classifications (Golden, 1982; McCutcheon, 1987; Young, 1983).

In recent years, a number of studies have employed LCA to address nosological issues in psychopathology. For example, LCA has been used to examine the criteria for major depression (Eaton, Dryman, Sorenson,

& McCutcheon, 1989), the validity of the melancholic subtype (Parker et al., 1990; Young, Scheftner, Klerman, Andreasen, & Hirschfeld, 1986), and the validity of diagnostic criteria for schizophrenia (Young, Tanner, & Meltzer, 1982) and mania (Young, Abrams, Taylor, & Meltzer, 1983).

Several factors should be considered in using LCA. First, although this procedure can be used to determine whether data are consistent with a particular hypothesized latent class structure, it cannot actually prove that the latent classes are discrete, rather than comprising ordinal levels of an underlying continuum (McCutcheon, 1987).

Second, it is generally recommended that cell sizes be at least equal to five. Thus, relatively large samples are required for latent class analyses using more than a handful of variables.

Third, the assumption of local independence may not always be tenable in psychopathology (Golden, 1991). Although much of the association between indicators of a diagnostic category may be due to an underlying latent process, it is likely that many of these indicators are also correlated with other disorders for different reasons. For example, whereas impaired smooth pursuit eye-tracking and schizophrenic symptomatology may both be expressions of a single dominant gene (Holzman et al., 1988), deviant eye-tracking is also common in bipolar patients taking lithium (Levy et al., 1985).

Finally, as with mixture analysis, few Monte Carlo studies of LCA are available. Hence, the performance of these models has not been extensively evaluated in empirical tests.

Meehl and Golden have developed a closely related group of taxometric methods based on Meehl's MAXCOV–HITMAX procedure (Golden, 1982, 1991; Meehl, 1973; Meehl & Golden, 1982). Their approach differs from LCA primarily in its eschewal of maximum likelihood methods of statistical inference. Instead, Meehl and Golden have devised a series of more informal consistency tests, which are designed to test the validity of the assumptions underlying their models (Meehl, 1973; Meehl & Golden, 1982). These procedures have been applied to taxometric problems in the areas of schizotypy (Golden & Meehl, 1979), risk for schizophrenia (Erlenmeyer-Kimling, Golden, & Cornblatt, 1989), borderline personality disorder (Trull, Widiger, & Guthrie, 1990), tardive dyskinesia (Golden, Campbell, & Perry, 1987), and dementia (Golden, 1982). Early studies using known taxa (e.g., biological sex and simulated data) suggested that these models were relatively sensitive and produced few false-positive findings (Meehl & Golden, 1982). However, more recent work has indicated that these methods may be susceptible to Type I errors due to the psychometric artifacts described by Grayson (1987). As a result, Golden (1991) has developed a taxometric regression model, which may be more robust. However, empirical studies are necessary to evaluate this method.

Nonlinearity

Another approach to examining whether there are discrete boundaries between psychiatric syndromes is to determine whether there is a nonlinear relationship between symptomatology and another variable, such as outcome, treatment response, family history, or a psychobiological marker (Hicks, 1984; Kendell, 1982, 1989). In its simplest form, this involves plotting the relationship between a continuous measure of symptomatology (e.g., number of symptoms or scores on a discriminant function between two disorders) and another independent variable. If there is a point at which a relatively small change in symptomatology is associated with a relatively large change in the other variable, it would suggest that the two conditions are distinct and that the boundary lies at the point of discontinuity.[6] As with most of the other methods discussed here, failure to find discontinuity cannot rule out discreteness, as nonlinear relationships might be evident with other variables. However, if nonlinear relationships were demonstrated with several different independent variables and the discontinuities all appeared at the same point on the symptom index, it would provide strong evidence for discreteness.

This approach was introduced into the psychopathology literature by Kendell and Brockington (1980). It has been employed in only a few studies. Kendell and Brockington (1980) found no evidence of discontinuity in the relationship between a discriminant index of schizophrenic and affective symptomatology and outcome in samples of unselected psychotic and schizoaffective patients. Robins and McEvoy (1990) also failed to find evidence for a discontinuous relationship between number of childhood conduct problems and adult substance abuse. In contrast, D. N. Klein (1990) reported preliminary support for a nonlinear relationship between number of depressive symptoms in outpatients with major depression and rates of mood disorders in their first-degree relatives. Specifically, major depressives with six, seven, or more DSM-III major depression symptoms exhibited similar rates of mood disorders in their relatives, and major depressives with four and five symptoms were similar, and did not differ from outpatients with nonaffective disorders, on rates of mood disorders in relatives. However, the major depressives with six, seven, or more symptoms exhibited significantly higher rates of mood disorders in relatives than the major depressives with four and five symptoms and the outpatients with nonaffective disorders. These data support the possibility that DSM-III major depression is a discrete condition, but suggest that current criteria are too broad and that the optimal cutoff may be six, rather than four symptoms.

Disordinal Interactions

This approach was recently introduced by D. F. Klein and his colleagues (Fyer, Liebowitz, & Klein, 1990; D. F. Klein, 1989) as a means of using pharmacological dissection to distinguish between comorbidity and syndromal complexity. However, it can be generalized to other types of boundary problems and variables.

Klein and his colleagues were concerned with the difficulty of determining whether patients who appear to exhibit a second disorder (Y), along with a first disorder (X), have the same condition as patients who exhibit only X, or whether they suffer from a single, qualitatively different condition, which is manifested by features of both X and Y. For example, is the major depression in patients who also have panic disorder the same as the major depression in patients who do not, or is there a third, "syndromally complex" condition that is expressed as a combination of both major depression and panic disorder?

In order to address this issue, Klein argued, one could compare patients with condition X to patients with both X and Y on response to a pharmacological agent proven to be effective in treating X. If patients with both X and Y responded more poorly, the results would be inconclusive, as patients with both X and Y might simply have a more severe form of X. However, if patients with both X and Y responded better to a treatment designed for disorder X than patients with X alone, it would suggest that there is a qualitative difference between the pure and syndromally complex forms of the disorder. Klein and his colleagues termed this latter pattern of results a *disordinal interaction.*

Fyer and colleagues (1990) and D. F. Klein (1989) have reviewed evidence suggesting that such disordinal interactions may be apparent in several sets of conditions, including atypical and typical depression, generalized anxiety and panic disorder, and discrete and generalized social phobia.

This approach can be generalized beyond the question of comorbidity versus syndromal complexity and the pharmacological dissection strategy. Indeed, it is applicable to any case in which there is a question of whether two categories are distinct conditions, or different points on a severity continuum, using any dependent variable that is relevant to both categories. As D. F. Klein and colleagues (1989) have argued, finding greater pathology in what could be regarded as the more severe group is not particularly informative. However, finding greater pathology in the putatively less severe group does suggest a qualitative difference.

A recent illustration of this more general approach can be found in D. N. Klein, Riso, and Anderson (1993). These investigators explored whether there was a qualitative distinction between dysthymia and major depression, as is implied by DSM-III-R. They compared 22 dysthymic outpatients without superimposed major depressions to 46 nonchronic major depressive outpatients on 18 depressive symptoms and argued that if dysthymics exhibited higher rates of specific symptoms, it would support a qualitative distinction. In fact, the two groups exhibited similar rates of all symptoms, which suggests that there are no qualitative differences between dysthymia and major depression, at least with regard to depressive symptomatology.

Conclusions

In summary, there are a number of approaches with some potential to elucidate the issue of discreteness in psychiatric disorders, although it is unlikely that any one of these methods can yield conclusive findings on its own. These approaches vary along a number of lines, including whether the data employed are categorical or continuous, the number of variables that can be accommodated in the analysis, whether an independent diagnostic classification is needed prior to the analysis, and the availability of statistical models to evaluate the findings. Each method has its own particular limitations. In addition, all are dependent on reliable measures and a perspicacious choice of variables, and are susceptible to sampling, referral, and rater biases and to psychometric artifacts (Grayson, 1987). Although some of these approaches (e.g., multimodality) appear to have outlived their usefulness, most continue to be viable.

Unfortunately, there are few clear theoretical and conceptual grounds for choosing among these techniques. There is also little empirical basis for preferring one method to another. The degree of convergence between these approaches is unclear, although it is somewhat disquieting that the few studies that have applied several different techniques to the same, or highly overlapping, data sets have tended to yield different results (Eaton & Bohrnstedt, 1989; Grove, Andreason, Young, et al., 1987; Young et al., 1986). It would be particularly useful to have Monte Carlo studies available, where the performance of several different methods in recovering groups from artificially constructed data was directly compared. Unfortunately, the few studies of this type that have been conducted have yielded inconsistent findings (Grove & Tellegen, 1987).

In view of the significant conceptual and methodological difficulties involved in establishing whether psychiatric disorders have discrete boundaries, it should not be surprising that little progress has been made on this issue despite decades of research and debate. Without detailed knowledge of etiology, it is possible that the choice of discrete versus continuous models of psychopathology may have to rest on subjective and pragmatic grounds, such as esthetic preference, familiarity and tradition, and efficiency of communication.

COMORBIDITY

The term *comorbidity* was introduced in the medical literature by Feinstein (1970) to refer to patients with two cooccurring diseases. In the past few years, numerous studies have documented extensive comorbidity among psychiatric disorders (Biederman, Newcorn, & Sprich, 1991; Boyd et al., 1984; Brady & Kendall, 1992; Caron & Rutter, 1991; Docherty, Fiester, & Shea, 1986; Gunderson & Phillips, 1991; Maser & Cloninger, 1990). This has a number of important clinical and research implications. First, the presence of comorbidity may affect the course and treatment response of the index disorder. Second, unless comorbidity is taken into account, it is unclear whether correlations between a disorder and other variables represent true associations or reflect the presence of comorbid conditions. Third, high levels of comorbidity may raise questions about the adequacy of particular diagnostic categories and suggest areas in need of revision. Finally, high rates of comorbidity may provide important clues to the etiology of both the index and comorbid disorders.

The concept of comorbidity presupposes the existence of discrete disorders. Otherwise, what appears to be the cooccurrence of two independent disorders may, in fact, reflect the arbitrary division of a single disorder. For example, it is likely that the frequent comorbidity between major depression and dysthymia really represents different phases of a single disorder (Keller & Lavori, 1984; D. N. Klein et al., 1993). In a dimensional system, the term *comorbidity* would have little meaning. However, it would still be important to study patterns of covariation between dimensions of psychopathology.

The Relationship between Nosological Conventions and Comorbidity

A nosological system's approach to establishing boundaries between disorders can affect comorbidity in a variety of ways. First, as the number of categories in a system increases, there is generally an increasingly larger opportunity for disorders to cooccur. Thus, splitting a large group of disorders into more specific conditions, rather then lumping them together under a single rubric, increases rates of comorbidity (Frances, Widiger, & Fyer, 1990). The creation of distinct categories for overlapping clinical syndromes (e.g., schizoaffective disorder), however, is an exception to this rule. Categories for overlapping syndromes reduce the rate of cooccurrences by substituting a single diagnosis for two cooccurring conditions (Frances et al., 1990).

Diagnostic thresholds (e.g., the number of symptoms required for a diagnosis) can also influence comorbidity. Low thresholds tend to increase the prevalence of disorder, whereas high thresholds tend to decrease prevalence. As the prevalence of a disorder increases, there is an increasing likelihood that it will cooccur with other conditions simply on the basis of chance (Frances et al., 1990). Similarly, comorbidity can be affected by the time frame adopted in considering a disorder to be present. The lifetime prevalence of a disorder is always equal to, or greater than, its current prevalence. Hence, comorbidity will be greater if it is defined as two disorders occurring at any point in an individual's life than if the disorders are required to overlap temporally.

Finally, comorbidity can be dramatically affected by the use of hierarchical exclusion criteria (First, Spitzer, & Williams, 1990; Frances et al., 1990). Diagnostic hierarchies, which have a long history in medical and psychiatric diagnosis, are based on both theoretical and practical considerations. From a theoretical perspective, they derive from the assumption that even very complex and heterogeneous clinical presentations are better understood as arising from a single underlying disorder than as multiple independent diseases (Caron & Rutter, 1991; Widiger & Trull, 1991). From a practical standpoint, hierarchical exclusionary rules limit the number of diagnoses given to patients and make communication simpler and more efficient. In light of the high comorbidity between psychiatric disorders, it appears that the advantage of categorical diagnostic systems with regard to simplicity and efficiency stems in large part from the use of hierarchical exclusionary rules. Without exclusion criteria, the attractiveness of a categorical system is attenuated.

Traditionally, most diagnostic systems in psychiatry have employed some kind of hierarchical exclusionary principles. The most common approach, implicit in Kraepelin's writings and explicitly formulated by Jaspers (First et al., 1990), is based on a combination of two principles: etiology and pervasiveness or severity. Disorders with an organic etiology are ranked at the top of the hierarchy, followed by schizophrenia, and then by severe mood disorders. Finally, at the bottom of the hierarchy, are neurotic and personality disorders. The presence of a disorder higher in the hierarchy excludes all lower diagnoses.

Although DSM-III-R does not employ a Jasperian hierarchy, it does utilize its underlying principles in a more limited fashion. Thus, when an organic factor can account for the clinical presentation, it preempts the diagnosis of any other disorder that could produce the same features. In addition, when a more pervasive disorder has associated symptoms that are the defining features of a more circumscribed disorder, only the more pervasive disorder is diagnosed when the essential features of both disorders are present (American Psychiatric Association, 1987).

A second commonly employed hierarchical exclusionary principle is based on the focus of treatment (Klerman, 1990). Thus, when multiple disorders are present, diagnostic priority is accorded to the disorder that led to the patient being evaluated and is likely to be the focus of treatment. This is similar to the concept of principal diagnosis in DSM-III-R, except that in DSM-III-R nonprincipal diagnoses are also recorded. In clinical practice, however, principal diagnoses are often used in an exclusionary fashion, with nonprincipal diagnoses being disregarded.

A third approach is to use chronology as a hierarchical principle. In the Feighner and associates (1972) system, which was designed to increase the homogeneity of research samples, when individuals present with two or more disorders, the condition that developed first is considered primary. Although secondary diagnoses are also made, they are frequently disregarded in the analysis and reporting of data.

Finally, one of the most explicit and detailed hierarchical systems was proposed by Foulds (e.g., Foulds & Bedford, 1975). It consists of four classes: delusions of disintegration (e.g., first-rank symptoms), integrated delusions (e.g., delusions of grandeur, persecution, and guilt), neurotic symptoms (e.g., phobic, obsessive–compulsive, conversion, and dissociative symptoms), and dysthymic states (e.g., anxiety, depression, and elation). Foulds postulated a nonreflexive inclusive relationship between classes, such that membership in a group higher in the hierarchy overrides membership in a lower group, and patients who exhibit symptoms from a particular class will manifest the features of all lower classes (Foulds & Bedford, 1975; Morey, 1987).

While DSM-III-R still retains a number of hierarchical exclusionary criteria, it eliminated many of the exclusion criteria that were present in DSM-III. This change was based on the lack of evidence for most exclusion criteria and data suggesting that some of these criteria resulted in the loss of important information. For example, DSM-III excluded a diagnosis of panic disorder when it was "due to" a mood disorder. However, Leckman, Weissman, Merikangas, Pauls, and Prusoff (1983) reported that probands with both major depression and panic disorder exhibited significantly higher rates of mood and anxiety disorders and alcoholism in their first-degree relatives than probands with major depression alone. Because of the elimination of many of the hierarchical exclusion criteria in DSM-III, rates of comorbidity tend to be much higher when DSM-III-R criteria are employed.

Models of Comorbidity

Comorbidity can exist for a number of reasons. In the following section, we outline 11 possible explanations for cooccurrences between psychiatric disorders (see Table 2.1). The first three models explain comorbidity

TABLE 2.1. Models of Comorbidity

Explanations based on sampling and base rates
 1. Comorbidity due to chance
 2. Comorbidity due to sampling bias
 3. Comorbidity due to population stratification

Explanations based on artifacts of diagnostic criteria
 4. Comorbidity due to overlapping criteria
 5. Comorbidity due to one disorder encompassing the other

Explanations based on drawing boundaries in the wrong places
 6. Multiformity
 7. Heterogeneity of the comorbid condition
 8. The comorbid condition is a third, independent disorder
 9. The pure and comorbid conditions are different phases or alternative expressions of the same disorder

Explanations based on etiological relationships
10. One disorder is a risk factor for the other
11. The two disorders arise from overlapping etiological processes

by sampling procedures and base rates. Models four and five view comorbidity as an artifact of the diagnostic criteria. Models six through nine attribute comorbidity to incorrect boundaries between disorders. The last two models view comorbidity as reflecting causal relationships between the comorbid conditions.

1. *Chance.* The first explanation of comorbidity is that it is a random event. Given two disorders with high prevalences, a significant number of individuals will experience both disorders simply on the basis of chance. The likelihood of comorbidity occurring by chance can be readily calculated by multiplying the base rate (or prevalence) of each of the relevant disorders. For example, if the 6-month prevalences of major depression and alcoholism are 3% and 5%, respectively, then 0.15% of the population would be expected to exhibit both major depression and alcoholism during the same 6-month period simply on the basis of chance.

2. *Sampling bias.* As noted by Berkson (1946), studies using clinical populations can produce artifactually high estimates of comorbidity. Berkson's fallacy is based on the following line of reasoning: Only a subset of individuals with a given disorder ever formally seek treatment. However, the likelihood of seeking treatment is higher for individuals with multiple disorders than for individuals with only one disorder because it is a function of the combined likelihood of referral for each disorder. As a result, studies using clinical samples are likely to overestimate the rate of comorbidity.

3. *Population stratification.* According to the third model, each of the two pure conditions is associated with a distinct set of risk factors, and

both sets of risk factors happen to have an increased prevalence in the same subgroups, or strata, of the population. Within these strata, the likelihood of the two disorders cooccurring is no greater than chance. However, because of the increased prevalence of both sets of risk factors within the same subgroups, the rate of comorbidity is higher than that expected by chance for the population as a whole. As a result, unless population stratification is taken into account, it will appear that the two disorders cooccur at a greater than chance frequency.

This can be illustrated using the comorbidity between depression and alcoholism and between depression and conduct disorder as examples. Thus, it appears that major depression and alcoholism arise from independent etiological processes. However, due to assortative mating between depressives and alcoholics, these sets of risk factors may be associated within families (Merikangas, 1982; Merikangas, Leckman, Prusoff, Pauls, & Weissman, 1985). As a result, offspring in these families often exhibit both major depression and alcoholism.

As a second example, parental depression is a powerful risk factor for depression in children (Hammen, 1991; Weissman, 1988), whereas marital discord is a risk factor for conduct disorder (Rutter & Quinton, 1984). Because depression and marital discord are commonly associated among adults (O'Leary & Beach, 1990), this may account for much of the comorbidity between depression and conduct disorder in children (Caron & Rutter, 1991; Downey & Coyne, 1990).

4. *Overlapping diagnostic criteria.* In Model 4, comorbidity is an artifact of the diagnostic criteria. It can occur when similar symptoms are included in the criteria sets for several different diagnoses (Widiger, 1989). There are a number of such instances in the DSM-III-R. For example, several of the criteria for borderline personality disorder are similar to those for major depression and dysthymia (affective instability, chronic feelings of emptiness or boredom, and recurrent suicidal behavior). It is likely that this contributes to the high comorbidity between these disorders (Kroll, 1988; Widiger, 1989). In addition, the degree of bias produced by overlapping criteria varies as a function of severity. More severely disturbed patients tend to exhibit a greater number of symptoms, including the nonspecific symptoms that are shared by several disorders, than less severely disturbed patients. As a result, the more severe group also exhibits greater comorbidity (Caron & Rutter, 1991).

One approach to addressing this issue is to delete the overlapping criteria from the two disorders and determine whether they are still associated. This strategy has several limitations, however. First, the deletion of criteria changes the original diagnostic construct (Widiger, 1989). For example, the construct of borderline personality is clearly altered by excluding affective lability, chronic feelings of emptiness or boredom, and recurrent suicidal behavior. In addition, this strategy makes it more difficult to meet criteria for the disorder, because there are fewer criteria. Of course, one could also reduce the number of criteria required or substitute new nonoverlapping criteria, but this would alter the construct even further. Finally, if the association between disorders disappeared after overlapping criteria have been eliminated, it is difficult to know whether this is a substantive finding or a result of altering the diagnostic threshold. However, if a significant association remained after the deletion of overlapping criteria, it would be a powerful argument in favor of the existence of real comorbidity.[7] Other approaches to testing this model are outlined later.

5. *One disorder is encompassed by the other.* Another way in which comorbidity can be produced artifactually is when one of the disorders is a part, or manifestation, of the other. This can be viewed as a special case of Model 6, multiformity, discussed next. Examples include diagnosing conversion disorder in a patient with somatization disorder, diagnosing both generalized anxiety and panic disorder in a patient who worries primarily about having panic attacks, and diagnosing both obsessive-compulsive disorder and major depression in a patient who is preoccupied with thoughts of guilt. As discussed previously, one of the major functions of the hierarchical exlusion criteria in DSM-III-R is to eliminate this type of artifactual comorbidity. However, there are cases in which a disorder that is a secondary manifestation of a more pervasive condition should be diagnosed, and the cooccurrence should be viewed as an example of one disorder being a risk factor for another disorder (see Model 10). For instance, a social phobia that develops as a result of body–image disturbance in anorexia nervosa may not be distinguishable from other social phobias but may require additional treatment that is not ordinarily indicated for anorexia (Widiger & Trull, 1991).

Another way of looking at this model is that it implies that the more circumscribed syndrome has a different meaning when accompanied by the symptoms of the more pervasive disorder than when it appears alone. Thus, individuals with both the pervasive and circumscribed conditions should be similar to individuals with only the pervasive syndrome, and different from individuals with only the circumscribed syndrome on relevant correlates such as course, treatment response, and familial transmission.

6. *Multiformity.* As noted previously, Model 5 can be viewed as a special case of a more general model, multiformity (Winokur, 1990). *Multiformity* refers to the fact that disorders can often assume phenomenologically heterogeneous forms, including symptoms that are typically associated with other disorders. Thus, according to Model 6, the comorbid condition is really an atypical form of one of the pure disorders and completely distinct from the other pure disorder, despite its phenomenological overlap. Rather than reflecting true comorbidity, multiformity

indicates that the boundaries of a disorder have been drawn in the wrong place.

In some cases, the comorbid condition may be a more severe form of one of the pure disorders (see the previous discussion of disordinal interactions). For example, several recent studies have suggested that major depression with concurrent panic attacks may represent a more severe form of mood disorder than major depression without panic (Coryell et al., 1988; Leckman et al., 1983).

7. *Heterogeneity of the comorbid condition.* A further variant of the multiformity model can be distinguished when the comorbid condition can be divided into atypical forms of both pure disorders. Hence, this can also be referred to as the *heterogeneity model.* For example, many investigators believe that schizoaffective disorder is a heterogeneous condition that consists of atypical forms of schizophrenia and the affective disorders (Harrow & Grossman, 1984; Tsuang & Simpson, 1984). Indeed, in the Research Diagnostic Criteria (RDC; Spitzer, Endicott, & Robins, 1978), schizoaffective disorder was divided into "mainly schizophrenic" and "mainly affective" subtypes. Similarly, many investigators believe that patients with major depression and substance abuse include subgroups of substance abusers with secondary depression and primary depressives who abuse substances in an attempt to self-medicate (Khantzian, 1985; Schuckit, 1986).

8. *The comorbid condition is a third, independent disorder.* Another possible explanation of comorbidity is that the comorbid condition is a third disorder that is distinct from both of the pure forms. This is similar to D. F. Klein's (1989) concept of syndromal complexity discussed earlier. Although there are few clear examples of it, such a model has been hypothesized for schizoaffective disorder (Harrow & Grossman, 1984; Tsuang & Simpson, 1984).

9. *The pure and comorbid conditions are different phases, or alternative expressions, of the same disorder.* According to Model 9, the two pure conditions and the comorbid condition are all different phases or alternative expressions of a single disorder. In some respects, this can be viewed as the most extreme possible variant of Model 6, multiformity. An example in which the two pure conditions and their comorbid state may all represent different phases of the same disorder is major depression, dysthymia, and double depression, as noted previously (D. N. Klein et al., 1993). An example in which two disorders and their comorbid state may represent different expressions of the same disorder is antisocial personality disorder and somatization disorder (Cloninger, 1978).

10. *One disorder is a risk factor for the other.* According to this model, one of the comorbid disorders functions as a risk factor for the other disorder. Examples of comorbidity that could plausibly be explained by a risk factor model include conduct disorder leading to an increased risk of

substance abuse (Robins & McEvoy, 1990) and obsessive–compulsive disorder giving rise to secondary major depression.

11. *The two disorders arise from overlapping etiological processes.* In this model, the risk factors that contribute to each of the two pure disorders overlap. Thus, each pure disorder is associated with both common and unique etiological processes. As a result, each disorder can appear in its pure form, but the two disorders have a high probability of cooccurring. Two plausible examples of shared risk factors that might contribute to comorbidity in depression include maltreatment in childhood increasing the risk of both major depression and alcoholism (Holmes & Robins, 1987) and serotonergic dysregulation contributing to the risk of major depression and impulsive–aggressive personality disorders (Cocarro et al., 1989).

From the perspective of this model, the traditional search for diagnostically specific correlates has been overemphasized. Identifying nonspecific factors that play a major role in the etiology of multiple disorders may be at least as important for understanding causality and developing more effective interventions.

Distinguishing between Models of Comorbidity

In the final section of this chapter, we outline a systematic approach to distinguishing between these competing explanations of comorbidity. We focus on epidemiological, longitudinal, and family studies, as these are the most commonly employed approaches to research on comorbidity (Maser & Cloninger, 1990). However, other strategies, particularly controlled treatment (Fyer et al., 1990) and twin (Torgerson, 1990) studies, can also make significant contributions. In addition, the methods for establishing boundaries between disorders that were discussed in the first part of this chapter could also be used to test the subset of models that view comorbidity as the result of drawing boundaries in the wrong places (i.e., Models 6 through 9).

Epidemiological Studies

Epidemiological studies of the prevalence of pure (or noncomorbid) and comorbid disorders are critical to understanding comorbidity, as they provide the only means of addressing the first two models, comorbidity due to chance and referral bias. Studies of representative community samples are particularly important, as they can determine whether the rate of cooccurrences between psychiatric disorders is greater than chance without being subject to referral bias.

Epidemiological studies can also be useful in other ways. For example, they may help to identify risk factors that might be shared between disorders (Model 11) or might contribute to population stratification (Model 3). These models could then be tested by determining whether comorbidity was still evident after controlling for the risk factors (Caron & Rutter, 1991).

Longitudinal Studies

A number of investigators have employed longitudinal studies to understand comorbidity (e.g., Angst, Vollrath, Merikangas, & Ernst, 1990; Hagnell & Grasbeck, 1990; Hirschfeld, Hasin, Keller, Endicott, & Wunder, 1990; Kovacs, Gatsonis, Paulauskas, & Richards, 1989). This approach can be used to examine both the course and stability of psychiatric disorders. In our opinion, studies of diagnostic stability have greater potential to elucidate the processes underlying comorbidity than studies focusing on course variables such as rates of recovery and relapse, levels of symptomatology, and social adjustment. A particularly important limitation of studies focusing on course variables is that the pure forms of the two index disorders and the comorbid group cannot be directly compared on most course measures. For example, in a study of comorbidity between major depression and panic disorder, comparisons of the rates of depressive recovery and relapse are necessarily limited to the pure depressive and comorbid groups, whereas comparisons of recovery and relapse of panic are restricted to the pure panic and comorbid groups. The three groups can be directly compared only on nonspecific indices such as social adjustment and global functioning.

Follow-up studies using diagnostic stability as a means of understanding comorbidity should include three groups: subjects with pure (noncomorbid) forms of each of the disorders of interest (Disorder A and Disorder B) and a comorbid group (with both A and B). Table 2.2 outlines five patterns of results that would be consistent with a number of the models of comorbidity outlined previously. In the following discussion, we will assume that the two index disorders can be diagnosed reliably, the sample size is large enough to provide adequate power, and the duration of the follow-up is appropriate for the disorders being considered. We will also assume that comorbidity is defined cross-sectionally, as the presence of two concurrent or intercurrent disorders, rather than on a lifetime basis. Finally, although recovery is a possible outcome for all three groups (A, B, and AB) in all models, it is not included in the following discussion because it cannot contribute to distinguishing between the various models.

This design cannot distinguish between all 11 models. The first two models, comorbidity due to chance and sampling bias, can be addressed only through epidemiological studies, as discussed before. Further, sev-

TABLE 2.2. Predictions of Comorbidity Models Regarding Diagnostic Stability

| | Diagnosis | |
Models	Index	Follow-up
3, 4, 8, and 11	A	A
	AB	AB
	B	B
5 and 6	A	A or AB
	AB	A or AB
	B	B
7	A	A
	AB	A, B, or AB
	B	B
9	A	A, B, or AB
	AB	A, B, or AB
	B	A, B, or AB
10	A	A, B, or AB
	AB	A, B, or AB
	B	B

eral patterns of findings are consistent with multiple models. However, this design is capable of narrowing the field of plausible hypotheses considerably. Finally, Table 2.2 does not provide an exhaustive listing of all possible patterns of results, as some findings would not be consistent with any of the models outlined previously.

The first pattern of results is consistent with Models 3, 4, 8, and 11, but cannot distinguish between them. This pattern consists of all three groups (A, B, and AB) exhibiting diagnostic stability over time. These findings are clearly consistent with the view of the comorbid condition (AB) as a third, independent disorder. However, both Models 3 (population stratification) and 11 (the two index disorders having overlapping etiological processes) would tend to predict stability for all three groups, assuming that the relevant risk factors exerted their impact before the period of maximal risk for the onset of both index disorders. Finally, if comorbidity was due to overlapping criteria (Model 4), the three groups would also be expected to exhibit diagnostic stability, provided that the symptom presentations of the two disorders were relatively stable over time.

The second pattern of findings would be most consistent with Model 6, multiformity. In this pattern, one of the pure groups (A) and the comorbid group (AB) both tend to exhibit A or AB at follow-up, whereas the second pure group (B) tends to exhibit diagnostic stability over time.

This indicates that Conditions A and AB are fundamentally similar, despite the presence of B in the comorbid group, and that Condition AB is probably an atypical form of Condition A. In addition, it suggests that AB and B are distinct conditions.

This pattern of results would also be consistent with Model 5 (one disorder encompassing the other) if Condition A was a relatively pervasive disorder and B was a more circumscribed syndrome that often accompanied A. As noted before, Model 6 is a more general case of Model 5, hence these should not be considered competing explanations. Rather, Model 5 would be the more appropriate explanation if B was an associated feature of Condition A.

Model 7, heterogeneity, would be suggested by the third pattern of findings. The heterogeneity hypothesis would be supported if both pure groups were stable over time, and the comorbid group was highly unstable and tended to evolve into either of the two pure forms of disorder. More specifically, at follow-up, the comorbid group should exhibit a significantly higher rate of pure Disorder A than subjects in pure Group B, and a significantly higher rate of pure Disorder B than subjects in pure Group A. In addition, it is likely that some subjects would continue to exhibit AB at follow-up. This pattern of results is similar to that expected with the multiformity model outlined previously, except that the comorbid group includes atypical forms of both pure disorders.

The fourth pattern would be most consistent with Model 9, the two disorders as different phases or alternative expressions of the same condition. In many, but not all cases, Model 9 would predict that the three conditions would exhibit considerable variability in the form that they assumed at any given point in time.[8] Thus, at follow-up, individuals in all three groups could exhibit Conditions A, B, or AB.

The last pattern would be most consistent with Model 10, one disorder as a risk factor for the other. This pattern assumes that Disorder A is associated with the subsequent development of Disorder B, after which Disorder A may persist or remit. If Disorder B is homogeneous, one might further hypothesize that patients in the pure B group should have previously manifested A, a conjecture that could be tested with retrospective data on clinical history. Specifically, Model 10 would predict that (1) patients with the pure form of A would tend to develop condition B during the follow-up period (in some cases, they might continue to exhibit A in addition to developing B, in other cases A could remit, and in still other cases some patients might not develop B at all); (2) patients with AB would tend to remain stable, although in some cases disorder A or B might remit, leaving just the other condition; and (3) patients with pure B would remain relatively stable over time.[9]

We have described these patterns in a very general manner and have not specified the pairwise comparisons that would be expected to differ significantly in a systematic way. Moreover, because of the general nature of the presentation, we have also failed to discuss a number of other important considerations in applying this approach to particular sets of disorders. Thus, the appropriate length of follow-up and the number and frequency of assessments will depend on the nature of the index disorders. For example, episodic disorders require more frequent assessments, and disorders with greater variability in the age of onset require longer follow-ups.

In addition, it is necessary to consider when in the course of the disorder the study should be initiated. Thus, it is critical to begin the follow-up before most of the comorbidity that might be expected has already developed. Ideally, the study should be restricted to patients in the very early stages of disorder (e.g., first-episode cases).

Furthermore, particular care must be taken in drawing inferences about temporal processes when one of the index disorders naturally tends to be more chronic than the other. In such instances, between-group comparisons (e.g., the stability of Disorder A in Group A versus Group AB, and the stability of Disorder B in Group B versus Group AB) may be more meaningful than within group comparisons (the stability of Disorder A versus B in the comorbid group).

Finally, the definition of *stability* should be consistent with the nature of the index disorders. For example, remission may suggest stability in an episodic disorder, but instability in a chronic disorder.

Family Studies

Family studies are probably the single most useful means of testing alternative models of comorbidity, as unique predictions regarding familial transmission can be generated for most of the 11 models. In fact, when family studies are used in conjunction with epidemiological studies, 10 of the 11 models of comorbidity can be distinguished.

Examples of recent family studies which have attempted to test two or more explanations of comorbidity include Biederman, Faraone, Keenan, and Tsuang (1991); Cloninger, Reich, and Wetzel (1979); Grove, Andreasen, Winokur, and colleagues (1987); Merikangas and associates (1985); and Pauls, Towbin, Leckman, Zahner, and Cohen (1986). However, no study to date has attempted to test the full range of models outlined here.

Ideally, family studies of comorbidity should include four groups: probands with a pure form of Disorder A (Group A), probands with a pure form of Disorder B (Group B), probands with comorbidity between A and B (Group AB), and controls with neither A nor B (Group C). All first-degree relatives should be systematically assessed for the pure forms of each of the index disorders and for their cooccurrence. The key assumption underlying this approach is that both of the index disorders are familial (although not necessarily genetic). In addition, we assume

adequate interrater reliability and statistical power. Comorbidity is assumed to be concurrent or intercurrent in probands. However, comorbidity in relatives is defined on a lifetime basis, as family studies generally
focus on morbid, or lifetime, risks.

Eight potential patterns of findings are outlined in Table 2.3. The first
column in Table 2.3 lists the models of comorbidity. The second column
indicates which dependent variable (i.e., the condition in *relatives*) is being
considered. Column 3 presents the predicted relationships among the
independent variables (i.e., the expected ordering of the *proband* groups
with respect to the rates of disorders in their relatives). Each pattern is
consistent with one or more of the 11 models of comorbidity. As before,
this is not an exhaustive list of all possible patterns of results. Also,
because this is offered as a generic approach, minor modifications may be
necessary, depending on the nature of the specific disorders being studied.
As noted earlier, epidemiological studies are required to test Models 1 and
2 (comorbidity due to chance and referral bias).

Model 3, population stratification, would be consistent with the first
pattern of findings. Thus, the rate of Condition A in the relatives of

**TABLE 2.3. Predictions of Comorbidity Models Regarding
Familial Transmission**

Models	Diagnosis in relatives	Relations of proband groups
3	A	A = AB > B = C
	AB	A = AB = B = C
	B	B = AB > A = C
4	A	A > AB > B = C
	AB	A = AB = B > C
	B	B > AB > A = C
5 and 6	A	A = AB > B = C
	AB	A = AB > B = C
	B	B > A = AB = C
7	A	A > AB > B = C
	AB	A = AB = B = C
	B	B > AB > A = C
8	A	A > AB = B = C
	AB	AB > A = B = C
	B	B > A = AB = C
9	A	A = AB = B > C
	AB	A = AB = B > C
	B	A = AB = B > C
10	A	A = AB = B > C
	AB	A = AB = B > C
	B	A = AB = B = C
11	A	A = AB > B > C
	AB	A = AB = B > C
	B	B = AB > A > C

probands in Groups A and AB should be significantly higher than that of the relatives of Group B and C probands. The rate of the comorbid Condition AB should be low, and similar in the relatives of all four proband groups. Finally, the rate of Condition B should be significantly higher in the relatives of probands in Groups B and AB than in the relatives of probands in Groups A and C.

Model 4, comorbidity due to overlapping diagnostic criteria, predicts the second pattern of findings in Table 2.3. Model 4 is similar to the heterogeneity model (Model 7), in that the comorbid proband group is a mixture of subjects with Disorder A and Disorder B. Their apparent comorbidity is an artifact of the overlap in criteria for the two index disorders. Thus, one would expect that the rate of pure Disorder A would be highest in the relatives of Group A, followed by the comorbid group, and that the rates would be lowest, and comparable, in the relatives of Groups B and C. Similarly, one would expect that the rate of pure Disorder B would be highest in the relatives of Group B, followed by the comorbid group, and that the rates would be lowest, and similar, in the relatives of Groups A and C. Finally, because the overlapping criteria would affect diagnoses in the relatives, as well as in the probands, we would expect higher rates of the comorbid condition (AB) in the relatives of all three patient groups (Groups A, B, and AB) compared to the relatives of controls.[10]

Models 5 (one disorder encompassing the other) and 6 (multiformity) both predict the third pattern of findings. As noted before, Model 5 is a special case of Model 6, and the two models generate similar predictions. Models 5 and 6 predict that the rate of pure Disorder A should be higher in the relatives of proband Groups A and AB than in the relatives of Groups B and C. Similarly, the rate of the comorbid Condition AB should be higher in the relatives of proband Groups A and AB than in the relatives of Groups B and C. Finally, the rate of pure Disorder B should be higher in the relatives of probands with B than in the relatives of probands in Groups A, AB, and C, who should not differ among themselves. If Condition AB was a more severe variant of Condition A, then the rates of A and AB in the relatives of probands with AB would be higher than those in the relatives of probands with A alone, but relatives of the latter group would still exhibit higher rates of both A and AB than the relatives of probands in Groups B and C.

Model 7, the comorbid group as a heterogeneous collection of patients with atypical forms of both A and B, generates the fourth pattern of predictions. This pattern is similar in many respects to the second pattern noted previously, which was generated by the overlapping criteria model. Thus, the rates of Condition A should be highest in the relatives of proband Group A, followed by the relatives of Group AB probands, and then by the relatives of probands in Groups B and C.

Similarly, the rates of Condition B should be highest in the relatives of proband Group B, followed by the relatives of Group AB probands, and then by the relatives of probands in Groups A and C. The only difference between the predictions generated by Models 4 and 7 is in the distribution of comorbid diagnoses in the relatives. Thus, the heterogeneity model would predict that the rate of comorbid Condition AB should be low and similar in the relatives of all four groups of probands.[11]

Model 8, the comorbid Condition as a third, independent disorder, generates the fifth pattern of predictions. According to Model 8, all three conditions should breed true. Thus, Condition A should be significantly more common in the relatives of probands in Group A than in the relatives of probands in Groups AB, B, and C. The comorbid Condition AB should be significantly more prevalent in the relatives of the comorbid probands than in the relatives of probands in Groups A, B, and C. Finally, the rate of Condition B should be significantly higher in the relatives of Group B probands than in the relatives of Group A, AB, and C probands.

Model 9, that the two disorders are different phases or alternative expressions of the same condition, generates the predictions in the sixth pattern. According to Model 9, the two pure disorders and the comorbid condition should all exhibit similar patterns of familial transmission. Thus, the rates of A, B, and AB should be similar in the relatives of all three groups of probands, and significantly greater than the rates of A, B, and AB in the relatives of controls (Group C).

Model 10, that one disorder is a risk factor for the other, leads to the predictions depicted in the seventh pattern. According to this model, Disorder A is the major cause of Disorder B. Hence, it predicts that the rates of Condition A in the relatives of probands in Groups A, AB, and B should be similar, and significantly greater than that in the relatives of controls. Similarly, because the increased rate of Disorder A should be associated with a subsequent increase in the rate of Disorder B, the rates of comorbid Condition AB should also be higher among the relatives of the three patient groups compared to the relatives of controls. Finally, the rates of pure Disorder B should be low, and similar among the relatives of all four groups of probands.[12]

The predictions generated by Model 11, the two disorders sharing overlapping etiological factors, are presented in the last pattern in Table 2.3. According to Model 11, Disorders A and B each have both unique and common risk factors. Thus, this model predicts that the rates of Condition A should be similar in the relatives of probands in Groups A and AB, and significantly higher than that in the relatives of Group B probands. In turn, the rate of A should be significantly higher in the relatives of Group B probands than in the relatives of controls. Model 11 also predicts that the rates of Condition AB should be similar in the relatives of probands in Groups A, AB, and B, and significantly higher than that in the relatives of controls. Finally, this model predicts that the rates of Condition B in the relatives of probands in Groups B and AB are similar, and significantly higher than that in the relatives of Group A probands. In turn, the rate of B in the relatives of probands in Group A should be significantly greater than that in the relatives of controls.

Conclusions

To summarize, the elimination of diagnostic hierarchies has sparked considerable interest in comorbidity. However, comorbidity can result from a variety of processes. Eleven potential explanations of comorbidity have been detailed in this chapter, and a systematic approach using a combination of epidemiological, follow-up, and family studies outlined in order to determine which explanation is most valid for a given pattern of comorbidity. According to the approach proposed here, 10 of the 11 models of comorbidity can be uniquely distinguished. Only two models, one of which (Model 5) is a special case of the other (Model 6), do not appear to be distinguishable on empirical grounds.

At this point, few systematic studies of comorbidity along the lines discussed here have been conducted. Thus, it is unclear whether the competing models outlined here will adequately cover the patterns of data that are observed empirically and whether the follow-up and family studies will converge on the same explanatory models. As more and higher-quality family and follow-up data become available, it should be possible to determine how useful this approach is to understanding the nature of comorbidity in psychopathology.

ACKNOWLEDGMENTS

Preparation of this chapter was supported by National Institute of Mental Health research grant RO1 MH-45757. Joseph E. Schwartz provided many helpful comments and suggestions both in discussions about, and on early drafts of, this chapter. We are also grateful to Charles G. Costello, Donald F. Klein, and Jack D. Maser for their comments on the manuscript.

NOTES

1. The term *entity* is somewhat misleading, as it implies that the disease is a concrete object lodged in the body that is distinct from, and causes, the clinical manifestations of the illness. Although this might be appropriate in certain cases (e.g., viruses), in most instances diseases are better conceptualized as a complex of processes occurring at multiple levels of the organism (Whitbeck, 1977).

2. As Kendell (1989) notes, the preeminent role assigned to etiology is based on more practical than theoretical considerations. Although the history of medicine provides many examples of effective treatments being developed without knowledge of etiology, as well as instances in which the elucidation of causal processes had minimal treatment implications, knowledge of etiology appears to be the single best means of developing effective forms of prevention and treatment.

3. Several additional techniques that may prove useful in exploring boundary issues have been introduced more recently. Grade of membership (GOM) analysis is a multivariate technique designed to identify and describe clinical symptom profiles. Unlike many of the approaches discussed in this chapter, it explicitly takes into account the fact that individuals often exhibit more than one syndrome and display the features of these syndromes to varying degrees. Moreover, GOM analysis can quantify *caseness,* based on the similarity between the individual's clinical profile and that of a prototypical case (George, Blazer, Woodbury, & Manton, 1988). GOM analysis has recently been applied to depression, somatization disorder, and antisocial personality (Blazer et al., 1988; George et al., 1989). Unfortunately, software for conducting GOM analysis is not generally available (Schoenberg & Arminger, 1989).

DeFries and Fulker (1988) recently developed a multiple regression technique that can be applied to twin data to determine whether deviant scores on a continuous measure (e.g., symptoms or personality traits) arise from distinctive etiological processes or simply reflect variation within the normal range. However, an important limitation is that it is extremely difficult to obtain large enough samples of twins to apply this technique to most forms of psychopathology.

A number of other multivariate statistical techniques, such as factor analysis, latent trait analysis, and multidimensional scaling, have been applied to the classification of psychopathology. Whereas these techniques are useful for certain purposes, they assume that the latent variables underlying psychopathology are continuous, rather than categorical, in nature. As a result, they cannot address the issue of boundaries between psychiatric conditions. For good discussions of the uses and limitations of factor analysis in the classification of psychopathology, see Grove and Andreasen (1986) and Maxwell (1972).

4. The notion of overlapping discrete clusters may appear paradoxical at first glance. In medicine, however, it is common to find individuals with multiple independent conditions (e.g., cancer and heart disease).

5. Mixture analysis can be applied to discrete data. In such cases, it can be viewed as equivalent to latent class analysis, discussed later in this chapter (Everitt & Hand, 1981).

6. A variant of this approach involves comparing the strength of the associations between continous and dichotomous versions of a diagnostic variable (e.g., number of symptoms versus above/below a cutoff score) and another variable. If the most important information is simply whether the individual is above or below the diagnostic threshold and distance from the cutoff is relatively unimportant, the dichotomous measure should yield reliability and validity coefficients that are equal to, or greater, than the continuous diagnostic index. If the individual's distance from the threshold conveys meaningful information, however, then the continuous diagnostic measure should exhibit higher reli-

ability and validity coefficients than the dichotomous index (Miller & Thayer, 1989).

7. Of course, the prevalence of comorbidity could not be determined because the diagnostic criteria were modified for the analysis.

8. The two major exceptions would be if Conditions A and B developed in an invariant sequence (e.g., separation anxiety evolving into agoraphobia) or remained relatively stable over time (e.g., antisocial personality and somatization disorder).

9. Because it is assumed that most patients with pure Disorder B exhibited Condition A at some point prior to the initiation of the follow-up study, it is conceivable that some individuals in Group B will experience a recurrence of A during the follow-up period. Thus, depending on whether they recover from B, some may exhibit AB or A alone at follow-up. The predictions generated by this model can be distinguished from those of Model 9 only if it is assumed that patients in Group B are significantly less likely to exhibit Condition A (in either its pure or comorbid form) during the follow-up period than patients in Group A or Group AB. In general, this appears to be a reasonable assumption, although it may not be tenable in specific cases.

One could also posit an interesting variant of Model 10 in which both Disorders A and B were risk factors for the other condition. In that case, one would expect that patients in all three groups (A, B, and AB) would tend to exhibit high rates of comorbidity at follow-up.

10. These predictions are predicated on the assumption that Disorders A and B contribute equally to the comorbid group. They would not hold if the overlapping criteria have a greater effect on one diagnosis than on the other, or if A and B have substantially different prevalences.

11. It is, of course, possible that the same factors that produced a mixed AB presentation in probands could produce the same mixed clinical picture in relatives. The predictions in Table 2.3 assume that this phenomenon is rare and that it could not be detected without huge samples. For example, the affected relatives of patients with schizoaffective disorder tend to suffer from mood disorders or schizophrenia, but rarely exhibit schizoaffective disorder themselves (Abrams, 1984). If this assumption is incorrect, the predictions generated by Model 7 would be similar to those of Model 4 (i.e., the relatives of patients with A, B, and AB would all exhibit higher rates of AB than the relatives of controls), although the two models could still be distinguished on the basis of follow-up studies (see Table 2.2).

12. Several aspects of this model require further explanation. First, the similar rates of pure Condition B in the relatives of Group B and control probands may appear inconsistent with the assumption that both index disorders are familial. However, in testing familiality, there is no distinction between cases in which Condition B occurs alone and cases in which it occurs in conjunction with Condition A. When both forms of Condition B are combined, the overall rate of B should be higher in the relatives of Group B than control probands because of their higher rate of AB.

Second, if A is the major cause of B, one might ask how a group of probands with only B can exist at all. In order to account for this, we have made the not-unreasonable assumption that in rare cases A can cause B without its full clinical manifestations being evident.

An alternative explanation of why B might be evident without A in probands is that Condition B is etiologically heterogeneous. If this were the case, it is likely that the rate of pure Condition B would be somewhat higher in the relatives of Group B probands than in the relatives of probands from Groups A, AB, and C, who should not differ among themselves. This modified set of predictions for Model 10 is still unique and can be distinguished from all the other patterns in Table 2.3.

REFERENCES

Abrams, R. (1984). Genetic studies of the schizoaffective syndrome: A selective review. *Schizophrenia Bulletin, 10,* 26–29.

Achenbach, T. M. (1985). *Assessment and taxonomy of child and adolescent psychopathology.* Beverly Hills, CA: Sage.

Akiskal, H. S., & McKinney, W. T. (1975). Overview of recent research in depression: Integration of ten conceptual models into a comprehensive clinical frame. *Archives of General Psychiatry, 32,* 285–305.

American Psychiatric Association. (1987). *Diagnostic and statistical manual of mental disorders* (3rd ed., rev.). Washington, DC: Author.

Andrews, G., Stewart, G., Morris-Yates, A., Holt, P., & Henderson, S. (1990). Evidence for a general neurotic syndrome. *British Journal of Psychiatry, 157,* 6–12.

Angst, J., Vollrath, M., Merikangas, K. R., & Ernst, C. (1990). Comorbidity of anxiety and depression in the Zurich cohort study of young adults. In J. D. Maser & C. R. Cloninger (Eds.), *Comorbidity of mood and anxiety disorders* (pp. 123–138). Washington, DC: American Psychiatric Press.

Baron, M., Endicott, J., & Ott, J. (1990). Genetic linkage in mental illness: Limitations and prospects. *British Journal of Psychiatry, 157,* 645–655.

Berkson, J. (1946). Limitations of the application of fourfold table analysis to hospital data. *Biometrics, 2,* 47–53.

Berrios, G. E. (1988). Depressive and manic states during the nineteenth century. In A. Georgotas & R. Cancro (Eds.), *Depression and mania* (pp. 13–25). New York: Elsevier.

Biederman, J., Faraone, S. V., Keenan, K., & Tsuang, M. T. (1991). Evidence of familial association between attention deficit disorder and major affective disorders. *Archives of General Psychiatry, 48,* 633–642.

Biederman, J., Newcorn, J., & Sprich, S. (1991). Comorbidity of attention deficit hyperactivity disorder with conduct, depressive, anxiety, and other disorders. *American Journal of Psychiatry, 148,* 564–577.

Blashfield, R. K. (1980). Propositions regarding the use of cluster analysis in clinical research. *Journal of Consulting and Clinical Psychology, 46,* 456–459.

Blashfield, R. K. (1990). Comorbidity and classification. In J. D. Maser & C. R. Cloninger (Eds.), *Comorbidity of mood and anxiety disorders* (pp. 61–82). Washington, DC: American Psychiatric Press.

Blashfield, R. K., & Aldenderfer, M. S. (1978). The literature on cluster analysis. *Multivariate Behavioral Research, 13,* 271–295.

Blashfield, R. K., & Morey, L. C. (1979). The classification of depression through cluster analysis. *Comprehensive Psychiatry, 20,* 516–527.

Blazer, D., Swartz, M., Woodbury, M., Manton, K. G., Hughes, D., & George, L. K. (1988). Depressive symptoms and depressive diagnoses in a community population: Use of a new procedure for analysis of psychiatric classification. *Archives of General Psychiatry, 45,* 1078–1084.

Boyd, J. H., Burke, J. D., Gruenberg, E., Holzer, C. E., Rae, D. S., George, L. K., Karno, M., Stoltzman, R., McEvoy, L., & Nestadt, G. (1984). Exclusion criteria of DSM-III. *Archives of General Psychiatry, 41,* 983–989.

Brady, E. U., & Kendall, P. C. (1992). Comorbidity of anxiety and depression in children and adolescents. *Psychological Bulletin, 111,* 244–255.

Brockington, I. F., Kendell, R. E., Wainwright, S., Hillier, V. F., & Walker, J. (1979). The distinction between the affective psychoses and schizophrenia. *British Journal of Psychiatry, 135,* 243–248.

Brockington, I. F., Roper, A., Copas, J., Buckley, M., Andrade, C. E., Wigg, P., Farmer, A., Kaufman, C., & Hawley, R. (1991). Schizophrenia, bipolar disorder, and depression: A discriminant analysis using "lifetime" psychopathology ratings. *British Journal of Psychiatry, 159,* 485–494.

Caine, E. D., Hunt, R. D., Weingartner, H., & Ebert, M. H. (1978). Huntington's dementia. *Archives of General Psychiatry, 35,* 377–384.

Cantor N., & Genero, N. (1986). Psychiatric diagnosis and natural categorization: A close analogy. In T. Millon & G. L. Klerman (Eds.), *Contemporary directions in psychopathology: Toward the DSM-IV* (pp. 233–256). New York: Guilford.

Carney, M. W. P., Roth, M., & Garside, R. F. (1965). The diagnosis of depressive syndromes and the prediction of ECT response. *British Journal of Psychiatry, 111,* 659–674.

Caron, C., & Rutter, M. (1991). Comorbidity in child psychopathology: Concepts, issues, and research strategies. *Journal of Child Psychology and Psychiatry, 32,* 1063–1080.

Clementz, B. A., Grove, W. M., Iacono, W. G., & Sweeney, J. A. (1992). Smooth-pursuit eye movement dysfunction and liability for schizophrenia: Implications for genetic modeling. *Journal of Abnormal Psychology, 101,* 117–129.

Clogg, C. C. (1977). *Unrestricted and restricted maximum likelihood latent structure analysis: A manual for users* (Working paper 1977-09). University Park: Pennsylvania State University, Population Issues Research Center.

Cloninger, C. R. (1978). The link between hysteria and sociopathy: An integrative model of pathogenesis based on clinical, genetic, and neurophysiological observations. In H. S. Akiskal & W. L. Webb (Eds.), *Psychiatric diagnosis: Exploration of biologic predictors* (pp. 189–218). New York: Spectrum.

Cloninger, C. R. (1989). Establishment of diagnostic validity in psychiatric illness: Robins and Guze's method revisited. In L. N. Robins & J. E. Barrett (Eds.), *The validity of psychiatric diagnosis* (pp. 9–18). New York: Raven.

Cloninger, C. R., Martin, R. L., Guze, S. B., & Clayton, P. J. (1985). Diagnosis and prognosis in schizophrenia. *Archives of General Psychiatry, 42,* 15–25.

Cloninger, C. R., Reich, T., & Wetzel (1979). Alcoholism and the affective disorders: Familial associations and genetic models. In D. Goodwin & C. Erickson (Eds.), *Alcoholism and the affective disorders* (pp. 57–86). New York: Spectrum.

Cloninger, C. R., Reich, T., & Yokoyama, S. (1983). Genetic diversity, genome organization, and investigation of the etiology of psychiatric diseases. *Psychiatric Developments, 3,* 225–246.

Cocarro, E. F., Siever, L. J., Klar, H. M., Maurer, G., Cochrane, K., Cooper, T. B., Mohs, R. C., & Davis, K. L. (1989). Serotonergic studies in patients with affective and personality disorders: Correlates with suicidal and impulsive aggressive behavior. *Archives of General Psychiatry, 46,* 587–599.

Coryell, W., Endicott, J., Andreasen, N. C., Keller, M. B., Clayton, P. J., Hirschfeld, R. M. A., Scheftner, W. A., & Winokur, G. (1988). Depression and panic attacks: The significance of overlap as reflected in follow-up and family study data. *American Journal of Psychiatry, 145,* 293–300.

Cronbach, L. J., & Meehl, P. E. (1955). Construct validity in psychological tests. *Psychological Bulletin, 52,* 281–302.

Crow, T. J. (1990). The continuum of psychosis and its genetic origins. *British Journal of Psychiatry, 156,* 788–797.

Day, N. E. (1969). Estimating the components of a mixture of normal distributions. *Biometrika, 56,* 463–474.

DeFries, J. C., & Fulker, D. W. (1988). Multiple regression analysis of twin data: Etiology of deviant scores versus individual differences. *Acta Geneticae Medicae et Gemellologiae, 37,* 205–216.

Depue, R. A., & Monroe, S. M. (1983). Psychopathology research. In M. Hersen, A. E. Kazdin, & A. S. Bellack (Eds.), *The clinical psychology handbook* (pp. 239–264). Elmsford, NY: Pergamon.

Docherty, J. P., Fiester, S. J., & Shea, T. (1986). Syndrome diagnosis and personality disorder. *Annual Review of Psychiatry, 5,* 315–355.

Dorus, E., Cox, N. J., Gibbons, R. D., Shaughnessy, R., Pandey, G. N., & Cloninger, C. R. (1983). Lithium ion transport and affective disorders within families of bipolar patients. *Archives of General Psychiatry, 40,* 545–556.

Downey, G., & Coyne, J. C. (1990). Children of depressed parents: An integrative review. *Psychological Bulletin, 108,* 50–76.

Eaton, W. W., & Bohrnstedt, G. (1989). Introduction. *Sociological Methods & Research, 18,* 4–18.

Eaton, W. W., Dryman, A., Sorenson, A., & McCutcheon, A. (1989). DSM-III major depressive disorder in the community: A latent class analysis of data from the NIMH Epidemiological Catchment Area Programme. *British Journal of Psychiatry, 155,* 48–54.

Erlenmeyer-Kimling, L., Golden, R., & Cornblatt, B. A. (1989). A taxometric analysis of cognitive and neuromotor variables in children at risk for schizophrenia. *Journal of Abnormal Psychology, 98,* 203–208.

Everitt, B. S. (1972). Cluster analysis: A brief discussion of some of the problems. *British Journal of Psychiatry, 120,* 143–145.

Everitt, B. S. (1981a). Bimodality and the nature of depression. *British Journal of Psychiatry, 138,* 336–339.

Everitt, B. S. (1981b). A Monte Carlo investigation of the likelihood ratio test for the number of components in a mixture of normal distributions. *Multivariate Behavioral Research, 16,* 171–180.

Everitt, B. S., Gourlay, J., & Kendell, R. E. (1971). An attempt at validation of traditional psychiatric syndromes by cluster analysis. *British Journal of Psychiatry, 119,* 399–412.

Everitt, B. S., & Hand, D. J. (1981). *Finite mixture distributions.* London: Chapman & Hall.

Eysenck, H. J., Wakefield, J. A., & Friedman, A. F. (1983). Diagnosis and clinical assessment: The DSM-III. *Annual Review of Psychology, 34,* 167–193.

Fawcett, J., Clark, D. C., Scheftner, R. D., & Gibbons, R. D. (1983). Assessing anhedonia in psychiatric patients. *Archives of General Psychiatry, 40,* 79–88.

Feighner, J. P., Robins, E., Guze, S. B., Woodruff, R. A., Winokur, G., & Munoz, R. (1972). Diagnostic criteria for use in psychiatric research. *Archives of General Psychiatry, 26,* 57–63.

Feinstein, A. R. (1970). The pre-therapeutic classification of co-morbidity in chronic disease. *Journal of Chronic Disease, 23,* 455–468.

First, M. B., Spitzer, R. L., & Williams, J. B. W. (1990). Exclusionary principles and the comorbidity of psychiatric diagnoses: A historical review and implications for the future. In J. D. Maser & C. R. Cloninger (Eds.), *Comorbidity of mood and anxiety disorders* (pp. 61–82). Washington, DC: American Psychiatric Press.

Fleiss, J. L. (1972). Classification of the depressive disorders by numerical taxonomy. *Journal of Psychiatric Research, 9,* 141–153.

Fleiss, J. L., & Zubin, J. (1969). On the methods and theory of clustering. *Multivariate Behavioral Research, 4,* 235–250.

Foulds, G. A., & Bedford, A. (1975). Hierarchy of classes of personal illness. *Psychological Medicine, 5,* 181–192.

Frances, A. J. (1982). Categorical and dimensional systems of personality diagnosis: A comparison. *Comprehensive Psychiatry, 23,* 516–527.

Frances, A. J., Widiger, T., & Fyer, M. R. (1990). The influence of classification methods on comorbidity. In J. D. Maser & C. R. Cloninger (Eds.), *Comorbidity of mood and anxiety disorders* (pp. 41–59). Washington, DC: American Psychiatric Press.

Fyer, A. J., Liebowitz, M. R., & Klein, D. F. (1990). Treatment trials, comorbidity, and syndromal complexity. In J. D. Maser & C. R. Cloninger (Eds.), *Comorbidity of mood and anxiety disorders* (pp. 669–680). Washington, DC: American Psychiatric Press.

George, L. K., Blazer, D. G., Woodbury, M. A., & Manton, K. G. (1989). Internal consistency of DSM-III diagnoses. In L. N. Robins & J. E. Barrett (Eds.), *The validity of psychiatric diagnosis* (pp. 99–125). New York: Raven.

Gershon, E. S., DeLisi, L. E., Hamovit, J., Nurnberger, J. I., Maxwell, M. E., Schreiber, J., Dauphinais, D., Dingman, C. W., & Guroff, J. J. (1988). A controlled family study of chronic psychoses: Schizophrenia and schizoaffective disorder. *Archives of General Psychiatry, 45,* 328–336.

Gershon, E. S., & Reider, R. O. (1980). Are mania and schizophrenia genetically distinct? In R. H. Belmaker & H. M. van Praag (Eds.), *Mania: An evolving concept* (pp. 97–109). New York: Spectrum.

Gibbons, R. D., Dorus, E., Ostrow, D. G., Pandey, G. N., Davis, J. M., & Levy,

D. L. (1984). Mixture distributions in psychiatric research. *Biological Psychiatry, 19*, 935–961.

Golden, R. R. (1982). A taxometric model for detection of a conjectured latent taxon. *Multivariate Behavioral Research, 17*, 389–416.

Golden, R. R. (1991). Bootstrapsing taxometrics: On the development of a method for detection of a single major gene. In W. M. Grove & D. Cicchetti (Eds.), *Thinking clearly about psychology: Vol. 2. Personality and psychopathology* (pp. 259–294). Minneapolis: University of Minnesota Press.

Golden, R. R., Campbell, M. D., & Perry, R. (1987). Taxometric method for diagnosis of tardive dyskinesia. *Journal of Psychiatric Research, 21*, 233–241.

Golden, R. R., & Meehl, P. E. (1979). Detection of the schizoid taxon with MMPI indicators. *Journal of Abnormal Psychology, 88*, 217–233.

Goodman, L. A. (1974). The analysis of systems of qualitative variables when some of the variables are unobservable. Part I: A modified latent structure approach. *American Journal of Sociology, 79*, 1179–1259.

Gorenstein, E. E. (1984). Debating mental illness: Implications for science, medicine, and social policy. *American Psychologist, 39*, 50–56.

Gould, S. J. (1989). *Wonderful life: The Burgess Shale and the nature of history.* New York: W. W. Norton.

Grayson, D. A. (1987). Can categorical and dimensional views of psychiatric illness be distinguished? *British Journal of Psychiatry, 151*, 355–361.

Grove, W. M. (1991). Validity of taxometric inferences based on cluster analysis stopping rules. In W. M. Grove & D. Cicchetti (Eds.), *Thinking clearly about psychology: Vol. 2, Personality and psychopathology* (pp. 313–329). Minneapolis: University of Minnesota Press.

Grove, W. M., & Andreasen, N. C. (1986). Multivariate statistical analysis in psychopathology. In T. Millon & G. L. Klerman (Eds.), *Contemporary directions in psychopathology: Toward the DSM-IV* (pp. 347–362). New York: Guilford.

Grove, W. M., & Andreasen, N. C. (1989). Quantitative and qualitative distinctions between psychiatric disorders. In L. N. Robins & J. E. Barrett (Eds.), *The validity of psychiatric diagnosis* (pp. 127–141). New York: Raven.

Grove, W. M., Andreasen, N. C., Winoker, G., Clayton, P. J., Endicott, J., & Coryell, W. H. (1987). Primary and secondary affective disorders: Unipolar patients compared on familial aggregation. *Comprehensive Psychiatry, 28*, 113–126.

Grove, W. M., Andreasen, N. C., Young, M., Endicott, J., Keller, M. B., Hirschfeld, R. M. A., & Reich, T. (1987). Isolation and characterization of a nuclear depressive syndrome. *Psychological Medicine, 17*, 471–484.

Grove, W. M., & Tellegen, A. (1987). Distinguishing types from continua: Not as easy as it looks. Unpublished manuscript, University of Minnesota, Department of Psychology, Minneapolis.

Grove, W. M., & Tellegen, A. (1991). Problems in the classification of personality disorders. *Journal of Personality Disorders, 5*, 31–41.

Gunderson, J. G., Links, P. S., & Reich, J. H. (1991). Competing models of personality disorders. *Journal of Personality Disorders, 5*, 60–68.

Gunderson, J. G., & Phillips, K. A. (1991). A current view of the interface between borderline personality disorder and depression. *American Journal of Psychiatry, 148,* 967–975.

Haberman, S. (1979). *Analysis of qualitative data* (Vol. 2). New York: Academic Press.

Hagnell, O., & Grasbeck, A. (1990). Comorbidity of anxiety and depression in the Lundby 25-year prospective study: The pattern of subsequent episodes. In J. D. Maser & C. R. Cloninger (Eds.), *Comorbidity of mood and anxiety disorders* (pp. 139–152). Washington, DC: American Psychiatric Press.

Hammen, C. (1991). *Depression runs in families: The social context of risk and resilience in children of depressed mothers.* New York: Springer-Verlag.

Hand, S., & Everitt, B. S. (1987). A Monte Carlo study of the recovery of cluster structure in binary data by hierarchical clustering techniques. *Multivariate Behavioral Research, 22,* 235–243.

Harris, H., & Smith, C. A. B. (1949). The sib–sib age of onset correlation among individuals suffering from the same hereditary syndrome produced by more than one gene. *Annals of Eugenics, 14,* 309–318.

Harrow, M., & Grossman, L. S. (1984). Outcome in schizoaffective disorders: A critical review and reevaluation of the literature. *Schizophrenia Bulletin, 10,* 87–108.

Hicks, L. E. (1984). Conceptual and empirical analysis of some assumptions of an explicitly typological theory. *Journal of Personality and Social Psychology, 46,* 1118–1131.

Hirschfeld, R. M. A., Hasin, D., Keller, M. B., Endicott, J., & Wunder, J. (1990). Depression and alcoholism: Comorbidity in a longitudinal study. In J. D. Maser & C. R. Cloninger (Eds.), *Comorbidity of mood and anxiety disorders* (pp. 293–304). Washington, DC: American Psychiatric Press.

Holmes, S. J., & Robins, L. N. (1987). The influence of childhood disciplinary experience on the development of alcoholism and depression. *Journal of Child Psychology and Psychiatry, 28,* 399–415.

Holzman, P. S., Kringlen, E., Matthysse, S., Flanagan, S. D., Lipton, R. B., Cramer, G., Levin, S., Lange, K., & Levy, D. L. (1988). A single dominant gene can account for eye tracking dysfunctions and schizophrenia in offspring of discordant twins. *Archives of General Psychiatry, 45,* 641–647.

Hudson, R. P. (1983). *Disease and its control: The shaping of modern thought.* Westport, CT: Greenwood.

Iacono, W. G., Moreau, M., Beiser, M., Fleming, J. A. E., & Lin, T.-Y. (1992). Smooth-pursuit eye tracking in first-episode psychotic patients and their relatives. *Journal of Abnormal Psychology, 101,* 104–116.

Jackson, S. W. (1986). *Melancholia and depression: From Hippocratic times to modern times.* New Haven: Yale University Press.

Keller, M. B., & Lavori, P. W. (1984). Double depression, major depression, and dysthymia: Distinct entities or different phases of a single disorder? *Psychopharmacology Bulletin, 20,* 399–402.

Kendell, R. E. (1968a). *The classification of depressive illness* (Maudsley Monograph No. 18). London: Oxford University Press.

Kendell, R. E. (1968b). An important source of bias affecting ratings made by psychiatrists. *Journal of Psychiatric Research, 6,* 135–141.

Kendell, R. E. (1969). The continuum model of depressive illness. *Journal of the Royal Society of Medicine, 62*, 335–339.

Kendell, R. E. (1975). *The role of diagnosis in psychiatry*. Oxford: Blackwell Scientific.

Kendell, R. E. (1982). The choice of diagnostic criteria for biological research. *Archives of General Psychiatry, 39*, 1334–1339.

Kendell, R. E. (1989). Clinical validity. *Psychological Medicine, 19*, 45–55.

Kendell, R. E., & Brockington, I. F. (1980). The identification of disease entities and the relationship between schizophrenia and affective psychoses. *British Journal of Psychiatry, 137*, 324–331.

Kendell, R. E., & Gourlay, J. (1970). The clinical distinction between psychotic and neurotic depression. *British Journal of Psychiatry, 117*, 257–266.

Kendler, K. S. (1985). Diagnostic approaches to schizotypal personality disorder: A historical perspective. *Schizophrenia Bulletin, 11*, 538–553.

Kendler, K. S., Heath, A. C., Martin, N. G., & Eaves, L. J. (1987). Symptoms of anxiety and symptoms of depression: Same genes, different environments? *Archives of General Psychiatry, 44*, 451–457.

Khantzian, E. J. (1985). The self-medication hypothesis of affective disorders: Focus on heroin and cocaine dependence. *American Journal of Psychiatry, 142*, 1259–1264.

Klein, D. F. (1989). The pharmacological validation of psychiatric diagnosis. In L. N. Robins & J. E. Barrett (Eds.), *The validity of psychiatric diagnosis* (pp. 203–216). New York: Raven.

Klein, D. N. (1990). Symptom criteria and family history in major depression. *American Journal of Psychiatry, 147*, 850–854.

Klein, D. N., Riso, L. P., & Anderson, R. L. (1993). DSM-III-R Dysthymia: Antecedents and underlying assumptions. In L. J. Chapman, J. P. Chapman, & D. C. Fowles (Eds.), *Progress in experimental personality and psychopathology research* (Vol. 16) (pp. 222–253). New York: Springer.

Klerman, G. L. (1990). Approaches to the phenomena of comorbidity. In J. D. Maser & C. R. Cloninger (Eds.), *Comorbidity of mood and anxiety disorders* (pp. 13–37). Washington, DC: American Psychiatric Press.

Kovacs, M., Gatsonis, C., Paulauskas, S. L., & Richards, C. (1989). Depressive disorders in childhood, IV: A longitudinal study of comorbidity with and risk for anxiety disorders. *Archives of General Psychiatry, 46*, 776–782.

Kroll, J. (1988). *The challenge of the borderline patient*. New York: W. W. Norton.

Lazarsfeld, P. F., & Henry, N. W. (1968). *Latent structure analysis*. Boston: Houghton Mifflin.

Leckman, J. F., Weissman, M. M., Merikangas, K. R., Pauls, D. L., & Prusoff, B. A. (1983). Panic disorder and major depression: Increased risk of depression, alcoholism, panic, and phobic disorders in families of depressed probands with panic disorder. *Archives of General Psychiatry, 40*, 1055–1060.

Lenzenweger, M. F., & Moldin, S. O. (1990). Discerning the latent structure of hypothetical psychosis proneness through admixture analysis. *Psychiatry Research, 33*, 243–257.

Lessing, E. E., Williams, V., & Gil, E. (1982). A cluster-analytically derived typology: Feasible alternative to clinical diagnostic classification of children? *Journal of Abnormal Child Psychology, 10*, 451–482.

Levy, D. L., Dorus, E., Shaughnessy, R., Yasillo, N. J., Pandey, G. N., Janicak, P. G., Gibbons, R. D., Gaviria, M., & Davis, J. M. (1985). Pharmacologic evidence for specificity of pursuit to schizophrenia: Lithium carbonate associated with abnormal pursuit. *Archives of General Psychiatry, 42,* 335–341.

Lorr, M., Klett, C. J., & McNair, D. M. (1963). *Syndromes of psychosis.* New York: Macmillan.

Maser, J. D., & Cloninger, C. R. (1990). *Comorbidity of mood and anxiety disorders.* Washington, DC: American Psychiatric Press.

Maxwell, A. E. (1972). Difficulties in a dimensional description of symptomatology. *British Journal of Psychiatry, 121,* 19–26.

McCutcheon, A. L. (1987). *Latent class analysis.* Newbury Park, CA: Sage.

Meehl, P. E. (1973). MAXCOV-HITMAX: A taxometric search method for loose genetic syndromes. In P. E. Meehl (Ed.), *Psychodiagnosis: Selected papers* (pp. 200–224). Minneapolis: University of Minnesota Press.

Meehl, P. E. (1977). Specific etiology and other forms of strong influence: Some quantitative meanings. *Journal of Medicine and Philosophy, 2,* 33–53.

Meehl, P. E. (1979). A funny thing happened to us on the way to the latent entities. *Journal of Personality Assessment, 43,* 564–577.

Meehl, P. E. (1986). Diagnostic taxa as open concepts: Metatheoretical and statistical questions about reliability and construct validity in the grand strategy of nosological revision. In T. Millon & G. L. Klerman (Eds.), *Contemporary directions in psychopathology: Toward the DSM-IV* (pp. 215–231). New York: Guilford.

Meehl, P. E. (1989). Schizotaxia revisited. *Archives of General Psychiatry, 46,* 935–944.

Meehl, P. E., & Golden, R. R. (1982). Taxometric methods. In P. C. Kendall & J. N. Butcher (Eds.), *Handbook of research methods in clinical psychology* (pp. 127–181). New York: Wiley.

Merikangas, K. R. (1982). Assortative mating for psychiatric disorders and psychological traits. *Archives of General Psychiatry, 39,* 1173–1180.

Merikangas, K. R., Leckman, J. F., Prusoff, B. A., Pauls, D. L., & Weissman, M. M. (1985). Familial transmission of depression and alcoholism. *Archives of General Psychiatry, 42,* 367–372.

Miller, M. L., & Thayer, J. F. (1989). On the existence of discrete classes in personality: Is self-monitoring the correct joint to carve? *Journal of Personality and Social Psychology, 57,* 143–155.

Milligan, G. W., & Cooper, M. C. (1987). Methodology review: Clustering methods. *Applied Psychological Measurement, 11,* 329–354.

Moldin, S. O., Gottesman, I. I., & Erlenmeyer-Kimling, L. (1987). Searching for the psychometric boundaries of schizophrenia: Evidence from the New York high-risk study. *Journal of Abnormal Psychology, 96,* 354–363.

Moldin, S. O., Rice, J. P., Gottesman, I. I., & Erlenmeyer-Kimling, L. (1990). Psychometric deviance in offspring at risk for schizophrenia: Resolving heterogeneity through admixture analysis. *Psychiatry Research, 32,* 311–322.

Moran, P. A. P. (1966). The establishment of a psychiatric syndrome. *British Journal of Psychiatry, 112,* 1165–1171.

Morey, L. C. (1987). The Foulds hierarchy of personal illness: A review of recent research. *Comprehensive Psychiatry, 28,* 159–168.

Morey, L. C. (1988). The categorical representation of personality disorder: A cluster analysis of DSM-III-R personality features. *Journal of Abnormal Psychology, 97,* 314–321.

Morey, L. C., & Blashfield, R. K. (1981). A review of cluster analysis studies of alcoholism. *Journal of Studies on Alcohol, 42,* 925–937.

Murphy, E. A. (1964). One cause? Many causes? The argument from the bimodal distribution. *Journal of Chronic Disease, 17,* 301–324.

O'Leary, K. D., & Beach, S. R. H (1990). Marital therapy: A viable treatment for depression and marital discord. *American Journal of Psychiatry, 147,* 183–186.

Parker, G., Hadzi-Pavlovic, D., Boyce, P., Wilhelm, K., Brodaty, H., Mitchell, P., Hickie, I., & Eyers, K. (1990). Classifying depression by mental state signs. *British Journal of Psychiatry, 157,* 55–65.

Pauls, D. L., Towbin, K. E., Leckman, J. F., Zahner, G. E. P., & Cohen, D. J. (1986). Gilles de la Tourette's syndrome and obsessive–compulsive disorder: Evidence supporting a genetic relationship. *Archives of General Psychiatry, 43,* 1180–1182.

Paykel, E. S. (1981). Have multivariate statistics contributed to classification? *British Journal of Psychiatry, 139,* 357–362.

Pearson, K. (1894). Contribution to the mathematical theory of evolution: 1. Dissection of frequency curves. *Philosophical Transactions of the Royal Society of London* (A), *185,* 71–110.

Pies, R. (1979). On myths and countermyths: More on Szaszian fallacies. *Archives of General Psychiatry, 36,* 139–144.

Rindskopf, D., & Rindskopf, W. (1986). The value of latent class analysis in medical diagnosis. *Statistics in Medicine, 5,* 21–27.

Robins, E., & Guze, S. B. (1970). Establishment of diagnostic validity in psychiatric illness: Its application to schizophrenia. *American Journal of Psychiatry, 126,* 983–987.

Robins, L. N., & McEvoy, L. (1990). Conduct problems as predictors of substance abuse. In L. Robins & M. Rutter (Eds.), *Straight and devious pathways from childhood to adulthood* (pp. 182–204). New York: Cambridge University Press.

Rosch, E., & Mervis, C. B. (1975). Family resemblances: Studies in the internal structure of categories. *Cognitive Psychology, 7,* 573–605.

Rosenberg, R., & Knight, R. A. (1988). Determining male sexual offender subtypes using cluster analysis. *Journal of Quantitative Criminology, 4,* 383–410.

Roth, M., & Mountjoy, C. Q. (1982). The distinction between anxiety states and depressive disorders. In E. S. Paykel (Ed.), *Handbook of affective disorders* (pp. 70–92). New York: Guilford.

Rutter, M., & Quinton, D. (1984). Parental psychiatric disorder: Effects on children. *Psychological Medicine, 14,* 853–880.

Schneider, K. (1958). *Psychopathic personalities.* London: Cassell.

Schoenberg, R., & Arminger, G. (1989). Latent variable models of dichotomous data: The state of the method. *Sociological Methods & Research, 18,* 164–182.

Schuckit, M. A. (1986). Genetic and clinical implications of alcoholism and affective disorder. *American Journal of Psychiatry, 143,* 140–147.

Sigvardsson, S., Bohman, M., von Knorring, A. L., & Cloninger, C. R. (1986). Symptom patterns and causes of somatization in men. I: Differentiation of two discrete disorders. *Genetic Epidemiology, 3,* 153–169.

Sims, A. (1986). Perspectives in the study of neuroses in contemporary psychiatric practice. *Psychiatric Developments, 4,* 273–287.

Skinner, H. A. (1981). Toward the integration of classification theory and methods. *Journal of Abnormal Psychology, 90,* 68–87.

Skinner, H. A. (1986). Construct validation approach to psychiatric classification. In T. Millon & G. L. Klerman (Eds.), *Contemporary directions in psychopathology: Toward the DSM-IV* (pp. 307–330). New York: Guilford.

Sneath, P. H. A., & Sokal, R. R. (1973). *Numerical taxonomy.* San Francisco: W. H. Freeman.

Sokal, R. R. (1974). Classification: Purposes, principles, progress, prospects. *Science, 185,* 1115–1123.

Sokal, R. R., & Sneath, P. H. A. (1963). *Principles of numerical taxonomy.* San Francisco: W. H. Freeman.

Spitzer, R. L., Endicott, J., & Robins, E. (1978). Research Diagnostic Criteria: Rationale and reliability. *Archives of General Psychiatry, 35,* 773–782.

Stein, D. J. (1991). Philosophy and the DSM-III. *Comprehensive Psychiatry, 32,* 404–415.

Strauss, J. S. (1975). A comprehensive approach to psychiatric diagnosis. *American Journal of Psychiatry, 132,* 1193–1197.

Strauss, J. S., Bartko, J. J., & Carpenter, W. T. (1973). The use of clustering techniques for the classification of psychiatric patients. *British Journal of Psychiatry, 122,* 531–540.

Taylor, M. A. (1992). Are schizophrenia and affective disorder related? A selective literature review. *American Journal of Psychiatry, 149,* 22–32.

Titterington, D. M., Smith, A. F. M., & Makov, U. E. (1985). *Statistical analysis of finite mixture distributions.* Chichester, England: Wiley.

Torgerson, S. (1990). A twin-study perspective of the comorbidity of anxiety and depression. In J. D. Maser & C. R. Cloninger (Eds.), *Comorbidity of mood and anxiety disorders* (pp. 367–378). Washington, DC: American Psychiatric Press.

Trull, T. J., Widiger, T. A., & Guthrie, P. (1990). Categorical versus dimensional status of borderline personality disorder. *Journal of Abnormal Psychology, 99,* 40–48.

Tsuang, M. T., & Simpson, J. C. (1984). Schizoaffective disorder: Concept and reality. *Schizophrenia Bulletin, 10,* 14–25.

Tyrer, P. (1989). *Classification of neurosis.* Chichester, England: Wiley.

Wakefield, J. C. (1992). The concept of mental disorder. *American Psychologist, 47,* 373–388.

Weiner, H. (1978). The illusion of simplicity: The medical model revisited. *American Journal of Psychiatry, 135* (Suppl.), 27–33.

Weissman, M. M. (1988). Psychopathology in the children of depressed parents: Direct interview studies. In D. L. Dunner, E. S. Gershon, & J. E. Barrett (Eds.), *Relatives at risk for mental disorders* (pp. 143–159). New York: Raven.

Whitbeck, C. (1977). Causation in medicine: The disease entity model. *Philosophy of Science, 44,* 619–637.

Widiger, T. A. (1989). The categorical distinction between personality and affective disorders. *Journal of Personality Disorders, 3,* 77–91.

Widiger, T. A. (1991). Personality disorder dimensional models proposed for DSM-IV. *Journal of Personality Disorders, 5,* 386–398.

Widiger, T. A., & Trull, T. J. (1991). Diagnosis and clinical assessment. *Annual Review of Psychology, 42,* 109–133.

Winokur, G. (1990). The concept of secondary depression and its relationship to comorbidity. *Psychiatric Clinics of North America, 13,* 567–583.

Young, M. A. (1983). Evaluating diagnostic criteria: A latent class model. *Journal of Psychiatric Research, 17,* 285–296.

Young, M. A., Abrams, R., Taylor, M. A., & Meltzer, H. Y. (1983). Establishing diagnostic criteria for mania. *Journal of Nervous and Mental Disease, 171,* 676–682.

Young, M. A., Scheftner, W. A., Klerman, G. L., Andreasen, N. C., & Hirschfeld, R. M. A. (1986). The endogenous sub-type of depression: A study of its internal construct validity. *British Journal of Psychiatry, 148,* 257–267.

Young, M. A., & Tanner, M. A. (1983). Recent advances in the analysis of qualitative data with applications to diagnostic classification. In R. D. Gibbons & M. Dysken (Eds.), *Statistical and methodological advances in psychiatric research* (pp. 149–180). New York: Spectrum.

Young, M. A., Tanner, M. A., & Meltzer, H. Y. (1982). Operational definitions of schizophrenia: What do they identify? *Journal of Nervous and Mental Disease, 170,* 443–447.

Zubin, J. (1938). A technique for measuring likemindedness. *Journal of Abnormal and Social Psychology, 33,* 508–516.

3

Psychopathology in the Clinic and in the Community

CHARLES G. COSTELLO

In the second half of this century, there have been an increasing number of community investigations of psychopathology. Some investigators have simply obtained data on prevalences of psychopathological disorders for different time periods ranging from lifetime to current (e.g., Robins & Regier, 1991). Others have investigated psychosocial factors associated with psychopathology (e.g., Bebbington et al., 1981; Bebbington, Tennant, & Hurry, 1981; Brown & Harris, 1978a; Costello, 1982; Surtees, Sashidharan, & Dean, 1986). In both kinds of investigations, random samples of the community have been interviewed, and standardized psychiatric interviews, ratings, and computational procedures have been used to identify individuals who satisfy one or another set of criteria for a psychopathological disorder.

There are the following advantages to researching psychopathology as it exists in the community:

1. Epidemiological studies that provide prevalence data are of value because they provide public health professionals with an indication of the extent of the problem of psychopathological disorders and therefore the adequacy of available and planned health services.

2. Only a small proportion of those with psychopathological disorders are seen by mental health professionals. Studies by Goldberg and Huxley (1980) and Giel, Koeter, and Ormel (1990) indicate that, whereas the annual rates per 1,000 of such disorders identified in the community is

67

250 and 303, respectively, the rates seen by psychiatrists are 23 and 44, respectively. Tansella and Williams's (1989) findings indicated that the weekly prevalence in the community was 227 per 1,000, whereas the weekly rate of patients seen by psychiatrists was 4.7 per 1,000. Shapiro and colleagues (1984) found that in three sites of the epidemiological catchment area investigation less than 20% of individuals with psychiatric disorders in the previous 6 months had contacted a mental health professional: 15.6% in Baltimore, 17.8% in St. Louis, and 19.5% in New Haven.

3. Experimental and quasi-experimental studies of cases of psychopathology identified in the community may, in some instances, provide more unequivocal data than those obtained from patients in clinics because (1) as Eysenck (1970b) has noted, the selection processes that bring people into clinics may give rise to unreal associations between symptoms; (2) factors that are associated with the onset of psychopathological disorders may not be identified in patient samples because they are also associated with a decreased likelihood of entry into the health system (for instance, Brown and Harris [1978a] found that women with small children at home were at increased risk for depression and were also less likely to seek professional help than women without such children at home); and (3) investigations of patients are often confounded by factors such as medication;

4. Investigations of psychopathology in the community might enable one to study the early development of symptoms.

These advantages of community investigations rest on the assumption that cases of psychopathology identified in the community do not differ in the nature of their disorders from cases in clinics. Otherwise, one would not be able to generalize to clinic cases the research findings obtained in studies of community cases. This assumption has been questioned in relation to depression, which is the disorder that has most often been investigated by those interested in obtaining data beyond simple prevalences of the disorder and also the disorder on which I focus in this chapter. For instance, Thase, Frank and Kupfer (1985) wrote: "Far too much research pertaining to the psychosocial aspects of depression has been conducted with milder subclinical samples rather than actual patient populations. . . . Therefore, it is difficult, if not impossible, to generalise findings from such investigations to the samples of major depressives studied in biological research settings" (p. 879). Similar concerns have been expressed by Tennant and Bebbington (1978), Richman and Barry (1985), Akiskal (1987), and Snaith (1987).

Those who believe that depression found in the community is different from depression found in clinics argue that community depressions, compared with clinic depressions, (1) have fewer symptoms, which are less severe and which are different in kind; (2) are of shorter duration; (3) are less incapacitating; (4) are more environmentally and less biologically caused; and (5) are more responsive to psychological intervention and less responsive to pharmacological intervention.

In this chapter I examine the degree to which there is empirical support for these arguments. The studies reviewed have all used established, standardized psychiatric interviews such as the Present State Examination (PSE) (Wing, Cooper, & Sartorius, 1974; Wing, Mann, Leff, & Nixon, 1978), as well as established symptom rating procedures and diagnostic algorithms.

NUMBER, SEVERITY, AND KINDS OF SYMPTOMS

Published Data

A rough indication of differences in symptomatology between community and clinic cases of depression can be obtained by comparing the PSE Indices of Definition (IDs) for community and clinic cases. The ID program associated with the PSE allocates each individual to one of eight levels that indicate the degree of confidence that sufficient symptoms are present to allow a clinical classification. Level 5 represents the threshold category. Individuals at Levels 6, 7, and 8 are considered to be definite cases of psychopathology (Wing et al., 1974, 1978). Calculations based on the data presented in Table 6.6 of Wing, Bebbington, Hurry, and Tennant (1981) indicate that whereas 40% of 35 community cases of depression had above-threshold IDs (i.e., ID = 6 or more) 82% of 45 depressed outpatients had IDs that were above threshold. Insufficient data were presented in the article to permit similar calculations for the depressed inpatients. Surtees and Sashidharan (1989) found that 18% of 50 community cases with a variety of affective disorders had above-threshold IDs, compared with 54.4% of a similar sample of 46 clinic cases.

The difficulty presented by any data on the difference in IDs between community and outpatient depressions is that one does not know the source of the difference. The ID is more than simply a sum of symptoms reported. The rules for determining the ID level operate both on total PSE scores and on type, severity, and combination of symptoms present (Wing and Sturt, 1978).

There appear to be only three published studies (Brown, Craig, & Harris, 1985; Surtees & Sashidharan, 1989; Wing, 1976) that have compared the total number of symptoms in their community and clinic cases. Brown and colleagues (1985) interviewed a community sample of 363 working-class women at two points 12 months apart, using the PSE.

Most of the data relevant to the present review were collected at the first interview. Symptom data collected at the time of this first interview indicated that 64 women had suffered from depression during the previous 12 months and that the average total number of PSE symptoms for these depressed women was 19. Wing (1976) reported an average total PSE score of 15 for 19 cases of depression identified in a random community sample. The means for 55 depressed inpatients and 24 depressed outpatients reported in Wing (1976) were, 26 and 24 respectively. The mean PSE score for the heterogeneous clinic sample of 46 cases in the Surtees and Sashidharan (1989) study was 20.3 and for the heterogeneous community sample of 50 cases it was 17.6.

These data do appear to provide support for the hypothesis that clinic cases of depression and of affective disorder have more symptoms than community cases. However, two important methodological problems cast doubt on the meaningfulness of the data. First, the short form of the PSE, which includes 40 items, mostly symptoms, was used in the community studies and the long form, which includes 140 items, mostly symptoms, was used in the clinic studies. Second, there is evidence (e.g., Shapiro et al., 1984) that individuals with more than one diagnosable psychiatric condition are more likely to seek or be referred to psychiatric clinics. Both of these differences might be expected to result in a higher total PSE score in the clinic samples than in the community samples. Then again, it is not true that cases identified in community samples always meet criteria for only one diagnosis. The published data of Brown and associates (1985) (Table 2, p. 617) suggest that, although there were 64 depressed women, only 29 were "pure" depressives; the remaining 35 women also had an anxiety condition. Examination of the data for the 29 apparent pure cases of depression, made available by. G. W. Brown (personal communication, November 15, 1988), indicated that, in actuality, 2 of the 29 cases were not pure in that they both had substance use disorders. Furthermore, 2 of the 27 pure cases of depression had contacted outpatient psychiatric services, so that only 25 cases were both true community cases *and* pure depressives. The average total number of PSE symptoms for this group of true community, pure depressives was 16.

The above two problems arise because the data concern the *total* number of symptoms in the cases. The problems would be avoided in comparisons of the number of *depressive symptoms.* Comparing community and clinic cases of depression in relation to the number of depressive symptoms rather than total symptoms would also seem to be more relevant to the question of the similarity or dissimilarity of the depressions per se in the two settings. Some new data of this sort is reported later in this chapter.

Data comparing the severity of symptoms in community and clinic cases of depression do not appear to have been reported. In any case, one would have to interpret cautiously any data on symptom severity. If it were shown that clinic cases had more severe symptoms than community cases, some of this greater severity might be due to the fact that the patients in clinic samples are usually interviewed on admission when they are at or near the peak of their disorders. Brown and Harris (1978a) measured overall severity of illness in 41 depressed outpatients and 73 depressed inpatients using a five-point scale ranging from 1 (marked) to 5 (mild). There was little change in severity from onset of illness ($M = 2.93$) to admission ($M = 2.54$) for outpatients but the severity for inpatients changed from 2.73 at onset to 1.86 at admission. When assessments in random community samples are based on the month before interview, some of the cases, although they meet diagnostic criteria, may not be close to the peak of their disturbances. When assessments in community samples are made for onsets earlier than 1 month before the time of interview, the passage of time may result in some symptoms being recalled at a different intensity than they actually were at the time of illness. Aneshensel, Estrada, Hansell, and Clark (1987) found that individuals tended to fail to report documented past episodes of depression when they were currently asymptomatic or when current life circumstances were positive or had improved over past circumstances.

Only two published studies appear to have provided data concerning differences between community and clinic cases in the nature of their depressive symptoms. The investigators in the first study, different aspects of which were reported in Wing and associates (1981) and Hurry and Sturt (1981), processed the PSE symptom data through the Index of Definition (ID) and CATEGO computer programs (Wing et al., 1974, 1978). The CATEGO program allocates each individual with an ID equal to 5 or greater to one of a number of categories that are approximately equivalent to the diagnostic categories of the International Classification of Diseases (World Health Organization, 1978). Calculations based on the tables reported in Wing and colleagues (1981) and Hurry and Sturt (1981) indicate that of 81 depressed inpatients 19% were in CATEGO Class D (that is, they suffered from delusions and/or hallucinations); 43% were in Class R (retarded depression) characterized by symptoms such as motor retardation, pathological guilt, and self-depreciation; and 38% were in Class N, (neurotic depression.) The distribution of cases for the 45 depressed outpatients was Class D = 4%, Class R = 27%, and Class N = 69%. The comparable figures for the 35 depressed community cases were 6%, 24%, and 71%, respectively. The distribution of cases over the three classes of depression is not different for the outpatients and community cases, but a greater proportion of the inpatients are in Classes D and R. Nevertheless, the data obtained from the R and N community depressions, that is, 95% of the cases, might be generalizable to the class R and N depressed inpatients, 81% of the cases.

TABLE 3.1. Description of Samples for Which Symptom Patterns Were Analyzed

Investigator or site	n	Age range	Mean age (SD)	Interview	Population from which sample was drawn	References
Belsher	40	19–57	33.8(10.1)	DIS	Referrals to a psychiatric assessment clinic attached to a general hospital	Belsher & Costello (1991)
Piper	118	16–57	32.9(9.8)	DIS	Day patients in a hospital department	Unpublished data
Wittchen	32	28–62	41.3(9.9)	DIS	Subjects in a follow-up study of former psychiatric inpatients	Wittchen (1987)
Edmonton, AB	29	20–66	35.4(11.9)	DIS	Identified in a community survey	Orn et al. (1988)
Munich	10	32–54	44.1(6.6)	DIS	Identified in a community study	Wittchen (1987)
New Haven	49	20–85	46.3(19.5)	DIS	Identified in epidemiological catchment area (ECA) study	Robins & Regier (1991)
St. Louis	48	19–76	41.7(15.9)	DIS	ECA study	Robins & Regier (1991)
Los Angeles	35	19–68	39.5(12.3)	DIS	ECA study	Robins & Regier (1991)
Durham, NC	28	18–92	45.8(19.9)	DIS	ECA study	Robins & Regier (1991)
Baltimore	33	21–80	44.2(17.3)	DIS	ECA study	Robins & Regier (1991)
Hooley						
Complete sample	23	19–70	49.3(13.3)			
Retarded	13	27–63	44.9(13.5)	PSE	Psychiatric inpatients	Hooley (1986)
Neurotic	10	38–70	55.0(11.3)			

Sample	N	Age range	Age mean (SD)	Assessment	Description	Source
Shapiro						
Complete sample	74	24–61	39.4(9.3)		Referrals to specialist clinic offering psychological therapy to professional, managerial and white-collar workers suffering from depression and/or anxiety	Shapiro et al. (1990)
Retarded	58	24–61	40.3(9.6)	PSE		
Neurotic	16	27–50	36.4(7.0)			
Veiel						
Complete sample	57	19–59	39.1(10.5)			
Retarded	29	19–56	38.3(10.5)	PSE	Psychiatric inpatients	Veiel et al. (1992)
Neurotic	28	25–59	39.9(10.3)			
Otago, NZ						
Complete sample	48	18–65 +	44.3(approx.)[a]			Romans-Clarkson et al. (1990)
Retarded	24	18–65 +	44.4(approx.)[a]	PSE	Identified in community survey	
Neurotic	24	18–65 +	44.2(approx.)[a]			
Great Britain						
Complete sample	81	All patients were 36 years old				
Retarded	23			PSE	Identified in community survey	Rodgers & Mann (1986)
Neurotic	58					
Camberwell, London	63	18–65	40.8(13.6)	PSE	Identified in community survey	Brown & Harris (1978a)
Hebrides, Scotland	68	20–65	42.4(12.9)	PSE	Identified in community survey	Brown & Prudo (1981)
Islington, London	124	20–49	33.7(7.0)	PSE	Identified in community survey	Brown et al. (1986)

[a]For the Romans-Clarkson sample age data were not available for each patient.

Sashidharan, Surtees, Kreitman, Ingham, and Miller (1990) compared thirteen CATEGO syndromes in 39 PSE clinic cases of depression and 35 PSE community cases of depression. With respect to the CATEGO syndromes of depression, namely, pathological guilt, subjective anergia, loss of interest and concentration, and somatic depressive symptoms, my analyses of the data presented in their Table 2 indicated that there was a significantly ($p < .05$) greater prevalence of subjective anergia and loss of interest and concentration in the clinic cases. It is noteworthy that there was not a significant difference in somatic depressive symptoms. When the RDC criteria for a major depressive disorder were applied to the subjects in the study, there were 43 clinic cases and 24 community cases. The authors noted that 64% of the clinic cases had at least three of the RDC "endogenous depressive disorder" symptoms, whereas only 46% of the community cases had at least three of these symptoms. Their wording suggests that the difference is significant whereas, in actuality, it is not a significant difference.

I shall now present some new data comparing community and clinic cases on specific symptoms of depression.

Symptom Data in 6 Clinic Samples and 12 Community Samples

Symptom data using the Diagnostic Interview Schedule (DIS; Robins, Helzer, Croughan, & Ratcliff, 1981) were obtained for three clinic samples and seven community samples. Present State Examination (PSE) symptom data were obtained for three clinic samples and five community samples. Brief descriptions of the samples are presented in Table 3.1. References to articles that present more details concerning the procedures that were used to access the subjects are also provided where available in Table 3.1. It should, however, be noted that because of the different, usually more restrictive, criteria used to select the study samples in the studies reported they do not match exactly the samples examined here.

In the case of the DIS samples, all of the subjects were female and satisfied DIS/DSM criteria for a current unipolar major depressive episode. DSM exclusion criteria were not applied. All of the subjects in the PSE samples were female. In all of the PSE samples, except George Brown's three samples (labeled Camberwell, Hebrides, and Islington), the subjects had an Index of Definition equal to 5 or greater and satisfied CATEGO criteria for a recent episode of neurotic depression or retarded depression. The subjects in the Brown samples satisfied Bedford criteria for a recent episode of borderline or case depression (Finlay-Jones et al., 1980).

The symptoms of the DIS may be coded 1 = symptom not present; 2 = symptom present at below a critical level; 3 = symptom present but due to a medical condition; 4 = symptom present but due to the effects of

TABLE 3.2. Mean *(SD)* Number of DIS Symptoms for Worst Episode of Women with a Current Major Depressive Episode

	Clinic samples	
Belsher	Piper	Wittchen
7.43(2.4)*a*	9.19(2.6)*b*	9.13(2.9)*bc*

		Community samples				
Edmonton, AB	Munich	New Haven	St. Louis	Los Angeles	Durham, NC	Baltimore
7.9(2.5)*ac*	6.4(2.1)*a*	7.1(2.5)*a*	6.9(1.7)*a*	7.5(2.5)*a*	7.0(2.3)*a*	6.8(2.3)*a*

Note. Groups with no overlapping letters differ significantly ($p < .01$).

alcohol or drugs; and 5 = symptom present at a critical level. The mean number of DIS symptoms with a code of 5 for the subjects in the ten samples examined are presented in Table 3.2.

With two exceptions, the symptoms of depression in the PSE may receive ratings of 0 = symptom not present; 1 = symptom present at a moderate level but at a severe level half the time; and 2 = symptom present at a severe level more than half the time. The mean total number of PSE symptoms, moderate symptoms, and severe symptoms for three clinic samples divided into neurotic depressives and retarded depressives and two community samples, similarly divided, are presented in Table 3.3.

The mean total, moderate, and severe PSE symptoms for three clinic samples and five community samples are presented in Table 3.4.

In general, it is quite clear that clinic cases of depression have significantly more symptoms of depression than community cases of depression. With respect to the DIS symptoms, the average number of symptoms for the seven community samples was seven. The average number of symptoms for the cases of one of the clinic samples (Piper) was 9.19 and

TABLE 3.3. Mean *(SD)* Number of Moderate, Severe, and Total PSE Symptoms in Women with Neurotic and Retarded Depression

	Clinic samples			Community samples	
	Hooley	Shapiro	Veiel	Otago, NZ	Great Britain
Neurotic depressives					
Moderate	8.1(1.4)*a*	8.9(2.3)*ab*	7.6(2.4)*ab*	6.5(2.03)*ab*	5.8(2.6)*b*
Severe	3.4(1.8)*a*	2.3(1.4)*ab*	3.0(2.4)*a*	2.2(1.9)*ab*	1.9(1.6)*b*
Total	11.5(2.1)*a*	11.1(2.8)*a*	10.6(3.1)*a*	8.7(2.7)*b*	7.7(3.0)*b*
Retarded depressives					
Moderate	7.9(2.2)*acd*	9.7(2.5)*b*	8.8(2.4)*abc*	7.6(3.0)*cd*	6.9(2.7)*d*
Severe	5.4(2.7)*a*	3.3(2.2)*b*	3.8(3.0)*ab*	2.2(2.0)*bc*	1.8(1.7)*c*
Total	13.4(2.9)*a*	13.0(2.9)*a*	12.6(3.3)*a*	9.8(3.3)*b*	8.7(3.9)*b*

Note. Groups with no overlapping letters differ significantly ($p < .01$).

TABLE 3.4. Mean *(SD)* Number of Moderate, Severe, and Total PSE Symptoms in Depressed Women

	Clinic samples		
	Hooley	Shapiro	Veiel
Moderate	8.0(1.9)*bc*	9.5(2.4)	8.2(2.5)
Severe	4.6(2.5)	3.1(2.1)	3.4(2.7)*b*
Total	12.6(2.7)	12.6(3.0)	11.6(3.8)

	Community samples				
	Otago, NZ	Great Britain	Camberwell, London	Hebrides, Scotland	Islington, London
Moderate	7.0(2.6)*abc*	6.1(2.6)*abc*	6.0(2.6)*ax*	6.7(2.9)*ax*	6.9(2.9)*cx*
Severe	2.2(1.9)*bc*	1.9(1.6)*abc*	1.4(1.5)*ax*	2.4(2.0)*bx*	2.0(1.8)*cx*
Total	9.2(3.1)*bc*	8.0(3.1)*abc*	7.4(3.4)*ax*	9.1(3.6)*bxy*	8.9(3.2)*cy*

Note. Groups with no overlapping letters differ significantly ($p < .01$). For comparison of Brown's three samples with the remaining samples, the letters *a, b,* and *c* are used. For comparison of Brown's three samples with one another, the letters *x* and *y* are used. No comparisons were made after combining the neurotic and retarded subjects in the Hooley, Shapiro, Veiel, Romans-Clarkson, and Rodgers samples.

was significantly larger than the average for any of the seven community samples. The average for the Wittchen clinic sample was 9.13, which was significantly larger than the average for all of the community samples except the Edmonton sample. The average number of symptoms for one of the three clinic samples (Belsher) was 7.43. This did not differ significantly from the means of any of the seven community samples and did differ significantly from the means for the other two clinic samples. There is no obvious reason for this difference.

With respect to the PSE symptoms of depression, when all the cases of depression in each sample were considered, irrespective of their CATEGO classification into retarded or neurotic depressives, the mean total number of symptoms for each of the clinic samples was significantly greater than the mean number for each of the five community samples. The means for the three clinic samples did not differ significantly from one another, and the average of these three means was 12.3. The Camberwell community sample had a significantly lower mean number of symptoms (7.4) than two of the other community samples (Otago, 9.2; Islington, 8.9). None of the other differences between the community samples were significant. The average number of symptoms for the 4 community samples other than the Camberwell sample was 8.8.

Considering the moderate and severe symptoms separately for all of the cases in each sample, two of the clinic samples (Shapiro and Veiel) had a higher mean number of moderate symptoms than any of the community samples. The average for these two samples was 8.85 moderate symptoms compared with an average of 6.5 for the five community samples, the means of which did not differ significantly from one another. Two of the clinic samples (Hooley and Shapiro) had a significantly higher mean number of severe symptoms than any of the five community samples. The average for the two clinic samples was 3.9, compared with an average of 1.98 for the five community samples, the means of which did not differ significantly from one another.

Considering the data for the retarded depressives and neurotic depressives separately, the mean total number of symptoms for both the neurotic depressives and retarded depressives in each of the three clinic samples was significantly greater than the mean total numbers for the two kind of depressives in the two community samples. The average total number for the neurotic depressives for the three clinic samples was 11.06, compared with the average total number for the neurotic depressives in the two community samples, which was 8.2. The average total number for the retarded depressives for the three clinic samples was 13, compared with the average total number for the retarded depressives in the two community samples, which was 9.25. When one considers the moderate and severe symptoms separately for the neurotic depressives, the picture is not so clear. None of the clinic samples had a significantly higher mean number of either moderate or severe symptoms than both of the community samples. Only one of the clinic samples of retarded depressives (Shapiro) had a significantly higher mean number of moderate symptoms than both the community samples. But the mean for the Shapiro sample was also significantly higher than the mean for one of the clinic samples (Hooley). With respect to the severe symptoms in the retarded depressives, one of the clinic samples (Hooley) had a significantly higher mean number than the two community samples, but the Hooley mean was also significantly larger than the mean for one of the clinic samples (Shapiro).

To recapitulate, and rounding off the means in doing so, cases of major depressive episodes in the clinic appear to have on average nine DIS symptoms of depression compared with seven DIS symptoms in the community cases. When assessed with the PSE, clinic cases have on average 12 symptoms and community cases 9 symptoms. There would seem to be no clear difference between clinic cases and community cases in the relative proportions of moderate and severe symptoms. The differences between the clinic cases and community cases when neurotic depressives and retarded depressives are considered separately seem to parallel the differences found when all of the cases are considered together.

The only conclusion that can be made with any confidence is that clinic cases of major depressive episodes have more symptoms of depression than community cases. What is the significance of this difference? First of all, it should be noted that the actual number of symptoms of depression that will be revealed in assessments depends on the total possible number allowed by the assessment interview used. The average number of PSE symptoms for both clinic and community cases was found to be higher than the average number of DIS symptoms. But there are 20 symptoms of depression in the PSE compared with 16 in the DIS. Furthermore, there seems to be a greater redundancy in the list of symptoms in the DIS. For instance, 4 of the 16 symptoms deal with thoughts of death and suicide and suicide attempts, whereas only one symptom covers this matter in the PSE. Three of the DIS symptoms deal with eating problems, whereas only one PSE symptom does so. It might be argued that the redundancy in the DIS should serve to inflate the number of symptoms reported by an individual. Then again, having reported a symptom in response to one question, an individual may feel no need to report the same symptom in response to similar questions.

There are other possible reasons for the differences in the number of DIS and PSE symptoms that were reported. For many of the DIS symptoms, in order for an individual's particular experience or behavior to receive a code of 5 in the DIS, the individual must have told a physician or another health professional about the problem or have taken medication for the problem, or the problem must have interfered a lot with the individual's life or activities. Help-seeking behaviors and social impairment do not play so large a role in the rating of the PSE symptoms. This difference between the two procedures might have resulted in the larger number of PSE symptoms being reported.

Another possible reason for the difference in the numbers of symptoms is that the DIS symptoms that were examined are those for the worst episode of depression experienced by the subjects. If the worst episode was earlier than the current episode, some of the symptoms may have been forgotten. Still, one might expect the memory problem to be counteracted by the fact that a worst episode is likely to have involved more symptoms than other episodes.

Whatever the explanation is for the difference between the two procedures, the fact remains that, on average, clinic cases with major depressive episodes have more symptoms of depression in their worst episode or in their current episode than community cases.

Another way of examining the DIS data is to calculate the number of the eight groups of DSM-III symptoms covered by the DIS. The likely importance of such an analysis is indicated by Klein's (1990) finding that the relatives of patients with major depression who had six, seven, or eight symptom groups had similar rates of mood disorders and significantly higher rates of these disorders than the relatives of patients with major depression who had four or five groups of symptoms and the relatives of patients with nonaffective disorders. The latter two groups did not differ from one another in this respect. Klein also found that the depressed patients with six or more groups of symptoms had a significantly higher rate of DSM-III melancholia than those with four or five symptoms. Sargeant, Bruce, Florio, and Weissman (1990) found that the more of the eight symptom groups assessed by the DIS that were exhibited in cases of current unipolar major depression identified in the community samples of the ECA study, the greater the likelihood of their being cases of depression 1 year later. The percentages of those exhibiting symptoms from four groups who were cases at follow-up was 15.3%; for those exhibiting symptoms from five groups, 24.5%; six groups, 30.7%; and seven or eight groups, 36.2%.

The mean number of groups of DIS symptoms and the proportion of subjects who had six or more groups of symptoms in three clinic samples and seven community samples are presented in Table 3.5. It can be seen that for two of the clinic samples, namely, Piper and Wittchen, the mean number of groups of symptoms was greater than six. It was less than six for all of the seven community samples. The difference between two clinic samples, namely, Belsher and Piper was significant at the $p < .01$ level. The Piper clinic sample and the Wittchen clinic sample both had significantly ($p < .01$) more groups of symptoms than six of the seven community samples. The exception in both cases was the Edmonton community sample. The Belsher clinic sample did not differ significantly from any of the community samples.

The average proportion of clinic cases who had six or more groups of symptoms was 64%, and the average proportion of community cases was 35%. When each clinic sample was compared in this respect with the seven community samples, none of the differences was significant at the .01 level. However, at the .05 level of significance, the Wittchen clinic

TABLE 3.5. Mean *(SD)* Number of Groups of DIS Symptoms and Proportion of Subjects with Six or More Groups of Symptoms with Current Major Depressive Episode

Clinic samples		
Belsher	Piper	Wittchen
5.55(1.13)*a*	6.17(1.35)*b*	6.25(1.32)*ab*
53%*a*	72%*a*	66%*a*

		Community samples				
Edmonton, AB	Munich	New Haven	St. Louis	Los Angeles	Durham, NC	Baltimore
5.76(1.41)*ab*	4.9(1.20)*ab*	5.24(1.15)*ab*	5.17(1.02)*ab*	5.40(1.31)*ab*	5.20(1.20)*ab*	5.30(1.31)*ab*
55%*a*	10%*a*	39%*a*	40%*a*	40%*a*	32%*a*	30%*a*

Note. Groups with no overlapping letters differ significantly ($p < .01$).

sample differed from all of the community samples except the Edmonton sample, and the Piper clinic sample differed from all of the community samples. The Belsher clinic sample differed significantly at the .05 level from only one community sample (Munich).

The percentages of depressed women in three clinic samples and seven community samples who had specific DIS symptoms of depression in their worst period are presented in Table 3.6. The percentages of depressed women who had specific PSE symptoms at a moderate level in three clinic samples and five community samples are presented in Table 3.7. The PSE data for symptoms at a severe level are presented in Table 3.8. The PSE data for two clinic samples and three community samples considering neurotic depressives and retarded depressives separately and moderate and severe symptoms separately are presented in Tables 3.9 through 3.12.

The significant differences between the percentages are indicated in the tables. In general, there were as many significant differences between the clinic samples and between the community samples as there were between the clinic samples and the community samples. The few exceptions to this pattern for the DIS data were worthlessness where the percentages of cases reporting the symptoms in the clinic samples were on average 88.3% compared with 60% in the community cases; poor concentration, clinic cases, 84% and community cases, 60%; and thoughts of suicide, clinic cases, 74% and community cases, 47.7%. The exceptions for the PSE data, when all the cases were considered, were self-depreciation at a moderate level, clinic cases, 56.3% and community cases, 33%; and pathological guilt at a moderate level, clinic cases, 42% and community cases, 14%. When neurotic depressives are considered separately, loss of interest at a moderate level appears to have occurred more often in the clinic cases (53% on average) than in community cases (15%). When retarded depressives are considered separately, loss of interest appears to have occurred more often in clinic cases than in community cases at a moderate level (48.7% vs. 10.5%) and at a severe level (27.6% vs. 0%).

What is perhaps more noteworthy, in view of the belief of some psychopathologists that clinic cases are more biological in nature than community cases, is that what are usually considered the more biological symptoms, such as loss of appetite, loss of sleep, psychomotor retardation, and loss of libido, did not occur in a significantly greater percentage of clinic cases than of community cases.

DURATION OF THE
PSYCHOPATHOLOGICAL CONDITION

Brown and Harris (1986) noted that in all of their community studies there were as many women with episodes of depression that lasted 12

TABLE 3.6. Percentages of Currently Depressed Women with Specific DIS Symptoms in Worst Episode

	Clinic samples[a,b]			Community samples[a,b]						
DIS number/Symptom	Belsher (40)	Piper (118)	Wittchen (32)	Edmonton, AB (58)	Munich (10)	New Haven (49)	St. Louis (48)	Los Angeles (35)	Durham, NC (28)	Baltimore (33)
74. Loss of appetite	50*ab*	61*a*	44*ac*	57*a*	60*ac*	47*a*	31*bc*	51*ab*	46*ab*	39*ab*
75. Loss of weight	26(39)*a*	42*a*	40*a*	38*a*	40*a*	31*a*	25*a*	35(34)*a*	41(27)*a*	27*a*
76. Weight gain	10*a*	31*bc*	13*ab*	24*ad*	10*ad*	10*a*	42*cd*	17*ac*	29*abd*	24*abd*
77. Loss of sleep	88*a*	80*a*	81*a*	83*a*	80*a*	73*a*	71*a*	66*a*	79*a*	76*a*
78. Increased sleep	28*abc*	41*a*	25*ac*	28*ac*	0*bc*	22*ab*	19*bc*	38(34)*abd*	14*cd*	15*bc*
79. Tiredness	69(39)*a*	79*a*	75*a*	76*a*	70*a*	73*a*	62(47)*a*	66*a*	79*a*	79*a*
80. Retardation	20*a*	36*ab*	50*b*	26*ab*	10*ab*	39*ab*	27*ab*	26*ab*	40(25)*ab*	36*ab*
81. Restlessness	21(39)*a*	37*a*	34*a*	26*a*	10*a*	29*a*	31*a*	29*a*	30(27)*a*	42*a*
82. Loss of libido	46(39)*ab*	37(115)*ab*	53*a*	45*ab*	40*acd*	22*bc*	22(46)*bd*	29*ad*	36*ad*	45*acd*
83. Worthlessness	90*ac*	91*a*	84*ad*	66*def*	50*bef*	65*bd*	75*cde*	74(34)*cdef*	43*bf*	47(32)*be*
84. Poor concentration	80*ac*	84(117)*a*	88*ad*	79*ae*	30*bf*	71*af*	56*cef*	63*cdef*	64*af*	48*bf*
85. Inefficient thinking	48*a*	61*a*	69*a*	55*a*	40*a*	63*a*	44*a*	49*a*	48(27)*a*	61*a*
86. Thoughts about death	45*ad*	72(117)*bc*	75*ac*	64*acd*	50*acd*	55*acd*	73*bce*	71*ace*	70(27)*ace*	42*de*
87. Death wishes	38*a*	66(117)*bc*	63*ab*	47*ab*	50*ab*	45*ab*	54*ac*	63*ab*	36*a*	45*ab*
88. Thoughts of suicide	65*acde*	74(117)*a*	84*ac*	47*df*	80*ad*	33*bf*	40*def*	57*adf*	41(27)*def*	36*def*
89. Suicide attempts	25*ab*	27(117)*a*	34*a*	28*a*	20*ab*	8*b*	19*a*	17*a*	19*a*	15*ab*

Note. Groups with no overlapping letters differ significantly ($p < .01$).
[a]Number in parentheses after name of investigator or site is the maximum *n* of the sample.
[b]Number in parentheses after a percentage is the *n* on which the percentage is based.

TABLE 3.7. Percentages of Currently Depressed Women with Moderate PSE Symptoms

	Clinic samples[a,b]			Community samples[a,b]				
PSE number/Symptom	Hooley(23)	Shapiro(74)	Veiel(57)	Otago, NZ(54)	Great Britain(81)	Camberwell, London(63)	Hebrides, Scotland(68)	Islington, London(124)
19. Inefficient thinking	45(22)*abc*	59*c*	56*c*	24*abc*	33*abc*	25*ax*	28*bx*	51(123)*c*
20. Poor concentration	70*ac*	78	63*ac*	11*c*	37*abc*	42(62)*ax*	35*bx*	47*cx*
21. Neglect due to brooding	45(20)*abc*	49(71)*abc*	44*abc*	22*a*	23*ac*	30*ax*	50*bx*	34(122)*cx*
22. Loss of interest	48(21)*ab*	58(73)*abc*	47*abc*	9*c*	17*a*	34(62)*ax*	50*bxy*	57(120)*cy*
23. Depressed mood	78*abc*	82*abc*	67*ab*	89*abc*	86*ab*	86*ax*	82*bx*	85(123)*cx*
24. Hopelessness	87	61(71)*bc*	54*abc*	26*ac*	27*a*	37*ax*	53*bx*	55*cx*
25. Suicidal plans	17*abc*	16(73)*abc*	18*abc*	28	11*abc*	8*ax*	4*bx*	7(122)*cx*
27. Morning depression	43(21)*abc*	70*abc*	49*abc*	12*abc*	44*bc*	70*ax*	54*bx*	57(114)*cx*
28. Social withdrawal	70(20)*ab*	59(73)*ab*	42*abc*	56*abc*	38*abc*	44(62)*ax*	41*bx*	37(123)*cx*
29. Self-depreciation	52*abc*	56(73)	61	39*abc*	40*abc*	27*ax*	25*bx*	34(123)*cx*
30. Lack of confidence	64(22)*abc*	56(73)*bc*	47*abc*	41*abc*	43*abc*	33*ax*	38*bx*	40(123)*cx*
31. Simple ideas of reference	27(22)*abc*	20*abc*	25*abc*	33(49)*bc*	21*abc*	8*ax*	13*bx*	34(122)*c*
32. Guilty ideas of reference	17*b*	31(67)	5*abc*	20	15*b*	2*ax*	3*bx*	3(104)*cx*
33. Pathological guilt	43*b*	48(66)	33	50	11*bc*	0*ax*	5*bx*	5(97)*cx*
34. Loss of weight	15(20)*abc*	18(72)*abc*	5*abc*	11*abc*	10*abc*	19*ax*	18*bx*	12(114)*cx*
35. Delayed sleep	9(22)*abc*	14*abc*	21*abc*	24*abc*	19*abc*	25*ax*	18*bx*	18(120)*cx*
36. Anergia/retardation	59(22)*abc*	58(73)*bc*	61*bc*	48*abc*	38*abc*	34*ax*	59*by*	50(119)*cx*
37. Early waking	5(21)*abc*	15(73)*abc*	14*abc*	13*abc*	12*abc*	19*ax*	19*bx*	7(122)*cx*
38. Loss of libido	20(10)*abc*	25(69)*abc*	19*abc*	11(46)*ab*	21*abc*	9*ax*	12*bx*	32(88)*c*
40. Irritability	26*abc*	36(72)*ab*	33*ab*	30*ab*	12*abc*	27*ax*	28*bx*	10(123)*c*

Note. Groups with no overlapping letters differ significantly ($p < .01$). For comparison of Brown's three samples with the remaining samples, the letters *a, b,* and *c* are used. For comparison of Brown's three samples with one another, the letters *x* and *y* are used. No comparisons were made on moderate symptoms for retarded depressives and neurotic depressives combined in the Hooley, Shapiro, Veiel, Romans–Clarkson, and Rodgers samples.
[a]Number in parentheses after name of investigator or site is the maximum *n* of the sample.
[b]Number in parentheses after a percentage is the *n* on which the percentage is based.

TABLE 3.8. Percentages of Currently Depressed Women with Severe PSE Symptoms

	Clinic samples[a,b]			Community samples[a,b]				
PSE number/Symptom	Hooley(23)	Shapiro(74)	Veiel(57)	Otago, NZ(54)	Great Britain(81)	Camberwell, London(63)	Hebrides, London(68)	Islington, London(124)
19. Inefficient thinking	18(22)*b*	12*b*	16*b*	0*abc*	1*abc*	0*ax*	3*bx*	2(123)*cx*
20. Poor concentration	17*ab*	8*abc*	16*ab*	0*abc*	4*abc*	5(62)*ax*	10*bx*	3*cx*
21. Neglect due to brooding	15*b*	14(71)*b*	19	6*abc*	0*abc*	0*ax*	3*bx*	2(122)*cx*
22. Loss of interest	38(21)	7(73)*abc*	26*b*	2*abc*	1*abc*	0(62)*ax*	10*by*	3(120)*cxy*
23. Depressed mood	22*bc*	16*abc*	23*bc*	7*abc*	10*abc*	3*ax*	13*bx*	10(123)*cx*
24. Hopelessness	4*abc*	1*abc*	7*abc*	2*abc*	0*abc*	2*ax*	1*bx*	6*cx*
25. Suicidal plans	26	0(73)*abc*	0*abc*	4*abc*	2*abc*	3*ax*	1*bx*	3(122)*cx*
27. Morning depression	52(21)*b*	26*abc*	39*b*	13*abc*	19*abc*	17*ax*	24(67)*bx*	12(114)*cx*
28. Social withdrawal	15(20)*bc*	7(73)*abc*	25*bc*	6*abc*	1*ab*	0(62)*ax*	10*by*	12(123)*cy*
29. Self-depreciation	9*abc*	16(73)	9*abc*	4*abc*	4*abc*	0*ax*	1*bx*	3(123)*cx*
30. Lack of confidence	14(22)*abc*	12(73)*abc*	23	7*abc*	2*abc*	2*ax*	1*bx*	5(123)*cx*
31. Simple ideas of reference	9(22)*abc*	9*abc*	5*abc*	4(49)*abc*	4*abc*	2*ax*	1*bx*	3(122)*cx*
32. Guilty ideas of reference	4*abc*	1(67)*abc*	2*abc*	4*abc*	1*abc*	0*ax*	0(66)*bx*	0(104)*cx*
33. Pathological guilt	0*abc*	17(66)	11*ab*	4*abc*	5*abc*	2*ax*	1*bx*	0(97)*cx*
34. Loss of weight	45(20)*bc*	13(72)*abc*	5(56)*ab*	20*abc*	12*abc*	10*ax*	18*bx*	21(114)*cx*
35. Delayed sleep	36(22)*abc*	28*abc*	18*ab*	26*abc*	21*ab*	29*ax*	34*bx*	38(120)*cx*
36. Anergia/retardation	23*b*	10(73)*abc*	14*bc*	7*abc*	4*abc*	0(62)*ax*	6*bx*	6(119)*cx*
37. Early waking	62(21)	23(73)*abc*	12*abc*	15*abc*	11*abc*	13*ax*	13*bx*	11(122)*cx*
38. Loss of libido	60(10)	22(69)*c*	30*c*	13(46)*abc*	9*abc*	4*ax*	2(57)*bx*	20(88)*c*
40. Irritability	35*abc*	44(72)*ac*	17*ab*	22*ab*	41*abc*	35*ay*	22*b*	52(123)*cxy*

Note. Groups with no overlapping letters differ significantly (*p* < .01). For comparison of Brown's three samples with the remaining samples, the letters *a, b,* and *c* are used. For comparison of Brown's three samples with one another, the letters *x* and *y* are used. No comparisons were made on severe symptoms for retarded depressives and neurotic depressives combined in the Hooley, Shapiro, Veiel, Romans–Clarkson, and Rodgers samples.

[a]Number in parentheses after name of investigator or site is the maximum *n* of the sample.
[b]Number in parentheses after a percentage is the *n* on which the percentage is based.

TABLE 3.9. Percentages of Women with Specific PSE Symptoms at a Moderate Level of Severity of Neurotic Depression

	Clinic samples[a,b]			Community samples[a,b]	
PSE number/Symptom	Hooley(10)	Shapiro(16)	Veiel(28)	Otago, NZ(30)	Great Britain(58)
19. Inefficient thinking	22(9)a	56a	54a	23a	34a
20. Poor concentration	70ac	81a	68ac	10b	40c
21. Neglect due to brooding	50a	50a	32a	20a	24a
22. Loss of interest	60a	56a	43ac	10b	20bc
23. Depressed mood	90a	94a	79a	93a	91a
24. Hopelessness	90a	47(15)ab	50ab	30b	24b
25. Suicidal plans	40a	13a	18a	30a	14a
27. Morning depression	56(9)a	69a	43a	67a	38a
28. Social withdrawal	70a	56a	43a	63a	40a
29. Self-depreciation	56(9)a	13(15)a	46a	27a	22a
30. Lack of confidence	70a	44a	43a	33a	38a
31. Simple ideas of reference	20a	19a	14a	27(26)a	17a
32. Guilty ideas of reference	0a	7(14)a	4a	0a	7a
33. Pathological guilt	0ab	31(13)a	11ab	30a	3b
34. Loss of weight	11(9)a	29(14)a	4a	7a	9a
35. Delayed sleep	20a	6a	18a	27a	22a
36. Anergia/retardation	40a	69a	64a	47a	40a
37. Early waking	11(9)a	19a	21a	20a	14a
38. Loss of libido	50(4)a	38a	14a	8(25)a	21a
40. Irritability	30a	38(15)a	29a	37a	14a

Note. Groups with no overlapping letters differ significantly ($p < .01$).
[a]Number in parentheses after name of investigator or site is the maximum *n* of the sample.
[b]Number in parentheses after a percentage is the *n* on which the percentage is based.

months as those with new episodes that had their onsets in the year before interview. Other studies have reported a lower proportion of chronic depressions. For instance, Costello (1982) found a 17% rate. However, because of the difficulties of studying the etiology of chronic conditions (Brown & Harris, 1986; Depue & Monroe, 1986), community investigations of the psychosocial correlates of depression have concentrated on episodes that have had their onset during the period covered by the interview. Only one of the studies followed the subjects to obtain data on the duration of these episodes. Brown and colleagues (1985) reported that, when 32 women who had had onsets of depression during the 12 months before their first interview were interviewed a second time 12 months later, it was found that 47% of the depressions had lasted for at least 6 months. However, it is not clear from the published article how

TABLE 3.10. Percentages of Women with Specific PSE Symptoms at a Severe Level of Neurotic Depression

	Clinic samples[a,b]			Community samples[a,b]	
PSE number/Symptom	Hooley(10)	Shapiro(16)	Veiel(28)	Otago, NZ(30)	Great Britain(58)
19. Inefficient thinking	22(9)*a*	13*ab*	11*ac*	0*bc*	2*b*
20. Poor concentration	20*a*	6*a*	11*a*	0*a*	3*a*
21. Neglect due to brooding	10*ab*	6*ab*	18*a*	8*ab*	0*b*
22. Loss of interest	30*a*	6*ac*	21*a*	3*ab*	2*bc*
23. Depressed mood	10*a*	6*a*	18*a*	7*a*	7*a*
24. Hopelessness	0*a*	0(15)*a*	4*a*	3*a*	0*a*
25. Suicidal plans	10*a*	0*a*	0*a*	0*a*	0*a*
27. Morning depression	44(9)*ab*	31*ab*	50*a*	20*ab*	21*b*
28. Social withdrawal	10*ab*	6*b*	7*a*	7*ab*	2*ab*
29. Self-depreciation	0*a*	0(15)*a*	4*a*	3*a*	3*a*
30. Lack of confidence	0*a*	6*a*	18*a*	7*a*	3*a*
31. Simple ideas of reference	0*a*	0*a*	0*a*	4(26)*a*	3*a*
32. Guilty ideas of reference	0*a*	0(14)*a*	0*a*	0*a*	2*a*
33. Pathological guilt	0*a*	0(13)*a*	4*a*	0*a*	0*a*
34. Loss of weight	56(9)*a*	7(14)*bc*	7*bc*	23*abc*	16*c*
35. Delayed sleep	30*a*	19*a*	14*a*	23*a*	21*a*
36. Anergia/retardation	20*a*	0*a*	11*a*	7*a*	5*a*
37. Early waking	44(9)*a*	25*ab*	18*ab*	7*b*	12*ab*
38. Loss of libido	25(4)*a*	19*a*	29*a*	20(25)*a*	12*a*
40. Irritability	40*ab*	50*a*	21*b*	27*ab*	41*ab*

Note. Groups with no overlapping letters differ significantly ($p < .01$).
[a]Number in parentheses after name of investigator or site is the maximum *n* of the sample.
[b]Number in parentheses after a percentage is the *n* on which the percentage is based.

many of these 32 cases were pure cases of depression. Examination of the data made available by Brown (personal communication, November 15, 1988) for the 25 pure cases of depression who had not had contact with outpatient services indicated that 13 (52%) had been depressed for more than a year. The duration of illness for the remaining 12 pure cases ranged from 2 months to 9 months, with an average of 5.5 months. Hollon's (1986) review of data obtained from studies conducted before the introduction of antidepressants indicated that the average duration of untreated episodes of depression for outpatients was 3 to 6 months and for inpatients 6 to 9 months.

These data suggest that the duration of depression in community cases is comparable to that found in clinic cases. In any case, with regard to this issue of the duration of depression, Brown and Harris (1978b) have

TABLE 3.11. Percentages of Women with Specific PSE Symptoms at a Moderate Level of Severity of Retarded Depression

PSE number/Symptom	Clinic samples[a,b]			Community samples[a,b]	
	Hooley(13)	Shapiro(58)	Veiel(29)	Otago, NZ(24)	Great Britain(23)
19. Inefficient thinking	62*ab*	60*ab*	59*ab*	25*b*	30*ab*
20. Poor concentration	69*acd*	78*a*	59*ad*	13*b*	30*cd*
21. Neglect due to brooding	40(10)*a*	49(55)*a*	55*a*	25*a*	22*a*
22. Loss of interest	36(11)*ab*	58(57)*a*	52*a*	8*b*	13*b*
23. Depressed mood	69*a*	79*a*	55*a*	83	74*a*
24. Hopelessness	85*a*	64(56)*ac*	59*a*	21*b*	35*bc*
25. Suicidal plans	0*a*	18(57)*a*	17*a*	25*a*	4*a*
27. Morning depression	33(12)*a*	71*ab*	35*ab*	79*b*	61*ab*
28. Social withdrawal	70(10)*a*	60(57)*a*	41*a*	46*a*	35*a*
29. Self-depreciation	54*a*	67(57)*a*	76*a*	54*a*	83*a*
30. Lack of confidence	58(12)*a*	60(57)*a*	51*a*	50*a*	57*a*
31. Simple ideas of reference	33(12)*a*	21*a*	34*a*	39(23)*a*	30*a*
32. Guilty ideas of reference	31*ab*	38(53)*a*	7*b*	46*a*	35*ab*
33. Pathological guilt	77*a*	53(53)*ab*	55*ab*	75*a*	30*b*
34. Loss of weight	18(11)*a*	16*a*	0(28)*a*	17*a*	13*a*
35. Delayed sleep	0(12)*a*	16*a*	24*a*	21*a*	9*a*
36. Anergia/retardation	75(12)*a*	54(57)*a*	59*a*	50*a*	35*a*
37. Early waking	0(12)*a*	14(57)*a*	7*a*	4*a*	9*a*
38. Loss of libido	0(6)*a*	21(53)*a*	24*a*	4(21)*a*	22*a*
40. Irritability	23*a*	36(56)*a*	38*a*	21*a*	9*a*

Note. Groups with no overlapping letters differ significantly (*p* < .01).

[a]Number in parentheses after name of investigator or site is the maximum *n* of the sample.

[b]Number in parentheses after a percentage is the *n* on which the percentage is based.

made two noteworthy observations. First, they suggested that to use duration as a criterion for distinguishing true clinic depression from community depression is conceptually suspect until empirical study can show that duration is an indication of some other difference in the conditions. They pointed out that when someone is ill for 3 days with meningitis and then recovers one does not then dismiss the episode as unreal just because patients can often go on to deteriorate from similar symptoms. Second, they noted that, even if community depressions do not generally last as long as clinic depressions, it is obviously important to include short-lived conditions in our investigations if we are to understand more about the factors that help to perpetuate depressive disorders.

TABLE 3.12. Percentages of Women with Specific PSE Symptoms at a Severe Level of Retarded Depression

PSE number/Symptom	Clinic samples[a,b]			Community samples[a,b]	
	Hooley(13)	Shapiro(58)	Veiel(29)	Otago, NZ(24)	Great Britain(23)
19. Inefficient thinking	15a	12a	21a	0a	0a
20. Poor concentration	15a	9a	21a	0a	4a
21. Neglect due to brooding	20(10)a	16(55)a	21a	4a	0a
22. Loss of interest	45(11)a	7(57)bc	31ab	0c	0c
23. Depressed mood	31a	19a	28a	8a	17a
24. Hopelessness	8a	2(56)a	10a	0a	0a
25. Suicidal plans	38a	0(57)b	0b	8ab	9ab
27. Morning depression	58(12)a	24ab	28ab	4b	13b
28. Social withdrawal	20(10)abc	7(57)ab	41c	4ab	0at
29. Self-depreciation	15a	21a	14a	8a	4a
30. Lack of confidence	25(12)ab	14(57)ab	28a	8ab	0b
31. Simple ideas of reference	17(12)a	12a	10a	4(23)a	4a
32. Guilty ideas of reference	8a	2(53)a	3a	8a	0a
33. Pathological guilt	0a	21(53)a	17a	8a	17a
34. Loss of weight	36(11)a	14ab	4(28)b	17ab	4ab
35. Delayed sleep	42(12)a	31a	21a	29a	22a
36. Anergia/retardation	25(12)a	12(57)a	28a	8a	0a
37. Early waking	75(12)a	23(57)b	7b	25b	9b
38. Loss of libido	83(6)a	23(53)bc	31ab	5(21)bc	0c
40. Irritability	31ab	41(15)a	14b	17ab	39ab

Note. Groups with no overlapping letters differ significantly ($p < .01$).
[a]Number in parentheses after name of investigator or site is the maximum *n* of the sample.
[b]Number in parentheses after a percentage is the *n* on which the percentage is based.

SOCIAL INCAPACITATION

Hurry and Sturt (1981), used the Social Performance Schedule (Creer & Wing, 1974) to investigate the social performance of 35 community cases of depression and 45 depressed outpatients. The data reported in their Tables 19.4 and 19.5 indicated that 18% of the community cases had scores of 0 on the schedule; the scores were between 1 and 10 for 27%, between 11 and 20 for 18%, between 21 and 30 for 23%, and between 31 and 100 for 15%, with higher scores indicating greater social incapacitation. The comparable figures for the depressed outpatients were 4%, 11%, 22%, 18%, and 44%, respectively. These data do suggest that clinic cases are more socially incapacitated than community cases. But it would be premature to conclude that the difference between the two groups in the degree of social incapacitation was a direct result of a difference in the severity or nature of their depressions. It might have been a consequence of differences in a variety of factors, including personality, coping style, and life circumstances. In general, it is well known that referral to clinics is complex and controlled by a number of factors, only one of which is the presence of a psychopathological condition (Brown & Harris, 1978a; Brown et al., 1985; Goldberg & Huxley, 1980; Mechanic, 1972; Shapiro et al., 1984). Among the nondepressive illness factors that these researchers have found to be associated with the referral of depressed individuals to psychiatrists are the presence of anxiety symptoms, alcoholism, and drug addiction. With respect to nonillness factors, it has been found that single, separated, divorced, and widowed individuals are more likely to be referred. More specifically, Hurry and Sturt (1981) referred to unpublished data that showed that, when individuals with a similar level of symptomatology were compared, those with a poor level of social performance, as measured by the Social Performance Schedule, were more likely to contact or be referred to outpatient services.

ENVIRONMENT VERSUS BIOLOGY

To support their argument that community depressions are more environmentally caused than are clinic depressions, Bebbington, Tennant and Hurry (1981) reported data from an investigation of a random community sample of 310 individuals and 74 psychiatric outpatients. The community sample was interviewed on two occasions with the PSE and Brown's Life Events and Difficulties Interview Schedule (Brown, 1978). The ID and CATEGO programs were applied to the PSE data. Those who were at level 5 or over on the ID at the first or second interview were defined as cases. However, the authors appear to be doubtful about the reliability of some of the data collected at the first interview. Therefore, they used two definitions to identify cases. The *broad definition* included cases identified at both interviews, and the *narrow definition* included only the cases identified at the second interview. They found that whereas 47% of 19 female community cases (narrow definition) had a severe life event in the previous 3 months, only 18% of 33 female outpatients had a severe event. They concluded that these data and similar data obtained for males were in favor of their claim that

> disorders seen in patients differ from (at any rate, acute) disorders seen in the community in their relationship to adversity. This difference supports the suggestion that disease theories are more likely to be required to explain the occurrence of the more severe affective disorders, whilst less severe

disorders often have a ready explication as understandable and unmysterious responses to adversity. (p. 364)

Brown and Harris (1982), in a critique of the Bebbington and colleagues (1981) article, reviewed seven studies of depressive inpatients and outpatients and noted that these studies found that 44% to 73% of patients reported a severe event before onset, with an average of 56%. Brown and associates (1985), in a further commentary on the discrepancy between these rates, proposed that the low rate of stressors in the Bebbington and colleagues (1981) study could be accounted for by three aspects of their design: (1) counting events over only a 3-month period before onset; (2) the exclusion of "possibly independent" events, that is, events over which the patients might have had some control; and (3) the inclusion, in their small sample of patients, of cases of anxiety without depression.

The belief that community cases may be more environmentally caused than clinic cases appears to rest on (1) the belief that a greater proportion of clinic patients than community cases are of an endogenous or melancholic nature and (2) the continued acceptance of the hypothesis that endogenous depressions are less environmentally caused than nonendogenous depressions. As Bebbington and associates (1988) noted in their recent review of the literature, a number of multivariate studies did find that presence of adversity discriminated neurotic from endogenous depressives. However, two methodological problems with these studies suggest that the findings may be an artifact: (1) comparisons were made between endogenous and neurotic groups that had been diagnosed by clinicians who usually make the distinction on grounds of both characteristic symptoms and the presence or absence of potential psychosocial stressors, and (2) age was not statistically controlled, which presents a problem because depression in older people is more likely to be of an endogenous type, and life events are rarer in older people. When Paykel (1971) did control for age in a multivariate study, the discriminant power of adversity was lost.

There are now a considerable number of studies reporting no differences between endogenous and nonendogenous types of depression in the rates of severe events. For instance, Benjaminsen (1981) used five different ways of defining neurotic depression and investigated the differences between the neurotic and nonneurotic depressives in the occurrence of stressful life events during the 6 months before the onset of illness. Paykel's scale of life events (Paykel, Prusoff, & Uhlenhuth, 1971) was used to record the events. Adopting Paykel's classification of types of events, Benjaminsen found no difference in rates of "severely upsetting events" for neurotic depressives ($M = 83\%$) and nonneurotic depressives ($X = 90\%$), or in the rates of "undesirable events" ($Ms = 91\%$ and 84%, respectively) or the rates of "severe losses" ($Ms = 65\%$ and 58%, respectively). Bebbington and colleagues (1988) found that 38% of a group of 63 psychiatric outpatients and inpatients classified by CATEGO as endogenous depressives had had a severe event during the 3 months before onset, and 39% of 61 neurotic depressives had had a severe event during the same period before onset. When chronic difficulties were included with events to constitute the variable "provoking agent," 48% of the endogenous patients and 49% of the neurotic patients had a provoking agent before onset of illness. Paykel, Rao, and Taylor (1984) found that the relationship between the absence of life stress and the presence of endogenous symptoms was weak because only 18 of 105 correlations reached the 5% level of significance. Calloway, Dolan, Fonagy, DeSouza, and Wakeling (1984a, 1984b) found that depressed patients with the clearest signs of biological involvement (i.e., nonsuppression on the dexamethasone suppression test [DST] and blunted thyroid-stimulating hormone [TSH] response to thyrotropin-releasing hormone [TRH] were as likely to have had an antecedent stressor as the remaining depressed patients. In actuality, patients with blunted TSH responses and high free thyroxine index (FTI) levels were more likely to report long-term environmental difficulties than patients with blunted responses and normal FTI values.

Bebbington (1984) suggested, "A biological basis for depressive illness is best sought through genetic studies, as biological markers such as the dexamethasone suppression test may merely be correlates of symptoms rather than correlates of the causes of symptoms" (p. 71). There do not appear to be any studies directly comparing the heritability of community and clinic cases of depression. Of indirect relevance, however, are the findings reported by Torgersen (1986). Data obtained from 151 index twins, all of whom were depressed inpatients, and their cotwins indicated that hereditary factors were important in the etiology of depression. The frequency of major depression in monozygotic (MZ) cotwins of patients with major depression was 27% compared with 12% among dizygotic (DZ) cotwins. This MZ/DZ difference was not statistically significant. But when all affective disorders in the cotwins were considered, the concordance rate for the MZ twin pairs was 45% compared with 22% in the DZ pairs, and this difference was statistically significant. Of greater importance, however, is Torgersen's finding that the concordance rates for subtypes of major depression differentiated into (1) those with melancholic or nonmelancholic features and (2) those with or without an antecedent severe event were not changed from those obtained for the total group.

If environmentally caused depressions do not have significant biological determinants, then one might expect little in the way of a family history of depression in those who have a severe event preceding their onsets of depression. However, McGuffin, Katz, and Bebbington (1987,

1988) noted that the difference is statistically insignificant between the 21% lifetime rate of depression in the relatives of probands whose onset of depression followed life events or chronic difficulties and the 13% rate in the relatives of probands whose onset was not associated with adversity. Furthermore, the trend, although insignificant, is in the opposite direction to that which is required by the hypothesis.

A recent study by Monroe, Thase, and Simons (1992) suggests that the presence or absence of stress before the onset of depression may be related to the degree of biological involvement *within* groups of endogenous depressives. As a biological marker, they used latency to the onset of the first rapid-eye-movement sleep period (REM latency). They found that patients diagnosed as nonpsychotic, major depressives who did not have severe stress before onset had reduced REM latency values, whereas similar depressed patients who did have a severe stress before onset had normal REM latency values. However, two considerations suggests the possibility that the findings may not be replicable: (1) As the authors noted, "Several tests with correlated variables were performed and the overall magnitude of the effect was relatively modest"; and (2) both life stress before onset and longer REM latencies were significantly associated with increased severity of depression. These findings, particularly the one relating to REM latency, are not in line with previous findings reported (see Thase & Kupfer, 1988).

RESPONSE TO PHARMACOLOGICAL INTERVENTION

Akiskal (1987) asked, "How, then, does one draw the line between, for example, an adaptive response to loss and clinical depression?" and answered, "Measurement of pharmacologic response is one useful approach. Morbid depression is often alleviated by tricyclic antidepressants, whereas ordinary sadness is unaffected. By contrast, stimulants with immediate mood-elevating properties have no long term benefit in clinical depression" (pp. 64–65).

There do not seem to have been any studies that have compared the response of community depressives to psychological and pharmacological intervention, and only one study (Nandi et al., 1976) has investigated the response of community cases to pharmacological treatment. It was found that the 17 cases identified in the community responded as well to imipramine as 20 cases of depression treated in a clinic. The authors noted that there was no significant difference between the two groups in the mean score on the Hamilton Depression Rating Scale (Hamilton, 1967) either before or after treatment. Akiskal (1987) wrote about this study: "At least one study has shown some response to tricyclic antidepressants in these 'non-cases' of so-called minor or intermittent depression (Nandi et al., 1976), suggesting some affinity with morbid depression" (p. 65). Akiskal's use of the term *non-cases* is surprising because, in actuality, Nandi and his colleagues were clearly searching for major depressions. The diagnostic criteria to be satisfied were described as follows:

> An affective disorder characterized essentially by morbid changes of mood in the form of depression which is unprovoked by any physical or environmental cause, and expressed [*sic*] the feeling of misery, gloom and wretchedness often tinged with anxiety, self-reproach, moral worthlessness (guilt feeling) and suicidal tendency are quite common. When occurring for the first time in late forties, strong paranoid component may be present. Hypochondriacal ideas which in extreme cases may be nihilistic and bizarre are frequent. The mood seems to be worse in the morning. Biological symptoms like disturbances of sleep patterns, early morning waking seem to be the rule, loss of weight, appetite and libido are almost invariably present. There is retardation of thinking and action which may proceed to the level of stupor. (pp. 526–527)

In the previous section on social incapacitation in this chapter, I noted that researchers have found the presence of a number of nondepressive illness factors such as anxiety, alcoholism, and drug addiction to be associated with referral of depressed individuals to psychiatrists. Therefore, any comparisons of the response to treatment of community and clinic cases of depression would have to take into account the possible modification of the response to treatment in clinic depressions resulting from the presence of other nondepressive psychiatric conditions. In general, as noted throughout this paper, any comparisons between community and clinic cases of depressions that aim to uncover the similarities and dissimilarities between the natures of the depressions per se must ensure that the two samples do not differ on other illness and nonillness variables.

DISCUSSION

There would seem to be little evidence that unequivocally demonstrates that community cases of depression differ from clinic cases. Where the research data do suggest the possibility of differences, for instance, with respect to the greater number of symptoms and greater social impairment in clinic cases, it may be argued that these differences could be due to the fact that community samples will be diluted because of the variable types and degrees of depression in such samples, whereas the clinic samples will be of a more distilled, selected nature. On the basis of this argument, it might be proposed that these differences could be reduced if one were to adopt a higher threshold for caseness in the community samples. However, the argument would appear to beg the question of the differences between cases of depression in the two settings, and the proposal that is based on the argument would appear to defeat the whole purpose of the development of instruments such as the Diagnostic Interview Schedule and procedures such as J. K. Wing's Index of Definition. As Wing (1976) noted, the use of the ID to identify community cases according to a specifiable and repeatable procedure makes it possible to investigate questions as to whether theories of etiology, symptom maintenance, and treatment that have been tested on the clinic cases can also be applied to the community cases. It may be that a number of yardsticks will have to be used in the investigation of the similarities and dissimilarities between community and clinic cases of depression. But each yardstick should be used in the same manner and with the same thresholds in each setting. Whereas threshold points on first-stage screening instruments may have to be changed from sample to sample in order to predict cases on some gold standard, as argued, among others, by Tarnopolsky, Hand, McLean, Roberts, and Wiggins (1979), thresholds on the gold standard itself should not differ from sample to sample if the nature of the psychiatric cases in the two samples are to be compared or findings from one sample are to be generalized to the other sample.

When one uses the same threshold, for instance, an ID of 5, to identify cases in a random community sample and a clinic sample, a larger proportion of the community sample than the clinic sample will be below threshold. Wing and associates (1981) found that 89% of a random community sample, including males and females, were below threshold, and Dean, Surtees, and Sashidharan (1983) found that 91% of a random sample of 576 women were below threshold. In both instances the data were obtained with the 40-item PSE. Wing and colleagues (1981), using the 140-item PSE, found that 12% of 74 outpatients and 5% of 162 inpatients were below threshold. Sashidharan (1985), using the 140-item PSE, found that 25% of his clinic cases, which included outpatients and inpatients, were below threshold. Comparisons between the community and clinic samples are made difficult because the PSEs used in the two settings are of different lengths. It is noteworthy that when data from a 40-item PSE were examined, Sashidharan (1985) found that 45% of the clinic cases were below threshold. Although the use of the full PSE in the community studies might have resulted in a lower proportion of individuals with below-threshold IDs, and although a considerable proportion of clinic cases are below threshold, there is no doubt that the community samples are more diluted than the clinic cases. However, no matter how much more diluted community samples may be than clinic samples, as a result of the greater proportion of individuals in the community sample who will be below case thresholds but who may show varying degrees of distress and symptoms of depression, this does not present a problem for those interested in comparing *cases* in the two settings. Individuals who are below case thresholds may be of interest for some research purposes but are not of interest for those who wish to investigate the similarities and dissimilarities between *cases defined and identified in the same manner* in community and clinic populations. Whether the community individuals above threshold show more variable degrees and types of depression than the clinic patients is an empirical question that this review of the literature suggests has not yet been adequately investigated.

Regardless of whether cases of depression from the two settings differ, an argument can be made for the importance, from a public health point of view, of investigating community cases. For instance, Wing and associates (1981) reported that, in a random community sample, those identified as cases had twice as many consultations with their family physicians as the remaining people. Brown and Davidson (1978) found in a random community sample of 458 women that the accident rate per year for children under 16 living with mothers who did not have a psychopathological condition was 10%. The accident rate for children whose mothers were cases (mostly depression) was 17%, and the rate for children whose mothers were borderline cases (ID = 5) was 14%. Brown and Davidson (1978) noted that the comparable data for a sample of psychiatric patients and a series of women attending family physicians because of depression were almost identical to those obtained from the community sample. Brown's raw data (personal communication, November 15, 1988) indicated that the accident rate for patients was 16%. Other evidence of the importance of identifying community cases of depression in terms of public health was reported by Murphy, Monson, Olivier, Sobol, and Leighton (1987), who found that depressed individuals identified in a community survey have a 50% increased mortality over the following 16 years and an 82% chance of poor outcome in terms of persisting affective symptoms. It may even be that from a public health point of view it would be unwise to neglect investigating people with depressive symptoms who do not meet current criteria for a diagnosis of depression. Wells and colleagues (1989) in a study of 11,242 outpatients in three U.S. health care systems found that patients with depressive symptoms but without a depressive disorder had poor physical functioning, such as remaining for long periods in bed, that was comparable or worse than that associated with eight major chronic medical conditions.

But recognition of community depressions as phenomena worthy of investigation in their own right does not permit us to skirt the problem of the similarity or dissimilarity between such depressions and clinic depressions. There are some who advocate an approach to community studies that sidesteps completely the issue of the comparability of psychopathology in community and clinic samples. They suggest that using measuring techniques that are used in clinics and taking a categorical, diagnostic approach to psychopathology in the community may not be fruitful. For instance, a sociologist reviewing Brown and Harris's (1978a) *Social Origins of Depression* wrote:

> Simply to assert the necessary utility of psychiatric diagnostic concepts and procedures in such a way as to exclude from consideration the possibility that they are reflections of institutional practices and ideological divisions, is to imbue them with a facticity that renders them unproblematic. A clear assumption of this study is that if sociologists are to be of use to psychiatrists then they must make use of existing psychiatric knowledge, and must further develop their own knowledge in ways that are acceptable to psychiatrists. While not wishing to decry the desire to be of assistance to psychiatrists, it is being suggested that the underlying methodology and perspective of this study has limited the extent to which a more sociological understanding of a phenomenon such as depression might be developed. (Goldie, 1979, p. 354)

Some psychiatrists have also expressed a similar view. For instance, Williams, Tarnopolsky, and Hand (1980) wrote:

> At the present time, epidemiologists face the challenge of disengaging themselves from preoccupations with methods of measurement derived from hospital psychiatry, and of facing up to the difficulties involved in conceptualizing and measuring forms of pathology more relevant to the description of the depressed person in the community. If this challenge can be met, it will result in a more realistic and human view of mental functioning than has been achieved so far. (p. 112)

Acknowledging the possibility that these views concerning the need for new approaches to the measurement of depression in the community are valid, it may be that a categorical, case-finding approach should be supplemented with a dimensional approach in community settings. But then an argument could also be made for increased exploration of the value of dimensional measurements in clinic settings. Since 1950, Eysenck has consistently argued for a dimensional approach to the measurement of psychopathology (e.g. Eysenck, 1970a, 1986). There is also some evidence for the usefulness of Eysenck's dimensional measures. Weissman, Prusoff, and Klerman (1978) and Hirschfeld, Klerman, Andreasen, Clayton, and Keller (1986) found that, of a large number of variables assessed, only scores on the neuroticism (N) scale of the Maudsley Personality Inventory (MPI; Eysenck & Eysenck, 1964) predicted the course of unipolar depression. High N scores have also been found to predict poor response to behaviour therapy (Lazarus, 1963; Morgenstern, Pearce, & Rees, 1965; Schmidt, Castell, & Brown, 1965; Wolpin &

Raines, 1966). However, any data on the similarities and dissimilarities between community and clinic cases of depressions in the utility of scores on personality scales such as Eysenck's Neuroticism Scale would not provide an answer to the question concerning the similarities and dissimilarities between the depressions themselves in the two settings. Research concerned with the latter question would need to keep its primary focus on the symptoms of depression. It is the latter symptoms that should be measured and analyzed with both categorical and dimensional models.

In general, research designed to compare the nature of depression in the community and the clinic should satisfy the following criteria:

1. Cases of depression in both settings should be identified by using well-established, standardized psychiatric interviews and by applying in both settings the same algorithms for diagnosis.

2. Interviewers in both settings should have reached the same standard in their interviewing and rating skills as indicated by the reliability of the data they produce. Where possible, the same interviewers should assess both the community and clinic individuals.

3. The cases of depression identified in both settings should be further classified with classification procedures (e.g., endogenous versus nonendogenous depression, acute versus chronic cases) that have shown promise in investigations of the nature of clinic depressions.

4. Classes and subclasses of individuals should be as homogeneous as possible. Although, for instance, it is extremely difficult to identify individuals who satisfy criteria for a depressive disorder but not for an anxiety disorder (Costello, Devins, & Ward, 1988; Stavraki & Vargo, 1986), the nature of depression will not be understood unless we find procedural and statistical strategies that enable us to determine the similarities and dissimilarities between community and clinic cases of pure depression unconfounded by other psychopathological conditions. Although depressions in both the community and clinic are likely to be complex conditions that, among other complexities, show coexistence with other psychiatric conditions, this does not mean that we should investigate them in all their complexity. As Banaji and Crowder (1989) have noted: "The more complex a phenomenon, the greater the need to study it under controlled conditions, and the less it ought to be studied in its natural complexity" (p. 1192).

5. Quantitative data concerning the number, severity, and duration of symptoms should be obtained, as well as categorical data concerning the number of individuals who meet criteria for classification as cases. Care should be taken to analyze separately quantitative data for the depressive and the nondepressive symptoms.

6. In order to obtain comparable data on the number and severity of symptoms, these data should be obtained for the peak of the depressive

disorder. Because of the difficulty of conducting prospective studies designed to enable concurrent assessments of the onset of a depressive disorder, these assessments will probably have to been made through careful, thorough retrospective interviews. However, when the depression identified in the community is not in remission, that individual should be followed up at regular intervals in case the peak of the disorder had not been reached at the first interview. Such follow-up assessments of clinic cases are not likely to produce useful data in a study comparing community and clinic cases because most of the clinic cases will be in a treatment program shortly after contact with the clinic. The best an investigator can probably do is to be sure that the assessments of the clinic cases are done before the treatment program starts and to do sufficient retrospective probing to obtain at least data on the course of the depression up to the point of entry into the clinic.

7. If measures of nonillness variables such as social performance are obtained, and given that the goal of an investigator is to determine how similar community and clinic cases of depression are, an effort should be made to demonstrate that differences on the nonillness variables are functionally related to the depression variable. Examining the correlations between scores on the depression and nonillness variables would provide some data that at least would suggest such a functional relationship. More convincing data might be obtained by interview probing as to the reasons for an individual's score on the nonillness variables.

The most general principle that should guide research into the similarities and dissimilarities between community and clinic depression is that one must not lose sight of the fact that it is the nature of the depression itself, unconfounded with other illnesses and unconfounded with nonillness variables, that one must investigate as thoroughly as possible.

ACKNOWLEDGMENTS

This chapter, which was written with the assistance of an Alberta Mental Health Grant, presents a further development of arguments that were originally presented in the article "The similarities and dissimilarities between community and clinic cases of depression" published in the *British Journal of Psychiatry,* 1990, *157,* 812–821.

I wish to acknowledge the kindness of the following researchers who made their raw data available to me: Gayle Belsher, George W. Brown, Jill Hooley, Steve Newman, William Piper, Bryan Rodgers, Sarah Romans-Clarkson, David Shapiro, Hans O. F. Veiel, and Hans-Ulrich Wittchen.

The assistance of Roger Bryant and others at Shell Canada Limited in Calgary, Alberta, and of Karen Colburne in the analyses of the new symptom data presented in this chapter is also gratefully acknowledged.

REFERENCES

Akiskal, H. S. (1987). The boundaries of mood disorders: Implications for defining temperamental variants, atypical subtypes, and schizoaffective disorder. In G. L. Tischler (Ed.), *Diagnosis and classification in psychiatry: A critical appraisal of DSM-III* (pp. 61–85). New York: Cambridge University Press.

American Psychiatric Association. (1980). *Diagnostic and statistical manual of mental disorders* (3rd ed.). Washington, DC: Author.

Aneshensel, C. S., Estrada, A. L., Hansell, M. J., & Clark, V. A. (1987). Social psychological aspects of reporting behaviour: Lifetime depressive episode reports. *Journal of Health and Social Behaviour, 28,* 232–246.

Banaji, M. R., & Crowder, R. G. (1989). The bankruptcy of everyday memory. *American Psychologist, 44,* 1185–1193.

Bebbington, P. E. (1984). Inferring causes: Some constraints in the social psychiatry of depressive disorders. *Integrative Psychiatry, 2,* 69–72.

Bebbington, P. E., Brugha, T., MacCarthy, B., Potter, J., Sturt, E., Wykes, T., Katz, R., & McGuffin, P. (1988). The Camberwell Collaborative Depression Study: I. Depressed probands: Adversity and the form of depression. *British Journal of Psychiatry, 152,* 754–765.

Bebbington, P., Hurry, J., Tennant, C., Sturt, E., & Wing, J. K. (1981). Epidemiology of mental disorders in Camberwell. *Psychological Medicine, 11,* 561–579.

Bebbington, P. E., Tennant, C., & Hurry, J. (1981). Adversity and the nature of psychiatric disorder in the community. *Journal of Affective Disorders, 3,* 345–366.

Belsher, G., & Costello, C. G. (1991). Do confidants of depressed women provide less social support than confidants of non-depressed women? *Journal of Abnormal Psychology, 100,* 516–525.

Benjaminsen, S. (1981). Stressful life events preceding the onset of neurotic depression. *Psychological Medicine, 11,* 369–378.

Brown, G. W. (1978). *Notes on the depression study.* Mimeograph. Bedford College, London.

Brown, G. W., Andrews, B., Harris, T. O., Adler, Z., & Bridge, L. (1986). Social support, self-esteem and depression. *Psychological Medicine, 6,* 813–831.

Brown, G. W., Craig, T. K. J., & Harris, T. O. (1985). Depression: Distress or disease? Some epidemiological considerations. *British Journal of Psychiatry, 147,* 612–622.

Brown, G. W., & Davidson, S. (1978). Social class, psychiatric disorder of mother and accidents to children. *Lancet, 1,* 378–381.

Brown, G. W., & Harris, T. (1978a). *Social origins of depression: A study of psychiatric disorder in women.* London: Tavistock.

Brown, G. W., & Harris, T. (1978b). Social origins of depression: A reply. *Psychological Medicine, 8,* 577–588.

Brown, G. W., & Harris, T. O. (1982). Disease, distress and depression: A comment. *Journal of Affective Disorders, 4,* 1–8.

Brown, G. W., & Harris, T. (1986). Establishing causal links: The Bedford College studies of depression. In H. Katschnig (Ed.), *Life events and psychi-*

atric disorders: Controversial issues (pp. 107–200). New York: Cambridge University Press.

Brown, G. W., & Prudo, R. (1981). Psychiatric disorder in a rural and urban population: I. Aetiology of depression. *Psychological Medicine, 11,* 581–599.

Calloway, S. P., Dolan, R. J., Fonagy, P., DeSouza, V. F. A., & Wakeling, A. (1984a). Endocrine changes and clinical profiles in depression: 1. The dexamethasone suppression test. *Psychological Medicine, 14,* 749–758.

Calloway, S. P., Dolan, R. J., Fonagy, P., DeSouza, V. F. A., & Wakeling, A. (1984b). Endocrine changes and clinical profiles in depression: 2. The thyrotropin-releasing hormone test. *Psychological Medicine, 14,* 759–765.

Costello, C. G. (1982). Social factors associated with depression: A retrospective community study. *Psychological Medicine, 12,* 329–339.

Costello, C. G., Devins, G. M., & Ward, K. W. (1988). The prevalence of fears, phobias and anxiety disorders and their relationship with depression in women attending family physicians. *Behaviour Research and Therapy, 26,* 311–320.

Creer, C., & Wing, J. K. (1974). *Schizophrenia at home.* London: National Schizophrenia Fellowship.

Dean, C., Surtees, P. G., & Sashidharan, S. P. (1983). Comparisons of research diagnostic systems in an Edinburgh community sample. *British Journal of Psychiatry, 142,* 247–256.

Depue, R. A., & Monroe, S. M. (1986). Conceptualization and measurement of human disorder in life stress research: The problem of chronic disturbance. *Psychological Bulletin, 99,* 36–51.

Eysenck, H. J. (1970a). A dimensional system of psychodiagnostics. In A. R. Mahrer (Ed.), *New approaches to personality classification* (pp. 169–207). New York: Columbia University Press.

Eysenck, H. J. (1970b). The classification of depressive illnesses. *British Journal of Psychiatry, 117,* 241–250.

Eysenck, H. J. (1986). A critique of contemporary classification and diagnosis. In T. Millon & G. L. Klerman (Eds.), *Contemporary directions in psychopathology: Towards the DSM-IV* (pp. 73–98). New York: Guilford.

Eysenck, H. J., & Eysenck, S. B. G. (1964). *The manual of the Eysenck Personality Inventory.* London: University of London Press.

Finlay-Jones, R. A., Brown, G. W., Duncan-Jones, P., Harris, T. O., Murphy, E., & Prudo, R. (1980). Depression and anxiety in the community: Replicating the diagnosis of a case. *Psychological Medicine, 10,* 445–454.

Giel, R., Koeter, M. W. J., & Ormel, J. (1990). Selection and referral of primary care patients with mental health problems: The second and third filter. In D. Goldberg & D. Tantam (Eds.), *The public health impact of mental disorder* (pp. 25–34). Lewiston, NY: Hogrefe & Huber.

Goldberg, D., & Huxley, P. (1980). *Mental illness in the community: The pathway to psychiatric care.* London: Tavistock.

Goldie, N. (1979). [Review of *The social origins of depression*]. *Sociology of Health and Illness, 1,* 352–357.

Hamilton, M. (1967). Development of a rating scale for primary depressive illness. *British Journal of Social and Clinical Psychology, 6,* 278–296.

Hirschfeld, R. M. A., Klerman, G. L., Andreasen, N. C., Clayton, P. J., & Keller,

M. B. (1986). Psycho-social predictors of chronicity in depressed patients. *British Journal of Psychiatry, 148,* 648–654.

Hollon, S. D. (1986, October 16). *Deconfounding cognitive vulnerability from symptom suppression: What we can learn from differential risk following treatment of depression.* Paper presented at the 20th annual convention for the Association for the Advancement of Behaviour Therapy, Chicago.

Hooley, J. (1986). Expressed emotion and depression: Interaction between patients and high- versus low-expressed-emotion spouses. *Journal of Abnormal Psychology, 95,* 237–246.

Hurry, J., & Sturt, E. (1981). Social performance in a population sample: Relation to psychiatric symptoms. In J. K. Wing, P. E. Bebbington, & L. Robins (Eds.), *What is a case? The problem of definition in psychiatric community surveys* (pp. 202–213). London: Grant McIntyre.

Klein, D. N. (1990). Symptom criteria and family history in major depression. *American Journal of Psychiatry, 147,* 850–854.

Lazarus, A. A. (1963). The results of behaviour therapy in 126 cases of severe neurosis. *Behaviour Research and Therapy, 1,* 69–79.

McGuffin, P., Katz, R., & Bebbington, P. (1987). Hazard, heredity and depression: A family study. *Journal of Psychiatric Research, 21,* 365–375.

McGuffin, P., Katz, R., & Bebbington, P. (1988). The Camberwell Collaborative Depression Study: III. Depression and adversity in the relatives of depressed probands. *British Journal of Psychiatry, 152,* 775–782.

Mechanic, D. (1972). Social psychological factors affecting the presentation of bodily complaints. *New England Journal of Medicine, 286,* 1132–1139.

Monroe, S. M., Thase, M. E., & Simons, A. D. (1992). Social factors and the psychobiology of depression: Relationships between life stress and rapid eye movement sleep latency. *Journal of Abnormal Psychology, 101,* 528–537.

Morgenstern, F. S., Pearce, J. F., & Rees, L. W. (1965). Predicting the outcome of behaviour therapy by psychological tests. *Behaviour Research and Therapy, 3,* 191–200.

Murphy, J., Monson, R., Olivier, D., Sobol, A., & Leighton, A. (1987). Affective disorder and mortality. *Archives of General Psychiatry, 44,* 473–479.

Nandi, D. N., Ajmany, S., Ganguli, H., Banerjee, G., Boral, G. C., Ghosh, A., & Sarkar, S. (1976). A clinical evaluation of depressives found in a rural survey in India. *British Journal of Psychiatry, 128,* 523–527.

Orn, H., Newman, S. C., & Bland, R. C. (1988). Design and field methods of the Edmonton survey of psychiatric disorders. *Acta Psychiatrica Scandinavica, 77* (Suppl. 338), 17–23.

Paykel, E. S. (1971). Classification of depressed patients: A cluster analysis derived grouping. *British Journal of Psychiatry, 118,* 275–288.

Paykel, E. S., Prusoff, B. A., & Uhlenhuth, E. H. (1971). Scaling of life events. *Archives of General Psychiatry, 25,* 340–347.

Paykel, E. S., Rao, B. M., & Taylor, C. N. (1984). Life stress and symptom pattern in out-patient depression. *Psychological Medicine, 14,* 559–568.

Richman, A., & Barry, A. (1985). More and more is less and less: The myth of massive psychiatric need. *British Journal of Psychiatry, 146,* 164–168.

Robins, L. N., Helzer, J. E., Croughan, J., & Ratcliff, K. S. (1981). National Institute of Mental Health Diagnostic Interview Schedule: Its history, characteristics and validity. *Archives of General Psychiatry, 38,* 381–389.

Robins, L. N., & Regier, D. A. (1991). *Psychiatric disorders in America: The Epidemiologic Catchment Area Study.* New York: Free Press.

Rodgers, B., & Mann, S. A. (1986). The reliability and validity of PSE assessments by lay interviewers: A national population survey. *Psychological Medicine, 16,* 689–700.

Romans-Clarkson, S., Walton, V., Herbison, P., & Mullen, P. (1990). Anxiety and depression in urban and rural New Zealand women. In N. McNaughton & G. Andrews (Eds.), *Anxiety* (pp. 19–30). Dunedin: University of Otago Press.

Sargeant, J. K., Bruce, M. L., Florio, L. P., & Weissman, M. M. (1990). Factors associated with 1-year outcome of major depression in the community. *Archives of General Psychiatry, 47,* 519–526.

Sashidharan, S. P. (1985). Definitions of psychiatric syndromes: comparison in hospital patients and general population. *British Journal of Psychiatry, 147,* 547–551.

Sashidharan, S. P., Surtees, P. G., Kreitman, N. B., Ingham, J. G., & Miller, P. McC. (1990). Affective disorders among women in the general population and among those referred to psychiatrists: Clinical features and demographic correlates. *British Journal of Psychiatry, 157,* 828–834.

Schmidt, E., Castell, D., & Brown, P. (1965). A retrospective study of 42 cases of behaviour therapy. *Behaviour Research and Therapy, 3,* 9–19.

Shapiro, D. A., Barkham, M., Hardy, G. E., & Morrison, L. A. (1990). The second Sheffield psychotherapy project: Rationale design and preliminary outcome data. *British Journal of Medical Psychology, 63,* 97–108.

Shapiro, S., Skinner, E. A., Kessler, L. G., Von Korff, M., German, P. W., Tischler, G. L., Leaf, P. J., Benham, L., Cottler, L., & Regier, D. A. (1984). Utilization of health and mental health services. *Archives of General Psychiatry, 41,* 971–978.

Snaith, R. P. (1987). The concepts of mild depression. *British Journal of Psychiatry, 150,* 387–393.

Stavraki, C., & Vargo, B. (1986). The relationship of anxiety and depression: A review of the literature. *British Journal of Psychiatry, 149,* 7–16.

Surtees, P. G., & Sashidharan, S. P. (1989). The epidemiology of affective disorders: National secular trends and local findings. *Psychiatry and Psychobiology, 4,* 287–298.

Surtees, P. G., Sashidharan, S. P., & Dean, C. (1986). Affective disorder amongst women in the general population: A longitudinal study. *British Journal of Psychiatry, 148,* 176–186.

Tansella, M., & Williams, P. (1989). The spectrum of psychiatric morbidity in a defined geographical area. *Psychological Medicine, 19,* 765–770.

Tarnopolsky, A., Hand, D. J., McLean, E. K., Roberts, H., & Wiggins, R. D. (1979). Validity and use of a screening questionnaire (GHQ) in the community. *British Journal of Psychiatry, 134,* 508–515.

Tennant, C., & Bebbington, P. (1978). The social causation of depression: A critique of the work of Brown and his colleagues. *Psychological Medicine, 8,* 565–575.

Thase, M. E., Frank, E., & Kupfer, D. J. (1985). Biological processes in major depression. In E. C. Beckham & W. R. Leber (Eds.), *Handbook of depression: Treatment, assessment and research* (pp. 816–913). Homewood, IL: Dorsey.

Thase, M. E., & Kupfer, D. J. (1988). Current status of EEG sleep in the assessment and treatment of depression. In G. D. Burrows & J. S. Werry (Eds.), *Advances in human psychopharmacology* (Vol. 4, pp. 93–148). Greenwich, CT: JAI.

Torgersen, S. (1986). Genetic factors in moderately severe and mild affective disorders. *Archives of General Psychiatry, 43,* 222–226.

Veiel, H. O. F., & Kühner, Ch., Brill, G., & Ihle, W. (1992). Psychosocial correlates of clinical depression after psychiatric in-patient treatment: Methodological issues and baseline differences between recovered and non-recovered patients. *Psychological Medicine, 22,* 415–427.

Weissman, M. M., Prusoff, B. A., & Klerman, G. L. (1978). Personality and the prediction of long-term outcome of depression. *American Journal of Psychiatry, 135,* 797–800.

Wells, K. B., Stewart, A., Hays, R. D., Burnham, N. A., Rogers, W., Daniels, M., Berry, S., Greenfield, S., & Ware, J. (1989). The functioning and well-being of depressed patients: Results from the medical outcomes study. *Journal of the American Medical Association, 262,* 914–919.

Williams, P., Tarnopolsky, A., & Hand, D. (1980). Case definition and case identification in psychiatric epidemiology: Review and assessment. *Psychological Medicine, 10,* 101–114.

Wing, J. K. (1976). A technique for studying psychiatric morbidity in in-patient and out-patient series and in general population samples. *Psychological Medicine, 6,* 665–671.

Wing, J. K., Bebbington, P., Hurry, J., & Tennant, C. (1981). The prevalence in the general population of disorders familiar to psychiatrists in hospital practice. In J. K. Wing, P. Bebbington, & L. N. Robins (Eds.), *What is a case? The problem of definition in psychiatric community surveys* (pp. 45–61). London: Grant McIntyre.

Wing, J. K., Cooper, J., & Sartorius, N. (1974). *The measurement and classification of psychiatric symptoms.* Cambridge: Cambridge University Press.

Wing, J. K., Mann, S. A., Leff, J. P., & Nixon, J. M. (1978). The concept of a "case" in psychiatric population surveys. *Psychological Medicine, 8,* 203–217.

Wing, J. K., & Sturt, E. (1978). *The PSE-ID-CATEGO system: A supplementary manual.* London: Institute of Psychiatry.

Wittchen, H.-U. (1987). Chronic difficulties and life-events in the long-term course of affective and anxiety disorders: Results from the Munich follow-up study. In M. C. Angermeyer (Ed.), *From social class to social stress: New developments in psychiatric epidemiology* (pp. 176–196). New York: Springer-Verlag.

Wolpin, M., & Raines, J. (1966). Visual imagery, expected roles and extinction as possible factors in reducing fear and avoidance behaviour. *Behaviour Research and Therapy, 4,* 25–37.

World Health Organization (1978). *Mental disorders: Glossary and guide to their classification in accordance with the ninth revision of the international classification of disorders.* Geneva: Author.

4

Similarities and Dissimilarities between Child and Adult Disorders: The Case of Depression

RICHARD HARRINGTON

Until relatively recently, the prevailing view was that depressive disorders rarely occurred in children or that if they did occur they took a "masked" form. In the last 15 years, however, there has been an increasing recognition that depressive conditions resembling adult depression can and do appear in childhood (see reviews by, for example, Angold, 1988; Harrington, 1990; Rutter, 1986a). Indeed, it has been suggested that they are quite common in clinical samples. Nevertheless, there are continuing uncertainties about the comparability of depressive disorders in children with the major depressive disorders of adults, and many writers remain doubtful about the true frequency of depressive syndromes in prepubertal children (Graham, 1981; Lefkowitz & Burton, 1978; Shaffer, 1985).

This chapter is concerned with the similarities and dissimilarities between child and adult depressive disorders. The chapter begins with a review of concepts of depression in young people. Next, the current practice of using unmodified adult criteria to diagnose depression among the young is considered. Finally, the evidence for links between child and adult depressive disorders is examined.

CONCEPTS OF DEPRESSION IN YOUNG PEOPLE

Current concepts of depression in young people use criteria that are closely comparable to those in adults. However, as we shall see later, these do not necessarily solve all the problems. Accordingly, it is helpful to consider earlier views briefly in order to highlight the key dilemmas and issues.

Masked Depression

During the 1960s the predominant view in the psychoanalytic literature was that depressive conditions resembling adult depression could not occur in children because the personality structure of the child was too immature (Rie, 1966). Rochlin (1959), for example, considered that depression was impossible in middle childhood because children do not have sufficiently formulated superegos to direct aggression against their own egos.

However, middle childhood has also been seen as a time when depression does occur, but in a masked form. In this formulation, children between roughly the ages of 6 and 10 years are in a transition period. They are able to experience adultlike depressive conditions, but they express these feelings in a different way. Frommer (1968), for example, hypothesized that there were three types of depression in childhood: uncomplicated or pure depression, enuretic depression, and phobic depression. Children with uncomplicated depression were the only group in which spontaneous complaints of depression were common. Cytryn and Mc-Knew (1972) proposed that the most common type of depression in childhood was masked depression, which could be diagnosed on the basis of features such as facial expression and fantasy content.

There is no doubt that the notion of masked depression has proved useful in some clinical settings in drawing attention to modes of presentation of depression that are easily missed. Moreover, it is not unreasonable to think that if depressive disorders do occur in prepubertal children then they may assume a different form. After all, children differ from adults in their ability to experience many of the so-called cognitive features of depression, such as hopelessness (Rutter, 1986b).

However, the idea that depression in young children is mostly expressed through nondepressive symptoms, with few obvious signs of a primary mood state, has proved very difficult to put into practice. The problem is that no one has been able to devise a set of criteria that can reliably distinguish between symptoms that are due to depression and identical symptoms that occur as part of a different underlying disorder. When, for example, is enuresis "true enuresis" and when is it a "depressive equivalent"? Furthermore, the symptoms that were thought to be due to masked depression included practically all the possible psychiatric symptoms of childhood (Puig-Antich & Gittelman, 1982). Because our current classification systems are mostly specified in descriptive rather than etiological terms, it is somewhat confusing to classify as depressed individuals who show few overt signs of depression.

Finally, as Kovacs and Beck (1977) pointed out, the term *masked depression* is not only misleading but also probably unnecessary. They noted that many of the behaviors listed as masking depression in children were often a prominent part of the clinical picture in adults. Moreover, several investigators have found that other psychiatric symptoms did not usually mask depressive symptoms. Careful clinical examination would usually reveal the underlying depression (Carlson & Cantwell, 1980a; Kolvin et al., 1991).

Operational Criteria for Syndromes Resembling Adult Depression

The next major development in the field was the attempt by several authors to specify operational diagnostic criteria for depression in children that resembled the criteria used to diagnose depression in adults (Ling, Oftedal, & Weinberg, 1970; McConville, Boag, & Purohit, 1973; Pearce, 1974, 1978; Weinberg, Rutman, Sullivan, Penick, & Dietz, 1973). These early operationalized systems stemmed from the idea that depression in children had many similarities with depression arising in adults, as well as a number of features seen only in childhood. Weinberg and colleagues (1973), for instance, used criteria that were broadly similar to the adult criteria of Feighner, Robins, Guze, Woodruff, and Winokur (1972).

Pearce (1974, 1978) devised a similar set of criteria for depression in children. Pearce (1974) used a variety of statistical techniques to identify symptoms that discriminated between depressed and nondepressed children and that were positively associated with the symptom of depressed mood. On the basis of these statistical analyses, he proposed that childhood depressive disorder should be defined by the symptom of depressed mood plus at least two of the following symptoms: suicidal and morbid thoughts, disturbance of sleep, disturbance of appetite, obsessions, irritability, hypochondriasis, alimentary symptoms, school refusal, and altered perception, such as delusions or overvalued ideas of guilt and worthlessness. The symptoms must represent a change in the child's usual functioning and be persistent and severe enough to be a handicap (Pearce, 1978).

These operationalized diagnostic criteria represented an important advance in the evolution of the current concept of depression in children. However, both sets of criteria were rather nonspecific to the extent that a depressive disorder could still be diagnosed in the absence of a majority of symptoms of depression. For example, in the Pearce system, it was possible to diagnose depression on the basis of depressed mood, school refusal, and hypochondriasis. Moreover, in order to make assessments more applicable for children, certain assumptions had to be made about the equivalence of child and adult symptoms. For example, in the Weinberg criteria, "desire to run away from home" was taken as evidence of self-depreciatory ideation. Furthermore, the existence of several different sets of criteria for childhood depression meant that there was little uniformity within the field.

THE USE OF UNMODIFIED CRITERIA

Several authors suggested that depressive disorders among children should be diagnosed with the standardized criteria that were used with adults, such as DSM-III. According to this viewpoint, the essential features for major depression were identical for prepubertal children, adolescents, and adults. Puig-Antich, Blau, Marx, Greenhill, and Chambers (1978), for example, identified 13 prepubertal children who met Research Diagnostic Criteria for major depressive disorder for at least 1 month. All were able to describe depressed mood, and 11 had suicidal thoughts. These children appeared to have a severe form of depression as judged by the fact that three of them had an endogenous symptom pattern and three had depressive hallucinations. Since then, there have been reports that such syndromes may be relatively common in children referred to psychiatrists (Carlson & Cantwell, 1980b; Kolvin et al., 1991), and it has been suggested that major depressive disorders can occur in preschoolers (Kashani, Holcomb, & Orvaschel, 1986).

Indeed, the main current classification systems make no distinction in the diagnostic criteria for prepubertal, adolescent, or adult depression. DSM-III-R (American Psychiatric Association, 1987) does state in the text that there may be age-specific associated features that differ across these age periods. For instance, irritable mood may substitute for depressed mood in both children and adolescents. In prepubertal children with major depression somatic complaints, agitation and mood-congruent hallucinations are said to be particularly frequent. In adolescence, wanting to leave home, restlessness, grouchiness, and aggression are common, and school difficulties are likely. In addition, withdrawal from social activities and a reluctance to cooperate in family ventures are said to be frequent. However, none of these features is actually part of the diagnostic criteria in DSM-III-R. Major depressive disorders are seen as occurring at any age, including infancy. In the draft version of the tenth edition of the International Classification of Diseases (World Health Organization, 1989), no mention is made of the features of major depression as they occur in children. Presumably, therefore, the criteria are identical across the age span.

Thus, in the space of a few years, the field has advanced from the position that depressive disorders cannot occur in children or that they occur in a masked form to the point where childhood disorders with features similar or identical to adult depression are part of our classification systems. Indeed, as Shaffer (1985) pointed out, for a time the idea of depression as a psychiatric disease affecting children became so popular that papers on it dominated scientific journals and meetings. Moreover, in that there seems to be little doubt that disorders meeting the full criteria for adult major depression can and do occur in children, it might be thought that the issue of the validity of childhood depression has been resolved. However, this is very far from being the case, and many uncertainties still exist about the concept.

Some Problems of Using Adult Criteria for Depression in Children

Some of these uncertainties apply equally to depressive disorders arising in adulthood. For instance, in neither age period is it clear where the boundaries lie between depressive disorder and, on the one hand, normal sadness and, on the other hand, nondepressive psychiatric disorders such as anxiety. Moreover, it is unclear whether depressive disorders in young people should be distinguished from depression that occurs in the context of environmental adversity. Thus, for example, Graham (1981) considered that depression as a biologically determined disorder occurs only rarely in children. In line with many critics of the biological model of adult depression, he believed that depression in children was usually a social response to stress. He proposed that childhood depressive disorders should be viewed as reactions until proved otherwise.

Perhaps more importantly, however, the strategy of applying unmodified adult criteria to children has also been criticized because it fails to take into account developmental research on age changes in the frequency and expression of affective phenomena. Three developmental issues are especially relevant here. First, there are substantial age differences in the occurrence of depressive phenomena (Angold, 1988; Rutter, 1986a). Depressive symptoms in the community are considerably more prevalent in adolescence than in childhood, and these changes seem to show an association with puberty (Rutter, Tizard, & Whitmore, 1970; Rutter, Graham, Chadwick, & Yule, 1976; Rutter, 1980). Data on depressive disorders in clinical samples (Pearce, 1978) and in the general population (Fleming, Offord, & Boyle, 1989) show the same trend. Moreover, suicide rates rise dramatically after puberty (McClure, 1988; Shaffer, 1986, 1988), and it seems that the same is true of mania (Strober, Hanna, & McCracken, 1989). Furthermore, there is some evidence of a change in sex ratio at around the time of puberty. Among prepubertal children, it seems that depressive symptoms and depressive disorders are more common in boys, whereas after puberty they are more common in girls (Fleming et al., 1989; Rutter, 1986a, 1988).

Second, children differ from adults in their ability to experience some of the cognitive features said to characterize adult depression (Rutter, 1986b). For example, if children are to experience guilt and a sense of failure, it is necessary that they can understand the concept of failure. It seems that children as young as 4 or 5 years old are aware that other people may feel ashamed of them, but not until around the age of 8 years do most children talk of being ashamed of themselves (Harter, 1983).

Third, the valid application of adult criteria to children requires not only that they are capable of experiencing the features said to be characteristic of adult depression but also that they can report them accurately. It seems that children have limitations in this last respect. Kovacs (1986), for example, reported that young children had difficulties differentiating basic emotions and often mislabeled emotions such as sadness and anger. Moreover, the young child's capacity to give an account of duration of problems and past events is limited. This may pose problems for the diagnosis of some categories of depressive disorder, such as recurrent depression, in which historical data are required to make the diagnosis.

Developmental Perspectives on Classification

These difficulties have led a number of authors to question the current trend of using adult-based diagnostic criteria to diagnose depressive disorders in children. Because the nature of the symptoms expressed at different ages may differ greatly, perhaps it is futile to try to define criteria that can be applied across the age span. According to this viewpoint, it might be better to identify age-appropriate signs and symptoms that take into account the child's level of functioning in the various cognitive and affective domains (Carlson & Garber, 1986).

To some extent, it is probably already the case that many clinicians who apply adult criteria for depression to young children draw upon their knowledge of child development to adapt these criteria to the developmental levels of their patients (Cicchetti & Schneider-Rosen, 1986). Indeed, early attempts to define adultlike operational criteria for childhood depression often made assumptions about the equivalence of child and adult symptoms. For instance, the criteria devised by Weinberg and his colleagues (1973) treated the symptom of being "negative and difficult to please" as a sign of "dysphoric mood." Moreover, DSM-III-R in effect advocates the notion of using age-specific criteria for depression when it lists the ways in which the manifestations of depression vary with age.

However, the problem with both the intuitive approach of the clinician and the more formal approach of DSM-III-R is that neither specifies exactly how the "developmental perspective" should be put into practice. It is all very well to suggest that the manifestations of depression may vary with age, but it is quite another thing to operationalize this idea in the form of criteria that can be used reliably and that will be widely accepted. Thus, one of the first attempts to classify childhood depression (Malmquist, 1971) was based on both etiology and developmental level. There were five major groups. Two were classed according to etiology (depressions associated with organic disease and deprivation syndromes) and three according to developmental stage (individuation, latency, and adolescent types). However, no systematic studies were done on the validity of these distinctions, and as a result the criteria were never widely used. Similarly, McConville and associates (1973) proposed that there were three types of depression in childhood: "Affectual" type occurred in children aged 6 to 8 years and was thought to be characterized by expressions of sadness, hopelessness, and helplessness. The second form was said to be more common after the age of 8 and was characterized by low self-esteem. In the third type, which occurred in children of 11 years or older, feelings of guilt were common. Once again, however, there has been little published research on the relationship between the various proposed subtypes.

More recently, Carlson and Garber (1986) have suggested that current diagnostic systems such as DSM could be revised to take into account developmental differences. They proposed a set of diagnostic rules involving a two-tiered process that takes into account different base rates at different ages. The first tier would consist of a set of core indicators that occur at roughly the same rate across the age span. A certain number would be required for the diagnosis of depression. A second set of indicators would consist of those symptoms found rarely in children, such as suicidal ideation. These symptoms would contribute to the diagnosis if present, but would not alter the diagnosis if absent. The third set would consist of symptoms highly associated with depression in children, such as social withdrawal, which would also contribute to the diagnosis if present. In essence, then, this classification scheme proposes that depression in children could be conceptualized as having a basic similarity with adult-onset depression, but with some age-specific features. The system has merit, but it remains to be seen whether it will become widely used. In any event, it is unlikely that a developmental approach to the description of depressive disorders will find its way into DSM-IV (Shaffer et al., 1989).

SIMILARITIES AND DISSIMILARITIES BETWEEN CHILD AND ADULT DEPRESSION

It would appear that the application of concepts borrowed from studies of depressed adults to the study of affective phenomena in children has generated much research and has led to some progress in recent years. Nevertheless, the classification and diagnosis of depression in children with unmodified adult criteria remain a matter of controversy. Accordingly, a variety of different research approaches have been undertaken in order to examine the similarities and dissimilarities between child and adult depressions.

Comparisons of Phenomenology across Ages

Several investigators have systematically compared the symptoms of depressed children with those of depressed adolescents or adults (Carlson & Kashani, 1988; Kovacs & Paulauskas, 1984; Mitchell, McCauley, Burke, & Moss, 1988; Ryan et al., 1987). In the largest such study (Ryan et al., 1987), symptom frequency and severity were compared in two clinically referred samples of 95 children and 92 adolescents with major depression. There was no difference between children and adolescents with major depressive disorders in the overall severity of depressive symptoms, or in the severity of the majority of individual depressive symptoms, including depressed mood, insomnia, irritability, and suicidal ideation. However, prepubertal children had more somatic complaints, psychomotor agitation, separation anxiety, phobias, and hallucinations. Adolescents had greater hopelessness/helplessness, anhedonia, hypersomnia, and use of alcohol and illicit drugs. Although prepubertal children seemed to have just as much suicidal ideation as depressed adolescents, the potential lethality of their suicidal attempts was lower.

Carlson and Kashani (1988) compared the symptom profiles of the children and adolescents from the study of Ryan and colleagues (1987) with the symptomatology of 9 preschool children with DSM-III major depression and with 100 adults who had been hospitalized with unipolar depression. Anhedonia, diurnal variation, hopelessness, psychomotor retardation, and delusions increased with age. Depressed appearance, low self-esteem, and somatic complaints decreased with age. In a similar study, however, Mitchell and associates (1988) found very few differences between the symptomatology of depressed children and adolescents. Moreover, their combined group of children and adolescents differed little in symptom presentation from adults with major depression.

Because all these studies were based on children who had previously been diagnosed as having DSM-III major depression, and because this diagnosis was based on the number and type of depressive symptoms, the amount of variation in depressive symptomatology was necessarily very limited. Nevertheless, even with this constraint, the findings of the systematic study of Ryan and colleagues (1987) point not only to substantial similarities between child and adult depression but also to important dissimilarities. Indeed, as these authors commented, some symptoms that are not part of the adult criteria for depression, such as somatic complaints and social withdrawal, were so common among depressed children and adolescents that consideration should be given to including them in the criteria for depression in this age group. Perhaps development may alter some of the features of depression. As we shall see in the next section, mathematical studies produce a similar pattern of phenotypic continuities and discontinuities between child and adult depressive disorders.

Mathematical Studies

Several types of mathematical approaches have been used to study the symptomatology of depressed children and to examine the degree of similarity with depressive disorders arising in adulthood. *Principal components analysis,* which forms groups of *symptoms* based on the cooccurrence of those symptoms in individuals, was used by Ryan and associates (1987) with the Pittsburgh sample described earlier. These authors found five clinically interpretable factors: an endogenous factor, a negative cognitions factor, an anxiety factor, an appetite and weight factor, and a disturbed conduct factor. The group was then divided into prepubertal children and adolescents. The adolescent group gave essentially the same factor structure. However, in the child group the endogenous factor combined with the negative cognition factor, and the other three factors remained basically unchanged.

Similar component structures were identified by Kolvin and colleagues (1991), who applied the same statistical techniques in a study of successive referrals to a university child psychiatry unit in Newcastle, England. In their principal components analyses, four clinically interpretable components were identified: (1) depression, anhedonia, increased fatigue, and psychomotor retardation; (2) negative cognitions and thoughts of suicide; (3) an anxiety component (including separation anxiety and fear); and (4) an anger, agitation, and irritability component. In contrast to Ryan and associates (1987), neither a conduct nor an appetite–weight component was identified. The smaller size of the Newcastle sample did not allow separate analysis of prepubertal and postpubertal groups.

It should be borne in mind that whereas principal component analysis permits the exploration of relationships between *attributes* (such as symptoms) it does not permit conclusions about the classification of *individuals.* Another mathematical technique, *cluster analysis,* is better suited for this task because it works by grouping like patients together. In the Pittsburgh research the results of a cluster analysis were rather inconclusive. However, Kolvin and associates (1991) were able to identify distinct clusters. Thus, when combined child–parent data were used, three clusters were obtained: depressive cognitions, endogenous depression, and a mixture of conduct disturbance and neurotic disorder.

All in all, these two studies provide some support for the concept of an endogenous form of depression occurring in older children and adolescents that is phenomenologically distinct from other forms of the disorder in this age group. This finding parallels the results from a large number of factor and cluster analysis studies conducted with samples of depressed adults. Indeed, probably the most consistent finding from these studies has been the identification of a group of patients with an endogenous depression characterized by symptoms such as nonreactivity of mood in the face of pleasurable events, terminal sleep disturbance, diurnal variation, and distinct quality of mood (Kendell, 1976; Nelson & Charney, 1981). Similarly, there is also support for the validity of an anxious factor, which again has been identified in several of the adult mathematical studies. Paykel (1971), for instance, produced four groups from a cluster analysis of the ratings of 165 adult patients with depression: psychotic depressives, anxious depressives, hostile depressives and young depressives with personality disorder. Similar factors were produced in Overall, Hollister, Johnson, and Pennington's study (1966) of adult depression.

However, the syndrome of depressive cognitions, which was found in both the Pittsburgh and Newcastle studies, is less easy to relate to adult typologies. Perhaps, as some cognitive theories of depression postulate, these cognitions are the precursors of later depression. Or, could it be that they are simply the result of a previous episode? This group certainly warrants further study and probably follow-up into late adolescence. In either event, the implication is that depression in young people may not have the same underlying factor structure as depression in adults. It may be that depression in childhood shows developmental heterogeneity, with some varieties being more or less specific to children, whereas others are isomorphic with depressions arising in later age periods.

Longitudinal Studies

The natural history of a psychopathological disorder has long been regarded as an important validating feature of that condition. Depressive disorders in adult life tend to be recurrent conditions (Outcome of depression, 1989). Thus, the validation of depressive syndromes in childhood relies, at least in part, on the demonstration that depressed children are more likely than children with other psychiatric disorders to develop depression in adulthood.

Most short-term follow-up studies of preadolescent children meeting DSM-III criteria for depression have shown that depression in childhood often recurs (Asarnow et al., 1988; Kovacs, Feinberg, Crouse-Novak, Paulauskas, & Finkelstein, 1984; Kovacs, Feinberg, Crouse-Novak, Paulauskas, Pollock, et al., 1984; McGee & Williams, 1988). For example, Kovacs and her colleagues (Kovacs, Feinberg, Crouse-Novak, Paulauskas, & Finkelstein, 1984; Kovacs, Feinberg, Crouse-Novak, Paulauskas, Pollock, et al., 1984) undertook a systematic follow-up of child patients with major depressive disorder, dysthymic disorder, adjustment disorder with depressed mood, and some other psychiatric disorder. The development of subsequent episodes of depression was virtually confined to children with major depressive disorders and dysthymic disorders. However, the follow-up assessments in the study of Kovacs and her colleagues were not made blind to the original diagnosis, and none of these follow-up studies of depressed children extended beyond adolescence.

Several longitudinal studies of depressed adolescents have extended into late adolescence or early adult life (Garber, Kriss, Koch, & Lindholm, 1988; Garrison, Jackson, Marsteller, McKeown, & Addy, 1990; Kandel & Davies, 1986; King & Pittman, 1970; Strober & Carlson, 1982). These studies have suggested both that self-ratings of depression in adolescent community samples predict similar problems in early adulthood (Kandel & Davies, 1986) and that adolescent patients with depressive disorders are at high risk of subsequent major affective disturbance (Garber et al., 1988; Strober & Carlson, 1982). The findings of these studies are limited by issues such as the uncertainty regarding the connection between depression questionnaire scores and clinical depressive disorder (Kandel & Davies, 1986), high rates of sample attrition (Garber et al., 1988), and a lack of blindness to earlier diagnosis (Strober & Carlson, 1982). Nevertheless, in our 18-year longitudinal study of depressed Maudsley patients, in which there was an 80% follow-up rate and in which outcome measures were obtained blind to child diagnosis, there were also strong temporal continuities between depression in young people and depression in adult life (Harrington, Fudge, Rutter, Pickles, & Hill, 1990). Thus, subjects who had suffered from an operationally defined depressive disorder in childhood were nearly four times more likely to suffer from some form of depressive disorder in adulthood. This risk was highly specific for depressive disorder: No disorder other than depression was increased in adulthood. Interestingly, continuity to major depression in adulthood was stronger in the postpubertal depressed group than in the prepubertal depressed group. In addition, children with depression and conduct disorder had lower rates of depression in adulthood than children with pure depression (Harrington, Fudge, Rutter, Pickles, & Hill, 1991).

All in all, these longitudinal studies provide strong support for the idea that depression in young people does represent the same psychiatric condition as depression in adulthood. It seems, however, that the continuities are stronger between adolescent and adult depression than between child and adult depression, and that the child-to-adult links are weaker when there is comorbidity with conduct disorder.

Family Studies

It will be appreciated that the course of a disorder may be influenced by many extraneous factors and should therefore not have overwhelming weight in studying the links between child and adult conditions. Another way of examining the links between child and adult depression is through the family study method, which has traditionally been an important tool for psychiatric nosologists wishing to study the links between psychiatric conditions (Robins & Guze, 1970). There are three main reasons for thinking that family studies of depressed children could provide a powerful way of investigating the links with depression in adulthood. First, depression in adults tends to run in families (Gershon et al., 1982; McGuffin, Katz, Aldrich, & Bebbington, 1988). Second, there are high rates of psychiatric disorders, including depression, in the children of depressed parents (Earls, 1987; Weissman et al., 1987). Third, several family studies of depressed adults have reported that an earlier age of onset was associated with an increased familial loading for depression (Mendlewicz & Baron, 1981; Weissman et al., 1984).

If these findings are valid, and depression in children is the same disorder as depression in adulthood, then rates of depression should be greater in the adult relatives of depressed children than in the relatives of controls. Several family history and family interview studies of the relatives of depressed children have found high rates of affective disorders among relatives (Dwyer & Delong, 1987; Harrington et al., in press; Kutcher & Marton, 1991; Livingston, Nugent, Rader, & Smith, 1985; Mitchell, McCauley, Burke, Calderon, & Schloredt, 1989; Puig-Antich et al., 1989). For example, in our family interview study of depressed child and adolescent patients, the lifetime prevalence of RDC depression was significantly higher in the interviewed relatives of the childhood depressed subjects than in the relatives of closely matched child psychiatric controls (Harrington et al., in press). Higher rates of depression were found among the female relatives of both the depressed and control probands. These findings suggest that depression in young people resembles depression in adults in two key respects: (1) It tends to run in families, and (2) there are higher rates of depression among female than among male first-degree relatives. This tendency for depression to run in the families of depressed child probands was specific, to the extent that no other disorder was increased in the relatives of the depressed group.

What does this familial aggregation mean? Clearly, the finding of specificity in the familial transmission of affective disorders points to a specific etiological process that may well be distinct from the numerous nonspecific factors that can link adult and child disorders (such as family discord; see Earls, 1987). Because there is now substantial evidence of an important genetic component in the major affective conditions of adults (see Rutter et al., 1990), one possible candidate is some kind of genetic mechanism. Indeed, the finding of very high rates of affective disorders among the relatives of child and adolescent probands with affective conditions (Puig-Antich et al., 1989; Strober et al., 1988) has led to the suggestion that depression in young people is actually the most severe form of these disorders (Puig-Antich et al., 1989) with a particularly high genetic component.

However, that there is specificity of familial transmission does not necessarily mean that transmission is due to a genetic process. Moreover, even if it is assumed that early-onset cases of depressive disorder with a strong family history have a genetic component (which remains unproven), no extrapolation to the broader range of affective disorders in young people is warranted. Indeed, it must once again be borne in mind that juvenile depressive disorders may be heterogeneous. For instance, there is evidence that children with depression and conduct disorder have lower rates of depression among relatives than children with depression and no conduct disorder (Puig-Antich et al., 1989). Once more, the implication is that the degree of similarity between child and adult depression depends on the type of childhood depression that is studied.

Biological Markers

Another approach to the investigation of the links between child and adult depression is provided by the study of the biological correlates of depression, as measured by such tests as the Dexamethasone Suppression Test. Potentially, these approaches offer not only the possibility of a trait marker of depression but also the prospect of studying the psychobiological mechanisms of the disorder. However, so far these correlates have but moderate specificity to depression in adults. Moreover, the available data on children suggest that age and puberty have substantial effects in most psychobiological markers of depressive disorder, such as the sleep electroencephalograph and the Dexamethasone Suppression Test (Casat & Powell, 1988; Ferguson & Bawden, 1988; Puig-Antich, 1986). These age-related changes are likely to complicate the comparison between child and adult depression, but are in themselves of considerable interest.

Response to Antidepressant Treatment

Response to antidepressant treatment is not a good indicator of the degree of nosological similarity between child and adult depression. A lack of drug response in children is no indication that they are not depressed. It could simply reflect age-related differences in drug response or inadequate drug dosage. Moreover, antidepressants such as imipramine have a very broad range of pharmacological actions such as their anxiolytic properties, sedative effects, and impact on disorders such as nocturnal enuresis. Thus, a beneficial response to treatment would not necessarily mean that the subject was depressed.

Nevertheless, although these problems limit the usefulness of drug response in the study of the nosological relationship between depression in children and adults, the question of whether depressed children respond to antidepressants is of great clinical interest. In depressed adults, the most thoroughly studied form of treatment has been administration of the tricyclic antidepressants (TCAs), which have been evaluated in numerous comparative trials against a placebo. The results have been impressive, with about three quarters of these trials showing that the drug was superior (Elkins & Rapoport, 1983). It seems that the best results occur in depressions of moderate severity. Severe psychotic depressions do not respond well to TCAs (Abou-Saleh & Coppen, 1983), but seem to do better with electroconvulsive therapy (Scott, 1989).

Much less is known about the efficacy of antidepressants in childhood depression. The results of early trials were encouraging, with most studies reporting that the TCAs were an effective form of treatment for clinically depressed children (see, for example, Petti, 1983; Weinberg et al., 1973). However, the findings of these studies were limited by issues such as diagnostic heterogeneity (Lucas, Locket, & Grimm, 1965) and a lack of blindness to clinical ratings (Weinberg et al., 1973).

The results from double-blind controlled trials, traditionally the best way of assessing drug efficacy, have been less encouraging. In one of the first systematic studies, Puig-Antich and colleagues (1987) compared imipramine with a placebo. There were no significant differences between the groups in clinical response rates, which were high in both groups (68% vs. 56%, respectively). However, there was a linear relationship between the size of response and imipramine and desipramine plasma levels. Indeed, two other studies have reported that plasma levels are a better predictor of clinical response than dosage levels in childhood depression (Geller, Cooper, Chestnut, Anker, & Schluchter, 1986; Preskorn, Weller, & Weller, 1982). The implication is that the inability to demonstrate a consistent effect of imipramine in early placebo-control trials such as that of Puig-Antich and associates (1987) may have been the result of methodological issues such as high placebo response rates and/or inadequate drug dosage.

In a recent study that was specifically designed to address these issues, Geller, Cooper, McCombs, Graham, & Wells (1989) compared nortriptyline with placebo in children (aged 5 to 12 years) with major depression. The design included a 2-week single-blind, placebo washout phase before the main trial so that subjects who responded rapidly to placebo could be excluded, and patients were then begun at a dose based on their 24-hour plasma level that would ensure steady-state nortriptyline plasma levels of 60 to 100 ng/ml. Eight of the 26 patients (31%) on active drug responded during the double-blind phase of the trial, compared with 4 of the 24 patients (17%) on placebo, the difference falling short of statistical significance. However, Preskorn, Weller, Hughes, Weller, and Bolte (1987) reported superiority of imipramine over placebo, particularly in dexamethasone-nonsuppressing children. Clearly, more work is needed to identify the characteristics of children who are likely to respond to antidepressants.

To turn to the treatment of adolescent major depression, the few systematic studies of the efficacy of TCAs have been unable to show either superiority over placebo or a relationship between plasma level and response. Thus, one small study of amitriptyline versus placebo failed to find any significant difference between the groups (Kramer & Feiguine, 1983). Similarly, Geller, Cooper, Graham, Marsteller, and Bryant (1990) stopped their study when 31 depressed adolescents (12 to 17 years old) had completed the 8-week double-blind, placebo-controlled phase because only one patient of 12 on nortriptyline had responded. Ryan and associates (1986) gave a fixed, weight-adjusted dose of imipramine in adolescent depression, but failed to find a plasma level–response relationship. Only 44% were rated as significantly improved. Strober, Freeman, and Rigali (1990) found an even lower response rate (one third) in adolescent inpatients with nondelusional major depression treated with imipramine in an "open" design.

Why is it that the TCAs seem to be less efficacious in the treatment of major depression in adolescents than in the apparently similar condition in adults? A variety of different types of explanations have been put forward (reviewed by Ryan, 1990). It could be, for example, that the low response rate in adolescents is accounted for by some methodological feature of the studies carried out so far, such as difficulties in establishing the correct drug dosage. It is also possible that depression in adolescence, although phenotypically similar to adult depression, differs in some important respect that might affect drug responsiveness. For instance, perhaps as the data from some family studies suggest, early-onset depressive disorders are more severe. Alternatively, it has been suggested that adolescents differ from adults both in the relative balance of the cerebral neurotransmitters on which antidepressants are thought to act (Strober et al., 1990) and in the hormonal milieu of the brain (Ryan et al., 1986).

It is, however, important to remember that research on the clinical utility of antidepressants in juvenile depressive conditions is necessarily at an early stage, if only because of the relatively recent identification of depressive disorders among the young by using standardized methods of assessment. It could be that the next wave of controlled studies will provide more pointers on which depressed young people are likely to respond to TCAs.

CONCLUSIONS

In conclusion, the available data suggest that there are both similarities and dissimilarities between juvenile-onset and adult depressions. The results of follow-up studies suggest that depressed adolescents quite commonly go on to develop depression later in life and are at risk of episodes of depression in adulthood. Family studies suggest that a sub-group of depressed young people has a strong familial loading of depression. So, it would seem that some depressed young people suffer depressive disorders that are isomorphic with the major depressions of adulthood. However, the finding of temporal and familial continuities has not been matched by similar findings in respect of response to antidepressant treatment. Depressive disorders in young people do not seem to respond to antidepressants in the same way that they do in adults.

Finally, it should be borne in mind that juvenile depression, like adult depression, probably comprises a heterogeneous group of disorders and that the correlates and response to treatment of the various subgroups may be different. For instance, there is growing evidence that depressions occurring in conjunction with conduct disorder should be distinguished from pure depressions. The presence of conduct disorder seems to indicate a form of childhood depression that has relatively low temporal and familial continuities with depression in adulthood. Doubtless, future research will delineate other subgroups. It may be that some of these groups are strongly linked with adult depression, and others much less so.

REFERENCES

Abou-Saleh, M. T., & Coppen, A. (1983). Classification of depression and response to antidepressive therapies. *British Journal of Psychiatry, 143,* 601–603.

American Psychiatric Association. (1987). *Diagnostic and statistical manual of mental disorders* (3rd ed., rev.). Washington, DC: Author.

Angold, A. (1988). Childhood and adolescent depression: I. Epidemiological and aetiological aspects. *British Journal of Psychiatry, 152,* 601–617.

Asarnow, J. R., Goldstein, M. J., Carlson, G. A., Perdue, S., Bates, S., & Keller, J. (1988). Childhood-onset depressive disorders. A follow-up study of rates of rehospitalization and out-of-home placement among child psychiatric inpatients. *Journal of Affective Disorders, 15,* 245–253.

Carlson, G. A., & Cantwell, D. P. (1980a). Unmasking masked depression in children and adolescents. *American Journal of Psychiatry, 137,* 445–449.

Carlson, G. A., & Cantwell, D. P. (1980b). A survey of depressive symptoms, syndrome and disorder in a child psychiatric population. *Journal of Child Psychology and Psychiatry, 21,* 19–25.

Carlson, G. A., & Garber, J. (1986). Developmental issues in the classification of depression in children. In M. Rutter, C. E. Izard, & P. B. Read (Eds.), *Depression in young people: Developmental and clinical perspectives* (pp. 399–434). New York: Guilford.

Carlson, G. A., & Kashani, J. H. (1988). Phenomenology of major depression from childhood through adulthood: analysis of three studies. *American Journal of Psychiatry, 145,* 1222–1225.

Casat, C. D., & Powell, K. (1988). The dexamethasone suppression test in children and adolescents with major depressive disorder: A review. *Journal of Clinical Psychiatry, 49,* 390–393.

Cicchetti, D., & Schneider-Rosen, K. (1986). An organizational approach to childhood depression. In M. Rutter, C. E. Izard, & P. B. Read (Eds.), *Depression in young people: Developmental and clinical perspectives* (pp. 71–134). New York: Guilford.

Cytryn, L., & McKnew, D. H. (1972). Proposed classification of childhood depression. *American Journal of Psychiatry, 129,* 149–155.

Dwyer, J. T., & Delong, G. R. (1987). A family history study of twenty probands with childhood manic–depressive illness. *Journal of the American Academy of Child Psychiatry, 26,* 176–180.

Earls, F. (1987). On the familial transmission of child psychiatric disorder. *Journal of Child Psychology and Psychiatry, 28,* 791–802.

Elkins, R., & Rapoport, J. L. (1983). Psychopharmacology of adult and childhood depression: An overview. In D. P. Cantwell & G. A. Carlson (Eds.), *Affective disorders in childhood and adolescence* (pp. 363–374). Lancaster, England: MTP.

Feighner, J. P., Robins, E., Guze, S. B., Woodruff, R. A., & Winokur, G. (1972). Diagnostic criteria for use in psychiatric research. *Archives of General Psychiatry, 26,* 57–63.

Ferguson, H. B., & Bawden, H. N. (1988). Psychobiological measures. In M. Rutter, A. H. Tuma, & I. S. Lann (Eds.), *Assessment and diagnosis in child psychopathology* (pp. 232–263). New York: Guilford.

Fleming, J. E., Offord, D. R., & Boyle, M. H. (1989). Prevalence of childhood and adolescent depression in the community: Ontario child health study. *British Journal of Psychiatry, 155,* 647–654.

Frommer, E. A. (1968). Depressive illness in childhood. In A. Coppen & A. Walk (Eds.), *Recent developments in affective disorders* (pp. 117–136). Ashford, Kent: Headley Brothers.

Garber, J., Kriss, M. R., Koch, M., & Lindholm, L. (1988). Recurrent depression in adolescents: A follow-up study. *Journal of the American Academy of Child Psychiatry, 27,* 49–54.

Garrison, C. Z., Jackson, K. L., Marsteller, F., McKeown, R., & Addy, C. (1990). A longitudinal study of depressive symptomatology in young adolescents. *Journal of the American Academy of Child Psychiatry, 29,* 581–585.

Geller, B., Cooper, T. B., Chestnut, E. C., Anker, J. A., & Schluchter, M. D.

(1986). Preliminary data on the relationship between nortriptyline plasma level and response in depressed children. *American Journal of Psychiatry, 143,* 1283–1286.

Geller, B., Cooper, T. B., Graham, D. L., Marsteller, F. A., & Bryant, D. M. (1990). Double-blind placebo-controlled study of nortriptyline in depressed adolescents using a "fixed plasma level" design. *Psychopharmacology Bulletin, 26,* 85–90.

Geller, B., Cooper, T. B., McCombs, H. G., Graham, D. L., & Wells, J. (1989). Double-blind placebo-controlled study of nortriptyline in depressed children using a "fixed plasma level" design. *Psychopharmacology Bulletin, 25,* 101–108.

Gershon, E. S., Hamovit, J., Guroff, J. J., Dibble, E., Leckman, J. F., Sceery, W., Targum, S. D., Nurnberger, J. I., Goldin, L. R., & Bunney, W. E. (1982). A family study of schizoaffective, bipolar I, bipolar II, unipolar, and normal control probands. *Archives of General Psychiatry, 39,* 1157–1167.

Graham, P. J. (1981). Depressive disorders in children: A re-consideration. *Acta Paedopsychiatrica, 46,* 285–296.

Harrington, R. C. (1990). Depressive disorder in children and adolescents. *British Journal of Hospital Medicine, 43,* 108–112.

Harrington, R. C., Fudge, H., Rutter, M., Pickles, A., & Hill, J. (1990). Adult outcomes of childhood and adolescent depression: I. Psychiatric status. *Archives of General Psychiatry, 47,* 465–473.

Harrington, R. C., Fudge, H., Rutter, M., Bredenkamp, D., Grootheus, C., & Pridham, J. (in press). Child and adult depression: A test of continuities with family-study data. *British Journal of Psychiatry.*

Harrington, R. C., Fudge, H., Rutter, M., Pickles, A., & Hill, J. (1991). Adult outcomes of childhood and adolescent depression: II. Risk for antisocial disorders. *Journal of the American Academy of Child Psychiatry, 30,* 434–439.

Harter, S. (1983). Developmental perspectives on the self-system. In E. M. Hetherington (Ed.), *Handbook of child psychology (4th ed.): Vol. 4. Socialization, personality, and social development* (pp. 275–385). New York: Wiley.

Kandel, D. B., & Davies, M. (1986). Adult sequelae of adolescent depressive symptoms. *Archives of General Psychiatry, 43,* 255–262.

Kashani, J., Holcomb, W. R., & Orvaschel, H. (1986). Depression and depressive symptoms in preschool children from the general population. *American Journal of Psychiatry, 143,* 1138–1143.

Kendell, R. E. (1976). The classification of depressions: A review of contemporary confusion. *British Journal of Psychiatry, 129,* 15–28.

King, L. J., & Pittman, G. D. (1970). A six-year follow-up study of 65 adolescent patients: Natural history of affective disorders in adolescence. *Archives of General Psychiatry, 22,* 230–236.

Kolvin, I., Barrett, M. L., Bhate, S. R., Berney, T. P., Famuyiwa, O., Fundudis, T., & Tyrer, S. (1991). The Newcastle Child Depression Project: Diagnosis and classification of depression. *British Journal of Psychiatry, 159* (Suppl. 11), 9–21.

Kovacs, M. (1986). A developmental perspective on methods and measures in the assessment of depressive disorders: The clinical interview. In M. Rutter, C. E. Izard, & P. B. Read (Eds.), *Depression in young people: Developmental and clinical perspectives* (pp. 435–468). New York: Guilford.

Kovacs, M., & Beck, A. T. (1977). An empirical clinical approach toward definition of childhood depression. In J. G. Schulterbrandt (Ed.), *Depression in childhood: Diagnosis, treatment and conceptual Models* (pp. 1–25). New York: Raven.

Kovacs, M., Feinberg, T. L., Crouse-Novak, M. A., Paulauskas, S. L., & Finkelstein, R. (1984). Depressive disorders in childhood: I. A longitudinal prospective study of characteristics and recovery. *Archives of General Psychiatry, 41,* 229–237.

Kovacs, M., Feinberg, T. L., Crouse-Novak, M. A., Paulauskas, S. L., Pollock, M., & Finkelstein, R. (1984). Depressive disorders in childhood: II. A longitudinal study of the risk for a subsequent major depression. *Archives of General Psychiatry, 41,* 643–649.

Kovacs, M., & Paulauskas, S. L. (1984). Developmental stage and the expression of depressive disorders in children: An empirical analysis. In D. Cicchetti & K. Schneider-Rosen (Eds.), *Childhood depression* (New directions for child development No. 26, pp. 59–80). San Francisco: Jossey-Bass.

Kramer, A. D. & Feiguine, R. J. (1983). Clinical effects of amitriptyline in adolescent depression: A pilot study. *Journal of the American Academy of Child Psychiatry, 20,* 636–644.

Kutcher, S. & Marton, P. (1991). Affective disorders in first degree relatives of adolescent onset bipolars, unipolars, and normal controls. *Journal of the American Academy of Child Psychiatry, 30,* 75–78.

Lefkowitz, M. M. & Burton, N. (1978). Childhood depression: A critique of the concept. *Psychological Bulletin, 85,* 716–726.

Ling, W., Oftedal, G., & Weinberg, W. (1970). Depressive illness in childhood presenting as severe headache. *American Journal of Diseases of Childhood, 120,* 122–124.

Livingston, R., Nugent, H., Rader, L., & Smith, G. R. (1985). Family histories of depressed and severely anxious children. *American Journal of Psychiatry, 142,* 1497–1499.

Lucas, A. R., Locket, H. J., & Grimm, F. (1965). Amitriptyline in childhood depressions. *Diseases of the Nervous System, 26,* 105–110.

Malmquist, C. P. (1971). Depressions in childhood and adolescence. *New England Journal of Medicine, 284,* 887–893.

McClure, G. M. G. (1988). Suicide in children in England and Wales. *Journal of Child Psychology and Psychiatry, 29,* 345–349.

McConville, B. J., Boag, L. C., & Purohit, A. P. (1973). Three types of childhood depression. *Canadian Psychiatric Association Journal, 18,* 133–138.

McGee, R. & Williams, S. (1988). A longitudinal study of depression in nine-year-old children. *Journal of the American Academy of Child Psychiatry, 27,* 342–348.

McGuffin, P., Katz, R., Aldrich, J., & Bebbington, P. (1988). The Camberwell Collaborative Depression Study: II. Investigation of family members. *British Journal of Psychiatry, 152,* 766–774.

Mendlewicz, J. & Baron, M. (1981). Morbidity risks in subtypes of unipolar depressive illness: Differences between early and late onset forms. *British Journal of Psychiatry, 139,* 463–466.

Mitchell, J., McCauley, E., Burke, P., & Moss, S. J. (1988). Phenomenology of depression in children and adolescents. *Journal of the American Academy of Child Psychiatry, 27,* 12–20.

Mitchell, J., McCauley, E., Burke, P., Calderon, R., & Schloredt, K. (1989). Psychopathology in parents of depressed children and adolescents. *Journal of the American Academy of Child Psychiatry, 28,* 352–357.

Nelson, J. C. & Charney, D. S. (1981). The symptoms of major depressive illness. *American Journal of Psychiatry, 138,* 1–13.

Outcome of depression. (1989). *Lancet, 1,* 650–651.

Overall, J. E., Hollister, L. E., Johnson, M., & Pennington, V. (1966). Nosology of depression and differential response to drugs. *Journal of the American Medical Association, 195,* 946–950.

Paykel, E. S. (1971). Classification of depressed patients: A cluster analysis derived grouping. *British Journal of Psychiatry, 118,* 275–288.

Pearce, J. B. (1974). *Childhood depression.* Unpublished master's thesis, University of London.

Pearce, J. B. (1978). The recognition of depressive disorder in children. *Journal of the Royal Society of Medicine, 71,* 494–500.

Petti, T. A. (1983). Imipramine in the treatment of depressed children. In D. P. Cantwell & G. A. Carlson (Eds.), *Affective disorders in childhood and adolescence: An update* (pp. 375–415). Lancaster, England: MTP.

Preskorn, S. H., Weller, E. B., Hughes, C. W., Weller, R. A., & Bolte, K. (1987). Depression in prepubertal children: Dexamethasone nonsuppression predicts differential response to imipramine vs. placebo. *Psychopharmacology Bulletin, 23,* 128–133.

Preskorn, S. H., Weller, E. B., & Weller, R. A. (1982). Depression in children: Relationship between plasma imipramine levels and response. *Journal of Clinical Psychiatry, 43,* 450–453.

Puig-Antich, J. (1986). Psychobiological markers: Effects of age and puberty. In M. Rutter, C. E. Izard, & P. B. Read (Eds.), *Depression in young people: Developmental and clinical perspectives* (pp. 341–382). New York: Guilford.

Puig-Antich, J., Blau, S., Marx, N., Greenhill, L. L., & Chambers, W. (1978). Prepubertal major depressive disorder: A pilot study. *Journal of the American Academy of Child Psychiatry, 17,* 695–707.

Puig-Antich, J. & Gittelman, R. (1982). Depression in childhood and adolescence. In E. S. Paykel (Ed.), *Handbook of affective disorders* (pp. 379–392). Edinburgh and London: Churchill-Livingstone.

Puig-Antich, J., Goetz, D., Davies, M., Kaplan, T., Davies, S., Ostrow, L., Asnis, L., Twomey, J., Iyengar, S., & Ryan, N. D. (1989). A controlled family history study of prepubertal major depressive disorder. *Archives of General Psychiatry, 46,* 406–418.

Puig-Antich, J., Perel, J. M., Lupatkin, W., Chambers, W. J., Tabrizi, M. A., King, J., Goetz, R., Davies, M., & Stiller, R. L. (1987). Imipramine in prepubertal major depressive disorders. *Archives of General Psychiatry, 44,* 81–89.

Rie, H. E. (1966). Depression in childhood: A survey of some pertinent contributions. *Journal of the American Academy of Child Psychiatry, 5,* 653–685.

Robins, E. & Guze, S. B. (1970). Establishment of diagnostic validity in psychiatric illness: Its application to schizophrenia. *American Journal of Psychiatry, 126,* 107–111.

Rochlin, G. (1959). The loss complex. *Journal of the American Psychoanalytic Association, 7,* 299–316.

Rutter, M. (1980). *Changing youth in a changing society: Patterns of adolescent development and disorder.* Cambridge, MA: Harvard University Press.

Rutter, M. (1986a). The developmental psychopathology of depression: issues and perspectives. In M. Rutter, C. E. Izard, & P. B. Read (Eds.), *Depression in young people: Developmental and clinical perspectives* (pp. 3–32). New York: Guilford.

Rutter, M. (1986b). Depressive feelings, cognitions, and disorders: A research postscript. In M. Rutter, C. E. Izard, & P. B. Read (Eds.), *Depression in young people: Developmental and clinical perspectives* (pp. 491–519). New York: Guilford.

Rutter, M. (1988). Epidemiological approaches to developmental psychopathology. *Archives of General Psychiatry, 45,* 486–495.

Rutter, M., Graham, P., Chadwick, O. F., & Yule, W. (1976). Adolescent turmoil: Fact or fiction? *Journal of Child Psychology and Psychiatry, 17,* 35–56.

Rutter, M., Macdonald, H., Le Couteur, A., Harrington, R. C., Bolton, P., & Bailey, A. (1990). Genetic factors in child psychiatric disorders: II. Empirical findings. *Journal of Child Psychology and Psychiatry, 31,* 39–83.

Rutter, M., Tizard, J., & Whitmore, K. (1970). *Education, health, and behaviour.* London: Longmans.

Ryan, N. D. (1990). Pharmacotherapy of adolescent major depression: Beyond TCAs. *Psychopharmacology Bulletin, 26,* 75–79.

Ryan, N. D., Puig-Antich, J., Cooper, T., Rabinovich, H., Ambrosini, P., Davies, M., King, J., Torres, D., & Fried, J. (1986). Imipramine in adolescent major depression: Plasma level and clinical response. *Acta Psychiatrica Scandinavica, 73,* 275–288.

Ryan, N. D., Puig-Antich, J., Ambrosini, P., Rabinovich, H., Robinson, D., Nelson, B., Iyengar, S., & Twomey, J. (1987). The clinical picture of major depression in children and adolescents. *Archives of General Psychiatry, 44,* 854–861.

Scott, A. I. F. (1989). Which depressed patients will respond to electroconvulsive therapy? The search for biological predictors of recovery. *British Journal of Psychiatry, 154,* 8–17.

Shaffer, D. (1985). Depression, mania and suicidal acts. In M. Rutter & L. Hersov (Eds.), *Child and adolescent psychiatry: Modern approaches* (pp. 698–719). Oxford: Blackwell Scientific.

Shaffer, D. (1986). Developmental factors in child and adolescent suicide. In M. Rutter, C. E. Izard, & P. B. Read (Eds.), *Depression in young people: Developmental and clinical perspectives* (pp. 383–398). New York: Guilford.

Shaffer, D. (1988). The epidemiology of teen suicide: An examination of risk factors. *Journal of Clinical Psychiatry, 9* (Suppl.), 36–41.

Shaffer, D., Campbell, M., Cantwell, D., Bradley, S., Carlson, G., Cohen, D.,

Denckla, M., Frances, A., Garfinkel, B., Klein, R., Pincus, H., Spitzer, R. L., Volkmar, F., & Widiger, T. (1989). Child and adolescent disorders in DSM-IV: Issues facing the working party. *Journal of the American Academy of Child Psychiatry, 28*, 830–835.

Strober, M. & Carlson, G. (1982). Bipolar illness in adolescents with major depression: Clinical, genetic and psychopharmacologic predictors in a three- to four-year prospective follow-up investigation. *Archives of General Psychiatry, 39*, 549–555.

Strober, M., Freeman, R., & Rigali, J. (1990). The pharmacotherapy of depressive illness in adolescence: I. An open label trial of imipramine. *Psychopharmacology Bulletin, 26*, 80–84.

Strober, M., Hanna, G., & McCracken, J. (1989). Bipolar disorder. In C. G. Last & M. Hersen (Eds.), *Handbook of child psychiatric diagnosis* (pp. 299–316). New York: Wiley.

Strober, M., Morrell, W., Burroughs, J., Lampert, C., Danforth, H., & Freeman, R. (1988). A family study of bipolar I disorder in adolescence: Early onset of symptoms linked to increased familial loading and lithium resistance. *Journal of Affective Disorders, 15*, 255–268.

Weinberg, W. A., Rutman, J., Sullivan, L., Penick, E. C., & Dietz, S. G. (1973). Depression in children referred to an educational diagnostic centre: Diagnosis and treatment. *Journal of Pediatrics, 83*, 1065–1072.

Weissman, M. M., Gammon, D., John, K., Merikangas, K. R., Warner, V., Prusoff, B. A., & Sholomskas, D. (1987). Children of depressed parents: Increased psychopathology and early onset of major depression. *Archives of General Psychiatry, 44*, 847–853.

Weissman, M. M., Wickramaratne, P., Merikangas, K. R., Leckman, J. F., Prusoff, B. A., Caruso, K. A., Kidd, K. K., & Gammon, G. D. (1984). Onset of major depression in early adulthood: Increased familial loading and specificity. *Archives of General Psychiatry, 41*, 1136–1143.

World Health Organization. (1989). *I.C.D.—10. First draft of revision 4 of chapter V, categories F00–F99. Mental and behavioural disorders. Clinical descriptions and diagnostic guidelines.* Geneva: Author.

II

ETIOLOGICAL ISSUES

5

Biological and Environmental Processes in Nonpsychotic Psychopathology: A Neurobehavioral Perspective

RICHARD A. DEPUE

DAVID H. ZALD

There is a major limitation to much of the current neurobiological research on nonpsychotic psychopathology. Neurobiological research almost invariably focuses on the integrity of functioning of a single biologic variable in the absence of a theoretical or conceptual framework. Therefore, selection of variables for study is usually based on what are currently "hot" variables, usually suggested by biological correlates of pharmacological treatments or on new basic research findings and technologies, rather than on the theoretically predicted relevance of the variable for the behavioral syndrome under study. As a result, as has so often occurred in biological psychopathology, the hot variables become cold because of their complexity, and the researcher is left with little theoretical guidance for further investigation. For us to present a review of these hot variables in isolation from any framework would simply be a process of extending this limitation. Thus, we shall attempt to provide a conceptual framework for the variables and disorders discussed in our analysis, and in so doing, our orientation will be more on the basic issues related to psychopathological disorder (consistent with the theme of this volume) than on exhaustive reviews of clinical literature.

There are at least two levels on which conceptual frameworks could be generated when we consider the biology of nonpsychotic psychopathology. The first level concerns the functional role played by a biological variable within the central nervous system. This is particularly relevant to the biogenic amines, which are most often studied in the nonpsychotic disorders (Depue & Iacono, 1989), because, based on the evidence accumulated from studies on different brain regions and on different behaviors, a new, more integrative perspective on the functional role of the amines has evolved. This perspective proposes that there is a specific functional principle for the action of an amine throughout the central nervous system irrespective of the nucleus of origin, the brain region innervated, or the behavior subserved (Cools, 1980; Oades, 1985; Robbins & Everitt, 1982). This idea is based on the notion that biogenic amines modulate the flow of information in a specific and similar manner across all brain regions innervated, and that the qualitative nature of output phenomena is determined by the function of the brain region in question rather than by the amine per se (Kravitz, 1988; Louilot, Taghzouti, Deminiere, Simon, & Le Moal, 1987). That is, amines may be viewed as modulators of information flow rather than as all-or-none mediators of specific output phenomena.

This development on the functional role of biogenic amines provides a powerful analytical tool in examining their effects on behavior, especially when considering the complex behaviors embodied in the notions of personality traits and psychopathological syndromes. The major problem facing an examination of amines and complex behavior is that their role has not been empirically defined in many of the brain regions receiving substantial innervation from the amine cell groups. Hence, the power of a general functional principle of amines is that, if the function of a particular brain region is known in adequate detail, the role that an amine may play in that function may be logically derived. This strategy, then, allows not only a more comprehensive, if speculative, analysis of the effects of an amine on behavior than would be strictly possible from available data, but it also would raise specific hypotheses to guide research on the effects of the amine on complex functions.

A second level of conceptual framework generation is at the behavioral level (Depue, in press). Ethologists and psychologists have long been concerned with the structure of behavior, that is, the manner in which behavior may be categorized into coherent patterns or systems (Fonberg, 1986; Fowles, 1980; Gray, 1973, 1982; MacLean, 1986, 1990; Panksepp, 1986; Ploog, 1986; Rolls, 1986; Schneirla, 1959). From an evolutionary biology perspective, such systems represent neurobehavioral mechanisms that have evolved as a means of adapting to stimuli that are critical to the organism's survival and to the preservation of the species (Fonberg, 1986; Gray, 1973; Levi, 1975; MacLean, 1986). For instance, defensive aggression serves as an adaptive neurobehavioral response to pain and potential destruction, whereas in the case of appetitive behaviors, such as sex and feeding, specific olfactory cues serve as critical stimuli in signaling a suitable mate or appropriate food. As is evident in these examples, a system is defined by the class of stimuli that engages it, as well as by the response patterns expressed by it. The importance of delineating such systems at the behavioral level is that they provide a framework for discovering the neurobiological systems that mediate the interface between classes of stimuli and specific response patterns.

Because their development has been closely tied to critical stimulus conditions, behavioral systems must be tightly linked with brain structures responsible for recognition of stimulus significance, on the one hand, and for subsequent activation of effector systems, on the other. Collectively, this group of interrelated brain functions has been referred to as emotion, or emotional evaluation and emotional expression, respectively (Depue, in press; LeDoux, 1987). Thus, adaptive behavioral systems, in the broadest sense, are really emotional systems that motivate and, in a general way, guide behavior in response to critical stimuli. Indeed, *emotion* derives from the Latin verb *emovere:* "to move, to push." Emotional systems, then, not only elicit certain patterns of behavior to particular stimuli but also provide a motivational state and subjective emotional experience that is concordant with the affective nature or reinforcement qualities of critical stimuli (Fonberg, 1986; Gray, 1973, 1982; MacLean, 1986; Ploog, 1986; Rolls, 1986). Concordant with this view, analyses of the basic types of emotion (Levi, 1975; Plutchik, 1980; Plutchik & Kellerman, 1986), combined with ethological descriptions of mammalian behavioral systems (MacLean, 1969,1970, 1990), suggest that the emotions of desire, anger, fear, sorrow, joy, and affection are elicited by particular classes of stimuli and subsequently motivate six main forms of behavior, including searching, aggressive, protective, dejected, gratulant, and caressive, respectively (MacLean, 1986). Gray (1973, 1982) has added to this list a system of behavioral inhibition that is associated with anxiety and activated by conditioned signals of punishment, nonreward, and novelty. Thus, a particular class of stimuli, the emotion generated, and the behavior patterns expressed all form integral components of a coherent emotional system.

The importance of this perspective for understanding the structure of *human* behavior has not been generally recognized. However, as Gray (1973) and others (Fonberg, 1986; Zuckerman, 1983) have cogently argued, behavioral systems that are closely linked to emotional mechanisms are largely unchanged along the pathway of mammalian evolution and, hence, are probably subject to strong genetic influence in our own species. Such systems are likely, therefore, to provide a foundation for individual differences in human emotional patterns (Plutchik, 1980). When viewed from a broad temporal perspective, emotional systems may be conceptualized not simply as phasic response patterns but rather as emotional dispositions with respect to particular classes of stimuli. That is to say, humans have individual differences in their sensitivity to particular classes of stimuli, and these differences are evident as trait variation both in subjective emotional experience and in overt patterns of emotional expression. Thus, it is possible to view emotional systems as major components of the structure of human personality (Ervin & Martin, 1986; Gray, 1973; Plutchik, 1980; Tellegen, 1985; Zuckerman 1983).

The relevance of the behavioral–emotional systems framework for nonpsychotic psychopathology lies in the possibility that several of these syndromes appear to represent manifestations of extreme values or of dysregulation within a particular system. This seems most plausible, for instance, in the case of disorders of affect, anxiety, and some personality disorders, which we shall discuss in more detail later. If such disorders are viewed within a behavioral systems perspective, and if the neurobiology of these systems is known from basic animal research, then specific hypotheses based on this knowledge can be generated to guide biological psychopathology research. Thus, we believe that in order for neurobiological models to provide a truly integrative framework for understanding the nature of nonpsychotic disorders, they must have as their foundation a comprehensive *interface* between neurobiological structure and function, on the one hand, and major behavioral systems, on the other.

In that which follows, the relation of three biogenic amines—dopamine (DA), serotonin (5HT), and norepinephrine (NE)—to nonpsychotic psychopathology is explored. Each of the amine sections addresses similar issues, including (1) an overview of the anatomy of the amine system, (2) the generalized functional role of the amine in information processing in the brain, (3) the behavioral effects of variation in the functional level of the amine and its role in behavioral systems, and (4) the contribution of the amine to certain forms of nonpsychotic psychopathologies.

Finally, it has become customary in the psychopathology literature, when the influence of environment on disorder is considered, to review the life events studies involving the population of interest. Several recent reviews on different psychopathological disorders have summarized this work (Monroe, 1992; Monroe & Depue, 1992). Conclusions stemming from these reviews are almost always based on correlational levels of analysis, and, accordingly, the studies shed little light on the *processes* by which environmental experiences *across the lifespan* influence vulnerability to, and onset or maintenance of, disorder (Depue & Monroe, 1986). In keeping with the theme of this chapter, we, instead, focus on the processes that may mediate the effects of the environment on neurobiology. In so doing, we take a broad perspective on these processes in that they would apply to the mediation of life experiences of various kinds, rather than just major life stressors. Moreover, these processes would apply to psychopathology in general, although specificity plays a role with respect to the neurobiological system under consideration. We, however, use a specific behavioral system associated with dopamine functioning as a convenient example to illuminate the processes decribed. The potential relation of these processes to disorders of affect are discussed in a subsequent section.

DOPAMINE, BEHAVIORAL FACILITATION, MEDIATION OF ENVIRONMENTAL EXPERIENCE, AND DISORDERS OF AFFECT

A Functional Principle of Dopamine Activity

DA neurons of the mesencephalon appear to have the general function of facilitating neural processes in brain regions they innervate (Cools, 1980; Louilot et al., 1987; Oades, 1985; Robbins & Everitt, 1982). The exact manner in which this facilitation is achieved is not known, but available evidence, comprehensively reviewed by Oades (1985), suggests that the mechanism underlying facilitation is one of switching. That is, an increase of DA activity is thought to promote the likelihood of switching between alternative sources of information. The act of switching (1) increases the probability that a new input to a given neural circuit influences the output of that circuit and/or (2) may result in an ongoing input being shut off from influencing a circuit's output. This implies that DA activity does not simply represent a Go or Stop signal, but rather a signal that may alter the form or temporal characteristics of an ongoing sequence of behavior. It is worth emphasizing that a switching function pertains to all forms of neural information. Thus, DA would be expected to facilitate various levels of complexity of motor behavior, from limb movements such as lever presses to whole body movements involved in drinking, eating, rearing, and exploring alleyways, to behavioral sequences requiring a strategy (e.g., a search for food or safety) (Oades, 1985). DA would also be expected to facilitate the flow of information between cortical areas that is required for working memory and for the entertainment of alternate hypotheses in complex, changing environments (Luciana, Depue, Arbisi, & Leon, 1992). Moreover, DA would be expected to facilitate the access of mnesic traces for comparator functions of the brain, which are important for evaluating the context of contemporaneous sensory information.

The behavioral manifestations of switching are complex because they depend on the prevailing response tendencies of the individual and on the existing basal level of DA activity. However, these factors tend to create at least two conceptually meaningful, if somewhat artificial, categories of behavioral outcomes. First, in the case where there is low basal DA activity and no prevailing, predominant response tendency, the effect of switching (increased DA activity) is to increase the probability of a new response or, put differently, to initiate a new response. This seems to be particularly the case in the initiation of motivated behavior, where DA appears to play a role in facilitating specific motivational states and in switching or gating motivational signals from the limbic system to the motor system. Thus, neurotoxic lesions resulting in DA reductions of 90% or more result in major deficits of motivated behavior associated with incentive motivation or other types of specific motivational systems, including social interaction (Bloom, 1979), sexual behavior, food hoarding (Kehr, 1981), maternal nursing behavior (Gaffori & LeMoal, 1979), acquisition and performance of approach and active avoidance responses (Beninger, 1983; Oades, Rea, & Taghzouti, 1984), exploratory activity (Fink & Smith, 1980), and locomotor activity (Fishman, Feigenbaum, Yanaiz, & Klawans, 1983). The nucleus accumbens (NAS) is a critical structure for relaying motivational information from the limbic system to the motor system (Depue & Iacono, 1989; Mogenson, Jones, & Yim, 1980), and thus it is not surprising that bilateral neurotoxic lesions of the NAS result in impaired initiation of locomotor activity in situations associated with incentive conditions (Fishman et al., 1983) and of exploratory behavior in a range of novel stimulus situations (novelty is thought to inherently induce incentive motivation) (Oades et al., 1984; Louilot et al., 1987). Taken together, then, lesions of ascending DA cell bodies or DA terminals in some neural structures result in a condition where initiating signals appear to have been strongly switched off and thereby do not influence the output.

A second behavioral manifestation of DA switching is observed when basal DA acitivity is not low and when predominant response tendencies exist. In this case, an ongoing motor program or behavioral sequence (the predominant response tendency), which has been established as a result of prior environmental circumstances, is in effect, but a change in the environmental contingencies or context necessitates the development of and switching to a modified or entirely new motor program. The modification may involve little more than a change in the temporal patterning of a behavior (e.g., its frequency or duration), it may involve the same behavioral sequence but a change in the stimulus contingencies to which it is emitted, or a switch to an entirely new behavioral strategy may be required.

Experimental demonstration of this aspect of DA's switching function has focused on behavioral alternation and reversal, extinction effects, and the number of behavioral strategies attempted (Oades, 1985). For instance, bilateral neurotoxic lesions of the NAS (Taghzouti, Louilot, Herman, Le Moal, & Simon, 1985) reduce or completely abolish alternation and nonrepetitious-choice behavior, whereas amphetamine (a DA agonist) increases alternation behavior (Evenden & Robbins, 1983; Oades, Taghzouti, Simon, & LeMoal, 1985). Perhaps the most dramatic demonstration of this form of DA switching involves switching between behavioral strategies or sequences. Neostriatal treatment with DA antagonists or agonists can reduce or facilitate, respectively, the number of strategies rats may try in order to escape from drowning in a basin of water (Cools, 1980).

Thus, considering all of these findings together, the fact that a switching function is observed in an array of different neural structures and different behavioral functions suggests that DA does not mediate specific functions but rather facilitates functions that are processed within different areas of the brain. This has been demonstrated by examining the behavioral consequences of selective lesions of DA neurons both at the level of the cell bodies (Simon, Scatton, & LeMoal, 1980) and at the level of the terminals in the prefrontal cortex (Simon et al., 1980), in the NAS (Taghzouti, LeMoal, & Simon, 1985; Taghzouti, Louilot, et al., 1985), and in the lateral septum (Taghzouti, Simon, & LeMoal, 1986; Taghzouti, Simon, Louilot, Herman, & LeMoal, 1985; Taghzouti, Simon, Tazi, Dantzer, & LeMoal, 1985). This interpretation is also suggested by the fact that selective DA lesions in these various projection areas create behavioral deficits that are similar to the deficits produced by electrolytic lesions of those same areas (Louilot et al., 1987; Taghzouti, Louilot, et al., 1985; Taghzouti et al., 1986). Furthermore, deficits of spontaneous alternation produced by lesions of the lateral septum are subject to recovery of function under food-deprived conditions in spite of the continued DA depletion (Taghzouti et al., 1986), suggesting that the behavioral functions are mediated by the septum and not by DA activity per se. At a more general behavioral level, the functional principle of DA implies that DA is of critical importance for behavioral adaptation to complex, changing environments, where its switching function would subserve both overt behavioral modification and the serial testing of alternative hypotheses at the cognitive level.

The Behavioral Facilitation System

As we have outlined previously (Collins & Depue, 1992), the generalized facilitation role of dopamine suggests that this amine may contribute to a behavioral system involved in facilitating goal-oriented behavior, or, more simply, to a behavioral facilitation system (BFS). In fact, such a behavioral–emotional system has been consistently described in all animals across phylogenetic levels (Hebb, 1949; Schneirla, 1959). The BFS is an emotional system that has evolved to motivate forward locomotion and search behavior as a means of satisfying an animal's need for food, a sex partner, social interaction, a nesting place, and so on. That is, the BFS serves to bring the animal into contact with positive rewarding stimuli when such stimuli are not within close proximity. Thus, the BFS is a generalized or nonspecific emotional system that is activated by a host of positive rewarding stimuli.

There is general agreement on the class of stimuli that elicit activity in the BFS. Stimuli that elicit consummatory responses are primary positive reinforcers. These same stimuli, when perceived at a distance by the animal, may be referred to as primary incentive stimuli because they facilitate forward locomotion, alertness, and goal-oriented approach to the primary positive reinforcer. That is, the occurrence of the latter behavior suggests the existence of an internal state of incentive motivation (an intervening variable), and, indeed, activation of this internal state appears to be inherently rewarding in and of itself, as indicated by the occurrence of facilitated behavior in sated animals in the presence of incentive stimuli (Blackburn, Phillips, Jakubovic, & Fibiger, 1989; Konorski, 1967; Stewart, de Wit, & Eikelboom, 1984). Neutral stimuli occurring in close temporal contiguity with primary incentive stimuli can become conditioned incentive stimuli and thereby can activate the BFS (Beninger, 1983; Bindra, 1968; Bolles, 1972; Panksepp, 1986; Stewart et al., 1984). Conditioned incentive stimuli may be established in two ways: (1) as a result of association with the internal state of incentive motivation generated by a primary incentive stimulus, as discussed previously, or (2) by association with cues occurring in close proximity to the *termination* of a primary negative reinforcer. An example of the latter case is active avoidance learning in animals, where the conditioned incentive stimuli established by association with shock termination may be conceived of as cues denoting the reward of safety (Gray, 1973, 1982). These cues induce incentive motivation, and facilitated approach to safety subsequently occurs. The role of the BFS in determining an enduring emotional disposition in humans is most relevant in relation to conditioned incentive stimuli because of the generally predominant influence of symbolic processes in guiding human behavior in the absence of unconditioned stimuli.

The BFS also appears to facilitate (but not mediate) behavior in stimulus conditions associated with aggressive interaction. The opportunity to engage in affective attack has been found to be a goal-oriented behavior that is rewarding (Valzelli, 1981). Moreover, under conditions where reward acquisition is blocked, the BFS may facilitate aggressive behavior whose goal is removal of stimuli associated with frustrative nonreward. It may be that the BFS is elicited in this latter case by expectations of the reward acquisition that will result from removal of the obstacle to reward. Thus, whereas the BFS is activated by a broad array of stimulus contexts, these contexts share in common an incentive–reward component.

All of these stimulus condittons could be viewed as activating at least three major processes. First, incentive motivation, and the subjective feeling of desire, is a core element of the BFS. With respect to the specificity of incentive and desire to the BFS system, one view of emotional systems posits that the emotion associated with a system is distinct in quality from other forms of emotional experience; that is, the intrinsic attributes of fluctuating activities of the system mediate a specific emotion (MacLean, 1986; Panksepp, 1986; Ploog, 1986). Indeed, MacLean (1986) suggested that the inherent mechanisms underlying emotions and their conscious experience may be analogous to fixed action patterns: that is, stimulation of inherent neural circuitry evokes fixed affect patterns that have a specificity independent of peripheral feedback. Of importance, desire, or one of its variant expressions, is cited as one of the primary emotions in most classificatory systems of emotion (MacLean, 1986; Ploog, 1986; Plutchik, 1980; Plutchik & Kellerman, 1986).

A second core process involved in BFS activity is the initiation of locomotor activity as a means of supporting goal acquisition. This would be consistent with the fact that locomotor activity is the most reliable indicator of an animal's incentive state (Iversen, 1978). This suggests that neural structures associated with the BFS provide a link or interface between emotional evaluation processes, on the one hand, and the motor system, on the other. Put differently, the BFS may provide a mechanism for communicating the emotional state of incentive motivation to the initiatory structures of the motor system.

Third, active goal seeking facilitated by the BFS will increase interaction with, and hence the need to evaluate, the environment. To assure that approach behavior is adaptively related to stimulus events, there will be an increased need to construct maps of extrapersonal space, to identify objects in space, to organize behavioral strategies, and to evaluate the emotional significance of objects and the outcome of those behavioral strategies. These are complex cognitive functions. Their functional integrity requires the passage of information among distinct brain regions that serve as processing nodes in neural networks devoted to cognitive functions (Goldman-Rakic, 1987, 1988; Kosslyn, 1988; Mesulam, 1984, 1990; Posner, Petersen, Fox, & Raichle, 1988). Although a role for the BFS in cognitive processes has not been emphasized previously, Plutchik (1980) has argued compellingly that cognitive systems evolved for the purpose of increasing the adaptability of emotional behavior in complex environments.

A final perspective on the BFS is that it can be viewed, not simply as a passive response system to stimuli, but rather as a dynamic system that influences emotional evaluation of incentive stimuli. There is evidence suggesting that responsivity of the BFS to incentive stimuli is dependent on the current state of BFS activity (Beninger, 1983; Beninger, Hanson, & Phillips, 1980; Blackburn et al., 1989; Hill, 1970; Panksepp, 1986; Robbins, 1975). That is, the effective incentive value of a stimulus is a relative function of stimulus intensity and current BFS activity. As noted previously, it may also be supposed that the BFS is in reciprocal interaction with brain mechanisms that elaborate cognitive functions and central representations of incentives. The implications of these points is that variation in trait levels of BFS activity may influence sensitivity to incentive stimuli. This would have the effect of modulating the emotional evaluation of incentive stimuli (i.e., their perceived intensity), as well as the threshold for stimulus elicitation of subsequent responses.

Neurobiology of BFS Processes within the Framework of Emotion

To understand the BFS as an emotional system, it is necessary to locate it at the neurobiological level within the network of neural structures devoted to emotional processes. Because goal-directed behavior in humans is predominantly influenced by conditioned incentive stimuli, it is particularly important to delineate the manner in which conditioned stimuli are associated with emotional meaning and how this meaning comes to elicit BFS activity. The former refers to the process of emotional evaluation, the latter to the process of emotional expression, of which BFS activation is but one form. The neurobiological organization of these processes are discussed next in highly condensed form; interested readers are referred to Depue (in press) and LeDoux (1987) for more detailed reviews.

The Basolateral Limbic Forebrain and Emotion

Research over the past 50 years has indicated that all of the subcortical and cortical areas that came to be associated with the concept of the limbic system could not be viewed as an integrated system from a functional standpoint. Accordingly, Livingston and Escobar (1971) and Mesulam and Mufson (1982a, 1982b) have extended Yakovlev's (1948, 1959) proposal that the limbic lobe be divided into two divisions. The division that is associated most closely with emotional functions is referred to as the basolateral limbic division, and its location in the brain is illustrated as the less regularly stipled areas in Figure 5.1. This division encompasses forebrain areas that evolved phylogenetically around very old olfactory cortex located at the posterior end of the olfactory bulb, which, since Broca's (1878) initial emphasis on the olfactory bulb as an integral part of the limbic lobe, indicates a central role for olfaction in the evolution of vertebrate emotional processes (Fonberg, 1986; Kling, 1986; MacLean, 1975; Papez, 1937).

The forebrain areas evolving around olfactory cortex and comprising the basolateral limbic division include the insula, temporal pole

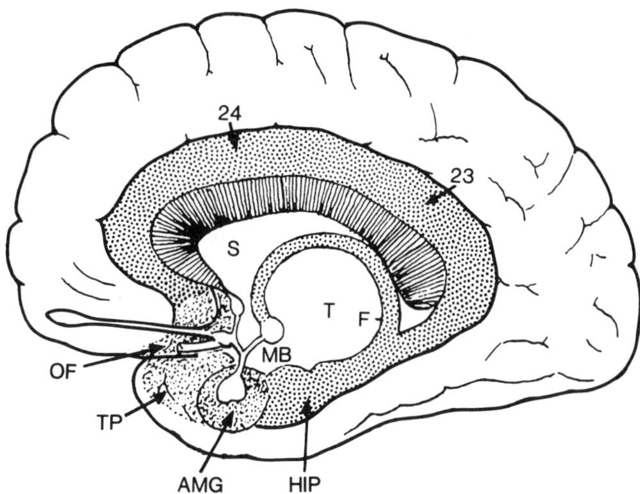

FIGURE 5.1. Medial view of brain showing two divisions of the limbic forebrain. The basolateral limbic division, which is most closely associated with emotional functions, is illustrated as the less regularly stipled areas. The dorsomedial division is illustrated as the regularly stipled areas. See text for discussion. AMG, amygdala; F, fornix; HIP, hippocampus; MB, mammillary bodies; OF, orbital frontal cortex; S, septal area; T, temporal lobe; TP, temporopolar cortex; 24, 23, Brodmann's designations for the anterior and posterior cingulate cortex, respectively.

(TP), and orbital frontal cortex (OFC), areas that Mesulam and Mufson (1982a, 1982b) refer to as paralimbic regions to distinguish them from core limbic structures such as the amygdala and hippocampus. The basolateral paralimbic regions evolved as a neural bridge to integrate unimodal sensory information into polymodal sensory representations that are then communicated to core limbic structures for emotional evaluation. For instance, the temporopolar cortex integrates visual and auditory sensory representations of an event, constructed in their respective temporal lobe regions, with olfactory information, whereas the insular cortex integrates autonomic, gustatory, and somatosensory input.

The amygdala, which is closely located to this olfactory core (see Figure 5.1), plays a central role in the basolateral limbic division. Sensory information from all unimodal sensory pathways and from polymodal paralimbic regions of the TP, OFC, and insular cortices converge in topographical order on the amygdala in the rhesus monkey (Aggleton & Miskin, 1986; Herzog & Van Hoesen, 1976; Jones & Powell, 1970; Kemp & Powell, 1970; Turner, Mishkin, & Knapp, 1980; Whitlock & Nauta, 1956). It has also been demonstrated that there are thalamic sensory neurons that project *directly* to the amygdala. Whereas the corticoamygdala pathways provide precise, highly processed information at the level of perceptual configurations (Aggleton & Mishkin, 1986; Turner et al., 1980), the thalamoamygdala projections appear to provide a rapid, crude representation of the sensory event (LeDoux, 1987). In that most sensory events in the natural environment are complex in character, perhaps the thalamoamygdala projections rapidly convey only essential features of critical events to which quick reaction is required.

The amygdala has a critical role in classical stimulus–reinforcement conditioning. That is, the process whereby neutral stimuli are associated with the reinforcing properties of primary positive and negative reinforcers, and the process of changing such associations when environmental conditions vary, appears to depend on normal amygdalar function (see Aggleton & Mishkin, 1986, for review). Thus, when specific central sensory representations of an event are activated, the amygdala (1) through a process of associative recall apparently activates an emotional representation of the event, (2) generates a subjective emotional experience appropriate to the emotional significance of the event (such as desire or anger), and (3) elicits neural, hormonal, and behavioral patterns that comprise the emotional response (Mishkin, 1982).

The OFC represents the highest level of hierarchical control within the basolateral limbic forebrain. It receives multimodal, integrated exteroceptive and interoceptive sensory information (Chavis & Pandya, 1976; Jones & Powell, 1970; LeDoux, 1987; Rolls, 1986; Van Hoesen, Pandya, & Butters, 1975), as well as emotional associations formed by the amygdala with respect to contemporaneous and recalled sensory events (Aggleton & Mishkin, 1986; Porrino, Crane, & Goldman-Rakic, 1981). The OFC holds these associations on-line in representational memory (Goldman-Rakic, 1987) and incorporates them into a larger, integrated structure of appetitive and aversive behavioral contingencies abstracted from the ongoing environment. Through its efferent projections, the OFC may initiate or inhibit motor, autonomic, and neurohumoral responses to specific sensory events (Kemp & Powell, 1970; Nauta, 1964, 1971, 1986; Rolls, 1986; Rosenkilde, 1979) depending upon the previous consequences of responses to similar events. When behavioral responses evoke unexpected reinforcement outcomes, the OFC actively encodes the new contingencies to avoid continued responding to nonrewarding or irrelevant events (Rolls, 1986, 1989; Thorpe, Rolls, & Maddison, 1983).

Integral to the capacity of the OFC to exert high-level regulation over behavioral responding is its connectivity with virtually all thalamic nuclei (Malakhova, Popovkin, & Gudina, 1989) and with the magnocellular basal forebrain cholinergic projection nuclei (Mesulam & Mufson, 1984; Russchen, Amaral, & Price, 1985). Through these connections, the OFC "orchestrates" a pattern of selective activation of cortical regions, against a background of signal-sharpening inhibition (Marczynski, 1986). By activating these modulatory feedback patterns, the OFC facilitates selection and initiation of appropriate behavioral responses within cortical nodes of neural networks devoted to emotional expression (Rolls, 1986, 1989).

An Anatomical–Functional Circuit Modulating Emotional Expression

Once the process of emotional evaluation has determined the significance of an event, complex neural processing must occur to determine (1) where in space and toward which objects a behavioral response is to be made and (2) whether such a response should be performed, given the expected outcome of the response under this particular set of environmental circumstances. As shown in Figure 5.2, these determinations are accomplished via partially closed loops that extend from frontal and other regions of the cortex, through striatal structures, midbrain dopamine areas, pallidal regions, thalamus, and back to the frontal cortex (Alexander, DeLong, & Strick, 1986). For example, the formulation of a program of motor movement (i.e., selection of motor movements required in making an emotional response) is accomplished in a motor circuit (Figure 5.3) that begins in motor (Brodmann's areas 8, 6, 4) and somatosensory (areas 3, 1, 2, 5) cortical regions, both of which are somatotopically organized precisely and can project information about specific body parts (e.g., the wrist) or specific movement of a body part (e.g., flex of the wrist). This information, which is clustered into leg, face, and arm fiber bundles, is projected to the putamen. In the putamen, there are somatotopically organized matrices of cell clusters located within leg, face, and arm sectors that represent specific movements of body parts. Thus, the matrices allow for specific representations of movements to be formed and activated, while irrelevant movements are inhibited. Only the relevant matrices or movements are activated by the putamen's activation of somatotopically relevant areas of the substantia nigra, which sends back dopamine projections to the relevant putamen matrices that switch this information through to the globus pallidus. Also somatotopically organized, the globus pallidus integrates the input from the putamen in relation to body parts; for example, all facial inputs are integrated to represent the facial expression that is relevant to the emotional response. This information is then passed on to several nuclei in the thalamus, which direct the information to the somatotopically organized supplementary motor area (SMA), which sequences and initiates the now programmed motor patterns by activating cortical motor regions that project to the spinal cord. The circuit is looped or partially closed so that a motor

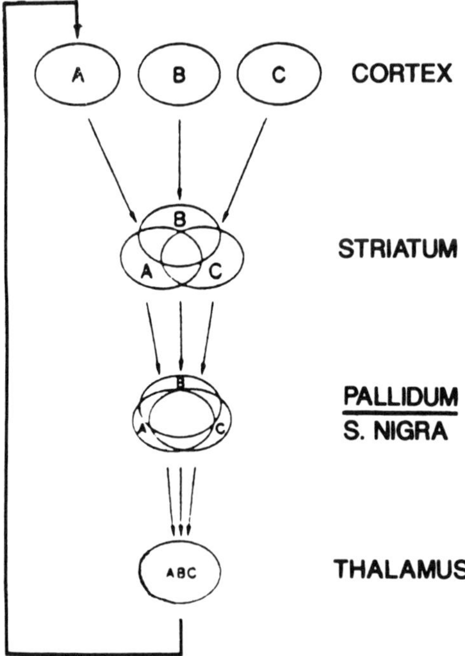

FIGURE 5.2. Skeleton diagram of the proposed basal ganglia–thalamocortical circuits. Each circuit receives output from several functionally related cortical areas (A, B, C) that send partially overlapping projections to a restricted portion of the striatum. These striatal regions send further converging projections to the globus pallidus and substantia nigra, which in turn project to a specific region of the thalamus. Each thalamic region projects back to one of the cortical areas that feeds into the circuit, thereby completing the closed loop portion of the circuit. From "Parallel Organization of Functionally Segregated Circuits Linking Basal Ganglia and Cortex" by G. E. Alexander, M. R. DeLong, and P. L. Strick, 1986, *Annual Review of Neuroscience, 9,* p. 361. Copyright 1986 by Annual Reviews, Inc. Reprinted by permission.

pattern can be maintained and/or updated (around the loop) for as long as is necessary.

Other, similarly organized circuits determine (1) a program for eye movements (the oculomotor circuit), (2) where in space the eyes and the previously formulated motor patterns should be directed (the dorsolateral prefrontal loop), and (3) toward which objects movements should be directed (the lateral orbital frontal loop). All of this information converges on the SMA for exact sequencing and initiation of movement.

This picture is incomplete in that a circuit is needed to determine whether, under current emotional outcome expectations, the previously formulated motor programs *should* be released to activate the muscula-

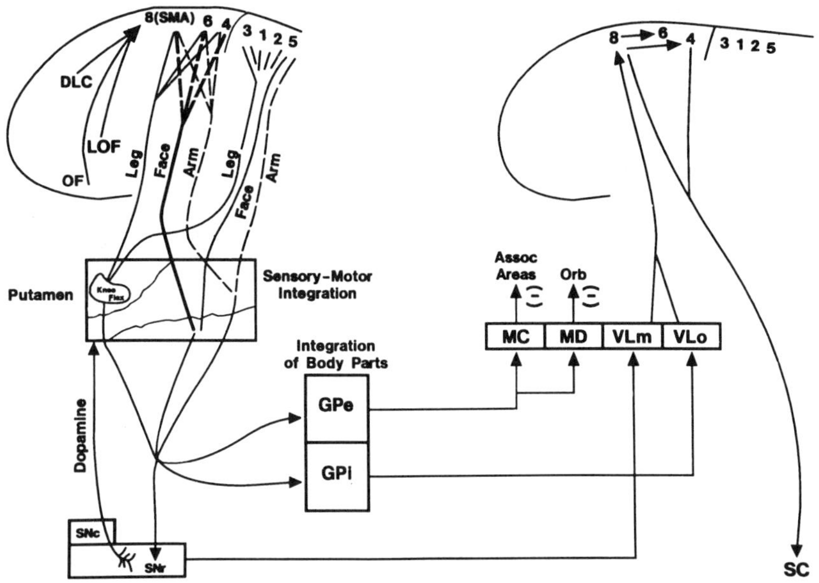

FIGURE 5.3. A schematic representation of the proposed basal ganglia–thalamocortical *motor circuit* of Alexander, DeLong, and Strick. See text for discussion. Assoc Areas, association areas of the cortex; DLC, dorsolateral prefrontal cortex; GPe, external segment of globus pallidus; GPi, internal segment of globus pallidus; LOF, lateral orbital prefrontal cortex; MC, MD, VLm, VLo, specific thalamic nuclei; OF and Orb, orbital frontal cortex; SC, spinal cord; SMA, supplementary motor area; SNc, substantia nigra, pars compacta; SNr, substantia nigra, pars reticulata. Numbers refer to Brodmann's designations for motor (8, 6, 4) and somatosensory cortical areas (3, 1, 2, 5).

ture. This is apparently the role of the neural network underlying the BFS, which we refer to as the medial orbital frontal circuit. The fundamental circuit originates in the reciprocally interconnected triad of medial OFC (Walker's area 13 in monkeys, Brodmann's area 13 in humans), temporal pole, and amygdala. Upon detection of an incentive stimulus, information regarding its appetitive associations is transmitted by the amygdala and temporal pole to the OFC. The OFC encodes this information within its ongoing representation of the structure of environmental reinforcement, which may be augmented by input from the hippocampal formation regarding similar stimuli experienced in the past. Assuming for the moment that an appropriate motor response is to be initiated in response to the incentive stimulus, the medial OFC transmits information related to initiation or alteration of locomotor activity to the ventral striatum (NAS). The NAS, like other striatal structures (e.g., putamen and caudate), may be a repository of phylogenetically old, species-specific response tendencies (McLean, 1986). The NAS, however, does not apparently formulate the actual motor program for these response tendencies, as in the motor circuit described previously. Rather, it apparently determines whether the motor program should be initiated at all and with what degree of vigor it should be performed. That is, the NAS integrates the motivational imperative associated with the current environmental conditions and transmits this imperative to the motor system. Thus, the NAS sends topographically organized inputs to the ventral tegmental area's (VTA) dopaminergic projections (as the putamen does to the substantia nigra), which return, in part, to the NAS. These VTA dopamine projections, in like manner to those of the substantia nigra in the motor circuit, (1) initiate the release of specific NAS information and (2) apparently code the relative vigor that each motor movement should have. The NAS information is passed to the ventral pallidum, which in turn relays output through the thalamus to the SMA, premotor, and motor cortices. In this way, the SMA not only receives the motor program but also information on the go–no go status of the motor program, and on the relative vigor with which specific movements should be made. The ventral pallidum also initiates a descending projection to the mesencephalic motor area that eventually terminates on motor pattern generators in the spinal cord that mediate, for instance, motor patterns that support forward locomotion, a major BFS component.

Dopamine Innervation of the Basolateral Limbic Forebrain: Implications for Behavioral Facilitation System Function

The preceding discussion on neural circuits involved in motor behavior indicates that dopamine (DA) plays a critical role in the functioning of the circuits. As we have discussed previously (Collins & Depue, 1992) in both the motor circuit and the medial orbital prefrontal loop, DA projections to the striatum (putamen and NAS, respectively) provide a means of facilitating the flow of specific information from the striatum to pallidal structures. That DA's facilitatory role in these circuits is critical is dramatically illustrated in the retarded motor behavior of Parkinson's disease, where the deterioration of DA cells in the substantia nigra result in a loss of DA facilitation in the putamen in the motor circuit. Similarly, bilateral 6-hydroxydopamine (6-OHDA) lesions in rats and monkeys resulting in DA reductions of 90% or more in the VTA or NAS produce major deficits in the initiation of behavior associated with incentive motivation, including social interaction, sexual behavior, food hoarding, maternal nursing behavior, approach and active avoidance responses, exploratory activity in novel environments, and locomotor activity.

Thus, as in the lack of facilitation of sensorimotor integration in Parkinson's disease due to DA deficiency, lesions of DA cells in the VTA appear to result in a generalized lack of facilitation of motivated, emotional behavior. This suggests that DA may play a critical modulatory role in the function of the BFS in motivational processes, and in the organization and initiation of goal-directed behavior.

The underlying neural network of the BFS (i.e., the basolateral limbic forebrain including the ventral striatum) is, indeed, strongly innervated by projections arising from the VTA A10 DA cells. We next briefly describe selective behavioral functions of two VTA DA ascending systems that innervate BFS structures, referred to as the mesolimbic and mesocortical systems (see Figure 5.4 for the location of structures described next).

Selected BFS Functions of the Mesolimbic Dopamine Projection System

Perhaps the largest VTA mesolimbic DA projection is to the ventral striatum, that is, the NAS, olfactory tubercle, and ventromedial caudate. There is substantial evidence that these structures, and in particular the NAS, serve as a functional interface between limbic structures, which integrate motivational processes, and the extrapyramidal motor system, which integrates motor responses (Mogenson, Jones, & Yim, 1980; Nauta, 1986; Oades & Halliday, 1987). As noted before in the discussion of the medial orbital prefrontal circuit, VTA DA projections to the NAS facilitate the flow of motivational information to the motor system, which informs the motor program as to the imperative value of the current situation. DA release in the NAS appears to be associated with two major BFS functions (incentive–reward motivation as a means of motivating approach to a goal; initiation of forward locomotion, which provides the means to reach a goal), whereas DA release in the amygdala may be related to the threshold of emotional expression.

Incentive–Reward Motivation. Several recent reviews have concluded that DA is integral to rewarding stimulation of mesencephalic and diencephalic loci (Bozarth, 1987; Fibiger & Phillips, 1987; Mason, 1984). Although the initial activation during intracranial self-stimulation (ICSS) occurs in non–DA, myelinated, fast-conducting neurons, at least some of which are cholinergic (Gallistel, Shizgal, & Yeomans, 1981), these first-stage fibers descend to transsynaptically activate a second-stage fiber system consisting of ascending mesolimbic DA projections (Bozarth, 1987). Fibiger and Phillips (1987) reported increased DA metabolism

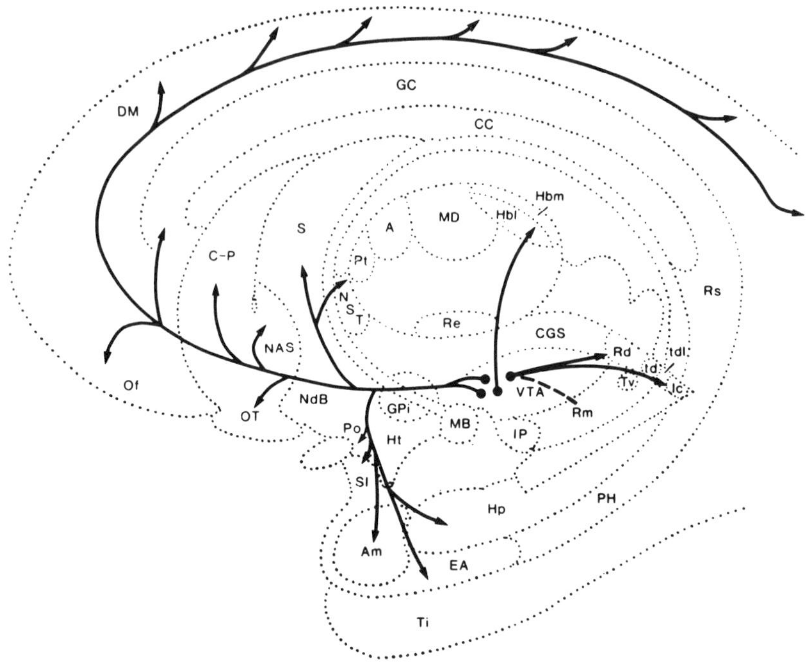

FIGURE 5.4. Dopaminergic projections ascending from the ventral tegmental area (shown as one mesolimbic-mesocortical bundle for clarity), as described in the text. A, nucleus anterior thalami; Am, amygdala; CC, corpus callosum; CGS, central gray substance; C-P, caudatoputamen; EA, entorhinal area; GC, gyrus cinguli; CPi, globus pallidus, internal segment; Hbl, lateral habenular nucleus; Hbm, medial habenular nucleus; Hp, hippocampal formation; Ht, hypothalamus; IP, interpeduncular nucleus; lc, locus ceruleus; MB, mammillary body; MD, nucleus mediodorsalis thalami; Nacc, nucleus accumbens; NdB, nucleus of the diagonal band of Broca; NST, bed-nucleus of stria terminalis; OF, orbitofrontal cortex; OT, olfactory tubercle; PH, parahippocampal gyrus; Po, preoptic area; Pt, nucleus parataenialis thalami; Rd, dorsal raphe nucleus; Re, nucleus reuniens thalami; Rm, median raphe nucleus; Rs, retrosplenial cortex; SI, substantia innominata; td, dorsal tegmental nucleus of Gudden; tdl, nucleus tegmenti dorsalis lateralis; Ti, interior temporal cortex. From "Ramifications of the Limbic System" by W. J. H. Nauta and V. B. Domesick, 1981. In S. Matthysse (Ed.), *Psychiatry and the Biology of the Human Brain* (p. 175). Amsterdam: Elsevier North Holland. Copyright 1981 by Elsevier North Holland. Adapted by permission.

during VTA ICSS confined to the structures of the ventral striatum (NAS, olfactory tubercle, ventromedial caudate) ipsilateral to the stimulating electrode. Furthermore, direct pharmacological evidence for specific DA involvement in VTA ICSS was obtained in a study employing unilateral microinjections of the DA receptor antagonist spiroperidol into the NAS (Mogenson, Takigawa, Robertson, & Wu, 1979). Microinjections into either the ipsilateral or contralateral prefrontal cortex did not affect VTA ICSS, suggesting that DA mediation of rewarding VTA stimulation does not require activation of telencephalic DA receptors.

In a related line of research, psychomotor stimulants such as amphetamine and cocaine have been shown to enhance responding during ICSS (Bozarth, 1987). Both drugs potentiate DA activity by blocking the reuptake process that normally terminates synaptic DA actions, whereas amphetamine may also increase DA release (Koob & Bloom, 1988). Moreover, humans, other primates, and rats readily perform operant responses to receive intravenous administrations or microinjections of these drugs (stimulant self-administration or SSA; Wise, 1978). Wise (1982) proposed that the VTA NAS pathway is activated by all forms of rewarding stimuli, and DA lesioning studies have indicated that an intact VTA NAS pathway is necessary for the rewarding effects of stimulants (Lyness, Friedle, & Moore, 1979; Roberts, Corcoran, & Fibiger, 1977; Roberts, Koob, Klonoff, & Fibiger, 1980). In contrast, lesions of other DA terminal fields (e.g., in the caudate) or of norepinephrine projections do not affect SSA (Roberts & Zito, 1987). Furthermore, studies using both ICSS and SSA have revealed an overlapping pattern of regional alterations in subcortical DA metabolism (Porrino, 1987; Seeger et al., 1984), leading Porrino (1987) to conclude that rewarding self-administration of electrical stimulation and psychomotor stimulants produce converging activation of VTA mesolimbic DA pathways. Thus, it seems clear that a neurobiological substrate for the mediation of reward, and presumably the generation of incentive motivation, is represented within BFS circuitry by the dopaminergic VTA NAS pathway. It is interesting to note in this context that, whereas the OFC plays an integral role in emotional evaluation and expression within the BFS, it does not directly participate in the mediation of the intervening state of incentive motivation (Mogenson, Takigawa, et al., 1979).

Initiation of Locomotor Activity (LA). Processes involved in the generation of volitional locomotion can be divided into three useful, albeit oversimplified, phases: initiation, programming, and execution. Processes involved in LA initiation have received comparatively least attention, but it is specifically this phase of locomotor generation that relates to the facilitation construct of the BFS because the initiation process is closely tied to affective/motivational input to the motor system.

There is a vast literature demonstrating that DA (but not norepinephrine) is the primary neurotransmitter in the initiation of LA (see reviews by Fishman et al., 1983; Iversen, 1978; Kelly, 1978; Oades, 1985). Importantly, LA initiation occurs via the action of DA and its agonists in the mesolimbic DA system, in general, and in the VTA A10 DA projection to the NAS, in particular. A recent review concluded that "a formidable number of studies have demonstrated that DA and its agonists injected into the NAS induce a greater arousal of LA than equivalent injections in the striatum; there are virtually no studies in the literature to the contrary" (Fishman et al., 1983, p. 61). Moreover, the quantity of spontaneous exploratory LA and magnitude of amphetamine-induced LA are both positively related to number of DA neurons (including those of the VTA cell group), to the relative density of innervation of DA terminals in target fields, and to DA content in the NAS in inbred mouse strains, effects perhaps related to the proportionately greater synthesis and release of DA in high–DA neuron strains (Fink & Reis, 1981; Oades, 1985; Sved, Baker, & Reis, 1984, 1985). Mesolimbic DA projections to the amygdala and olfactory tubercle do not account in a significant way for initiation of LA (Oades, 1985; Oades, Taghzouti, Rivet, Simon, & Le Moal, 1986).

Threshold of Emotional Expression. The VTA projects strongly to the amygdala. Indeed, approximately 90% of the DA in the amygdala is derived from VTA projections, which terminate in several nuclei of the amygdala, including the central, anterior lateral, posterior lateral, medial, and basal (Oades & Halliday, 1987; Moore & Bloom, 1978). The basolateral, medial, and central nuclei receive the densest DA innervation. The DA projections to the central and medial nuclei of the amygdala may have significance for BFS facilitation of emotional behavior, because these nuclei serve as important centers for output from the amygdala to brainstem and hypothalamic areas involved in the activation of vocal, gross motor, facial, hormonal, and autonomic aspects of emotional behavior. DA apparently influences the threshold of output from the amygdala, because increased DA activity in the central nuclei, for instance, facilitates remarkably the expression of aggressive behavior (Depue & Iacono, 1989).

Summary. Thus, activation of VTA DA projections to the limbic striatum and amygdala appears to facilitate behavioral functions that support emotional engagement of the animal with environmental goals. These functions include incentive motivation, forward locomotion, and enhanced emotional expression, and, as such, they in part define the functions proposed for the BFS construct.

Selected BFS Functions of the Mesocortical Dopamine Projection System

Active goal seeking facilitated by the BFS will increase interaction with, and hence the need to evaluate, the environment. To assure that approach behavior is adaptively related to stimulus events, there will be an increased need to design maps of extrapersonal space, to identify objects in space, to organize behavioral strategies, and to evaluate the emotional significance of objects and the outcome of those behavioral strategies. These are complex cognitive functions. We have suggested that the BFS, via the mesocortical DA projection system, plays a critical facilitatory role in these processes (Collins & Depue, 1992; Luciana, Depue, Arbisis, & Leon, 1992). An expansion of neocortical DA projections ascending from the VTA has paralleled the expansion of the neocortex itself in mammalian evolution. This connectivity can be observed in rat brain (Berger, Verney, Alvarez, Vigny, & Helle, 1985), but it is particularly extensive in primate brain, in which virtually all neocortical regions are innervated by VTA DA projections (Camps, Cortes, Queye, Probst, & Palacios, 1989; Lewis, Campbell, Foote, & Morrison, 1986). In relative terms, DA density is lowest in primary visual, auditory, and somatosensory regions, and highest in motor, premotor, and supplementary motor cortices. DA density is intermediate but variable within the temporal and parietal cortices. In the temporal lobe, DA density is low in the caudal portion of the superior gyrus (which includes primary auditory cortex), high in the rostral portion (auditory association cortex), and intermediate in the inferior gyrus (visual association cortex). In the parietal lobe, DA density is significantly higher in the inferior lobule.

The concentration of DA in prefrontal cortex (PFC) is among the highest in all cortical areas in monkeys (Brown, Crane, & Goldman, 1979), and both DA-containing terminals and DA receptors are prominent in the PFC of primates (Berger, Trottier, Gaspar, Verney, & Alvarez, 1988; Gaspar, Berger, Febvret, Vigny, & Henry 1989; Levitt, Rakic, & Goldman–Rakic, 1984a, 1984b; Lewis, Campbell, Foote, & Morrison, 1987; Lewis, Foote, Goldstein, & Morrison 1988; Lidow, Goldman–Rakic, Rakic, & Innis, 1989) and humans (Camps, Cortes, Gueye, Probst, & Palacios, 1989; Cortes, Gueye, Pazos, Probst, & Palacios, 1989). More specific innervation patterns were reported by Porrino and Goldman–Rakic (1982), where prefrontal areas on the ventral surface of the frontal lobe (inferior convexity, medial and lateral orbital cortex, frontal pole) were innervated preferentially by midline VTA nuclei. Dorsolateral and dorsomedial prefrontal areas were innervated by a band of cells that extends laterally from the midline VTA to the medial region of the substantia nigra.

In recent years there has been increasing interest in the neurobiology of higher-order cognitive functions. Much of this interest has focused specifically on the ability of the PFC to provide an association between events separated in time, that is, between environmental stimuli that are no longer present and the performance of motor responses based on those temporally separated stimuli (Funahashi, Bruce, & Goldman–Rakic, 1989; Fuster, 1973, 1980; Kubota & Niki, 1971; Niki 1974a, 1974b,

1974c; Sawaguchi, Matsumura, & Kubota, 1988, 1990a, 1990b; Watanabe & Niki, 1985). Goldman-Rakic (1987, 1988) has suggested that a critical prefrontal process for spanning the time period between stimuliand response is a special form of short-term memory, referred to as working memory. Working memory refers to the mnemonic process(es) by which information relevant for a correct response is temporarily maintained or held on-line to be reevaluated or updated on a trial-by-trial basis (Baddeley, 1986; Baddeley & Hitch, 1974; Friedman, Janas, & Goldman-Rakic, 1990; Olton, Becker, & Handelmann, 1979; Roitblat, 1987).

The functional importance of DA to one cognitive process, spatial mnemonic processes, has been demonstrated by several findings. First, 6-hydroxydopamine lesion of the dorsolateral convexity of the PFC has produced impaired spatial delayed alternation performance in rhesus monkeys that was reversed by DA agonists (Brozoski, Brown, Rosvold, & Goldman, 1979). Second, DA enhances the activity of PFC neurons of monkeys that show activity associated with mnemonic processes, including the spatial visual cue, the delay, and/or the response during the performance of delayed response tasks (Sawaguchi et al., 1988, 1990a, 1990b). Third, DA enhances spatial delayed performance in humans (Luciana et al., 1992), and, fourth, pharmacological blockade of DA receptors in monkeys has been shown to cause a reversible decrement in accuracy and latency of an oculomotor spatial delayed response task (Sawaguchi & Goldman-Rakic, 1991). Concordantly, Sawaguchi and colleagues (1988, 1990a, 1990b) concluded that "dopamine plays a role in the neuronal processes of facilitating . . . goal-directed behaviors associated with spatial cues of memory traces, as well as those associated with non-spatial cues used for environmental adaptation" (1988, p. 472).

Recent conceptualizations of the neurobiological basis of cognition have emphasized a network approach (Goldman-Rakic, 1987, 1988; Kosslyn, 1988; Mesulam, 1984, 1990; Posner, Petersen, Fox, & Raichle, 1988). The proposal is that complex cognitive functions are composed of many elementary operations, where each operation is localized in distinct, yet interconnected, cortical and subcortical regions. Collectively, these brain regions and their connections constitute an integrated network for that function. Coordination of such an integrated network would require communication between the distinct brain regions involved, as well as facilitation of neural processes within nodes of the network (Goldman-Rakic, 1987, 1988). As discussed previously, mesocortical DA projections appear to facilitate or enhance task-related processes within nodes of such a network (Sawaguchi & Goldman-Rackic, 1991; Sawaguchi et al., 1988, 1990a, 1990b). They may also initiate or gate the transfer of information across the different brain regions of a network, as suggested by Oades' review (1985), by facilitating long corticocortical, cortico-striatal (which may contribute to circuit loops discussed previously), and corticotectal neurons.

In general, then, mesocortical DA projections may serve to facilitate, as do mesolimbic DA projections, goal-directed activity, but they would facilitate neocortical, rather than limbic, processes that underlie cognitive functions necessary for behavioral flexibility. A similar conclusion was reached by others based on extensive reviews of DA's role in behaviors that require higher-order cognitive functioning, that is, behavioral responses to changing environmental contingencies, as in alternation, reversal, and extinction paradigms, and to tasks requiring changes in cognitive behavioral strategies (Cools, 1980; Louilot, Taghzouti, Deminiere, Simon, & LeMoal, 1987; Oades, 1985).

Overall, then, DA activity may be conceptualized as facilitating the OFC orchestration of neural excitation and inhibition within other cortical and subcortical structures, at least within environmental contexts that elicit incentive motivation. At the behavioral level, the VTA DA systems would facilitate emotional evaluation of rapidly occurring incentive events, particularly when such sequences signal a change in previous reward contingencies. Moreover, DA would facilitate continuous adaptation of motor sequences to ensure that the energizing influence of incentive motivation results in positive behavioral engagement. At the cognitive level, DA would facilitate the construction and serial testing of alternative strategies to obtain perceived, but initially distant, rewards. In humans, DA facilitation may be essential for goal-oriented behavior that requires delay of gratification because central representations of the ultimate reward must be continuously adapted to sequential revisions in long-term planning, presumably mediated by the PFC (Goldman–Rakic, 1987); moreover, DA activity would appear to be critical in maintaining incentive motivation throughout the period of delayed gratification.

Dopamine, the BFS, and the Structure of Personality

Because responsivity of the BFS to incentive stimuli is dependent on the current state of BFS activity (Beninger, 1983; Beninger et al., 1980; Blackburn et al., 1989; Hill, 1970; Panksepp, 1986; Robbins, 1975), the effective incentive value of a stimulus is a relative function of stimulus intensity and current BFS activity. The implication of this point for human personality is that variation in trait levels of BFS activity may influence sensitivity to incentive stimuli. That is, individual differences in the functioning of emotional systems (e.g., the BFS) may underly emotional dispositions (incentive, desire, positive emotion) to particular classes of stimuli (rewards or incentive stimuli). In the case of the BFS, such trait differences would have the effect of modulating (1) perceived intensity of incentive stimuli; (2) intensity and frequency of the resulting subjective experience of desire, incentive, and positive feelings; and (3) the threshold for stimulus–elicitation of overt emotional responses.

Variation in DA functioning could underly individual differences in BFS activity. In a 33-year-old man, there are approximately 690,000 cells in the VTA–substantia nigra complex, and this number may vary across individuals by as much as 20,000 cells (Oades & Halliday, 1987). Importantly, variation in DA cell number does affect BFS behaviors. For instance, the quantity of spontaneous exploratory locomotion and the magnitude of amphetamine-induced locomotion are both positively related to number of DA neurons (including those of the VTA cell group), the relative density of innervation of DA terminals in target fields, and to DA content in the NAS in inbred mouse strains (Fink & Reis, 1981; Oades, 1985; Sved, Baker, & Reis, 1984, 1985).

This conceptualization of a DA-BFS trait resembles existing personality "supertraits" or "superfactors," which represent a common influence across a number of individual, lower-order traits, just as the BFS is viewed as influencing a number of lower-order behaviors. Almost every trait theory of personality includes a dimension that encompasses positive affect, desire, incentive motivation, and a sense of personal efficacy. Numerous labels have been used, including *extraversion* (e.g., Eysenck & Eysenck, 1985), but because of the emotional aspects of the trait, we prefer *positive emotionality*.

In developing his Multidimensional Personality Questionnaire (MPQ), Tellegen has proposed an emotional systems approach to the structure of personality (see review by Tellegen & Waller, 1992). This structure includes a superfactor, labeled *positive emotionality* (PE), that corresponds to a BFS construct, correlates strongly (.62, $p < .01$) with Eysenck's (Eysenck & Eysenck, 1985) EPQ Extraversion Scale, and is subject to significant genetic influence. Tellegen systematically incorporated many subdomains into the item pool that makes up the emotional experience associated with the BFS, including sociability, social potency or dominance, positive emotional feelings, incentive or achievement motivation and its subjective aspect of a general sense of desire and excitement, and level of energy and activity. The affective interpretation of higher order MPQ PE is supported by its convergent–discriminant relations to the state dimensions of positive and negative affect, respectively, which dominate measures of current mood. Importantly, there is a strong emphasis on effectance motivation—for example, less on amount of socialization, more on one's perceived effectiveness and "power" in social interaction. This emphasis is more in keeping with the motivational aspect of the BFS construct.

A Preliminary Study of Dopamine Activity and Human Positive Emotionality

As outlined in Collins and Depue (1992), the validity of drawing comparisons between the personality construct of PE and the construct of the BFS developed from animal research may be addressed by assessing similarities in their neurobiology. To this end, we measured the effects of a specific DA receptor agonist on an index of central DA activity (prolactin inhibition) in subjects widely distributed along the dimension of MPQ PE (Collins & Depue, 1992; Depue, Luciana, Arbisi, Collins, & Leon, 1992).

The experimental manipulation involved administration of bromocriptine mesylate, a potent and specific agonist at D_2 receptor sites. Bromocriptine has a time-dependent biphasic effect, in which its initial agonist effect on presynaptic D_2 autoreceptors is inhibitory to DA function, whereas its subsequent postsynaptic D_2 effect, accompanying rising concentrations in blood activates DA function. Behaviorally, the biphasic effect may be seen in an initial dose-dependent immobility or hypomotility in rats, followed some time later, depending on dose, by hyperlocomotion. The latter effect suggests that bromocriptine activates DA terminals involved in initiating behaviors relevant to the BFS construct (i.e., forward locomotion and incentive–reward motivation).

Subjects were run from 11 A.M. to 6 P.M. with an indwelling catheter in a randomized, crossover design under double-blind conditions of identical bromocriptine (2.5 mg) or placebo (2.5 mg lactose) capsules ingested at 12 noon. Predrug samples for baseline serum prolactin (PRL) and ten postdrug samples were obtained every 30 minutes from 1:00 to 5:30 P.M.

Two variables, each reflecting the time required to achieve bromocriptine's postsynaptic inhibition of PRL secretion, assessed the efficacy of *pre*synaptic activation: (1) time until the first consistent drug-induced reduction in PRL values (PRL Descent) and (2) time until the point of maximum inhibition of PRL secretion (PRL TMax). Both PRL Descent and PRL TMax were strongly related to MPQ PE (Figure 5.5, A and B), suggesting that MPQ PE is related to the "sensitivity" of presynaptic D_2 autoreceptors to bromocriptine's agonist effects. These relations were specific to MPQ PE, as shown by the absence of significant correlations with MPQ Negative Emotionality (Ne, $r = .33, .43$, respectively, $p > .25$) and MPQ Constraint (C, $r = -.18 -.11$, respectively, $p > .5$).

We assessed postsynaptic D_2 receptor effects of bromocriptine by measuring the maximum inhibitory effect of the drug on PRL secretion (PRL Max). PRL Max was strongly related to MPQ PE (Figure 5.5 C), but not to MPQ NE ($r = .39, p < .25$) or MPQ C ($r = .02, p > .50$).

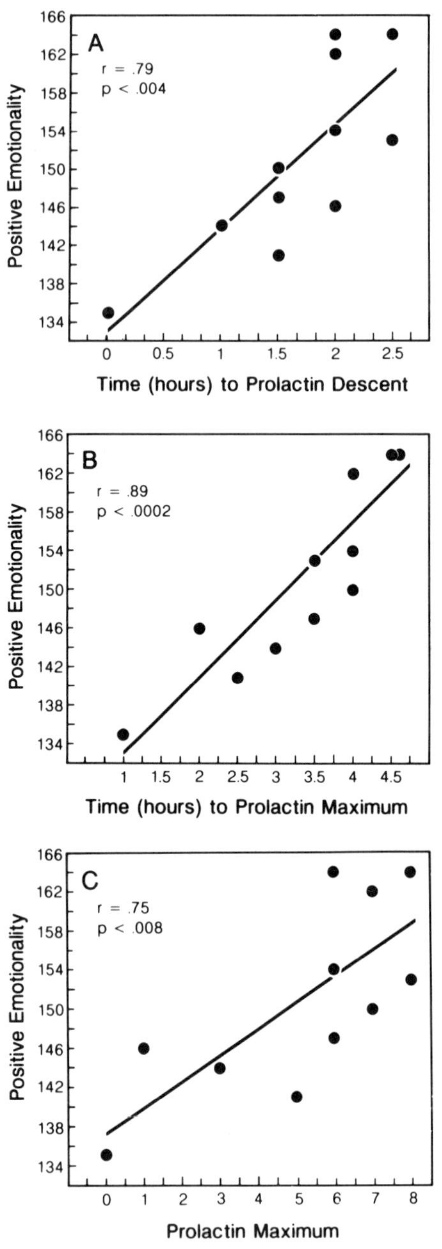

FIGURE 5.5. Individual subject plots of correlations between MPQ PE scores and (**A**) time to reach the initial point of consistent reduction in prolactin secretion due to bromocriptine (Time to Prolactin Descent), (**B**) time to reach the maximum inhibition of prolactin secretion by bromocriptine (Time to Prolactin Maximum), and (**C**) maximum inhibitory effect of bromocriptine on prolactin secretion (Prolactin Maximum).

Moreover, bromocriptine's postsynaptic receptor index (PRL Max) was significantly related to both presynaptic receptor indices (PRL TMax, $r = .88$, $p < .0004$; PRL Descent, $r = .68$, $p < .02$). Thus, presynaptic and postsynaptic PRL indices of bromocriptine's D_2 receptor effects were highly correlated, and both types of index were specifically related to MPQ PE.

Several points concerning interpretation of results must be noted. First, because the sample was selected along the diagonal of greatest behavioral variation between MPQ PE and MPQ C, the correlations between MPQ PE and DA response indices may be smaller in unrestricted samples. The goal of the current study was not to estimate the PE–DA relation in the population, however, but rather to demonstrate a specific and potentially important relation between PE and DA, if such existed. Second, because PRL is regulated by a variety of neurotransmitters and neuropeptides, associations between PRL indices and PE may be obscured under *basal* conditions, as indicated in our data by the lack of association between MPQ PE and baseline PRL ($r = .21$, $p > .3$) and pre-Descent PRL ($r = -.15$, $p > .3$) values. Interpretative clarity is increased in this study because the response to a DA receptor agonist was assessed. Thus, a PE–DA association emerged only after reactivity of DA systems was induced. Third, interpretation of the effects of bromocriptine on PRL as due solely to nonspecific processes unrelated to DA functioning seems unlikely. We have observed no significant magnitude or temporal effects ($p > .3$) of bromocriptine on biletter cancellation (attention) and spatial location (memory) tasks or on blood pressure (general arousal).

Taken together, the current findings suggest that the trait structure of personality is related to the responsivity of central DA projection systems. What is intriguing is that PRL variables, reflecting the action of DA in a hypothalamic DA system, were so strongly related to a set of personality behaviors that most likely reflect DA function in ascending projections arising from VTA DA cells. It is known that DA cell groups, including those in the substantia nigra, VTA, and hypothalamus, can manifest a common genetic influence that is reflected in their functional properties. For instance, DA agonist effects are correlated across PRL secretion, exploratory behavior, and locomotor activity in inbred strains of mice that differ in DA cell number in all DA cell groups. It is possible, therefore, that the heritability of MPQ PE is related to genetic influences on DA cell groups, and that unmeasured genetic variance in our subjects contributed substantially to the observed correlations between MPQ PE and drug response indices. In any case, the consistently strong and specific PE–DA associations indicate that the emotional–behavioral functions of DA derived from animal research may hold for humans as well.

Environmental Influence and BFS Functioning: Potential Mediation of the Effects of Stressors

If the BFS underlies or contributes to a major emotional trait dimension in humans, it must be subject to sources of variation that ultimately produce stable individual differences in levels of BFS responsivity. Whether genetic or environmental, these influences will converge within the adaptive neural circuitry of the BFS to produce functional variations, such as individual differences in DA responsivity, that correspond to variation in behavioral trait levels. Thus, one approach to understanding the origins of individual differences within the BFS is to examine genetic and environmental processes that shape its underlying neural system, that is, to focus upon a neurobiological interface between genotype and environment. At present, this approach is constrained by the relative paucity of neurodevelopmental data, but several sources of influence on mammalian neural systems have been studied in detail. Although this work has been applied primarily to perceptual and cognitive functioning, an extension to the development of emotional systems, if valid, would provide an organizational structure for future study of the origins of BFS trait levels. Accordingly, we here outline these neurodevelopmental influences, and describe how they might apply to the BFS. For a fuller discussion of these issues, see Collins and Depue (1992).

Within the neurobiology literature, Greenough and colleagues (e.g., Greenough & Black, in press; Black & Greenough, 1986; Greenough, Black, & Wallace, 1987) have proposed a framework in which three basic sources of input to the brain induce functional specialization across a variety of information processing pathways. Although the three types of processes undoubtedly overlap during the development of neural systems, it is useful to consider them separately in terms of their possible application to individual differences within the BFS.

Genotype–Driven Processes

Genotype-driven processes influence the basic structure and function of neuron populations in a manner that is largely insensitive to experiential input. One outcome of genotype-driven development is of obvious importance to individual differences in BFS responsivity: variation across individuals in DA cell number produced during prenatal development. In animals, variation in DA cell number is related strongly to differences in DA-regulated behaviors, such as locomotor reactivity to novel environments (Fink & Reis, 1981; Sved, Baker, & Reis, 1984, 1985). It is likely that differences in DA cell number will have similar functional consequences in humans; for example, variation in DA cell number may have contributed to the strong association between bromocriptine-induced

DA responsivity and PEM scores, as described previously. Thus, one simple but important source of individual differences in BFS responsivity may be genotype-driven variation in the number of DA cells produced during prenatal development.

Experience-Expectant Processes

Experience-expectant processes occur within sensitive periods in brain development, and they involve widespread overproduction of neuronal synapses that precedes environmental experience. Through selective preservation and strengthening of a subset of these synapses, species-typical patterns of neuronal cytoarchitecture are established during exposure to phylogenetically predictable forms of environmental experience. This type of development is regulated rather than driven by genotype; that is, the timing and regional location of experience-expectant synaptic overproduction are determined by genotypic influences, but the functional relations encoded by the preserved synapses vary in response to environmental experience. A primary feature of experience-expectant processes is widespread cortical synapse overproduction, which defines sensitive periods in brain development. The magnitude of synaptic overproduction at the cortical level is striking, as juvenile synaptic density values are 75–95% above adult values in nonhuman primates (Rakic, Bourgeois, Eckenhoff, Zecevic, & Goldman-Rakic, 1986; O'Kusky & Colonnier, 1982). Following overproduction, excess cortical synapses are pruned back gradually in response to stimulation provided by the environment; in simple terms, a particular synapse is eliminated, or regresses, if activity at an adjacent synapse is driven more strongly by environmental stimuli. This regressive competition among synapses occurs within a relatively discrete period of time and establishes a specific and organized pattern of functional synaptic connections within a developing cortical region. Clearly, such powerful neurodevelopmental processes are adaptive only if they are restricted to early experiences with both a predictable content and a relatively consistent timing for all young members of a species. Similar processes occur at subcortical levels, but they involve the overproduction and subsequent elimination of entire cells. Conversely, cortical synapse overproduction and elimination appear to occur only in mammals, and with greatest prominence in primates (Huttenlocker, 1990; Killackey, 1990). Accordingly, the remainder of this section will focus upon experience-expectant processes as they apply to the functional development of information-processing pathways within mammalian cortex.

The basic implication of experience-expectant processes for the development of individual differences in neural system functioning is shown schematically in Figure 5.6. During a period of experience-

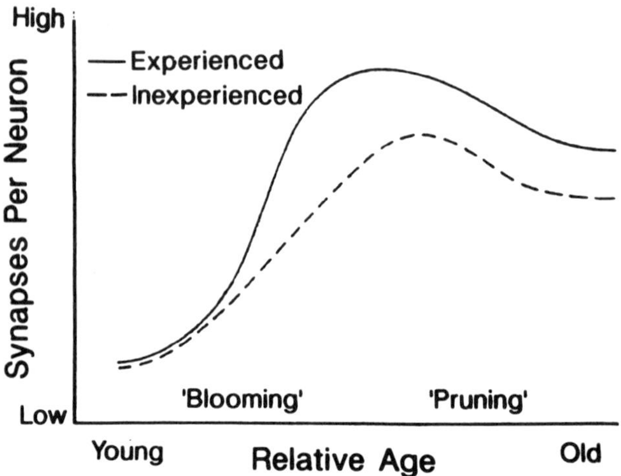

FIGURE 5.6. Schematic diagram of synapse overproduction ("blooming") and deletion ("pruning") during an experience-expectant process. From "Induction of Pattern in Neural Structure by Experience: Implications for Cognitive Development" by J. E. Black and W. T. Greenough, 1986. In M. E. Lamb, A. L. Brown, and B. Rogoff (Eds.), *Advances in Developmental Psychology* (Vol. 4, p. 28). Hillsdale, NJ: Erlbaum. Copyright 1986 by Lawrence Erlbaum Associates. Reprinted by permission.

expectant development, individuals exposed to a stimulation-rich environment ("experienced" curve) will encode that experience by retaining a large number of functional synaptic connections within relevant neural system pathways. In contrast, individuals exposed to a stimulation-impoverished environment ("inexperienced" curve) will retain a relatively small number of functional synaptic connections. As a lasting consequence, individual differences will be established in the functional capacity of the neural system to respond to subsequent environmental stimulation. Similar patterns of synaptic development may occur within the BFS. For example, if experience-expectant development were to occur within the reciprocal pathways connecting the amygdala and temporal pole, an individual exposed to a reward-rich environment may establish functional synaptic relations that provide an enhanced capacity to respond to conditioned signals of reward in the future. A degree of ecological validity may be incorporated into this scenario by considering the overlap between genotype-driven and experience-expectant processes: An individual born with a relatively large number of VTA–DA cells would seek engagement with potentially rewarding stimuli and thereby contribute actively to the development of enhanced synaptic connectivity among BFS structures during an experience-expectant sensitive period.

Experience-Dependent Processes

Experience-dependent processes modify neuronal cytoarchitecture to encode environmental experience that is unique to the individual and thus unpredictable on the basis of phylogeny. In contrast to experience-expectant development, experience-dependent processes involve localized synapse production that is initiated during the encoding of information arising from any significant form of experience, including mentation; thus, the timing and location of experience-dependent modifications are not influenced by genotype.

Whereas experience-expectant development may provide an early foundation for future neural system refinements, experience-dependent processes may mediate smaller scale synaptic modifications throughout the life-span. That is, it is these processes that may be responsible for encoding environmental influences, including life stressors, throughout life. One of the primary contributions of Greenough and colleagues is their empirical documentation of the production of new synapses, on demand, as a fundamental component of experience-dependent processes in postweanling animals. The most direct data are derived from studies in which differences in synaptic number were recorded in groups of post-weanling animals (usually rats) after extended exposure to three different environments: (1) group housing in cages filled with toys that were changed daily ("environmental complexity" or EC condition), usually accompanied by daily exploration of a separate, toy-filled playbox; (2) paired housing in standard laboratory cages ("social" or SC condition); and (3) individual housing in standard cages (IC condition). Although many researchers describe EC animals as housed within an "enriched" environment, Greenough and Black (in press) emphasized that all three conditions actually are impoverished relative to the feral environment, albeit in varying degrees. The distinction is not trivial becaise synaptic phenomena observed under the EC condition should be viewed as experimental analogs of what occurs in natural settings, rather than the unnatural products of laboratory manipulation.

At the behavioral level, EC animals have demonstrated consistently superior learning ability in many types of complex tasks involving potential rewards or punishers (e.g., Brown, 1968; Freeman & Ray, 1972; Greenough, Fulcher, Yuwiler, & Geller, 1970; Greenough, Wood, & Madden, 1972; Greenough, Yuwiler, & Dollinger, 1973; Morgan, 1973). At the neural level, several studies have described enhancement of various morphological features of EC animals, including a thicker visual cortex with enlarged cell bodies (Diamond, 1967) and a higher ratio of RNA and protein to DNA (i.e., altered gene expression; Rosenzweig & Bennett, 1978). Empirical data also suggest that preexisting synaptic connections may be strengthened in EC animals (e.g., Gerenough, West, & DeVoogd,

1978; Sirevaag & Greenough, 1985; West & Greenough, 1972). However, the most illuminating data are found in studies that reported a greater number of synapses within samples of brain tissue from EC animals. In visual cortex, EC rats have demonstrated approximately 20% to 25% more synapses per neuron than IC rats, with SC rats intermediate but somewhat closer to IC values (Volkmar & Greenough, 1972; Greenough & Volkmar, 1973; Turner & Greenough, 1983, 1985). Similar results have been reported in cats and monkeys (Beaulieu & Colonnier, 1987; Floeter & Greenough, 1979), as well as in other cortical regions, the hippocampus, and the cerebellum (Greenough, Volkmar, & Juraska, 1973; Juraska, Fitch, Henderson, & Rivers, 1985; Juraska, Fitch, & Washburne, 1989; Pysh & Weiss, 1979), although effect sizes have been smaller outside of visual cortex. Experience-dependent synapse production has no discernible association with sensitive periods, as it demonstrates a similar pattern (ECSCIC) and a nearly equivalent magnitude in adult or even middle-aged rats (Green, Greenough, & Schlumpf, 1983; Juraska, Greenough, Elliott, Mack, & Berkowitz, 1980; Uylings, Kuypers, & Veltman, 1978). Moreover, the synaptic patterns appear to have a specific association with learning and memory, in that they do not reliably covary with generalized hormonal or metabolic alterations related to differential housing or training (see Greenough & Black, in press; Greenough et al., 1987).

In recent reviews, Greenough and Black (in press; Greenough et al., 1987) have emphasized the importance of moving beyond experimental designs in which the effects of environmental manipulations are examined in only one brain region. Obviously, such designs are difficult to interpret with respect to complex tasks employed in developmental psychology research, but they also lack clear relevance for emerging models of parallel distributed pathways or networks in neural processing. Goldman-Rakic (1987) has outlined a general model in which specific areas of the prefrontal cortex modulate neural activity within diverse networks of cortical and subcortical structures, each subserving a separate class of complex behavioral functions. At a more detailed level, Rolls (1989; in press) has described task-specific correlations of single-unit activity across subsets of neurons in multimodal cortical regions, the hippocampal formation, and the amygdala. Rolls has extended these findings to a general computational model of neural networks, in which competitive learning contributes to the establishment of "ensemble encoded" associative memories, that is, information that is stored in a distributed fashion across subsets of neurons in task-relevant brain structures. With respect to this model, Greenough and Black (in press) suggested that experience-dependent processes may continuously modify the pattern of synaptic connectivity within neural networks in response to new learning experiences.

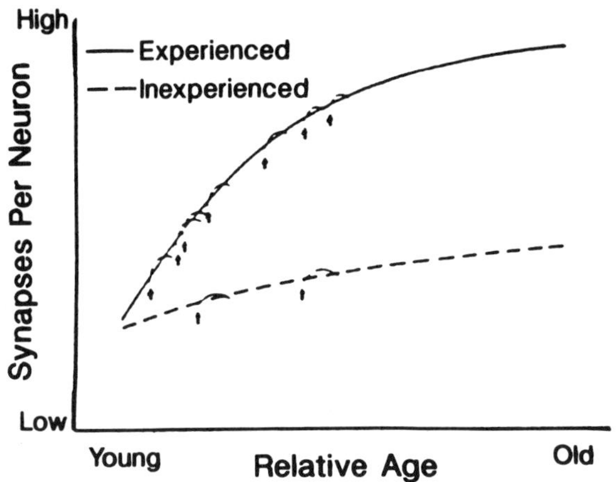

FIGURE 5.7. Schematic diagram of synapse formation and selective retention during an experience-dependent process. The arrowheads mark salient experiences that generate local synaptic overproduction and deletion (*small curves*). The cumulative effect of such synaptic blooms and prunes is a smooth increase in synapses per neuron, which is greater for the animals with more experience. From "Induction of Pattern in Neural Structure by Experience: Implications for Cognitive Development" by J. E. Black and W. T. Greenough, 1986. In M. E. Lamb, A. L. Brown, and B. Rogoff (Eds.), *Advances in Developmental Psychology* (Vol. 4, p. 38). Hillsdale, NJ: Erlbaum. Copyright 1986 by Lawrence Erlbaum Associates. Reprinted by permission.

These theoretical notions may be applied to the type of learning and memory that occurs in the BFS. Specifically, associative memories of positive behavioral engagements may be formed within the interconnected neural structures of the BFS, as they encode relations among the perceived incentive value of a stimulus, the incentive motivation experienced, and the rewarding consequences of the behavior expressed. Experience-dependent synaptic processes may mediate this ensemble encoding of emotional evaluation, experience, and expression, and thereby contribute over time to learning-related modifications in BFS responsivity. In this manner, experience-dependent processes may contribute substantially to individual differences in BFS responsivity, but unlike experience-expectant development, changes in neural system responsivity will accrue in a gradual, stepwise manner (see Figure 5.7).

Neurobiological Control of Synapse Production and Elimination

Although the synaptic alterations associated with experience-expectant and experience-dependent processes have been well documented, the underlying control of synaptic events remains poorly understood. By definition, the timing and magnitude of experience-expectant overproduction of synapses are controlled by specific, but largely unknown, genetic mechanisms. More data exist with respect to extrinsic neurochemical modulation of new synapses, which appears to follow a similar form in both experience-expectant and experience-dependent development. During early sensitive periods, the development of functional synaptic connections may be initiated and/or regulated by levels of thyroid and corticosteroid hormones, neurotrophic factors such as nerve growth factor, and classical neurotransmitters (reviewed by Lauder & Krebs, 1986; see also Greenough & Black, in press). More generally, the specific patterns of neuronal cytoarchitecture produced by experience-expectant and experience-dependent processes appear to be regulated by local interactions with diffuse neurotransmitter projection systems. As described recently by Mattson (1988), these local interactions may represent modulatory processes by which projection systems contribute to the organization of input–output relations within neural systems that they innervate. Accordingly, we outline here a possible role for diffuse neurotransmitter systems, such as the projections arising from VTA DA cells, that may be related inherently to their role in modulating the functional activity levels within neurobehavioral systems.

After axons have stopped their primary growth, a sequence of events occurs that leads to stabilization of functional synaptic contacts. During prenatal and early postnatal periods, this sequence features stages of neurite outgrowth (i.e., fine, hairlike processes that extend from the tip of the developing axon, referred to as the *growth cone*), cessation of outgrowth, and synaptogenesis. As described previously, a stage of regressive competition completes the sequence and provides a foundation for neural systems underlying the species-typical behavioral repertoire. Particularly at higher levels of the neuraxis (e.g., allocortex, cortex, and neocortex), the release of various neurotransmitters regulates the expression of each stage in the sequence (Mattson, 1988). As a distributed form of this regulation, activity within diffuse neurotransmitter systems may guide the development of basic patterns of synaptic connectivity (see Figure 5.8) and thereby elevate neural system development to a level of functional fine-tuning beyond the scope of genotype-driven processes (Mattson, 1988; see also Greenough & Black, in press).

Thus, mechanisms may exist within the growth cone for transducing the release of various neurotransmitters into signals that guide neurodevelopment at the synaptic level. Through these mechanisms, activity in neurotransmitter projection systems may regulate patterns of functional synaptic connectivity within the distributed structures of a particular neural system; for example, the activity of VTA DA cells during development may influence synaptic relations within critical neural pathways

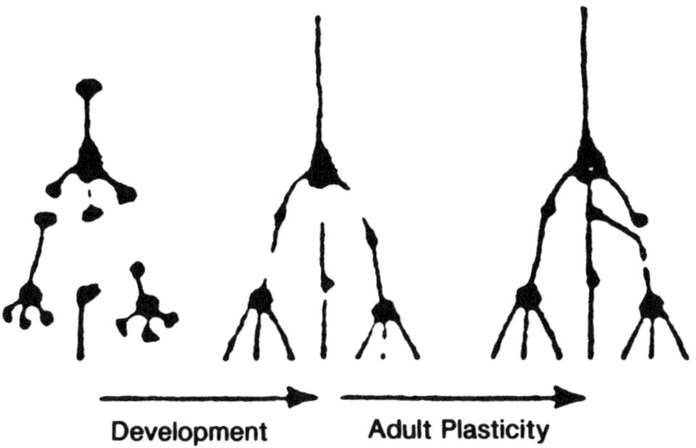

FIGURE 5.8. Neurotransmitter involvement in brain development and adult plasticity. As neurons extend axons and dendrites during development, axons releasing neurotransmitter stabilize the outgrowth of the dendritic fields they invade, and synapses form, establishing a functional circuitry. Throughout adult life, changes in neuronal circuitry may be mediated by the activity of neurotransmitters. From "Neurotransmitters in Regulation of Neuronal Cytoarchitecture" by M. P. Mattson, 1988. *Brain Research Review, 13,* 206. Copyright 1989 by Elsevier Science Publishers. Reprinted by permission.

of the BFS, such as the OFC–VTA–NAS loop. In addition, alterations in neurotransmitter levels may mediate regression of dendritic terminals (Mattson, 1988), perhaps as a tightly regulated and adaptive expression of the capacity of some neurotransmitters, such as excitatory amino acids, to produce selective cell death (Watkins & Evans, 1981) or dendritic loss (Mattson, Dou, & Kater, 1988). As Mattson (1988) noted, the potential is obvious for applying these cell-level neurotransmitter actions to the encoding of sensory experience within neuronal cyctoarchitecture because variation in the sensory environment will be reflected, ultimately, in alterations of neurochemical transmission at cortical synapses. Furthermore, there is direct empirical evidence of the persistence of neurotransmitter modulation of neuronal cytoarchitecture throughout the lifespan. Put simply, the transition of nerve cell endings from growth cones to presynaptic terminals appears to be a two-way street, and reversions to growth cone mode may occur in the adult brain when locally altered neural activity levels demand changes in dendritic fields (Mattson, 1988).

From this perspective, neurotransmitter projection systems may be viewed as modulators of synaptic structure as well as function, that is, as sources of influence over both cytoarchitectural and chemical encoding of information within neural pathways. In terms of the framework of Greenough and colleagues, neurotransmitter activity likely modulates dendritic outgrowth, synaptogenesis, and synaptic regression during both experience-expectant and experience-dependent development. Moreover, the regulation of neuroarchitecture by neurotransmitters may be one avenue for collaboration among all three forms of neurodevelopmental processes. As an illustration, consider the earlier suggestion that individual differences in the number of VTA DA cells may be viewed as an outcome of genotype-driven processes. If the number of cells is relatively large, an individual will possess the structural capacity to release high levels of DA at the terminals of VTA projections during experience-expectant sensitive periods. Such an individual would be predisposed to stabilize, and thereby retain, a large number of synaptic contacts within BFS structures, provided that a sufficient level of activity was maintained in the VTA source cells. Although this functional outcome would not occur if environmental experience were reward-impoverished, empirical findings in animal behavior genetics suggest that an individual with a rich genetic endowment of DA cells would actively explore the environment in search of rewarding stimulation (Fink & Reis, 1981; Sved, Baker, & Reis, 1984, 1985). Thus, the likely (but not inevitable) outcome of the sensitive period would be the emergence of a strong functional capacity in the VTA DA system to motivate and guide emotional responses to signals of reward, and this foundation for BFS responsivity would be resistant to large scale modification in the future. As neural system development proceeds, experience-dependent processes would likely provide incremental increases in the synaptic connectivity within BFS structures, in that an enduring predisposition to engage potentially rewarding stimuli would entail frequent demands for additional synapses in the terminal fields of VTA DA projections. By adulthood, the extensive synaptic arborization within BFS circuitry would consistently amplify responses of the VTA DA system to signals of reward, and the individual would exhibit a high and stable level of BFS responsivity.

Despite its simplicity, this hypothetical example illustrates how fundamentally distinct neurodevelopmental processes (i.e., genotype-driven, experience-expectant, and experience-dependent) may exert overlapping influences upon the development of neural systems by converging upon modulatory neurochemical systems. To the extent that modulatory neurotransmitters form an integral component of neurobehavioral systems, they will incorporate these influences within basic parameters of neural functioning, such as synaptic connectivity, that underlie variation in neurobehavioral traits. With respect to the origins of individual differences in the BFS, trends in the level of BFS responsivity will emerge as individuals experience stimulus contexts that modifiy earlier neurodevelopmental outcomes involving the structural and functional capacities of the VTA DA projection system. In view of the potential for collaboration among neurodevelopmental processes, it is likely that individuals will exhibit progressively discrepant outcome trajectories that ultimately stabilize as trait-level variation in BFS responsivity. However, it is important to emphasize that retention of mechanisms for functional alterations during later development is an inherent property of adaptive neural systems; through these mechanisms, developmental discontinuities in the BFS will be expressed over time if individuals are guided toward, or subjected to, a significantly altered reward environment.

Implications for Disorders of Affect

A natural extension of the BFS into the domain of psychopathology emerges upon examination of the symptoms associated with disturbances of positive emotionality, that is, affective disorders. When core affective symptoms are considered, they fall primarily within the locomotor, incentive–reward, and mood dimensions (see review by Depue & Iacono, 1989), and the relevance of the BFS construct becomes obvious. Space limitations preclude a full discussion of this issue, and many of the points have been discussed elsewhere (Depue, Krauss, & Spoont, 1987; Depue & Iacono, 1989). However, any BFS framework for disorders of affect probably needs to consider the following conditions.

Extreme BFS State Levels and Affective Disorders

As illustrated in Figure 5.9, symptoms of bipolar depression and hypomania/mania appear to represent opposite extremes of normal behavioral dimensions (Depue & Iacono, 1989; Post & Uhde, 1982) that describe extreme states of engagement (and disengagement) with both interpersonal and achievement-related environments. The poles of the core behavioral dimensions may be viewed as the products of extreme variations in the probability that incentive stimuli of all forms—exteroceptive, interoceptive, cognitive—will initiate or facilitate motor and affective responses. In these terms, the probability of initiating emotional behavior is excessively low in depression and excessively high in hypomania or mania. Both states, then, may be viewed along a single dimension representing the propensity to behavioral and affective reactivity to incentive stimuli (Depue & Iacono, 1989).

In the case of bipolar depression, low reactivity encompasses familiar behavioral features such as psychomotor retardation, as well as typical subjective features involving the lack of usual interest or enthusiasm for engagement in social, sexual, vocational, or recreational activities (Depue & Monroe, 1978; Post & Uhde, 1982). In addition, bipolar depressives frequently display general affective poverty or blunting, and the absence of positive affect is typically a far more prominent clinical feature than the

MOTOR			INCENTIVE REWARD ACTIVATION		MOOD	NONSPECIFIC AROUSAL						COGNITIVE	
Locomotion	Speech	Facies	Hedonia (Social, Sex, Food)	Desire for Excitement		Appetite	Energy	Sleep/Wake	Thought	Attention	Sensory Vividness	Optimism	Self-Worth
hyperactivity	rapid pressured	expressive	excessive interest and pleasure	excessive, creates new activities	elation, euphoria, reactive	decreased	excessive, boundless	< need for sleep	sharper, flight of ideas, witty > decisional power	concrete, distractible	extremely vivid	> self confidence, < estimation of negative outcomes, grandiosity	increased worth, grandiosity
retardation slowed delayed stupor	retardation slowed delayed mute	unchanging, unexpressive	no interest or pleasure (pervasive anhedonia)	avoidance of stimulation	devoid of emotion depression, lack reactivity	carbo-hydrate intake	easily fatigued, devoid of energy	hyper-somnia, naps	< decisional power, thoughts "dead," mind dull	poor concen-tration	senses dull, food tastes bland	pessimistic, persistent gloom, brood about past, hopeless about future outcomes, suicidal ideation	totally worthless, delusional

FIGURE 5.9. Categorization of the bipolar behavioral dimensions associated with bipolar affective disorder.

164

presence of negative affect. This observation is consistent with the higher-order structure of mood derived from research with normal subjects (Watson & Tellegen, 1985), which is modeled better by orthogonal positive and negative dimensions, each with "high" and "low" poles, than by a single positive–negative dimension. As noted previously, self-report ratings of positive affect (state) and positive emotionality (trait) correlate strongly (Tellegen & Waller, 1992), which again raises the possibility of a direct relation between bipolar depressive episodes and extreme reductions in BFS responsivity. Thus, the essential features of bipolar depression may be modeled parsimoniously as an extreme state-wise reduction in the effective value of rewarding stimuli to elicit the primary components of BFS activation: incentive motivation, psycho-motor activation, and positive mood.

The primary features of hypomania/mania may be viewed as analo-gous manifestations of excessively high BFS responsivity. In comparison with bipolar depression, however, the extreme status of DA's behavioral facilitation function is more transparent in hypomania/mania. Along with excessive levels of incentive motivation, locomotor activation, and posi-tive mood, distractibility and mixed affect are typically observed during hypomanic/manic episodes (Post & Uhde, 1982; Secunda et al., 1987). Distractibility in hypomania/mania appears to represent excessive re-sponsivity to stimuli that are rewarding or novel but task irrelevant, rather than a generalized and affectively neutral attentional impairment (Depue & Iacono, 1989). At a more detailed level, this type of inappro-priate reward responding reflects both attribution of exaggerated incen-tive value to stimuli during emotional evaluation and an extremely low threshold for initiating approach types of responses. With such extreme amplification of these fundamental BFS processes, sustained and focused behavioral responding is difficult to maintain; thus, the hypomanic/manic exhibits high levels of incentive motivation in the context of apparently purposeless behavior. In sum, when hypomania/mania is viewed as an episode of extreme behavioral and affective reactivity to incentive stimuli, its core symptoms emerge as polar opposites of those in bipolar depres-sion.

Extreme BFS Trait Level and Disorders of Affect: A Model for Gene–Environment Interaction

When less extreme trait levels of BFS responsivity are postulated, the previous formulation naturally extends to characterological expressions of affective disorder, such as hyperthymia and dysthymia (see Collins & Depue, 1992). Consistent with their classification as characterological entities, some forms of dysthymia and hyperthymia may reflect levels of DA responsivity that constitute minimum and maximum values, respectively, along a trait dimension underlying positive emotionality in the normal population.

One source of extreme BFS trait levels may be genotype driven in terms of the number of neurons per DA cell group formed during the prenatal period. As noted before, this variation can be substantial and strongly influences the range of functional expression of DA-modulated behaviors in rodents. From a developmental perspective, this influence could become manifest in several ways, and these are summarized in Figure 5.10. Consider low (vs. high) VTA DA cell number as an example that is most relevant to depressive conditions (Person B vs. Person A,

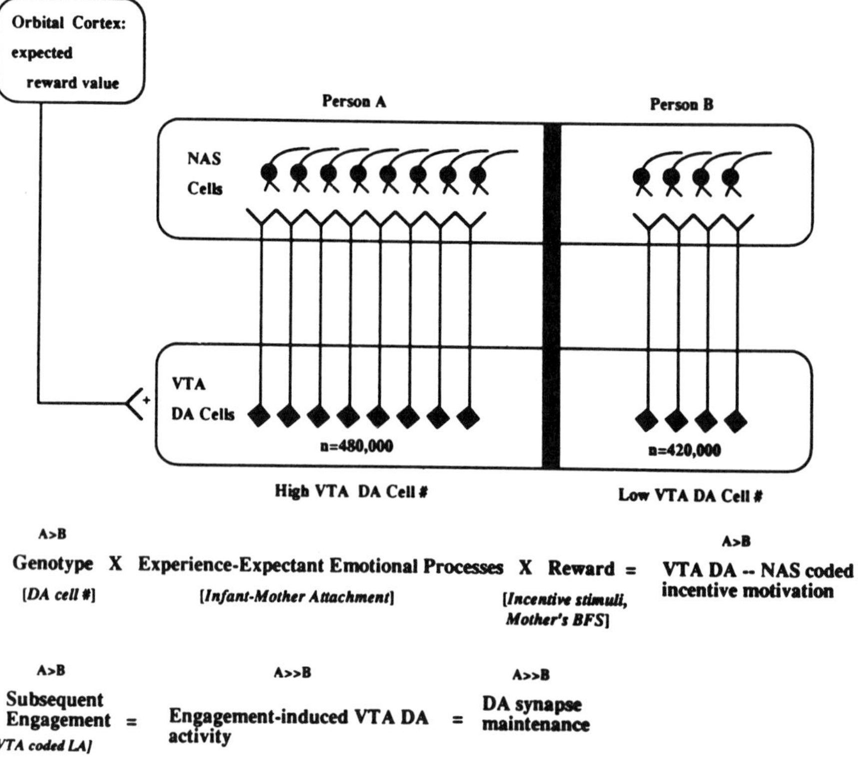

FIGURE 5.10. Schematic representation of how ventral tegmental area dopamine cell number (genotype) interacts with experience-expectant processes during environmental reward circumstances to determine the encoded reward value of a stimulus (first line of type), the subsequent level of engagement-induced dopamine activity (second line of type), and experience-dependent processes during rewarding environmental contexts (third line of type).

respectively, at the top of Figure 5.10). As shown across the first line in Figure 5.10, in experience-expectant emotional periods, a condition of a reduced number of VTA DA cells (i.e., genotype), and hence density of axon terminals in the NAS, would yield fewer possibilities for synaptogenesis in the NAS in Person B versus Person A (A > B). Thus, even adequate environmental reward experiences at the *expected* time would have a reduced neurological substrate in Person B on which to reinforce synaptic connections in the NAS. In this way, the ontological development of sensitivity to reward in Person B may begin in a diminished way; or, put differently, as indicated in Figure 5.10, VTA DA–NAS encoded incentive motivation would be less in Person B than in Person A.

This differential sensitivity to reward could have at least two major effects. First, as shown in the second line in Figure 5.10, subsequent rewarding experiences would result in differential incentive motivation via VTA DA–NAS mechanisms and, hence, differential approach to or engagement with reward. This condition, in turn, would result in differential engagement-induced DA activation, with Person B experiencing much less DA activation than Person A. Accordingly, the resulting decrease in DA synapse maintenance in the NAS in Person B would exacerbate an already diminished sensitivity to reward. That is, as shown on the third line of Figure 5.10, a progessively weakened experience-dependent process of synaptic growth in the NAS might be expected in Person B relative to Person A. By adulthood, this experience-dependent process of diminished DA release to reward, and hence diminished synaptic growth in DA terminal areas, in Person B could result in significantly reduced synaptic arborization within BFS circuitry. Behaviorally, this might appear as a quantitatively low trait position on the dimension of positive emotionality (à la Tellegen's model) or, more simply, as a form of characterological depression or pure dysthymia.

A second effect of reduced sensitivity to reward in Person B is that other traits that function *interactively* with DA in modulating emotional behavior would become dominant relative to BFS activity. For instance, a situation that presents signals of both reward and punishment may increasingly evoke constraint and behavioral inhibition rather than exploration and goal acquisition. Subjectively, the cumulative effect of reduced reward sensitivity and behavioral inhibition could be a sense of low self-efficacy in obtaining rewarding goals (a form of learned helplessness or passive avoidance?) and a persistent lack of positive affect or persistent dysphoria due to the low frequency of achieved rewards over time.

As suggested in the last line of Figure 5.10, the previous view of the ontology of some forms of characterological depression would be modified by the quality and quantity of environmental reward experience and perhaps by BFS trait level of caregivers, who are predominantly responsible in early years for providing reward and for encouraging exploration and goal acquisition. Importantly, however, the magnitude of effect of the interpersonal environment on the ontological development of BFS trait level will probably vary, depending on the individual's genotype driven DA trait level (e.g., DA cell number), as illustrated in the discussion of Figure 5.10. At extreme ends of a dimension of DA trait level, the effects of environmental reward are likely to be constrained in the direction of the extremity. For instance, in an individual at the low extreme of DA trait level, a reward-rich environment may increase DA function over time, but the effect of a rewarding stimulus will always be less in promoting experience-dependent plasticity (see Figure 5.10). Moreover, the effects of a reward-poor environment may be diminished because of the already low level of DA reactivity. The opposite effects would be predicted at the high extreme end of DA trait level. It is in the midrange values of DA cell number that variations in environmental reward would be predicted to have complementary effects in experience-dependent synaptic growth because rich and poor environments will have equally strong, but opposite, effects. This leads to the intriguing possibility that the effects of variation in rewarding environments on DA, and hence BFS, responsivity may be most powerfully demonstrated within less extreme or midrange values of DA or positive emotionality trait levels.

BFS Regulatory Strength as a Trait and Disorders of Affect

Unlike dysthymia and hyperthymia, bipolar and some forms of unipolar affective disorders cannot be modeled sufficiently with a single dimension of trait level of DA responsivity, as the symptomatology of these disorders reflects extreme *intra*individual alterations in BFS, and perhaps DA, functioning. Accordingly, we describe here briefly a second dimension of DA responsivity we refer to as regulatory strength, which is a summarizing construct for the variety of processes within a neurotransmitter system that modulate reactivity under functional challenge to the system (see full discussion in Depue et al., 1987). Regulatory strength is viewed as a dimension that is etiologically orthogonal to trait level of DA responsivity. However, weak regulatory strength, which may involve weak negative feedback processes that result in positive feedback snowball effects, would possibly interact with DA trait level. Under weak regulatory conditions, at low and high extremes of the dimension of DA trait level, strong functional (including environmental) challenges to the DA system may produce prolonged state DA levels that are sufficiently low or high, respectively, to be manifested as extreme BFS states, or simply as affective disorder.

The possibility that weak regulatory strength in some DA projection systems, leading to dysregulation, is present in bipolar disorders is supported by a growing literature (see review by Depue & Iacono, 1989). Importantly, dysregulation has not been observable in measures of metabolic turnover. For instance, both baseline and probenecid-induced accumulation measures of CSF HVA have not consistently or significantly differentiated manic, depressed (except occasionally retarded depressives), and normal or psychiatric control groups, or the manic state from the recovered state (Post, 1980). However, pharmacological data reviewed recently (Cookson, 1985; Post, 1980; Silverstone, 1985; Wood, 1985) do suggest a role for DA in mania and depression. The efficacy of neuroleptics (and their generally short clinical time course of 1 to 5 days, which correlates with the rise in DA-inhibited prolactin) and, in some patients, of low–dose DA receptor agonists (such as piribedil, which at a low dose preferentially stimulate DA autoreceptors and, thereby, inhibits DA turnover) in the treatment of mania, as well as the antidepressant effects in some depressed patients of the DA receptor agonists piribedil and bromocriptine, has raised the possibility of altered DA function in bipolar disorders. Accordingly, in view of the apparent insensitivity of DA turnover measures, hypotheses that focus more on the functional, regulatory dynamics of DA activity have been proposed (Bunney, Post, Anderson, & Kopanda, 1977). We focus here on the behavioral instability that occurs when the regulation of the DA system is challenged or altered in bipolar disorders. To the extent that symptomatic behavioral functioning reflects BFS functioning, the DA literature has implications for evaluating BFS instability in bipolar disorders.

Evidence related to behavioral (BFS?) instability concerns the effects of DA challenges and of unimodal treatments (treatments aimed at one phase—either depression or mania—of bipolar disorder), both of which are associated with an increased probability of extreme levels of engagement (i.e., hypomania/mania). Since manipulation (Cookson, 1985; Jimerson & Post, 1984; Post, 1980; Silverstone, 1985; Wood, 1985) and pharmacologic (Bunney, 1978; Pickar, Cowdry, Zis, Cohen, & Murphy, 1984; Post, 1980; Post & Udhe, 1982; Silverstone, 1985) studies were reviewed recently, they are only outlined here. In several studies, enhancement of DA activity by increasing synthesis (L-dopa), release (amphetamine), or postsynaptic receptor activation (piribedil or bromocriptine) was associated with hypomanic or, less frequently, manic behavioral disturbance, an effect more commonly found in bipolar than unipolar depressed patients. These studies do not, however, represent a large number of patients, and other studies using amphetamine or piribedil did not observe a manic response (Post & Uhde, 1982). Whether a DA-induced vulnerability to hypomania/mania exists in the remitted state is insufficiently tested, having been found with methylphenidate challenge in euthymic bipolar patients on lithium but not in medication-free (off drugs only 2 weeks on average) euthymic patients with amphetamine challenge.

As reviewed previously (Bunney, 1978; Pickar et al., 1984; Post, 1980), acute and chronic treatment with tricyclic antidepressants (TCAs) and monoamine oxidase inhibitors (MAOIs) is associated with an increased incidence of hypomanic/manic disturbance, an effect that is much more common in bipolar than unipolar depressed patients and in bipolar 1 versus 2 patients. When assessed from literature review (where patient subtype is not always specified), the proportion of patients experiencing disturbance with TCA usage is approximately 9%, whereas for MAOIs it varies from 11% to 27%, depending on type of MAOI. However, in several double-blind analyses where patient subtype was specified, rates of 30–60% have been reported for bipolar patients for both treatment and prophylactic studies of TCAs and for treatment studies of MAOIs.

Although the relevance of DA-agonist induction of hypomanic/manic behavioral disturbance to BFS function seems clear, TCA and MAOI effects require explanation. In the case of some TCAs (desipramine and iprindole but not fluoxetine), long-term (15 days) but not short-term (1 to 2 days) treatment enhanced DA-mediated behaviors in rats, such as amphetamine-induced LA (if moderate doses are used; Spyraki & Fibiger, 1981) and intracranial self-stimulation rate–intensity function from the VTA A10 region (a DA-mediated behavior) (Fibiger & Phillips, 1981). Neither amphetamine- nor apomorphine-induced stereotypy was enhanced by chronic TCA (Spyraki & Fibiger, 1981), suggesting that *chronic TCA administration affects the functional properties of the mesolimbic, but not the striatal, DA system.* Interestingly, electroconvulsive shock (ECS) also enhances amphetamine- and apomorphine-induced LA in rats (Fink, 1984).

Also possibly reflecting BFS instability are effects of the cholinesterase (the degrading enzyme of acetylcholine [ACh] in the synapse) inhibitor physostigmine, which has antimanic properties in some manic patients, especially those without a strong irritable–hostile component (reviewed by Risch & Janowsky, 1984). (This strategy is based on the notion that ACh and DA oppose each other in modulating motor behavior and possibly affect, so promotion or inhibition of ACh may reduce manic or increase depressive behavior, respectively.) Centrally active physostigmine has induced depressive symptoms in a subgroup of manic patients and in a majority of remitted bipolar patients on lithium, as well as rebound hypermania in a limited number of severe manics. Except for very small subgroups, normal and psychiatric controls do not manifest depressive symptoms, but rather show an anergic syndrome that can be antagonized in normal subjects by methylphenidate administration. If physostigmine-induced depression in manic patients is mediated primarily by inhibitory cholinergic effects in the NAS, rather than in the striatal system and cerebellar tracts, then the cholinergic data are of interest with respect to BFS regulation.

Although responses to amphetamine vary widely in normal controls, most frequently subjects experience elevated mood and arousal in a dose-related manner, affective lability and irritability, insomnia, and increased LA, speech rate, thoughts, and energy (Silverstone, 1985), all of which can be attenuated by pimozide (a DA postsynaptic receptor blocker) administration (Silverstone, 1985). Induction of hypomanic/ manic disturbance, however, has not been reported. Moreover, cholinergic activation induces an anergic syndrome in normal subjects, but only rarely a depressed state. Thus, DA and ACh challenges to behavioral regulation appear to set in motion a dynamic process that leads to either activation or inhibition of engagement in normal subjects, depending on the type of challenge.

As noted by others (Risch & Janowsky, 1984), bipolar patients show a qualitatively similar but quantitatively exaggerated behavioral response to these challenges, where the functional process set in motion may proceed until an extreme behavioral state opposite from the prechallenge level is achieved. This may indicate, as suggested by others (Mandell, Knapp, Ehlers, & Russo, 1984; Sitiram, Gillin, & Bunney, 1984), that behavior is inadequately regulated in bipolar disorders, and that this problem is most likely to become manifest under conditions of internal or external regulatory challenge. Concordantly, noting that lithium reduces behavioral instability in remitted bipolar patients, Mandell and colleagues (1984) demonstrated at both enzymatic and *behavioral* levels that one basic effect of lithium is to increase regulatory stability of variables. We suggest the possibility, particularly on the basis of the clinical DA-challenge and TCA studies and the animal TCA–DA interaction literature, that the inadequate regulation observed in bipolar disorder may be located in the BFS.

Overall, then, in comparison to normal controls, bipolar patients demonstrate qualitatively similar but quantitatively exaggerated BFS responsivity when functional activity in their DA system is challenged by either enhancement or antagonism (Depue & Iacono, 1989). Together with their naturally occurring fluctuation in extreme states of affective symptomatology, this biological characteristic suggests that bipolar patients possess a vulnerability to episodes of extreme engagement or disengagement (dysregulation) of DA-modulated processes within the BFS. Thus, a dimension of BFS regulatory strength may be conceptualized as independent of trait levels of BFS responsivity, as dysregulation of BFS activity may presumably occur at any trait level. With the introduction of a dysregulation threshold at the extreme, weak end of the regulatory strength dimension, the full neurobehavioral model of bipolar disorder emerges (see also Depue et al., 1987). The dysregulation threshold is displayed schematically in Figure 5.11, which also illustrates the manner in which BFS regulatory strength can vary independently while the level of traitwise BFS responsivity remains fixed. It should be emphasized that the positions along the regulatory dimension in Figure 5.11 represent the range of variation across, not within, individuals; that is, the strength of BFS regulation is itself a stable, traitlike characteristic. As Tellegen and Waller (1992) noted, this model may be viewed as incorporating two basic parameters of interindividual measurement with respect to a dimensional personality trait, namely, the relative level and the relative consistency of trait expression (also referred to as *traitedness*). Accordingly, the model departs from the domain of normal personality only in that it includes a dysregulation threshold to account for distinctly pathological trait expression within the BFS system.

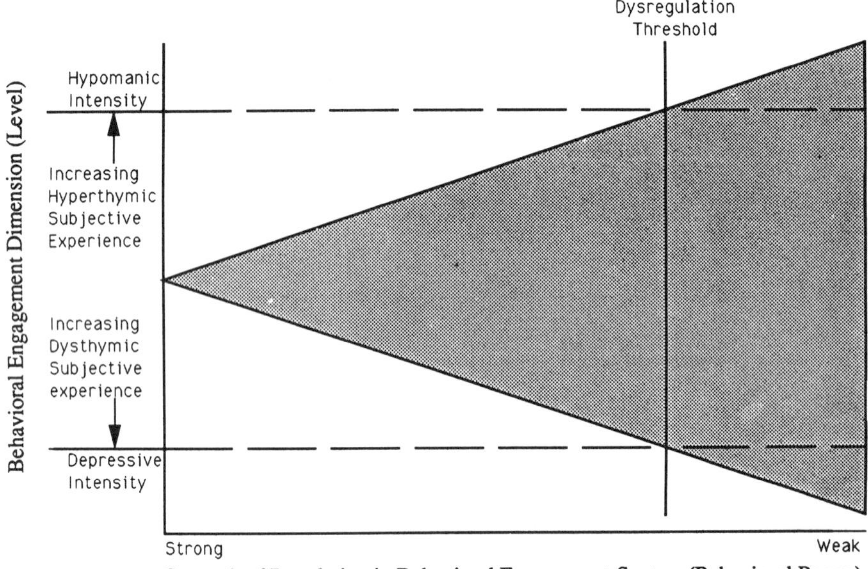

Strength of Regulation in Behavioral Engagement System (Behavioral Range)

FIGURE 5.11. Schematic model of one form of bipolar affective disorder. Bipolar disorder is hypothesized to occur at the weak end of a trait dimension of regulatory strength in the behavioral facilitation system. Disorder is hypothesized to occur when the system's regulatory strength is so weak that a dysregulation threshold is approached or surpassed. See text for details. From "A Two-Dimensional Treshold Model of Seasonal Bipolar Affective Disorder" by R. A. Depue, S. Krauss, and M. R. Spoont, 1987. In D. Magnusson and A. Ohman (Eds.), *Psychopathology: An Interactional Perspective* (p. 115). New York: Academic Press. Copyright 1987 by Academic Press, Inc. Reprinted by permission.

BFS Trait Level and Modification of Clinical Course in Affective Disorders

Whereas the last model suggests that vulnerability to bipolar disorder may be related to the level of BFS regulatory strength, the associated trait level of BFS responsivity may be a primary determinant of clinical course (Depue et al., 1987). In other words, a bipolar patient's traitwise BFS responsivity may determine which extreme of BFS state level is experienced most intensely at times of dysregulation. As shown in Figure 5.12, in which the strength of BFS regulation is held constant, descending trait levels of BFS responsivity are associated with a stepwise progression toward a predominantly depressive course of illness. For instance, individuals beyond the dysregulation threshold who have low trait levels of BFS responsivity would experience reductions of BFS activity during dysregulation as intense depression, whereas their experience of dysregulated increases in BFS activity would rarely, if ever, exceed the subjec-

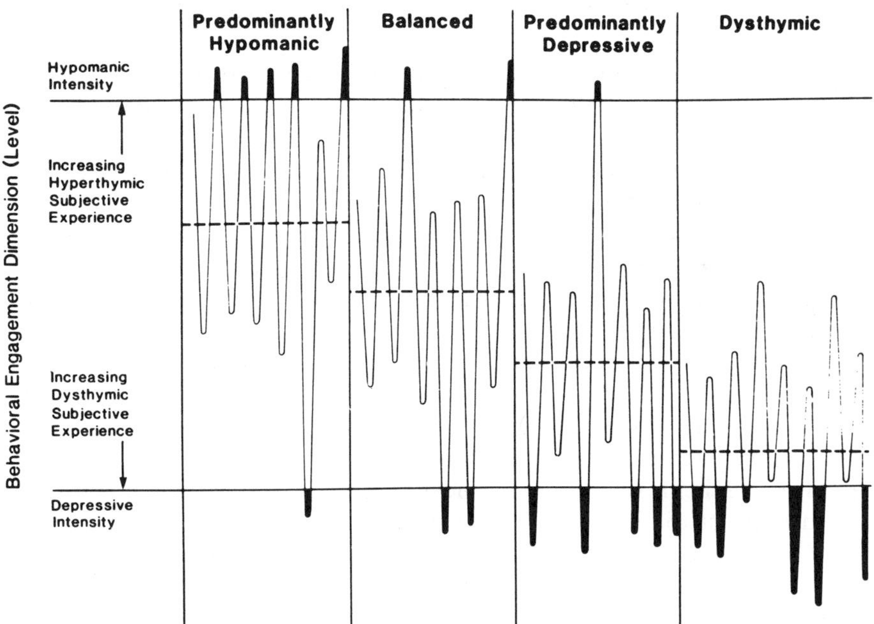

FIGURE 5.12. Variation in the predominant phenotypic picture of clinical course as a function of trait level in the behavioral facilitation system. See text for discussion. From "A Two-Dimensional Threshold Model of Seasonal Bipolar Affective Disorder" by R. A. Depue, S. Krauss, and M. R. Spoont, 1987. In D. Magnusson and A. Ohman (Eds.), *Psychopathology: An Interactional Perspective* (p. 117). New York: Academic Press. Copyright 1987 by Academic Press, Inc. Reprinted by permission.

tive intensity of normal positive emotionality or engagement. Indeed, dysthymics and chronically depressed unipolar depressives often describe their normal states of positive emotionality as "high" mood periods. Concordant with this hypothesis, we have recently found that MPQ PE, but not MPQ NE or C, correlates positively and significantly with the ratio (frequency) of hypomanic:depressive episodes in unipolar and bipolar affective disorder patients (Depue, Kraus, Spoont, & Arbisi, 1989).

Vulnerability to Disorders of Affect

As we outlined previously (Collins & Depue, 1992), the entirety of the above discussion suggests that vulnerability to disorders of affect, based on the DA neurotransmitter system, incorporates at least two variables that, no doubt, interact in complex ways. These variables can be represented in the following, oversimplistic model:

$$\text{vulnerability} = f(\text{DA trait level} + \text{DA regulatory strength})$$

The probability, type (characterological, unipolar, bipolar), and predominant course of affective disorder would depend on the value of these two variables. DA trait level presumably reflects, in part, genotype driven DA cell number, but it can be estimated by reactivity of the DA system to agonist challenge, as in the DA–MPQ PE study described previously. It is of particular importance with respect to depressive disorders that Davis and colleagues (1988) found in a multicenter study of NE, DA, and 5HT in a range of depressive conditions that a reduced DA level was the most significant, and most consistent, neurotransmitter deviation observed. Considering the second term in the model, DA regulatory strength needs validation as a construct, but variance, peak, and recovery rate of DA levels under agonist challenge conditions may be a place to begin this validation. Treatment of these biological variables within a multiple prediction scheme may provide a host of interesting relations. As more is learned about the interaction of these variables, more complex models may be entertained. For instance, other neurotransmitter (e.g., serotonin, which modulates DA activity) and enzyme (e.g., activity level of monoamine oxidase, which influences the degradation rate and storage levels of neurotransmitters) systems will undoubtedly modify vulnerability via their effect on the functional properties of DA (Depue & Iacono, 1989). Of course, what is missing from this model are environmental factors that interact with biological predispositions. It is our hope that this discussion of encoding of environmental influences in the brain will stimulate environmental research that moves beyond the epidemiological strategy of life events studies.

SEROTONIN, BEHAVIORAL STABILITY, AND DISORDERS OF AFFECT, IMPULSE CONTROL, AND MOTOR ACTIVITY

Anatomical Features of Ascending Serotonergic Projections

Of the nine serotonin (5HT) cell groups (labeled B1–B9), the median or central (MR or B8) and dorsal (DR or B7) raphe groups comprise approximately 80% of forebrain 5HT (Azmitia, 1978). The DR has at least five ascending tracts that densely innervate (1) limbic forebrain structures, such as the amygdala, NAS, olfactory cortex, cingulate cortex, hippocampus, and lateral and medial septum involved in emotional responding; (2) basal ganglia areas, such as the caudate, putamen, and globus pallidus involved in the integration of many aspects of the sensory environment and motor programming; (3) cortical lobes, including temporal, parietal, occipital, frontal, and prefrontal, involved in higher levels of information processing; (4) hypothalamic nuclei, such as the median eminence involved in endocrine control; and (5), along with the MR, thalamic nuclei, such as the nonspecific nuclei that serve as a diffuse system that projects broadly to CNS tissue to modulate arousal and sleep.

The MR provides two major ascending projections to (1) medial structures of the forebrain, including the hippocampus, medial septum, and cingulate cortex; and (2) the lateral hypothalamus, which is the major region involved in activating autonomic emotional responding.

Although 5HT innervates all cortical layers, with respect to cortical lobes, 5HT preferentially innervates sensory regions, especially primary visual and auditory cortical fields, but also provides intermediately dense innervation of primary somatosensory areas. In the primary sensory regions, the densest laminar distribution of 5HT is in layer IV (Azmitia & Gannon, 1986; Morrison, Foote, Molliver, Bloom, & Lidov, 1982), which is the layer in which sensory information from specific thalamic nuclei inputs the cortex. Thus, 5HT apparently plays an important role in modulating sensory input to the cortex.

Other anatomical features of ascending 5HT neurons suggest a tonic influence on the flow of information in the brain, an influence that, in most instances, appears to be inhibitory in nature. The 5HT terminals provide a widespread, diffuse pattern of innervation in the brain, and, in many cases, there is a lack of classical synapses (Tork, 1990). This pattern of innervation is more in keeping with a modulatory than a mediating role. Moreover, 5HT neurons display slow regular firing, have a long latency of exerting postsynaptic effects, have a long temporal postsynaptic effect, and manifest nonspecific changes in unit activity to a variety of afferent inputs arising from the cortex and limbic, reticular, motor, and arousal structures (Azmitia, 1978). Thus, the 5HT signal appears to be a tonic one that lacks differentiation as to the information being conveyed.

Behavioral Effects of Manipulations of Serotonin Neurotransmission

Behavioral neurobiology research with animals has demonstrated repeatedly that 5HT provides a tonic inhibitory influence over DA facilitatory effects. Hence, use of 5HT antagonists that block 5HT's inhibitory influence releases and potentiates DA's facilitation of emotional and motor behavior. Conversely, 5HT agonists tend to increase 5HT's inhibitory influence over DA facilitation. It is important to realize, however, that the effects of 5HT manipulation are usually most dramatically observed in studies that concurrently activate DA facilitation with a DA agonist. In any case, as illustrated by the following brief review, the effects of 5HT manipulation are significant for a diverse set of emotional and motor behaviors. The following review relies on several recent reviews to which the interested reader is referred for details (Depue, in press; Depue & Spoont, 1986; Soubrie, 1986; Spoont, in press).

Initiation of Locomotor Activity (LA)

As reviewed previously a vast literature indicates that DA plays a major role in the initiation of LA via its release from VTA projections to the NAS. There is also a large body of evidence indicating that increases in 5HT activity inhibit, whereas decreased activity potentiates, LA. Although the data are inconsistent with some forms of 5HT manipulation when *spontaneous* LA is assessed, consistency is much enhanced when the 5HT manipulation is complimented by the use of the DA agonists amphetamine (particularly in lower doses) or apomorphine. Also, the duration of the apomorphine effect on LA was found to be inversely related to increases in brain 5HT. By contrast, amphetamine- or apomorphine-induced LA is potentiated when decreased availability of 5HT is achieved by use of electrolytic lesions of the raphe nuclei, tryptophan-free diets, para-chlorophenylalanine (PCPA, which blocks synthesis of serotonin), 5HT anatagonists, or 5HT neurotoxic compounds. Importantly, 5HT injections directly into the NAS significantly attenuate or totally abolish DA-stimulated activity, which suggests that the 5HT input may be downstream from the DA synapse. Thus, overall, it appears that 5HT plays an inhibitory interactive role with DA in the NAS in the modulation of LA. The significance of these observations is that LA represents the strongest marker of the BFS (and of incentive motivational states in general), and its disinhibition by reduced 5HT activity provides a powerful conceptual model for the behavioral effects of 5HT.

Exploratory Activity

Responses to novelty are rather complex, because novel stimuli induce two conflicting inherent behavioral tendencies. From a temporal perspective, novelty first induces neophobia, which seems beneficial from a survival point of view, and this effect is followed, if no threat is detected, by activation of the BFS (e.g., incentive motivation and forward locomotion). Thus, response to novelty may be seen as reflecting a balance between approach and constraint, and this balance depends upon the properties inherent in the stimulus context and on the state and traits of the individual. Both DA activation and high trait levels of DA cells in the VTA reliably facilitate spontaneous exploratory behavior, perhaps by mediating incentive motivation (Depue & Iacono, 1989; Depue & Spoont, 1986). Conversely, both pharmacological enhancement of 5HT and intraamygdala injections of 5HT inhibit DA-stimulated exploration.

Response to Reward and Punishment

Reward responding in the absence of punishment is best observed when the DA system is concurrently stimulated. Although 5HT antagonism facilitates reward responding in an amphetamine dose-dependent manner—that is, there is a reduced threshold for responding to lower doses of amphetamine—5HT agonists inhibit amphetamine-stimulated intracranial self-stimulation (ICSS). In addition, 5HT antagonism increases resistance to extinction, especially during the first number of trials when reward is still anticipated. This has been interpreted as an effect of increased DA responsivity that occurs to the conditioned incentive cues in the environment during the early extinction phase (Beninger, 1983).

When both reward and punishment are introduced, as in a conflict task, the effects of 5HT manipulation are particularly strong. Several methods of decreasing 5HT functioning are associated with a release of suppression of reward responding to punishment, whereas 5HT agonists attenuate the release from punishment-induced suppression. Particularly in 5HT antagonist conditions, results are dramatic: Although control animals maintain the normally increased sensitivity to punishment relative to reward, "low"-5HT animals appear to overrespond to reward. That is, the low-5HT animals appear to be engaged in impulsive behavior that is insensitive to aversive characteristics of the environment.

Stimulus Reactivity

In primates and humans, 5HT innervation of the primary sensory receptive areas of the cortex and of visual nuclei of the thalamus is extensive, and, as noted before, is densest in layers IV a and c, where thalamic input of sensory information is targeted. Thus, it can be supposed that 5HT plays a major role in modulating sensory input to the cortex. This modulation, however, does not appear to be strongly phasic or specific, in that dorsal raphe cells do not differentiate between auditory and visual input. Moreover, these cells do not habituate to sensory signals and have a long response latency. Therefore, raphe cells apparently do not respond directly to sensory stimuli.

There are, nevertheless, several indications that 5HT plays a crucial role in stimulus reactivity. For instance, 5HT exerts a tonic inhibitory influence on (1) sensitization to auditory and tactile startle stimuli, (2) nociceptive sensitivity, and (3) escape latencies following periaqueductal gray stimulation. Thus, in animals and humans, lowered 5HT functioning has been associated with increased startle and increased pain sensitivity. Indeed, investigators have consistently noted an exaggerated reactivity in animals and humans with low 5HT functioning to all forms of stimulation, even stimulation of relatively low intensity. It is as if the individual has exquisite sensitivity to sensory input and finds this sensitivity to be aversive.

There are at least two major ways in which stimulus reactivity may be modulated by 5HT. First, extensive innervation of sensory receptive areas of the cortex and of specific sensory nuclei of the thalamus modulates stimulus intensity and controls sensory overload. Second, increased dorsal and median raphe activity has been found to result in reduced refractoriness of neural tissue to subsequent stressful stimuli for several hours. This effect appears to be due to a complicated negative feedback system during stress that incorporates 5HT as a critical component. Stress-induced release of cortisol results in increased cortisol binding in the hippocampus and amygdala. The hippocampal cortisol binding activates a pathway to the dorsal raphe and results in a 150% increase of dorsal raphe activity. The increased raphe activity has at least two important effects in this context: (1) The dorsal raphe pathway to the hypothalamus is activated, resulting in inhibition of corticotropic releasing factor (which normally initiates an increase in cortisol) and hence in reduction of cortisol release; and (2) the dorsal and median raphe pathways to the diffuse activation system of the thalamus, which is involved in modulating arousal and sleep, are activated. Both this latter system of controlling cortical arousal, as well as the 5HT inhibitory modulation of sensory input to the cortex, may relate, in part, to Pavlovian notions of protective inhibition, which play an important part in Eysenck's discussion of personality structure.

Aggression

One of the most pronounced effects of reduced 5HT functioning is increased aggression in animals, and again this is most evident under conditions of concurrent DA stimulation. DA activation shows a dose-dependent facilitation of irritable (goalless) and defensive aggression, and 5HT agonists suppress, whereas 5HT antagonists enhance, this DA effect dramatically. A large part of this 5HT modulation of aggression may occur via 5HT projections to the amygdala. Injections of 5HT antagonists into the amygdala facilitate affective aggression, whereas injection of 5HT agonists into the amygdala inhibits several forms of aggression. These 5HT effects may be exerted via dorsal raphe 5HT projections to the central and median nuclei of the amygdala, which represent the major 5HT input to these nuclei. Both the median and central nuclei are the major output nuclei of the amygdala through which emotional behavior (hormonal, autonomic, facial, and motor components), including aggression, is activated.

Emotional Reactivity

An implication of 5HT modulation in the amygdala is that the level of 5HT inhibitory modulation activity may affect the ease with which, threshold by which, DA facilitates emotional responding in general. Indeed, low 5HT animals are consistently described as emotionally hyperreactive or emotionally labile to most incentive–reward stimuli.

A Functional Principle of Serotonin

In practically every case where DA facilitates the flow of neural information, 5HT appears to modulate that facilitation in an inhibitory manner, an inhibitory effect that is usually tonic in nature. One way to conceptualize this influence is to view 5HT as a component of neural homeostasis, where 5HT raises a tonic threshold to signals both entering and exiting a neural circuit (Spoont, in press). Whereas DA facilitates entry and exit of neural information, 5HT raises a threshold or gate to DA's facilitatory influence. This threshold would be tonic in nature, but slowly modulated up or down as a function of environmental conditions. Thus, the low-5HT animal could be viewed as one that has a low threshold to the facilitation of neural processing or, in behavioral terms, of emotional responding, whereas the high–5HT animal would require a much stronger stimulus input to overide the higher threshold and thus elicit an emotional response. The low 5HT animal would appear emotionally labile, whereas the very-high-5HT animal may appear inflexible or as being characterized by behavioral rigidity in environmental circumstances that require modification of the ongoing behavioral program. Because 5HT appears to influence the ease of behavioral facilitation, 5HT may relate to a dimension of behavioral stability. Low 5HT would be associated with emotional instability, that is, facilitation of emotional responding under minimal intensity or even inappropriate stimulus conditions in which the cost of responding to reward is actually greater than nonresponding (i.e., a conflict situation). Then again, high 5HT would be associated with high emotional stability to the point of emotional flatness, or of emotional rigidity at the extreme.

A threshold model of 5HT with respect to emotional responding is illustrated in Figure 5.13. Down the left column in the figure are the various stimuli that induce emotional responding. The central column shows the nature of the fixed-affect patterns or emotional feelings associated with these stimuli, where the magnitude of the feelings elicited varies as a function of the biological sensitivity of the specific emotional system. Note that the resulting feelings to certain stimulus inputs depend

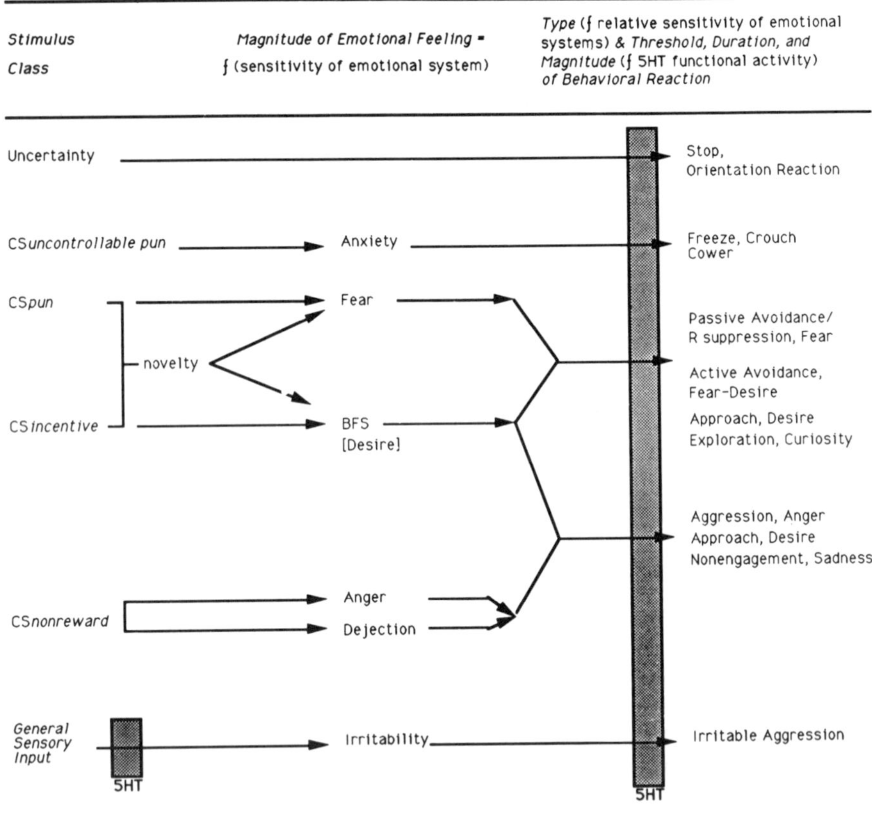

FIGURE 5.13. Model of how serotonin (5HT) provides a threshold (shaded vertical bar on right side of figure) for facilitation of responses across several emotional systems. See text for discussion.

in most cases on the balance between the strengths of at least two emotional systems. Thus, novelty will eventually elicit a predominant subjective response of fear or desire, depending upon the relative strength of the
BFS and the fear system. Also, nonreward may elicit frustration and anger
versus dejection and sadness, depending on the relative sensitivity of
those emotional systems to conditioned stimuli of nonreward. The ease
with which overt and biological emotional responses are facilitated,
largely through output from the amygdala, can be seen as a balance
between DA facilitation and a 5HT threshold for facilitation, the latter
threshold being represented by the shaded vertical bar toward the right of
the figure. At the right of the figure, the type of overt emotional behavioral response is indicated. The ease with which an individual expresses
emotional responses and the extent to which emotional responding alternates between different behavioral responses (lability) comprise, along
with strength of DA facilitation, the basic aspects of emotional stability or
of a 5HT behavioral trait.

Low Serotonin Activity and Behavioral Instability in Humans

The benefit of the preceding model of a 5HT behavioral trait based on
animal research is that clear predictions about 5HT's modulation of
human behavior are possible. Most animal behavioral research has focused on the effects of reduced 5HT conditions, which is fortunate
because there is a growing, impressive literature on the behavioral correlates of reduced 5HT in humana. With respect to human behavior, one
might expect the occurrence of behavioral conditions that reflect several
basic effects of low 5HT:

1. *Emotional instability:* A 5HT-produced low threshold for emotional expression should result in (1) easier elicitation of an emotional
response by a relatively low intensity stimulus, (2) an increased magnitude of the emotional response due to more slowly engaged negative
feedback mechanisms, and (3) emotional lability, that is, an increased
propensity to experience a variety of emotions per unit time; this would
reflect a reduced threshold to emotion–eliciting stimuli gaining access to,
and coming to dominate, output neural circuits, even when the circuits
are currently engaged in expression of another emotional response.

Emotions that are accompanied by strong BFS (and DA) activity as a
means of supporting the behavioral components of the emotional pattern
may be expressed with particularly high frequency and intensity. For
instance, this would be true of *affective aggression,* which is strongly
enhanced by DA administration (Valzelli, 1981). Affective aggression is a
goal-oriented response pattern that follows many principles of reward-

elicited behavior. An attack program must be facilitated in order to be effective. Therefore, it may be expected that low 5HT conditions in humans as in animals, are accompanied by a history of frequent, intense affective aggression and impulsive assault.

2. Exaggerated response to stimulus conditions eliciting DA facititation: A 5HT-produced low threshold to DA facilitation of behavior (i.e., to BFS reactivity) should result in an exaggerated response to stimulus conditions of incentive reward. If the animal literature can be taken as a model here, this exaggeration should be greatest in conflict situations that can be resolved by engaging the reward option or by actively avoiding punishment by engaging the reward of safety. The effects of this condition are at least fourfold:

a. The person's sensitivity to current reward stimuli would be greater than his or her sensitivity to (1) imagined, expected future rewards and (2) future, potential aversive outcomes (i.e., future punishment). This would seem devastating for adult levels of behavior, because it implies that the human ability to guide extensively delayed, long-term behavior programs, such as obtaining a degree at the end of completing 4 years of college, by repeatedly bringing and holding on-line rewarding expected outcomes of the program and aversive expected outcomes if the program is not followed, is compromised. Behavior would be oriented to chasing short-term rewards at the expense of achieving more enduring life goals.

b. An increased reactivity to the reward of safety—or in daily life circumstances, sanctuary from stress and conflict—may become manifest as strong active avoidance. When the conflict is intense, and no other means of dealing with it are apparent, active avoidance may be engaged in rather impulsively, as a means of gaining relief. Therefore, low 5HT conditions in humans may be associated with active avoidance at its most tragic level, *suicidal behavior.*

c. The combination of overreactivity to reward and of performance of active avoidance when conflict becomes unbearable suggests that low-5HT conditions in humana may be characterized by a general tendency to *impulsive behavior,* that is, a propensity to respond to reward when withholding or delaying a response may produce a more favorable long-term outcome.

d. A low-5HT condition may be accompanied by frequent, varied attempts to experience the increased magnitude and frequency of DA facilitation, or, rather, DA-related incentive reward. Thus, it may be expected that use and *abuse of DA-activating agents* would be a strong correlate of low-5HT conditions. This has been found to be the case in animal research (Depue & Spoont, 1986; Spoont, in press), where there is increased self-administration of DA-active drugs and an increased preference and tolerance for alcohol, whose initial incentive effects are due to increased DA release (Depue & Iacono, 1989).

3. *Irritability–hypersensitivity:* Low-5HT animals are excessively irritable to any environmental perturbation. They are described as hypersensitive and hyperreactive to stimulation in several sensory modalities, including tactile, auditory, and visual. As noted before, this may be due, in part, to reduced sensory modulation at several levels of the brain, as well as to reduced MR inhibition of the lateral hypothalamic region that activates autonomic reactivity under stressful conditions. Thus, one can expect irritability to be a central feature of low-5HT conditions in humans.

Research Findings on Low Serotonin Function in Humans

Most of the predictions from the animal research on low 5HT functioning appear to hold in humans as well. This work began with Brown's inventive studies on military recruits who had committed aggressive acts that led to discharge (Brown, Goodwin, & Ballenger, 1979; Brown, Ebert, & Goyer, 1982). Brown found that most of these men had personality disorders characterized by emotional instability and impulsivity, including impulsive, explosive, borderline, and antisocial personality disorders. That is, they had what now would be referred to as the unstable group of personality disorders. Quantitative estimates of aggressive life history derived from interview correlated highly ($-.78$) with the major metabolite of 5HT measured in CSF, CSF-5HIAA, as did the Minnesota Multiphasic Personality Inventiry (MMPI) psychopathic deviancy (Pd) scale ($-.77$). Other patterns of correlation among different scales helped to define the trait underlying the 5HT–aggression association. The aggressive life history index correlated highly with the overall Buss-Durkee Aggression Inventory (BDAI, .77), whereas the Pd scale correlated with the life history index only .57. Thus, whereas both the BDAI and Pd measures each contain a domain related to 5HT functioning, these domains may not be identical. Interestingly, the Pd scale does not relate significantly to the behavioral aggression subscale of the BDAI, but it does relate (.64) to the irritability subscale, indicating that irritable aggression may be accounting for the Pd–5HIAA correlation.

Numerous studies have since documented a strong relation between irritable, assaultive aggression and various indicators of low 5HT. For instance, in one of the most carefully performed investigations, Coccaro, Sirver, and Klar (1989) found that the maximum increase in prolactin stimulated by the 5HT agonist fenfluramine was most highly correlated with the irritability + assault scales of the BDAI ($-.77$), particularly in patients with unstable types of personality disorders, including border-line disorder. This confirms previous work showing that reduced levels of CSF-5HIAA are inversely related to impulsive violence (Linnoila, Virkkunen, & Scheinin, 1983), impulsive homicide (Lidberg, Tuck, & Asberg, 1985), impulsive arson (Virkkunen, Nuutila, & Goodwin, 1987), and outwardly directed hostility, as well as Eysenck's Psychoticism scale, in normal volunteers (Asberg, Schalling, & Traskman-Bendy, 1987; Coccaro et al., 1989; Roy, Adinoff, & Linnoila, 1988). Moreover, a 2-year prospective follow-up study of children and adolescents with disruptive behavior disorders at time 1 found that baseline CSF-5HIAA significantly predicted severity of physical aggression during follow-up (Kruesi et al., 1992). In addition, a significant inverse correlation between CSF-5HIAA and ranking of aggression was found for rhesus monkeys in their natural habitat (Higley et al., 1992). Thus, one of the strongest, most consistent findings in the human behavioral neurobiology area is between aggression of an impulsive type, rather than planned or attitudinal hos-tility forms, and reduced 5HT functioning.

Low indices of 5HT functioning have also been robustly related to suicidal behavior (including both attempters and completers) (Asberg et al., 1987; Brown, Goodwin, & Ballenger, 1979; Brown et al., 1982, 1985; Mann, Stanley, & McBride, 1986; Meltzer & Lowy, 1987; Stanley & Mann, 1986). Reduced 5HT in this case does not appear to be a marker of depressed state, depressive disorder, or suicide in general. It is particularly related to what is referred to as "violent" suicidal behavior, where the means of suicide include jumping off high places, gunshot, stabbing, gas poisoning, and multiple longitudinal wrist cuts (as opposed to drug overdose). This appears to be an impulsive suicidal behavior in that, on Beck's suicide scale, the only difference between high and low CSF-5HIAA suicide attempters (besides violence of method) was that the latter had a shorter period of planning for the attempt (Asberg et al., 1987). The relation of suicidal behavior and low 5HT functioning appears to be unrelated to type of psychopathology, having been found for depression, nondepressed schizophrenics, nondepressed alcoholics and personality disorder subjects, obsessive compulsive patients, schi-zoaffective subjects, and anxiety disorders (Asberg et al., 1987; Ballen-ger, Goodwin, & Major, 1979; Brown et al., 1982; Traskman, Asberg, & Bertilsson, 1981, 1984; van Praag, 1984, 1986). When reduced 5HT has been related to depression, it appears to bear a closer, inverse relation to frequency of episode as opposed to depressive disorder per se (van Praag, 1984, 1986).

It is likely that suicidal behavior and impulsive aggression represent two different indicators of a central (behavioral and biochemical) trait, such as a low threshold for emotional behavior (Depue & Spoont, 1986). This is supported by the fact that both indicators often cooccur, and by the fact that this cooccurrence is associated with the most extreme quantitative values of the trait (i.e., the lowest CSF–5HIAA values) (Brown et al., 1982; Linnoila et al., 1983). Moreover, other forms of disorder appear to be associated with reduced 5HT functioning, and these have a high incentive–reward sensitivity component. For instance, there is initial evidence that so-called type B alcoholics (Babor et al., 1992), which is characterized by childhood risk factors, early onset of alcohol-related problems, polydrug use, a more chronic treatment history, greater psychopathological dysfunction, and poorer treatment outcome, have reduced 5HT functioning that may serve as a vulnerability factor (Cloninger, 1987).

Although reduced 5HT functioning appears to be related, in general, to instability of emotional behavior and, formally, to the unstable group of personality disorders, the phenotype of the unstable personality disorders varies substantially. This may be due to other modifying traits that contribute to the behavioral profile. One such trait may be level of DA activity or, behaviorally, level of facilitation to incentive reward. For instance, the depressive patients that have a history of suicidal behavior, often referred to historically as *neurotic depression,* display not only reduced 5HT functioning but also reduced CSF and urinary levels of the major DA metabolite, HVA, when depressed (Roy, Pickar, & Linnoila, 1985; Roy, Karoum, & Pollack, 1992; Traskman et al., 1981) and at 5-year follow-up (Roy, DeLong, & Linnoila, 1989). However, it seems more difficult to imagine that other forms of unstable personality disorders would also have low HVA accompanying low 5HT, such as histrionic and antisocial personality disorders. It may be that the phenotype of unstable behavioral conditions associated with low 5HT varies depending on level of DA activity trait levels.

This speculative, but completely testable, suggestion is illustrated in Figure 5.14, where a stability behavioral trait associated with 5HT functioning is shown in interaction with a facilitation behavioral trait associated with DA functioning. Whereas level of 5HT functioning is related to degree of instability of emotional behavior, level of DA functioning is related to affective valence of the behavioral profile, ranging from dysthymia, through euthymia, to hyperthymia. One might predict that suicidal behavior is observed with similar frequency along the dimension of DA facilitation (although the impulsiveness of the attempt may increase with higher levels of DA); it may be that level of impulsive aggression increases with higher levels of DA, whereas persistence of depressed affect (dysphoria, dysthymia) increases as DA levels decrease.

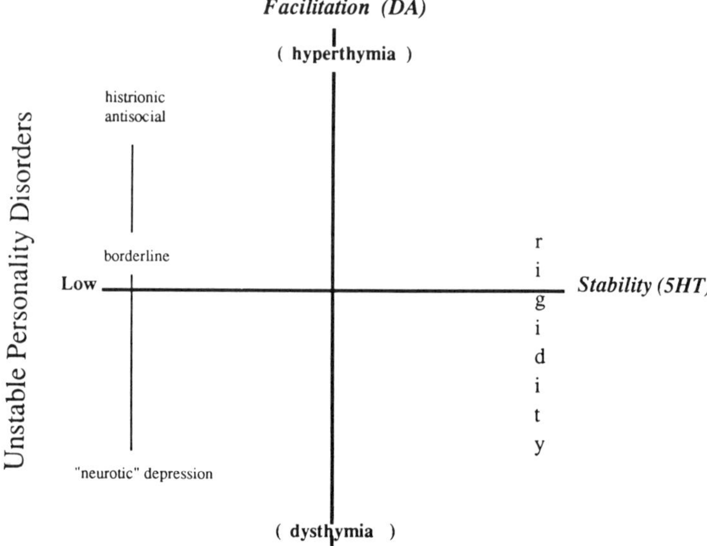

FIGURE 5.14. Illustration of the interaction of serotonin (5HT, stability) and dopamine (DA, facilitation) behavioral traits as contributors to the phenotype of different forms of unstable personality disorders. See text for discussion.

A Potentially Interactive Role for Serotonin in Obsessive–Compulsive Disorder

Dysfunction of a neurobehavioral network may arise from abnormalities in the structures involved in the network, from aberrant input to the network, or from extreme levels of the neurotransmitters that modulate the flow of information through the network. Because of the multiple levels (and often iterative pathways) of processing within a neural system and the inherent regulatory adaptation of neurotransmitter systems, a subtle, localized dysfunction in one component of a network may result in only minimal behavioral effects. However, extreme levels of neurotransmitter functioning due to environmental challenge, extreme trait values, or inherent regulatory weakness may permit or exacerbate the expression of the dysfunction throughout the entire neurobehavioral network. In such instances, the etiology of a disorder may be conceptualized along multiple interacting dimensions. Obsessive–compulsive disorder (OCD) is presented as a potential example of how altered values of a neurotransmitter (i.e., 5HT) may produce behavioral pathology by uncovering or exacerbating a dysfunctional neurobehavioral network.

Phenomenological accounts of OCD frequently focus on the role of intrusive thoughts (Rachman & Hodgson, 1980; Salkovskis, 1985). These thoughts may consist of images, words, or ideas that are experienced as intrusive and ego alien. It is well substantiated that intrusive thoughts are not unique to OCD, but rather occur regularly within the normal population, especially during negative emotional states (Horowitz, 1975; Parkinson & Rachman, 1981; Sutherland, Newman, & Rachman, 1982). OCD patients differ from normal subjects in the frequency, unacceptability, intensity, and resistance to dismissal of their intrusive thoughts (Rachman & Hodgson, 1980). Thus, the difference between the intrusive thoughts of normal and obsessive–compulsive subjects is apparently dimensional rather than categorical. The perseveration of these thoughts in consciousness (or where they have easy access to conciousness) is particularly distinguishing. It is as if this emotionally valenced information remains stuck on-line in working memory, resisting even extreme attempts to dismiss it. (*Working memory* refers to the process by which information is kept in a state of moment-to-moment awareness and of instant retrievability [Goldman-Rakic, 1990; Baddeley, 1986].)

Perseveration in OCD, however, is not limited to intrusive thoughts. The subjective emotional experience and behavioral impulse that occur in response to these thoughts are also strikingly perseverative. For instance, touching something dirty may result in a behavioral impulse to wash and a subjective feeling of anxiety related to a fear of contamination. The relative strength of the subjective component and the behavioral impulse may vary, depending upon the familiarity with the situation. Especially when well learned, stimuli may directly trigger a behavioral impulse without producing a strong subjective feeling. It is not uncommon for obsessive–compulsive patients to feel compelled to perform a stereotyped ritualized action, but be unable to report why they felt compelled to perform it. Because the goal of an emotional system is to select an adaptive response, it need not fully engage a subjective component when the behavioral set is strong enough to modulate behavior by itself. For example, in animals that have overlearned avoidance of shock, physiological signs of fear may no longer occurr, in spite of maintaining a strong avoidance impulse (Starr & Mineka, 1977). With or without the subjective component of fear, the emotional network utilizes the same output pathways to influence the selection of adaptive behavior. Perhaps by delineating the aspects of the emotional system engaged in holding information on-line, as well as the production of behavioral sets or impulses, it is possible to examine what factors may lead to the perseveration of behavioral impulses in OCD.

Orbital Frontal Cortical Loops and Behavioral Output

The OFC receives both integrated unimodal and multimodal sensory projections, as well as emotional associations based on contemporaneous and past reinforcement histories (Chavis & Pandya, 1976; Jones & Powell, 1970; LeDoux, 1987; Rolls, 1986; Van Hoesen, Pandya, & Butters, 1975). The OFC holds a representation of this sensory and emotional information on-line in working memory (Goldman-Rakic, 1987), and incorporates this information into a larger integrated structure of appetitive and aversive behavioral contingencies abstracted from the ongoing environment. It then actively encodes revised appetitive and aversive behavioral contingencies based on its recent reinforcement history (Rolls, 1986; Thorpe, Rolls, & Maddison, 1983).

OFC lesions leave animals unable to alternate their behavior based on changes in reward contingencies (Butter, 1964, 1969; Butter & Snyder, 1972). In humans, prefrontal lesions that include the OFC produce perseverative errors on the Wisconsin Card Sort, which requires a person to change behavioral set based on reinforcement contingencies (Milner, 1963, 1964). On such tasks, patients with OFC lesions may be able to verbalize the correct rules, but are unable to select the appropriate behavioral set (Milner, 1971; Rolls, 1986). Damage to the OFC also causes socially inappropriate behavior, a lack of behavioral inhibition, and an inability to match affective and motivational responses with environmental situations (Nauta, 1971; Struss & Benson, 1986). In summary, dysfunction of the OFC reduces the ability to modify behavioral sets based on environmental reinforcement contingencies.

The OFC facilitates the selection of appropriate behavioral responses through its extensive efferents to thalamic nuclei and the magnocellular basal forebrain cholinergic projection nuclei (Mesulam & Mufson, 1984). The OFC also contributes significantly to two loops through the basal ganglia. One loop originates from the medial region of the OFC (Walker's area 13 in monkeys and Brodmann's area 13 in humans) and courses through the NAS (see previous discussion). The more lateral aspects of the OFC (area 11 in humans and monkeys), which include the cortex of the inferior convexity (Walker's areas 12), project to the ventromedial caudate nucleus (Alexander, Crutcher, & DeLong, 1990; Alexander, DeLong, & Strick, 1986; Rolls, 1986; Selemon & Goldman-Rakic, 1985; Yeterian & Van Hoesen, 1978). We refer to this orbital–striatal circuit as the lateral OFC loop to emphasize its segregation from the medial orbital frontal circuit. A schematic representation of the lateral OFC loop may be seen in Figure 5.15. It remains difficult to entirely distinguish differential functions of medial and lateral OFC areas. However, neuroanatomical and neurobehavioral evidence suggests that they hold different information on-line in representational memory. Visual information is preferentially directed to the lateral OFC, whereas projections from the amygdala are focused more on the medial OFC. Consistent with their connectivity, lesions of the lateral OFC have been observed to cause a greater decrement in the inhibition of responses in visual discrim-

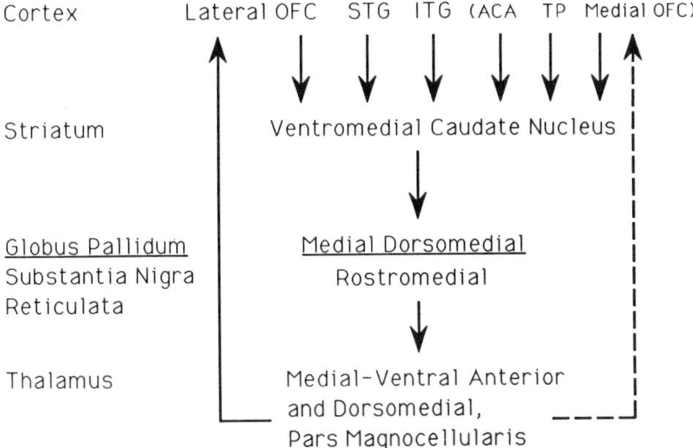

FIGURE 5.15. The components of the *lateral* orbital frontal cortical loop. The superior (STG) and inferior (ITG) temporal gyri and the lateral OFC project to a strip of the ventromedial caudate. A projection from the thalamus returns to the OFC to close the lateral OFC loop. Additional projections from the medial OFC, temporal pole (TP), and anterior cingulate area (ACA) also project to the extreme ventral edge of this region. These projections get focused on the mediodorsal thalamus, which also sends a projection (*dashed line*) to the medial OFC to close the caudate extension of the medial orbital loop.

ination tasks (e.g., go–no go tasks), whereas lesions to area 13 appear to play a greater role in specific extinction deficits and altered emotional and autonomic responses to stimuli (Rosenkilde, 1979; Iversen & Mishkin, 1970; Fuster, 1989).

A ventromedial strip of the caudate nucleus runs from head to tail of the caudate. In addition to lateral OFC projections, the ventromedial caudate receives efferents from the inferior and superior temporal association cortices (Selemon & Goldman-Rakic, 1985; Van Hoesen, Yeterian, & Lavizzo-Mourey, 1981). The anterior cingulate area (ACA), medial OFC, and the temporal pole (TP) also send minor projections into the ventral region of the caudate, but these projections may represent an extension of the medial OFC loop to the NAS. Even though these projections may be highly segregated from the other ventromedial caudate projections, they are structurally similar and equally subject to disruption in the presence of ventromedial caudate pathology. The ACA projection may be of particular relevance to OCD in that it is involved in the outflow of limbic computations to motor regions. Through its projections to the supplementary motor area (as well as the basal ganglia), the ACA helps to determine the readiness to perform a specific motoric act and may also help to specify the intensity of the motor movement (Goldberg, 1985). The ventromedial caudate thus receives integrated information from both sensory association areas and limbic output regions involved in the computation of behavioral contingencies and the readiness to perform motor acts. The ventromedial caudate projects to the internal pallidal segment and the rostromedial substantia nigra (Alexander, Delong, & Strick, 1986; Alexander, Crutcher, & DeLong, 1990). These two areas have efferents to the ventral anterior and dorsomedial nuclei of the thalamus (pars magnocellularis), the latter nuclei project back to the lateral OFC to close the loop.

Limbic and paralimbic areas, such as the amygdala, OFC, and ACA, are not involved in the execution of motor programs per se, but, through their projections to the basal ganglia, they significantly influence the choice and vigor of motor programs. As discussed previously, the medial OFC and VTA DA projections to the NAS may alter the sensitivity of the basal ganglia for facilitating a behavioral response. In contrast, projections to the ventromedial caudate appear to be more involved in the relay of information influencing the striatum's response selection. The head of the caudate nucleus is involved in the utilization of specific sensory cues for the preparation of particular behavioral responses (i.e., stimulus–motor habit formation) (Rolls, Thorpe, & Maddison, 1983; Rolls & Williams, 1987). The striatum thus allows the OFC access to motor patterns that have been paired to the behavioral contingencies that it computes.

Recent models of basal ganglia functioning suggest that response selection is accomplished through a gating process (Schneider, 1987; Seigel, 1987). By gating input, the striatum determines which information to allow access to motor areas. The information allowed through striatal gates triggers or releases stereotyped or modifiable responses (Seigel, 1987). Applying this same process to lateral OFC projections, the striatum may be able to gate which information regarding behavioral contingencies is allowed access to areas involved in the preparation of motor acts.

Experimental lesions of the ventromedial caudate in animals cause perseverative difficulties in which animals lose their ability to make appropriate switches in behavioral set (Divac, Rosvold, & Swarebart, 1967). The animals appear to receive information regarding reinforcement contingencies, but this information does not exert any influence over response selection. Humans with disorders of the basal ganglia, such as Parkinson's and Huntington's, make cognitive errors similar to those seen in humans with OFC lesions. They have particular difficulty on the Wisconsin Card Sort and other tasks that require a change in behavioral set (Seigel, 1987). Even when instructed as to which behavioral set to switch, Parkinson's patients are unable to modulate their behavior appropriately (Flowers & Robertson, 1985).

Because the loops running through the basal ganglia terminate, in part, in the same region from which they originate, there exists a potential for positive feedback to result whenever the circuit is activated. Penney and Young (1983) have proposed that a major role of basal ganglia loops (and positive feedback) is to allow cortical cells to maintain their firing. For instance, if the caudate associates a sensory cue with a motor response, it may then allow this information to be returned to the lateral OFC in order to maintain or update on-line information relevant to the computation of behavioral contingencies. If the relay of this information is disturbed, the lateral OFC may be unable to maintain or update what information it holds on-line, leaving it unable to appropriately select a behavioral set. Thus, lesions at the level of the striatum and pallidum may not only alter the output pathway of the OFC, but also alter the information held on-line and, hence, the computations made in the OFC.

Important to our discussion, without proper damping, positive feedback may evolve into indefinite reverberation of information. In the case of OCD, a positive feedback loop may continue to fire until the circuit is broken by the initiation of behavior or cognition that breaks the loop. Even when the appropriate behavior is activated, the OFC may be too dysregulated by aberrant subcortical feedback to properly encode that it is time to switch the behavioral set. OCD patients will wash their hands raw despite being able to see that their hands are, in fact, clean. The behavioral set or impulse, and possibly even the images or representations related to it, continue unmodulated. This is similar to what is seen with OFC lesions, where the sensory information indicating a change in behavior is received, but there is still an inability to initiate the change.

Neurological Findings in OCD Patients

Positron emission tomography of OCD patients reveals distinct brain regions with abnormal metabolic rates. OCD patients have elevated metabolism bilaterally in the orbital gyri and in the head of caudate nuclei (Baxter et al., 1987, 1988; Benkelfat et al., 1990; Nordahl et al., 1989). The left anterior and posterior putamen (Benkelfat et al., 1990) and the anterior cingulate region (Swedo et al., 1989) may also be abnormally elevated, but this has not been observed consistently. One study observed significantly smaller caudate nuclei bilaterally in OCD patients compared with control subjects, as measured by computerized tomography volumetric analysis (Luxenberg et al., 1988). Similarly, Weilburg and colleagues (1989) have reported a single case study of OCD in a patient with focal atrophy of the left head of the caudate, as revealed by magnetic resonance imaging.

Another line of evidence implicating the basal ganglia in the pathophysiology of OCD is the prevalence of obsessive–compulsive symptoms in the context of other neurological disorders known to involve the striatum. Gilles de la Tourette's syndrome, in which the primary symptoms are uncontrollable motor movements and vocal noises, has a high comorbidity with OCD (Nee, Caine, Polinsky, Eldridge, & Ebert, 1980; Pitman, Green, Jenike & Mesulam, 1987). There is also a high prevalence of OCD in relatives of Tourrette's probands and of tic disorders in the relatives of OCD probands (Pauls, Towbin, Leckman, Zahner, & Cohen, 1986; Pitman et al., 1987). Obsessive–compulsive symptoms have also been noted in cases of Sydenham's chorea (Swedo et al., 1989), in some cases of Parkinson's disease (Marks, 1987), and in patients with basal ganglia lesions caused by encephalopathy or carbon monoxide poisoning (Laplane, Bulac, Widlocher, & Dubois, 1984). On neuropsychological tests, OCD subjects also look similar to patients with OFC and basal ganglia lesions (Cox, Fedio, & Rapoport, 1989).

Although limited by methodological difficulties, further support for the involvement of the OFC and its striatal loops in OCD comes from the literature suggesting an efficacy of psychosurgical treatment of OCD. Surgical ablations of the OFC are associated with decreased obsessive–compulsive symptoms (Corsellis & Jack, 1973; Scoville & Bettis, 1977). A safer and apparently more effective procedure consists of bilateral stereotactic lesions of the anterior internal capsule, which contains the sole pathway between the OFC and the dorsomedial thalamus (Hassler & Dieckman, 1973; Mindus et al., 1987; Rylander, 1979).

A Potential Role of 5HT in the Pathophysiology of OCD

In the neuroanatomical structures that appear to be involved in OCD, 5HT plays a critical modulatory role. Interest in 5HT's role in OCD initially developed because of the antiobsessional effects of 5HT reuptake blockers, regardless of the presence or absence of depression. Clomipramine (Clomipramine Collaborative Study Group, 1991), fluvoxamine (Goodman et al., 1990), and fluoxetine (Pigott et al., 1990; Turner, Jacob, Beidel, & Himmelhoch, 1985) reduce obsessive–compulsive symptoms. All three medications are potent inhibitors of 5HT terminal and 5HT somatodendritic autoreceptors. Other antidepressants that do not specifically affect 5HT reuptake have minimal or no effect on obsessive–compulsive symptoms (Thoren, Asberg, Cronhom, Jornstedt, & Traskman, 1980).

Subsequent to the clinical success of 5HT reuptake inhibitors, several studies of 5HT functioning in untreated OCD patients were undertaken. The level of the major 5HT metabolite 5HIAA in cerebrospinal fluid (CSF) is an indicator of the overall rate of 5HT turnover in the CNS. CSF levels of 5HIAA were found to be 30% higher in OCD patients compared to normals in a small study (Insel, Mueller, Alterman, Linnoila, & Murphy, 1985) and 20% higher (although not statistically significant) in a larger study (Thoren et al., 1980). These early studies fueled speculation that OCD represented the extreme high end of a behavioral inhibition dimension (Insel, Zohar, Benkelfat, & Murphy, 1990). This would be the polar opposite of the impulsivity conditions characterized by low CSF-5HIAA described previously. However, well-controlled studies of CSF-5HIAA in OCD have consistently found no evidence of elevated CSF-5HIAA in adult (Altemus et al., 1992) or child (Swedo et al., 1992) patients. Moreover, theoretical placing of OCD at the low end of an impulsivity dimension does not match the phenomenology of the disorder. It is not that OCD subjects are blocked from acting on their impulses; rather, they have to expend great energy resisting and controlling these impulses. In this regard, their problems are similar to impulse-control disorders such as trichotillomania (hair pulling). Not surprisingly, like OCD, trichotillomania is effectively treated with 5HT reuptake blockers (Stanley, Bowers, Swann, & Taylor, 1991; Swedo et al., 1989).

CSF-5HIAA is a gross measure of CNS 5HT functioning and is incapable of demonstrating subtler abnormalities in neurotransmitter functioning, whereas neuroendocrinological responses to 5HT agonists are more specific measures of central 5HT *receptor* sensitivity. Robust increases in prolactin release are caused by a variety of 5HT agonists, 5HT precursors, and 5HT releasing agents that activate 5HT-1a and 5HT-1c receptors in the hypothalamus (Cowen, Anderson, & Gartside, 1990; Van De Kar, Lorens, Urban, & Bethea, 1989). OCD subjects have a blunted prolactin response to a single oral dose of the 5HT agonists m-chlorophenylpiperazine (m-CPP) (Charney et al., 1988; Hollander et al., 1992; Hollander, DeCaria, Cooper, & Liebowitz, 1989) and 6-chloro-2-[1-piperazinyl]-pyrazine (MK-212) (Bastani, Nash, & Meltzer, 1990). The m-CPP and MK-212 share a preferential affinity for 5HT-1c and 5HT-2 receptor subtypes (Hoyer, 1988). Fenfluramine, which releases neuronal stores of 5HT, has been observed to produce a blunted prolactin response in some studies (Hewlett, Agras, & Berman, 1989; Hollander, DeCaria, Fay, & Liebowitz, 1989) but not in others (Hollander et al., 1988; Hollander et al., 1992). Gender composition of control and patient groups may contribute to the inconsistency of these findings because females have greater responses to fenfluramine than males (Hewlett, Agras, & Berman, 1989). In contrast to their response to m-CPP and MK-212, OCD patients do not differ from normal subjects in response to the 5HT precursor L-tryptophan, which increases 5HT synthesis (Charney et al., 1988), or to the 5HT-1a agonist ipsapirone (Charney et al., 1988). This indicates that the 5HT abnormality in OCD is not related to differences in 5HT synthesis or in altered sensitivity at 5HT-1a sites.

Both m-CPP and MK-212 are 5HT-1c agonists. However, m-CPP is a pure 5HT-2 antagonist, whereas MK-212 is a partial 5HT-2 agonist (Conn & Sanders-Bush, 1987). As MK-212 and m-CPP have effects that are often opposite at 5HT-2 receptors, it would appear that the blunted prolactin response in OCD may be due to subsensitivity of the 5HT-1c receptors in the hypothalamus. It is possible that there is also an abnormality at the 5HT-2 site, but this remains to be adequately tested.

Blunted cortisol responses to m-CPP (Zohar, Mueller, Insel, Zohar-Kadouch, & Murphy, 1987), MK-212 (Bastani, Nash, & Meltzer, 1990), and fenfluramine (Hollander et al., 1989; Zohar et al., 1987) have also been observed, but these findings have been inconsistent or await replication (Charney et al., 1988; Hollander et al., 1992). Like prolactin, cortisol is released via 5HT-1a and 5HT-1c activation in the hypothalamus (Cowen, Anderson, & Gartside, 1990). The source of the inconsistencies in these findings remains unclear, but may reflect a greater involvement of 5HT-1a sites than 5HT-1c receptors in cortisol release, weakening the effect of a 5HT-1c abnormality on cortisol levels.

5HT receptor subtypes mediate different and sometimes opposite effects (Boante, 1991; Glennon, 1990). For instance, m-CPP elicits responses opposite to 5HT-1a activation (Murphy et al., 1989). The 5HT receptor subtypes also have distinct and often complementary cortical and subcortical distribution patterns, and 5HT-1c receptors, in particular, have a highly specific distribution pattern. The caudate nucleus, putamen, NAS, and globus pallidus all have high to very high densities of 5HT-1c and 5HT-2 receptors, but very low levels of 5HT-1a receptors (Pazos, Probst, & Palacios, 1987a, 1987b). The frontal cortices and limbic regions have relatively low levels of 5HT-1c receptors, with some specific regions such as the ventromedial hypothalamus possessing higher densities. Given the specificity of 5HT-1c distribution, it becomes possible to attribute the effects of low 5HT-1c sensitivity to specific anatomical regions. In particular, 5HT-1c receptors are situated in a position to modulate significantly the flow and integration of information moving through the basal ganglia.

OCD patients become markedly more anxious and obsessional following a single oral dose of m-CPP (Hollander et al., 1988, 1992; Zohar et al., 1987), whereas control subjects do not show a similar increase in either anxiety or obsessions. Hollander and colleagues (1992) demonstrated that obsessions increased independently of antecedent anxiety ratings, which lends support to the argument that m-CPP directly results in an increase in obsessions. The behavioral effects of m-CPP can be blocked by pretreatment with the potent 5HT antagonist metergoline (Pigott et al., 1991), indicating that the action of m-CPP is via a 5HT agonistic mechanism. However, it remains unclear if the increase in obsessions is a direct or indirect response to m-CPP, a similar increase in anxiety, but not in obsessions, is observed when m-CPP is administered to panic disorder patients (Kahn, Asnis, Wetzler, & van Praag, 1988).

In studies utilizing an intravenous injection of m-CPP, both OCD and normal control subjects develop a marked increase in anxiety, but do not show an increase in obsessive–compulsive behaviors (Charney et al., 1988; Murphy et al., 1989). It has been suggested that the lack of obsessive–compulsive behaviors may be due to the rapid, acute administration of m–CPP. The pathway through which oral m–CPP exacerbates symptoms in vulnerable individuals remains unknown. It might be hypothesized that the behavioral response is due to a 5HT-1c hypersensitivity. But if this were the case, other pharmacological challenges that activate the 5HT-1c receptor should also have an obsessional effect, and neither MK-212 (Bastani, Nash, & Meltzer, 1990), fenfluramine (Hollander et al., 1992; Insel, Mueller, Gillin, Siever, & Murphy, 1984), nor intravenous m–CPP reliably increases obsessions. Furthermore, m–CPP's 5HT-2 antagonism cannot account for its obsessional effect, because metergoline not only does not produce a behavioral response but also blocks the response to m–CPP (Piggot et al., 1991). It is possible that the combination of 5HT-1c agonism and 5HT-2 antagonism in the right proportion is capable of interfering with the regular flow of information in the basal ganglia in vulnerable individuals, but this hypothesis remains speculative. It may more definitively be stated that obsessive–compulsive behaviors are not caused by 5HT-1c activation, but selective activation and antagonism of 5HT receptor subtypes may induce obsessive–compulsive behavior in vulnerable individuals.

A Model of OCD Behavioral Disturbance

Neurotransmitters Involved in the Basal Ganglia Loop. Despite the variety of neurotransmitters present in the basal ganglia, the nature of most of the projections in the loop is becoming known. A schematic representation of a few neurotransmitter connections is illustrated in Figure 5.16. Cortical input into the striatum utilizes the excitatory amino acid glutamate and possibly aspartate (Graybiel, 1990; Haber, 1986). The striatal projections to the globus pallidus utilize the inhibitory transmitter GABA, as do the pallidal connections to the thalamus (DeLong & Georgopoulos, 1979; Haber, 1986; Penny & Young, 1983). The latter connections, then, provide a tonic inhibition of thalamic projections to the cortex that are largely excitatory in nature. Of particular significance in this circuit is the double GABAergic inhibition in the striatopallido-thalamic circuit. Because the pallidum tonically inhibits the thalamus, inhibitory firing from the striatum to the pallidus disinhibits the thalamus and allows it to fire back to the OFC (Chevalier & Deniau, 1990). Because the thalamus also receives reciprocal excitatory projections from the cortex, disinhibition of the thalamus allows the establishment of a positive cortical–thalamocortical feedback loop. At the same time that this cortical–thalamocortical loop is active, the loop through the basal ganglia

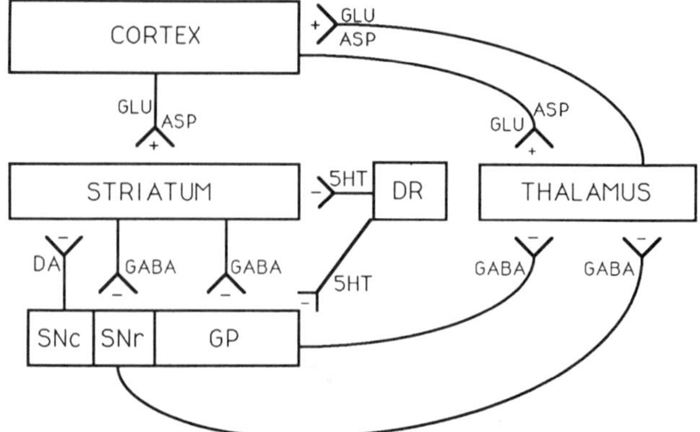

FIGURE 5.16. A simplified diagram of neurotransmitters involved in basal ganglia loops. For the sake of clarity, many of the neurotransmitters that play a role in this circuit are not included in the diagram, and only the dominant projections are shown. See text for discussion. GP, globus pallidus; SNr, substantia nigra, pars reticulata; SNc, substantia nigra, pars compacta; GLU, glutamate; ASP, aspartate.

may also continue to be active, thus allowing a continued disinhibition of the thalamus. Such feedback will produce rigidity in the flow of information from the thalamus to the OFC, forcing a perseveration of the information that can be held on-line in the OFC and, hence, a perseveration of the OFC's output as well.

The 5HT axons in this region are highly arborized, and 5HT-1c and 5HT-2 receptors in this region lack classical synaptic connections (Tork, 1990); they appear to innervate postsynaptic receptors through a drip irrigation method. The ventromedial head of the caudate receives some of the densest 5HT innervation in the forebrain (Haber, 1986). The 5HT produces a long-lasting postsynaptic effect on its target cells, and this fact, together with a widespread innervation pattern, suggests that 5HT does not carry specific information, but rather is consistent with a modulatory role. As elsewhere in the CNS, 5HT produces a threshold to a cell's firing in circuits like those passing through the basal ganglia; 5HT may dampen the circuit and prevent it from establishing a reverberating feedback loop. Because 5HT appears to diminish GABAergic firing in the striatum (Limberger, Späth, & Starke, 1986), chronically low 5HT thresholds in the striatum would produce a situation in which excitatory corticostriatal projections could cause a disinhibition of thalamocortical projections. Without a sufficiently high 5HT threshold, a positive feedback loop, from thalamus to cortex and back, may reverberate until an action is performed that disrupts it. Although a low 5HT threshold in the pallidum may increase the tonic firing rate of the pallidal GABAergic neurons, this effect is unlikely to compensate for the increased inhibition from striatal neurons.

Thus, overall, *the net effect of low 5HT-1c in the basal ganglia could be a low threshold for establishing positive feedback loops.* Receiving the reverberating feedback information, the lateral OFC would continue to code the same behavioral output perserveratively. Because of either the aberrant loop or an initial dysfunction in the OFC, the person may be unable to update and modulate the behavioral output pathways. Other components of the neurobehavioral network appear to function normally in OCD and are able to properly evaluate exteroceptive information. For instance, OCD patients are often able to see that their obsessions and compulsions are senseless and excessive. However, this knowledge appears to be unable to modulate the OFC or the striatum, and thus remains dissociated from the behavioral impulses.

Effects of 5HT Reuptake Blockers on OCD Patients. Consistent with the hypothesis that low 5HT-1c responsivity permits or exacerbates obsessive–compulsive behavior, medications that increase 5HT functioning reduce obsessions and compulsions. The mechanism through which clomipramine, fluvoxamine, and fluoxetine increase 5HT functioning is complex. Initially, stimulation of somatodendritic and terminal autoreceptors causes a dramatic decrease in the firing of 5HT raphe neurons (Blier, Chaput, & de Montigny, 1988; Chaput, de Montigny, & Blier, 1986) which may cause a decrease in net 5HT functioning. After long-term treatment, autoreceptors become down-regulated, and raphe firing returns to normal. The lack of negative feedback due to the down-regulated uptake sites allows more 5HT to be released per impulse, causing an increase in 5HT functioning (Blier et al., 1988; Chaput et al., 1986). Although many tricyclic antidepressants can cause a down-regulation of postsynaptic 5HT-2 receptors, 5HT reuptake blockers have usually not been found to down-regulate postsynaptic 5HT-1 or 5HT-2 receptors to any significant degree. Although it is still possible that some subtypes of 5HT receptors are down-regulated by 5HT reuptake blockers (for example, see Wong & Bymaster, 1980), the net effect of long-term administration is a marked increase in 5HT functioning. The delayed clinical efficacy of 5HT reuptake blockers in OCD is consistent with their delayed increase in 5HT functioning.

OCD patients medicated with clomipramine (Zohar, Insel, Zohar-Kadouch, Hill, & Murphy, 1988) or fluoxetine (Hollander, DeCaria, Fay, & Liebowitz, 1989) no longer demonstrate an exaggerated behavioral response or a blunted prolactin response when given an oral dose of m-CPP. Conversely, administration of the 5HT receptor antagonist metergoline over several days causes OCD patients who had shown improvement on clomipramine to become progressively more anxious and obsessional (Benkelfat et al., 1990). In blocking postsynaptic 5HT receptors, metergoline may attenuate the gain in 5HT functioning caused by clomipramine. Because 5HT-1c sites are not up-regulated by 5HT reuptake blockers, the increased endocrinological effect may largely be due to the subsensitivity of 5HT autoreceptors. Given acute administration of m-CPP, autoreceptor subsensitivity may block the normal down-regulation of raphe firing, allowing m-CPP and endogenous 5HT to have a sufficiently large combined effect to cancel out any preexisting postsynaptic subsensitivity.

While receiving long-term treatment with clomipramine, OCD patients have shown significant decreases in the metabolic rates of the inferomedial orbital frontal cortex and the left caudate nucleus, as well as a significant increase in the right anterior putamen (Benkelfat et al., 1990). This is consistent with the hypothesis that clomipramine is altering characteristics of the OFC loop. As increased serotonergic damping causes a decrease in striatal activity, the pallidus is disinhibited, which allows the pallidus to increase its tonic inhibition of the thalamocortical projections. Thus, by increasing serotonergic damping in the striatum, clomipramine may decrease the perseverative feedback in the lateral OFC loop.

Vulnerability to Perseverative Behavioral Impulses. Evidence from experiments utilizing pharmacological challenges in OCD patients and normal subjects indicates that a dysregulation of functional levels of 5HT by itself does not appear to be a sufficient cause of obsessive–compulsive behavior. In particular, manipulations of 5HT do not produce obsessive–compulsive behaviors in normal subjects, and, as reviewed previously, individuals with low 5HT as measured by CNS 5HIAA tend to demonstrate impulsivity rather than perseveration. As a modulator of information flow through the OFC–basal ganglia loops, 5HT is in a position to modulate the maintenance and updating of information in the OFC that is relevant to the construction of behavioral contingencies or impulses. When components of this circuit are not functioning properly, individuals appear to have difficulty altering their behavioral sets in accordance with information regarding reinforcement contingencies. The propensity to disorder probably depends on several factors. If the dysfunction in one component is subtle, it may not significantly alter computations made in other parts of the network. For instance, dysfunction of the lateral OFC loop due to striatal lesions may remain unexpressed behaviorally if 5HT activity is strong enough to prevent the appearance of aberrant positive feedback loops. However, as 5HT functioning decreases (perhaps, in particular, in 5HT-1c receptor activity), the striatal dysfunction is more likely to be expressed. The vulnerability to perseverative behavioral sets may be represented by the following (albeit oversimplistic) model:

$$\text{vulnerability} = f(\text{striatal dysfunction} \div \text{5HT-1c activity level})$$

This model implies that, as 5HT-1c activity increases, the effects of striatal dysfunction are reduced (see Figure 5.17). In addition, as latent dysfunction of the striatum decreases toward zero, vulnerability to perseveration will also decrease, even in the case of extremely low 5HT-1c activity. Conversely, when latent striatal dysfunction is large enough, even high 5HT activity may be unable to prevent positive feedback loops. This implies that subjects who are above a striatal dysfunction threshold may be nonresponders to serotonergic intervention, such as clomipramine. Moreover, these individuals may be more likely to express soft neurological signs or motor tics (see Hollander et al., 1990).

Functional levels of 5HT receptors, as well as the amount of 5HT present in the brain, vary in a dynamic manner (Roth, Hamblin, & Ciaranello, 1990; Sanders-Bush, 1990). Temporally, 5HT activity may vary greatly because of circadian rhythms or weak regulation, or in response to environmental challenge. This implies that the vulnerability to perseverative feedback loops may also vary dynamically over time, which may relate to the waxing and waning of obsessive–compulsive behaviors often exhibited by OCD patients.

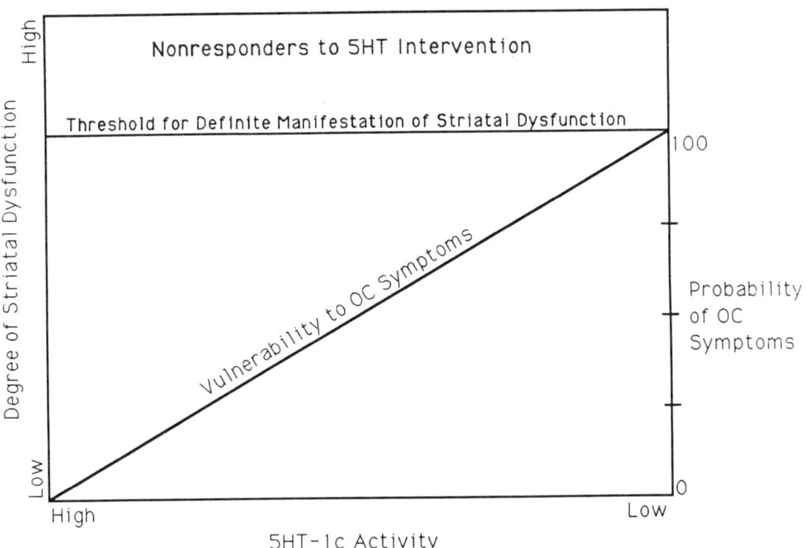

FIGURE 5.17. A schematic model of the interaction between serotonin (5HT) activity (perhaps, in particular, 5HT-1c activity) and local dysfunction of the ventromedial caudate nucleus. As 5HT activity decreases, the probability that a focal striatal dysfunction will result in a perseverative positive-feedback loop is increased. See text for discussion.

In summary, low levels of 5HT activity due to environmental challenge, extreme trait values, or inherent regulatory weakness may increase the impact of a restricted or localized dysfunction of the striatum on the functioning of the entire neurobehavioral network involved in the output of behavioral sets. Other neurotransmitters (in particular, DA) also appear capable of modifying the expression of pathology in the OFC–basal ganglia loops. As more is learned about the interaction of neurotransmitters in this region, and as the nature of the OFC/striatal pathology involved in OCD becomes clearer, more complex models may be put forward.

NOREPINEPHRINE, DIRECTED ATTENTION, NEGATIVE EMOTIONALITY, AND PANIC DISORDER

Research on the emotional and behavioral correlates of norepinephrine in humans does not lead in as clear directions as that on 5HT and DA. Therefore, we necessarily are required to provide more speculative associations than in the preceding discussion. We offer the following, then, as a means of stimulating further work in this important area of behavioral neurobiology.

Anatomical Features and Behavioral Functions of Ascending Noradrenergic Projections

Anatomy of the Locus Ceruleus

Among the seven norepinephrine (NE) cell groups, labeled A1–A7, lying below the midbrain in the pons region, there are two major ascending projections arising from the A6 and A7 cell groups. The A7 cell group gives rise to what is referred to as the ventral bundle of ascending NE projection fibers, which comprise part of the central tegmental tract and the ascending reticular system. Because of its widespread innervation pattern to the hypothalamus, nonspecific thalamus, midbrain nuclei, striatum, and cortex (densely to the orbital area), the A7 group is thought to be involved in modulating general levels of arousal of the brain. This would serve an important role in functions such as vigilance and perhaps sleep.

The A6 NE cell group lies in the dorsal part of the pons, gives rise to the dorsal fiber bundle, and forms part of the pontine reticular system. The A6 group is composed of at least four cell divisions in humans, but is referred to generally as the locus ceruleus or LC. The LC is composed of 20,000 neurons in humans, which is much less than the 690,000 DA cells of the VTA/SN region. These few neurons, nevertheless, project to many diverse brain regions, accounting for 80% of forebrain NE and providing the only source of NE to neocortical regions except for the orbital area. This diverse innervation is accomplished with few cells, because each NE fiber displays an extensive pattern of collateralization (or network), where no cortical cell is further than 30 μm from an NE–containing bouton. This type of nonspecific innervation pattern suggests that the LC does not convey specialized information to different brain regions, but rather that it widely transmits a uniform message.

This role for the LC is supported by the fact that the afferents reaching the LC come mainly from two large nuclei (nucleus prepositus hypoglossi, nucleus paragigantocellularis) located in the rostral medulla. The functions of these two nuclei are not well understood, but they are thought to be crossroads for circuitry pertaining to autonomic neuron integration as well as polymodal exteroceptive and interoceptive stimuli. Both of these nuclei have cells using 5HT, enkephalins, substance P, acetylcholine, neurotensin, corticotropin-releasing hormone, somatostatin, and epinephrine as transmitter. Hence, input to the LC is comprised of a host of transmitter systems.

This form of configuration of input to the LC has implications for LC function. The LC receives information via these nuclei on diverse sensory and behavioral events, to which the LC is responsive. However, the signals reaching the LC are apparently highly preprocessed in the cortex and by these medullary nuclei. Thus, the LC receives nondifferentiated, homogeneous information and perhaps, in turn, weighs input from these two nuclei in distributing a uniform message. This means that the LC may be under greater influence or control from the medulla than the forebrain and, therefore, is not likely to be required *in a primary way* in processes associated with the forebrain, such as learning, memory, and emotion. That is, the LC may be seen as modulating such processes as part of a more global function, such as behavioral orientation and directed attention.

Although these sources of afferent input to the LC greatly influence its activity, the major regulatory mechanism of LC NE is provided by presynaptic autoreceptors located on somas and terminals. These autoreceptors are of the alpha-2 type. Stimulation of these receptors by the alpha-2 agonist, clonidine, markedly decreases LC activity, whereas administration of the alpha-2 antagonist, yohimbine, results in a significant increase in LC activity. Pharmacological inhibition of the LC via the alpha-2 agonist clonidine has become a potent means of controlling the alarm response accompanying opiate, alcohol, and cigarette withdrawal, whereas use of clonidine and yohimbine as pharmacological probes of LC NE functioning offers a means of assaying central NE function in humans, as in the panic disorder research discussed later in this chapter.

Functions of Locus Ceruleus Norepinephrine Activity

Behavioral Orientation and Alertness. Studies of LC activity in behaving animals indicate that the LC displays slow spontaneous activity, which is more in keeping with a phasic rather than tonic neural system. Indeed, LC discharge rates correlate with spontaneous changes in levels of vigilance and alertness, where rates are very low in states of inattentive waking and during slow-wave sleep, but are increased in states of behavioral orientation and alertness. The greatest increases in rates of discharge occur when surveillance of the external environment was suddenly and dramatically increased, such as during sensory-evoked increases in behavioral arousal to unexpected or preferred stimuli. Intense LC reactivity occurs, in general, when stimuli disrupt any behavioral state and require increased vigilance and behavioral reorienting. The most intense reactivity occurred in monkeys in response to human imitations of primate agonistic social signals. This reactivity showed no evidence of habituation, and during long-term, highly significant exteroceptive stimulation, LC activity can be tonically enhanced. The type of stimulation seems to be less important: LC reactivity has been observed in response to simple (low-intensity tone, light flash, touch, 100-dB tone) and complex (food, but not when it is unaccessible and hence requires no attention; restraint, novel objects, entrance or exit of experimenters, signals of noxious stimulation) stimuli. Moreover, LC activity increases dramatically in response to threatening environmental stimuli (Grant & Redmond, 1984; Jacobs, 1986; Rasmussen, Morilak, & Jacobs, 1986). But in most of these cases, LC reactivity is homogeneous to some extent, where groups of LC cells increase and decrease in concert.

Of course, the LC is composed of subgroups of cells that may be grouped by termination region. It is known that LC turnover rates due to psychological stress are regionally specific (Tsuda & Tanaka, 1985). For instance, in rats psychological stress induced by exposure to other rats being shocked causes marked elevations of turnover in the hypothalamus, amygdala, and LC, but not in other regions (Tsuda et al., 1986). Furthermore, reexposure to an environment in which the animal has been shocked, or had observed other animals being shocked, caused significant elevations in NE turnover in the hypothalamus and amygdala. NE utilization in the amygdala induced by stress may facilitate rapid learning and retention of stimulus–reinforcer associations, and may aid in the rapid sensitization to environments associated with psychological distress.

Interoceptive Stimuli, Physiological Arousal, and Fear–Alarm Responses. The LC dramatically increases firing in response to peripheral somatosensory and autonomic stimuli. Loss of blood volume, hypercapnia, hypoxia, noxious mechanical stimuli, heat, and distension of the colon, stomach, or bladder all phasically increase LC firing (Elam, Svensson, & Thoren, 1986; Elam, Yao, Thoren, & Svensson, 1981; Svensson, 1987). Acute hyperventilation, which is associated with many symptoms found in panic disorder (Clark, 1986), such as shortness of breath, dizziness, faintness, palpitations, disorientation, derealization, depersonalization, tightness in the chest, nausea, flushing, and paresthesias (Gorman & Papp, 1989; Lum, 1976), produces several physiological changes that directly increase LC firing. For instance, hypocapnia induced by hyperventilation causes marked vascular constriction, which in turn reduces cerebral blood flow and creates a relative state of cerebral hypoxia (Hange, Thoresen, & Wallace, 1980; Kennealy, McLellan, London, & McLaurin, 1980). Chemoreceptors associated with hypoxia trigger LC firing (Elam et al., 1981). Not only does hyperventilation-induced hypoxia appear to play an active role in lactate-induced panic (Gorman et al., 1986), but also CO_2 inhalation causes dramatic increases in LC firing (Elam et al., 1981) and has proved to be a powerful tool for provoking panic attacks in the laboratory (Gorman et al., 1984; Gorman & Papp, 1989).

The importance of reactivity of the LC to interoceptive stimuli may stem from two factors. First, it is likely that such input to the LC serves as a means of "judging" the magnitude of the psychological significance of the situation at hand. As significance (coded by level of interoceptive input) increases, LC activity may react in kind and, hence, induce equivalent levels of alertness and orientation to the environment via its projections to the forebrain and neocortex. Second, the ventral aspect of the LC issues descending projections to the spinal cord and, thereby, influences in an inhibitory manner autonomic nervous system activity. Thus, interoceptive input would aid the LC in modulating autonomic arousal (Blizzard, 1988).

The interaction of the LC with autonomic processes may be important with respect to the experience of fear or alarm (Mason, 1981). Although bilateral lesions or pharmacological inhibition of the LC do not affect response to primary negative reinforcers, such as the efficacy of shock in the acquisition of an avoidance task, the amplitude of the fear or alarm responses in monkeys to social group situations, threatening confrontations with humans, lights, sounds, and rubber snakes is greatly reduced (Huang, Redmond, & Snyder, 1976; Redmond, Huang, & Snyder, 1972; Uhde et al., 1984). In these studies, the fear response was not eliminated, as indicated by the lack of effect on defecation and grooming; and, concordantly, LC lesions or chemical destruction of NE terminals in rats does not block conditioned emotional responses or active or passive avoidance performance. Only the amplitude of fear responding appears to be affected. Thus, it is not surprising that electrical stimulation or pharmacological activation of the LC enhances naturally occurring or experimentally induced fear states in monkeys (Redmond & Huang, 1979).

Clarification of the role of NE and epinephrine in the periphery is important in discussions of LC NE and arousal. The "fight–flight" system described by Cannon (1929) involves the sympathoadrenomedullary system, which reacts in emergency situations by releasing epinephrine and NE into the bloodstream. Cannon theorized that this system enabled the organism to rapidly prepare for emergency responses in crisis situations. These include tachycardia, hyperventilation, sweating, inhibition of the gastrointestinal tract, and changes in vasoconstriction and dilation (Kopin, Eisenhofer, & Goldstein, 1986). The LC appears to act as a central analog to the peripheral sympathoadrenomedullary system, preparing the organism to react in threatening situations. In fact, LC activity correlates highly with peripheral sympathoadrenal activation (Abercrombie & Jacobs, 1987; Reiner, 1986). In threatening situations, then, central NE may serve the function of adaptively increasing vigilance, accuracy of directed attention, and emotional evaluation, whereas the sympathoadrenal system prepares the organism to respond physically.

Stimulus Relevancy and Selective Attention. Mason (1981) and Jacobs (1986) have provided extensive reviews of the evidence on the effects of NE manipulations on behavior, and we shall only briefly summarize their conclusions. Reductions in NE most consistently result in an increased resistance to extinction, but only when the reductions are effected during the acquisition phase of learning. The results hold equally for positive and negative reinforcement tasks. Mason showed that this effect is due to NE's ability to increase the salience of relevant to irrelevant stimuli. Thus, reductions in NE result in poor selective attention to the most task-relevant stimuli; hence, many irrelevant stimuli become associated with reward during the phase of acquisition. That is, many irrelevant stimuli in the environment become associated with increased DA activity during goal acquisition and, thereby, become effective incentive stimuli (Beninger, 1983). In the extinction phase, more incentive stimuli need to be extinguished, leading to the overall effect of increased resistance to extinction. This explanation would apply to why partial reinforcement, where the relevant stimuli are more difficult to discriminate, also leads to increased resistance to extinction.

In view of a selective attention function for LC NE projections, it seems concordant that the LC is particularly reactive whenever environmental conditions require close scrutiny, such as when sudden changes occur, when the animal is more alert and actively exploring the environment, or when interoceptive cues indicate an aroused state induced by environmental change or threat.

A Functional Principle of Norepinephrine

In an extensive review of the role of NE in many different functions, Oades (1985) has concluded that what underlies the selective attention to relevant stimuli is NE's ability to tune neural information. Tuning occurs by NE's enhancement of the signal-to-noise ratio, which involves a reduction in spontaneous firing rates of neurons, accompanied by an increased response of the neuron when a stimulus of sufficient strength evokes an action potential. Conceptually, NE hyperpolarizes a field of cells, making it more difficult for them to respond to general (i.e., irrelevant) stimulus input. However, strong (i.e., relevant) stimuli will evoke a particularly large response in the neurons receiving stimulation. Thus, the relevant stimuli evoke a response, while the irrelevant stimuli have diminished effects. This effect would likely occur for signals derived from both external (environmental) and internal (memory retrieval, corticocortical input, interoceptive stimuli) sources.

This would mean that NE has the general effect of sharpening and enhancing the efficiency of information processing. For instance, in sensory modalities, NE increases the reliability and efficiency of feature extraction from sensory input (Foote, Bloom, & Aston-Jones, 1983), an effect that may also occur with interoceptive input. Interoceptive information is received by the basolateral limbic forebrain via projections from the nucleus of the solitary tract in the medulla (Sumal, Blessing, Joh, Reis, & Pickel, 1982). The nucleus of the solitary tract projects to the central nucleus of the amygdala, the bed nucleus of the stria terminalis, and several hypothalamic nuclei (Ricardo & Koh, 1978). This is one way in which cells in the amygdala are responsive to changes in respiration and cardiovascular functioning (Cechetto & Carlaresu, 1984; Cechetto, Ciriello, & Carlaresu, 1983; Pascoe & Kapp, 1985). As with other sensory information, the amygdala codes interoceptive stimuli for its emotional significance, and generates a subjective emotional experience (Collins & Depue, 1992). The LC projects to both the amygdala and the hippocampus, where it potentiates both excitatory and inhibitory responses (Foote, Bloom, & Aston-Jones, 1983; Segal & Bloom, 1976a, 1976b). NE may increase the efficiency with which the hippocampus and amygdala extract affective features from stimuli to produce a heightening of limbic mediated emotional associations and responses. Although no studies to date have specifically tested this hypothesis, NE injections into the amygdala have been shown to enhance the retention of amygdala-mediated associations (Liang, Juler, & McGaugh, 1986; Liang, McGaugh, Yao, 1990), whereas decreased NE activity impairs the functioning of the amygdala, as demonstrated by the ability of intraamygdaloid infusions of β-adrenergic antagonists to impair retention (Gallagher, Kapp, Pascoe, & Rapp, 1981; McGaugh, Introni-Collison, & Nagahara, 1988). Heightened efficiency of the LC NE projections to the amygdala may thus influence not only which stimuli are attended but also the magnitude of significance attributed to them.

Although well beyond the scope of this chapter, it is worth noting briefly that there is anatomical support for the LC NE system's role in directed attention. In the visual system, LC NE projections preferentially innervate structures associated with spatial analysis (e.g., medial pulvinar, inferior parietal lobe, and dorsolateral convexity of prefrontal cortex) and visuomotor (posterior parietal and primary motor cortices) response rather than feature extraction and pattern analysis (e.g., occipital and inferior temporal lobe). Sensory information coursing through the sensory nuclei of the thalamus must pass the gatelets of the reticular nucleus of the thalamus, which then passes the information to other thalamic nuclei having the function of directing the information to specific cortical areas (Stuss & Benson, 1986). LC NE projections densely innervate the reticular nuclei gatelets and hyperpolarize them. Thus, in the case of visual sensory information, visual signals converging on the gatelets are generally constrained from passing when LC NE activity is high; only the strongest or most relevant stimuli pass the gatelets. The information that does pass will go to the medial pulvinar, which then will direct it to the appropriate cortical areas, such as the inferior parietal lobe for mapping of extrapersonal space (Andersen, 1987). The important point here is that NE has helped to select the visual information that is from the relevant part of extrapersonal space that now requires mapping. Thus, in this example, the LC NE system plays a critical role, via its influence on reticular gatelets, in directing attention to the relevant regions of extrapersonal space or, put simply, to the relevant stimuli in space.

The Locus Ceruleus Norepinephrine System and Negative Emotionality

Tellegen (Tellegen & Waller, 1992; Watson & Tellegen, 1985) has demonstrated that one of the two major superfactors that consistently are discovered in factor analytic studies of personality structure is the trait of negative emotionality (NEM). NEM is composed of lower-order traits that convey a subjective experience of a variety of negative emotions, including anger and hostility, depression, anxiety, alienation, and feeling easily stressed by life circumstances. Tellegen conceives of the negative emotionality system, which has substantial genetic influence when considered as a trait, as producing a diffuse state of negative affect that serves to motivate the directing of attention under conditions of environmental uncertainty. For example, a deer at the threshold of a meadow must, for survival's sake, scan the environment for sources of potential threat before entering. Negative affect would motivate this scanning process.

When environmental uncertainty is reduced (in this case, no threat is perceived), negative affect would decrease, and forward locomotion and incentive motivation as a means of supporting exploratory behavior would ensue.

As this example suggests, the negative emotionality system may be linked neurologically with processes of directed attention (for instance, both processes appear to be right-hemisphere dominant) and, as such, may be modulated by or linked to the LC NE system. Blizzard (1988) has, on the basis of a large pharmacological, behavioral, and genetic literature, suggested just such an association between LC NE activity and negative emotionality. Blizzard hypothesizes that high trait negative emotionality may be related to traitwise low LC activity. According to our understanding of Blizzard's hypothesis, traitwise low LC activity would have two main effects. First, low LC NE activity in ascending projections would result in chronic inability to detect relevant from irrelevant, or threatening from nonthreatening, stimuli. That is, environmental uncertainty would be chronically high, overactivating the negative emotionality system. The latter would, in turn, continually provide a subjective sense of negative affect, accompanied by cognitions of worry, vague threat, and anticipatory fear. Second, the process would be aggravated by low activity in the ventral LC NE descending projections that provide inhibitory modulation over automonic reactivity. Thus, low LC functioning would result in elevated physiological activity that normally accompanies arousal and alarm.

Unfortunately, the source of the negative affect, physiological arousal, and environmental uncertainty would not be clear to the individual because the problem is not located externally in the environment, but rather is located internally within NE's signal-to-noise ratio function. Over time, assessment of such an individual's subjective emotional state would produce a picture consistent with a trait of elevated negative emotionality, as defined previously by Tellegen. The extent to which elevated levels of NEM are associated with anxiety conditions is not known, but this would appear to be an interesting direction for future research.

Norepinephrine and Panic Disorder

Panic is an extreme state of negative affect, characterized by intense physiological and psychological arousal. From an ethological perspective, it may be viewed as the product of an alarm system, mobilizing the organism in the face of imperative stimuli (Cannon, 1929). Elements of this system are ancient from a phylogenetic standpoint. Serving as a discrete intense burst of activity, it is able to markedly alter cognitive and physiological processes in order to react rapidly to threatening stimuli.

In panic disorder (PD), these alarm states often appear uncued, at times even occurring during sleep. This leads to the speculation that a central neural system involved in alarm is subject to states of hyperactivity or dysregulation such that it fires spontaneously. Recent models of PD have suggested that uncued attacks may be caused by changes in internal states (Clark, 1986). After the occurrence of one attack, recurrence of these same somatic signs is evaluated catastrophically as signs of impending loss of control or physical harm. Because the LC and its NE projections play a critical role in the way exteroceptive and interoceptive stimuli are processed and evaluated, we will examine the evidence related to NE function, and specifically dysregulation of the α_2-adrenergic receptor (α_2). The evidence suggests that NE function may serve as a vulnerability factor in PD.

Noradrenergic Levels in Panic Disorder

Studies of central NE functioning in psychiatric patients index central NE turnover by measuring the NE metabolite, 3-methoxy-4-hydroxyphenylglycol (MHPG), in plasma and urine. Ballenger et al. (1984) found small but statistically significant elevations of plasma MHPG in PD patients compared to normals. However, the majority of studies measuring baseline MHPG have found no significant elevation of MHPG in PD patients (Carr et al., 1986; Charney, Heninger, & Breier, 1984; Liebowitz et al., 1985; Woods, Charney, McPherson, Gradman, & Heninger, 1987). Although increased plasma MHPG levels have been observed following panic attacks induced by exposure to phobic stimuli (Ko et al., 1983; Woods et al., 1987), it is difficult to judge if the elevations represent the cause or the result of panic. Plasma and urinary MHPG are significantly increased in healthy controls in response to stress (Uhde et al., 1982), but these elevations are not significantly less than those found in PD subjects exposed to a stressor (Woods et al., 1987). Furthermore, increased MHPG has not always been observed in panicking subjects (Charney et al., 1984).

Noradrenergic Dysregulation in Panic Disorder

Inadequate modulation of a biological regulatory system may produce several effects. As discussed regarding the regulation of the BFS, weak regulation may cause (1) a persistent quantitative increase or decrease in a biological variable, (2) heightened intraindividual variability due to decreased efficiency of negative feedback responses to changing values of the biological variable, (3) a reduced postchallenge rate of recovery to prestress levels for similar reasons, and (4) heightened reactivity to exogenous or endogenous challenges to the homeostatic steady-state (Depue

& Monroe, 1986). In general, weak regulation is accompanied by lability of the system when challenged.

Because the α_2-autoreceptor is the major source of regulation of LC activity, this regulatory system has been evaluated in PD patients rather intensively. PD patients administered the α_2-antagonist yohimbine have demonstrated greater increases in anxiety, somatic symptoms, blood pressure, and plasma MHPG levels than healthy controls (Charney et al., 1984; Charney, Woods, Goodman, & Heninger, 1987). Moreover, a single oral (20 mg) or intraveneous (0.4 mg/kg) dose of yohimbine produced panic attacks in more than half of PD patients compared with 5% of healthy subjects (Charney et al., 1987). Importantly, the exaggerated yohimbine-induced anxiogenic/panicogenic and MHPG response appears to be specific to PD; it has not been observed in patients with generalized anxiety disorder (GAD), major depression, obsessive compulsive disorder, schizophrenia, or in normal controls (Charney et al., 1989; Glazer, Charney, & Heninger, 1987; Heninger, Charney, & Price, 1988; Rasmussen, Goodman, & Woods, 1987). Finally, in terms of interpatient variability, PD patients experiencing yohimbine-induced panic attacks show greater changes in MHPG than patients who are behaviorally unresponsive to yohimbine (Charney et al., 1987), and patients experiencing frequent panic attacks (> 2.5 per week) have significantly greater elevations in MHPG following yohimbine administration than patients with less frequent attacks (Charney et al., 1984).

Several responses to the α_2-agonist clonidine are similarly exaggerated in PD patients. Clonidine produces greater decreases in plasma MHPG in PD patients than in healthy subjects (Charney & Heninger, 1986; Nutt, 1989), and the hypotensive effects of clonidine are also more elevated in PD patients (Charney & Heninger, 1986; Nutt, 1986, 1989). PD patients also possess a decreased growth hormone (GH) response to clonidine as compared with controls (Charney & Heninger, 1986; Nutt, 1989; Uhde, Vittone, Siever, Kaye, & Post, 1986). It has been suggested that this blunting is the result of subsensitive postsynaptic α_2-receptors, in that NE mediates GH release through postsynaptic α_2-receptors located in the hypothalamus (Tuomista & Mannisto, 1985; Uhde et al., 1982). However, GH-releasing factor acts as an intermediate step between NE and GH, and GH response in panic disorder appears to be blunted in response, not just to clonidine, but to GH releasing factor as well (Rapoport, Risch, Gillin, Golshan, & Janowsky, 1989). The lowered GH response thus appears to be occurring at the level of the pituitary and may be the result of desensitization due to chronic stress-induced activation (Abelson et al., 1991). This may underly the fact that blunted GH responses are not specific to PD; they are also seen in some forms of depression (Amsterdam, Maislin, Skolnick, Berwish, & Winokur, 1989; Charney et al., 1982; Siever, Uhde, & Silberman, 1982) and GAD

(Ableson et al., 1991). In GAD patients, the best predictor of blunted GH response is ratings of stress and anxiety for the 6 months prior to testing (Abelson et al., 1991). Thus, blunted GH may be a marker of long-term stress and anxiety rather than a specific marker of PD.

The existence of excessive presynaptic responses to both α_2-agonism and antagonism is consistent with weak regulation of the α_2-receptors. A simple hyposensitive or hypersensitive receptor model cannot account for the exaggerated responses in both directions. Instead, these results are indicative of an inability to maintain or return to homeostasis when challenged. Charney and his colleagues (Charney et al., 1989; Charney, Woods, Price, et al., 1990) have suggested that PD may involve a dysregulation of the coupling of α_2 receptors to the effector systems that mediate their actions within cells. After a receptor binds with an agonist or antagonist, it activates a biological process intracellularly. This process is mediated through the ability of the receptor to interact or "couple" with intracellular effector components. Alpha$_2$- and β-adrenergic receptors are coupled to the adenylate cyclase effector system by guanine nucleotide regulatory proteins (G proteins) (Lefkowitz, Stadel, & Caron, 1983). Alpha$_2$-activation inhibits the adenylate cyclase system and its second messenger, cyclic adenosine monophosphate (cAMP), whereas β-adrenergic receptors activate cAMP (Lefkowitz, Caron, & Stiles, 1984). G protein deficiencies reduce the responsiveness of target cells by limiting the ability of receptors to activate or inhibit cAMP. This sort of dysregulation due to deficient G proteins has been observed in pseudohypoparathyroidism (Heinsimer et al., 1983).

Not only do G proteins couple the receptor with the adenylate cyclase effector system, but also they regulate the affinity level of the receptors themselves. Receptors modulate between states of high or low affinity for agonists. When a receptor is coupled with a G protein, its affinity for agonists is high. Coincident with activation of the adenylate cyclase system, the G protein dissociates from the receptor, returning the high affinity receptor to a low affinity state (Lefkowitz, Caron, & Stiles, 1984). The sensitivity to agonists may, therefore, change drastically following activation. Thus, PD may be characterized, for example, by a reduced rate of changing from high to low affinity states of the α_2-receptor following agonist or antagonist binding with the receptor.

G proteins are just one component of a complex and dynamic system that regulates the sensitivity of receptors. Receptors on a cell membrane are rapidly desensitized through a process of phosphorylation (Kobilka, 1992; Raymond, Hnatowich, Lefkowitz, & Caron, 1990). Receptor densities are also reduced through the functional removal of receptors from the cell membrane following activation. In some tissue cultures, up to 60% of receptors may be removed from the cell membrane within 5 minutes of exposure to an agonist (Chueng, Dixon, Hill, Sigal, & Strader,

1990). These receptors are sequestered, and may then be redistributed onto the cell membrane at a later time. Receptors may also be removed and destroyed through a slower process of down-regulation (Kobilka, 1992). Rates of receptor degradation and/or receptor assembly or processing, messenger RNA (mRNA) stability, and alterations in the rates of gene transcription may all affect the number of receptors at any given time (Collins, Bouvier, Bolanowski, Caron, & Lefkowitz, 1989; Raymond et al., 1990).

Dysregulation of receptors may have far-ranging effects, causing increases and decreases in the effects of a neurotransmitter in different tissues. Furthermore, different receptor subtypes may be differentially affected by dysregulation because they are coded by different genes. For instance, hypothyroidism and hyperthyroidism produce increases and decreases in the number of β-adrenergic receptors or the physiological responses they mediate, depending on the specific tissue site examined (Bilezekian & Loeb, 1983; Stiles, Stadel, DeLean, & Lefkowitz, 1981). In contrast, α_2-receptors are consistently decreased in number or unchanged (Bilezekian & Loeb, 1983). This may result in decreased inhibitory regulation of the LC and also in a mixture of increased and decreased NE sensitivity at postsynaptic sites.

The involvement of dysregulated NE functioning in PD suggests that the LC is a primary site of pharmacotherapeutic intervention. For instance, benzodiazepines facilitate GABAergic inhibition of the LC (Cedarbaum & Aghajanian, 1977; Grant, Huang, & Redmond, 1980), and the triazolobenzodiazepine, alprazolam (Xanax), is an effective antipanic agent (Ballenger et al., 1988) that also appears to regulate NE functioning. Long-term treatment with alprazolam blunts yohimbine-induced increases in plasma MHPG, anxiety, and blood pressure in PD patients (Charney & Heninger, 1985). It thus appears to be increasing the stability of NE systems.

In summary, a simple model of elevated NE functioning cannot account for the hypersensitivity of PD patients to *both* agonists and antagonists observed in the α_2-pharmacological challenge studies. Thus, NE dysregulation may be neither necessary nor sufficient for the development of PD. Perhaps (1) the mechanisms that maintain NE homeostasis in the LC system are dysfunctional or dysregulated in at least a *subset* of PD patients, or (2) regulatory strength in the LC system may be conceived of as a dimensional trait (ranging from strong to weak) that interacts with other etiological factors to create panic attacks. In this sense, degree of regulatory strength in the LC NE system may serve as a liability factor, where above a certain threshold of weakness, individuals possessing other etiological factors for PD are adversely affected. In terms of the latter case, for example, degree of regulatory strength may act as a modifier of course, where increasingly weak LC regulation is correlated with increasing frequency of panic attacks in PD patients. When the LC is triggered in these patients, they may produce excessive bursts of NE that cause an increase in the attention paid to, and the physiological impact of, exteroceptive and interoceptive stimulation.

CONCLUSIONS

We are aware that models of psychopathology based on only one neurotransmitter are clearly too simplistic and that they will rapidly require the addition of other factors. Indeed, in several of the models we presented, we indicated that the biogenic amine in question could not by itself account for the disorder. It appeared to be the case that amines frequently enter the etiological picture as interacting vulnerability variables, depending on their trait values. There is, however, good reason to entertain such models when the biogenic amines are involved. None of the amines appears to serve primarily a mediating role in the central nervous system. Rather, the amines each have a particular modulatory role in influencing the flow of information in neural networks. This fact, taken together with their broad distribution patterns in the brain, indicates that variation in a single amine can have widespread effects on behavior, as the animal research clearly shows experimentally. Thus, variation in the biogenic amines may come to provide a powerful predictor of behavioral variation. Because the amines are very old from a phylogenetic standpoint, moreover, they modulate brain structures associated with very basic forms of behavior relevant to personality and psychopathology, including the emotions, reward, and motor propensity, as well as important cognitive functions. Therefore, the currently simplistic biogenic amine models of behavior may be viewed as important building blocks for more complex future modeling of neurobehavioral systems.

ACKNOWLEDGMENTS

This work was supported by NIMH Research Grants MH37195 and MH48114 and NIMH Research Training Grant MH17069 awarded to R. A. Depue.

REFERENCES

Abelson, J. L., Glitz, D., Cameron, O. G., Lee, M. A., Bronzo, M., & Curtis, G. C. (1991). Blunted growth hormone response to clonidine in patients with generalized anxiety disorder. *Archives of General Psychiatry, 48,* 157–162.

Abercrombie, E. D., & Jacobs, B. L. (1987). Single-unit response of noradrenergic neurons in the locus coeruleus of freely moving cats: I. Acutely presented stressful and nonstressful stimuli. *Journal of Neuroscience, 7,* 2837–2843.

Aggleton, J. P., & Mishkin, M. (1986). The amygdala: Sensory gateway to the emotions. In E. Plutchik & H. Kellerman (Eds.), *Emotion: Theory, research, and experience: Vol. 3. Biological foundations of emotion* (pp. 281–299). New York: Academic Press.

Alexander, G. E., Crutcher, M. D., & DeLong, M. R. (1990). Basal ganglia–thalamocoritical circuits: Parallel substrates for motor, oculomotor, "prefrontal" and "limbic" functions. *Progress in Brain Research, 85,* 119–146.

Alexander, G. E., DeLong, M. R., & Strick, P. L. (1986). Parallel organization of functionally segreted circuits linking basal ganglia and cortex. *Annual Review of Neuroscience, 9,* 357–381.

Altemus, M., Pigott, T., Kalogeras, K. T., Demitrack, M., Dubbert, B., Murphy, D. L., & Gold, P. W. (1992). Abnormalities in the regulation of vasopressin and corticotropin releasing factor secretion in obsessive–compulsive disorder. *Archives of General Psychiatry, 49,* 9–20.

Amsterdam, J. D., Maislin, G., Skolnick, B., Berwish, N., & Winokur, A. (1989). Multiple hormone responses to clonidine administration in depressed patients and healthy controls. *Biological Psychiatry, 26,* 265–278.

Andersen, R. (1987). Anatomy and function of the inferior parietal lobe. In *Handbook of Physiology* (Vol. 5, pp. 221–273). Washington, DC: American Physiological Society.

Asberg, M., Schalling, D., & Traskman-Bendy, L. (1987). Psychobiology of suicide, impulsivity, and related phenomena. In H. Meltzer (Ed.), *Psychopharmacology of the third generation of progress* (pp. 665–668). New York: Raven Press.

Azmitia, E. C. (1978). The serotonin-processing neurons of the midbrain median and dorsal raphe neurons. In L. Iversen, S. Iversen, & S. Snyder (Eds.), *Handbook of Psychopharmacology* (Vol. 8, pp. 109–181). New York: Plenum Press.

Azmitia, E. C., & Gannon, P. J. (1986). The primate serotonergic system: A review of human and animal studies and a report on macaca fascicularis. In S. Fahn (Ed.), *Advances in Neurology, Vol. 43, Myoclonus* (pp. 407–468). New York: Raven.

Babor, T., Hofmann, M., DelBoca, F., Hesselbrock, V., Meyer, R., Dolinsky, Z., & Rounsaville, B. (1992). Types of alcoholics: I. Evidence for an empirically derived typology based on indicators of vulnerability and severity. *Archives of General Psychiatry, 49,* 599–608.

Baddeley, A. D. (1986). *Working memory.* Oxford: Oxford University Press.

Baddeley, A. D., & Hitch, G. (1974). Working memory. In G. H. Bower (Ed.), *The psychology of learning and motivation: Advances in research and theory* (Vol. 8, pp. 47–89). New York: Academic Press.

Ballenger, J. C., Burrows, G. D., DuPont, R. L., Lesser, I. M., Noyes, R. Jr., Pecknold, J. C., Rifkin, A., & Swinson, R. P. (1988). Alpazolam in panic disorder and agoraphobia: Results from a multicenter trial. I: Efficacy of short-term treatment. *Archives of General Psychiatry, 45,* 413–422.

Ballenger, J. C., Goodwin, F., & Major, L. (1979). Alcohol and central serotonin metabolism in man. *Archives of General Psychiatry, 36,* 224–227.

Ballenger, J. C., Peterson, G. A., Lararia, M., Hucek, A., Lake, C. R., Kimerson,

D., Cox, D. J., Trackman, C., Shipe, J. R., & Wilkinson, C. (1984). A study of plasma catecholamines in agoraphobia and the relationship of scrum, tricyclic levels to treatment response. In J. C. Ballenger (Ed.), *Biology of agoraphobia* (pp. 171–210). Washington, DC: American Psychiatric Press.

Bastani, B., Nash, J. F., & Meltzer, H. Y. (1990). Prolactin and cortisol response to MK-212, a serotonin agonist, in obsessive–compulsive disorder. *Archives of General Psychiatry, 47,* 833–839.

Baxter, L. R., Phelps, M. E., Mazziotta, J. C., Guze, B. H., Schwartz, J. M., & Selin, C. E. (1987). Local cerebral glucose metabolic rates in obsessive–compulsive disorder: A comparison with rates in unipolar depression and in normal controls. *Archives of General Psychiatry, 44,* 211–218.

Baxter, L. R., Schwartz, J. M., Mazziotta, J. C., Phelps, M. E., Pahl, J. G., Guze, B. H., & Fairbanks, L. (1988). Cerebral glucose metabolic rates in nondepressed obsessive–compulsives. *American Journal of Psychiatry, 15,* 1560–1563.

Beaulieu, C., & Colonnier, M. (1987). Effects of the richness of the environment on the cat visual cortex. *Journal of Comparative Neurology, 266,* 478–494.

Beninger, R. J. (1983). The role of dopamine in locomotor activity and learning. *Brain Research Reviews, 6,* 173–196.

Beninger, R. J., Hanson, D. R., & Phillips, A. G. (1980). The effects of pipradrol on the acquisition of responding with conditioned reinforcement: A role for sensory preconditioning. *Psychopharmacology, 69,* 235–242.

Benkelfat, C., Nordahl, T. E., Semple, W. E., King, C. A., Murphy, D. L., & Cohen, R. M. (1990). Local cerebral glucose metabolic rates in obsessive compulsive disorder: Patients treated with clomipramine. *Archives of General Psychiatry, 47,* 840–848.

Berger, B., Trottier, S., Gaspar, P., Verney, C., & Alvarez, C. (1988). Regional and laminar distribution of dopamine and serotonin innervation in the cynomolgus cerebral cortex. Major differences of dopamine input in the granular and agranular cortices. A radioautographic study. *Journal of Comparative Neurology, 273,* 99–119.

Berger, B., Verney, C., Alvarez, C., Vigny, A., & Helle, K. B. (1985). New dopaminergic fields in the motor, visual (area 18b) and retrosplenial cortex in the young and adult rat: Immunocytochemical and catecholamine histochemical analyses. *Neuroscience, 15,* 983–998.

Bilezekian, J. P., & Loeb, J. N. (1983). The influence of hyperthyroidism and hypothyroidism on α- and β-adrenergic receptor systems and adrenergic responsiveness. *Endocrinology Review, 4,* 378–388.

Bindra, D. (1968). Neuropsychological interpretation of the effects of drive and incentive-motivation on general activity and instrumental behavior. *Psychological Review, 75,* 1–22.

Black, J. E., & Greenough, W. T. (1986). Induction of pattern in neural structure by experience: Implications for cognitive development. In M. E. Lamb, A. L. Brown, & B. Rogoff (Eds.), *Advances in developmental psychology* (Vol. 4, pp. 1–50). Hillsdale, NJ: Erlbaum.

Blackburn, J. R., Phillips, A. G., Jakubovic, A., & Fibiger, H. C. (1989). Dopamine and preparatory behavior: II. A neurochemical analysis. *Behavioral Neuroscience, 103,* 15–23.

Blier, P., Chaput, Y., & de Montigny, C. (1988). Longterm 5-HT reuptake blockade, but not monoamine oxidase inhibition, decreases the function of terminal 5-HT autoreceptors: An electrophysiological study in the rat brain. *Naunyn Schmiedebergs Archives of Pharmacology, 337,* 246–254.

Blizzard, E. (1988). The locus coeruleus and emotional behavior. *Experientia, 44,* 491–495.

Bloom, F. E. (1979). Is there a neurotransmitter code in the brain? In P. Simon (Ed.), *Advances in pharmacology and therapeutics* (Vol. 12, pp. 205–213). Oxford: Pergamon.

Boante, P. L. (1991). Serotonin receptor subtypes: Functional, physiological, and clinical correlates. *Clinical Neuropharmacology, 14,* 1–16.

Bolles, R. C. (1972). Reinforcement, expectancy, and learning. *Psychological Review, 79,* 394–409.

Broca, P. (1878). Anatomie comparee des circonvolutions cerebrales. Le grand lobe limbique et la scissure limbique dans le serie des mammiferes. *Reviews in Anthropology, 1,* 385–498.

Brown, G., Ebert M., & Goyer, P. (1982). Aggression, suicide, and serotonin: Relationships to CSF amine metabolites. *American Journal of Psychiatry, 139,* 741–746.

Brown, G., Goodwin, F., & Ballenger, J. (1979). Aggression in humans correlates with cerbrospial fluid metabolites. *Psychiatry Research, 1,* 131–139.

Brown, R. M., Crane, A. M., & Goldman, P. S. (1979). Regional distribution of monoamines in the cerebral cortex and subcortical structures of the rhesus monkey: Concentrations and in vitro synthesis rates. *Brain Research,* pp. 133–150.

Brown, R. T. (1968). Early experience and problem solving ability. *Journal of Comparative and Physiological Psychology, 65,* 433–440.

Brozoski, T. J., Brown, R. M., Rosvold, H. E., & Goldman, P. S. (1979). Cognitive defict caused by regional depletion of dopamine in prefrontal cortex of rhesus monkey. *Science, 205,* 929–931.

Bunney, W. E. (1978). Psychopharmacology of the switch process in affective disorders. In M. A. Lipton, A. DiMascio, & K. F. Killam (Eds.), *Psychopharmacology: A generation of progress* (pp. 1249–1259). New York: Raven.

Bunney, W. E., Post, R. M., Anderson, A. E., & Kopanda, R. T. (1977). A neuronal receptor sensitivity mechanism in affective illness (a review of evidence). *Community Psychopharmacology, 11,* 393–406.

Butter, C. M. (1964). Habituation of responses to novel stimuli in monkeys with selective frontal lesions. *Science, 144,* 313–315.

Butter, C. M. (1969). Preseveration in extinction and in discrimination reversal tasks following selective prefrontal ablations in Macaca mulatta. *Physiology and Behavior, 4,* 163–171.

Butter, C. M., & Snyder, D. R. (1972). Alterations in aversive and aggressive behavior following orbitofrontal lesions in rhesus monkeys. *Acta Neurobiologiae Experimentalis, 32,* 525–565.

Camps, M., Cortes, R., Gueye, B., Probst, A., & Palacios, J. M. (1989). Dopamine receptors in human brain: Autoradiographic distribution of D2 sites. *Neuroscience, 28,* 275–290.

Cannon, W. B. (1929). *Bodily changes in pain, hunger, fear and rage: An account of recent research into the functions of emotional excitement* (2nd ed.). New York: Appleton-Century-Crofts.

Carr, D. B., Sheehan, D. V., Surman, O. S., Coleman, J. H., Greenblatt, D. J., Heninger, G. R., Jones, K. J., Levine, P. H., & Watkins, W. D. (1986). Neuroendocrine correlates of lactate-induced anxiety and their response to chronic alprazolam therapy. *American Journal of Psychiatry, 143,* 483–494.

Cechetto, D. F., & Carlaresu, F. R. (1984). Units in the amygdala responding to activation of carotid baro- and chemoreceptors. *American Journal of Physiology, 246 (Regulatory Integrative Comparative Physiology, 15),* R832–R836.

Cechetto, D. F., Ciriello, J., & Carlaresu, F. (1983). Afferent connections of cardiovascular sites in the amygdala: A horseradish peroxidase study in the cat. *Journal of the Autonomic Nervous System, 8,* 97–110.

Cedarbaum, J. M., & Aghajanian, G. K. (1977). Catecholamine receptors on locus coeruleus neurons: Pharmacological characterization. *European Journal of Pharmacology, 44,* 375–385.

Chaput, Y., de Montigny, C., & Blier, P. (1986). Effects of a selective 5-HT reuptake blocker, citalopram, on the sensitivity of 5-HT autoreceptors: Electrophysiological studies in the rat brain. *Naunyn Schmiedebergs Archives of Pharmacology, 333,* 342–348.

Charney, D. S., Goodman, W. K., Price, L. H., Woods, S. W., Rasmussen, S. A., & Heninger, G. R. (1988). Serotonin function in obsessive–compulsive disorder: A comparison of the effects of tryptophan and m-chloro-phenylpiperazine in patients and healthy subjects. *Archives of General Psychiatry, 45,* 117–185.

Charney, D. S., & Heninger, G. R. (1985). Noradrenergic function and the mechanism of action of antianxiety treatment: I. The effects of long-term alprazolam treatment. *Archives of General Psychiatry, 42,* 458–467.

Charney, D. S., & Heninger, G. R. (1986). Abnormal regulation of noradrenergic functioning in panic disorder: Effects of clonidine in healthy subjects and patients with agoraphobia and panic disorder. *Archives of General Psychiatry, 43,* 1042–1054.

Charney, D. S., Heninger, G. R., & Breier, A. (1984). Nonadrenergic function in panic anxiety: Effects of yohimbine in healthy subjects and patients with agoraphobia and panic disorder. *Archives of General Psychiatry, 41,* 751–763.

Charney, D. S., Heninger, G. R., Sternberg, D. E., Hafstad, K. M., Giddings, S., & Landis, H. (1982). Adrenergic sensitivity in depression. *Archives of General Psychiatry, 39,* 290–294.

Charney, D. S., Woods, S. W., Goodman, W. K., & Heninger, G. R. (1987). Neurobiologic mechanisms of panic anxiety: Biochemical and behavioral correlates of yohimbine-induced panic attacks. *American Journal of Psychiatry, 144,* 1030–1036.

Charney, D. S., Woods, S. W., Price, H. L., Goodman, W. K., Glazier, W. M., & Heninger, G. H. (1990). Noradrenergic dysregulation in panic disorder. In J. C. Ballenger (Ed.), *Neurobiology of panic disorder* (pp. 91–105). New York: Wiley-Liss.

Chavis, D. A., & Pandya, D. N. (1976). Further observations on corticofrontal connections in the rhesus monkey. *Brain Research, 117,* 369–386.

Chevalier, G., & Deniau, J. M. (1990). Disinhibition as a basic process in the expression of striatal functions. *Trends in Neuroscience, 13,* 277–280.

Chueng, A. H., Dixon, R. A. F., Hill, W. S., Sigal, I. S., & Strader, C. D. (1990). Separation of the structural requirements for agonist-promoted activation and sequestration of the b-adrenergic receptor. *Molecular Pharmacology, 37,* 775–779.

Clark, D. M. (1986). A cognitive model of panic attacks. In S. Rachman & J. D. Maser (Eds.), *Panic: Psychological perspectives* (pp. 71–91). Hillsdale, NJ: Erlbaum.

Clomipramine Collaborative Study Group. (1991). Clomipramine in the treatment of patients with obsessive–compulsive disorder. *Archives of General Psychiatry, 48,* 730–738.

Cloninger, R. (1987). Neurogenetic adaptive mechanisms in alcohol. *Science, 236,* 410–416.

Coccaro, E., Siever, L., & Klar, H. (1989). Sertonergic studies in affective and personality disorder patients. *Archives of General Psychiatry, 46,* 587–599.

Collins, P., & Depue, R. A. (1992). A neurobehavioral systems approach to developmental psychopathology. In D. Cicchetti & S. Toth (Eds.), *Developmental perspectives on depression* (vol. 4). Rochester, NY: University of Rochester Press.

Collins, S., Bouvier, M., Bolanowski, M. A., Caron, M. G., & Lefkowitz, R. J. (1989). cAMP stimulates transcription of b_2-adrenergic receptor gene in response to short term agonist exposure. *Proceedings of the National Academy of Science USA, 86,* 4853–4857.

Conn, P. J., & Sanders-Bush, E. (1987). Relative efficacies of piperazines at the phospoinositide hydrolysis-linked serotonergic (5-HT-2 and 5-HT-1c) receptors. *Journal of Pharmacology and Experimental Therapeutics, 242,* 552–557.

Cookson, J. C. (1985). The neuroendocrinology of mania. *Journal of Affective Disorders, 8,* 233–241.

Cools, A. R. (1980). The role of neostriatal dopaminergic activity in sequencing and selecting behavioral strategies: Facilitation of processes involved in selecting the best strategy in a stressful situation. *Behavioral Brain Research, 1,* 361–374.

Corsellis, J., & Jack, A. B. (1973). Neuropathological observation on yitrium implanted on undercutting in the orbito-frontal areas of the brain. In L. V. Laiitinen & K. V. Livingston (Eds.), *Surgical approaches in psychiatry* (pp. 90–95). Baltimore: University Park Press.

Cortes, R., Gueye, B., Pazos, A., Probst, A., & Palacios, J. M. (1989). Dopamine receptors in human brain: Autoradiographic distribution of D1 sites. *Neuroscience, 28,* 263–273.

Cowen, P. J., Anderson, I. M., & Gartside, S. E. (1990). Endicrinological responses to 5-HT. *Annals of the New York Academy of Sciences, 600,* 250–257.

Cox, C. S., Fedio, P., & Rapoport, J. L. (1989). Neuropsychological testing of obsessive–compulsive adolescents. In J. L. Rapoport (Ed.), *Obsessive–compulsive disorder in children & adolescents* (pp. 73–85). Washington, DC: American Psychiatric Press.

Davis, J., Koslow, S., Gibbons, R., Maas, J., Bowden, C., Casper, R., Hanin, I., Javaid, J., Chang, S., & Stokes, P. (1988). Cerebrospinal fluid and urinary amines in depressed patients and healthy controls. *Archives of General Psychiatry, 45,* 705–717.

DeLong, M. R., & Georgopoulos, A. P. (1979). Motor functions of the basal ganglia as revealed by studies of single cell activity in the behaving primate. *Advances in Neurology, 24,* 1331–1340.

Depue, R. A. (in press). *Neurobehavioral systems, personality, and psychopathology.* New York: Springer-Verlag.

Depue, R. A., & Iacono, W. G. (1989). Neurobehavioral aspects of affective disorders. *Annual Review of Psychology, 40,* 457–492.

Depue, R. A., Krauss, S., & Spoont, M. R. (1987). A two-dimensional threshold model of seasonal bipolar affective disorder. In D. Magnusson & A. Ohman (Eds.), *Psychopathology: An interactional perspective* (pp. 95–123). New York: Academic Press.

Depue, R., Krauss, S., Spoont, M., & Arbisi, P. (1989). Identification of unipolar and bipolar affective conditions in a university population with the General Behavior Inventory. *Journal of Abnormal Psychology, 98,* 117–126.

Depue, R. A., Luciana, M., Arbisi, P., Collins, P. F., & Leon, A. (1992). *Relation of agonist-induced dopamine activity to personality.* Manuscript submitted for publication.

Depue, R. A., & Monroe, S. M. (1978). The unipolar–bipolar distinction in the depressive disorders. *Psychological Bulletin, 85,* 1001–1029.

Depue, R. A., & Monroe, S. M. (1986). Conceptualization and measurement of human disorders in life stress research: The problem of chronic disturbance. *Psychological Bulletin, 92,* 35–36.

Depue, R. A., & Spoont, M. R. (1986). Conceptualizing a serotonin trait: A behavioral dimension of constraint. *Annals of the New York Academy of Sciences, 487,* 47–62.

Diamond, M. C. (1967). Extensive cortical depth measurements and neuron size increases in the cortex of environmentally enriched rats. *Journal of Comparative Neurology, 131,* 357–364.

Divac, I., Rosvold, H. E., & Szwarcbart, M. K. (1967). Behavioral effects of selective ablation of the caudae nucleus. *Journal of Comparative and Physiologic Psychology, 63,* 184–190.

Elam, M., Svensson, T. H., & Thoren, P. (1986). Locus coeruleus neurons and sympathetic nerves: Activation by cutaneous sensory afferents. *Brain Research, 366,* 254–261.

Elam, M., Yao, T., Thoren, P., & Svensson, T. H. (1981). Hypercapnia and hypoxia: Chemoreceptor-mediated control of locus coeruleus neurons and splanchnic, sympathetic nerves. *Brain Research, 222,* 281–287.

Ervin, F. R., & Martin, J. (1986). Neurophysiological bases of the primary emotions. In E. Plutchik & H. Kellerman (Eds.), *Emotion: Theory, research, and experience: Vol. 3. Biological foundations of emotion* (pp. 145–170). New York: Academic Press.

Evenden, J. L., & Robbins, T. W. (1983). Increased response switching, perseveration and perseverative switching following d-amphetamine in the rat. *Psychopharmacology, 80,* 67–73.

Eysenck, H. J., & Eysenck, M. W. (1985). *Personality and individual differences: A natural science approach.* New York: Plenum.

Fibiger, H. C., & Phillips, A. G. (1981). Increased intracranial self-stimulation in rats after long-term administration of desipramine. *Science, 214,* 683–685.

Fibiger, H. C., & Phillips, A. G. (1987). Role of catecholamine transmitters in brain reward systems: Implications for the neurobiology of affect. In J.

Engel & L. Oreland (Eds.), *Brain reward systems and abuse* (pp. 61–74). New York: Raven.

Fink, J. S., & Reis, D. J. (1981). Genetic variations in midbrain dopamine cell number: Parallel with differences in responses to dopaminergic agonists and naturalistic behaviors mediated by dopaminergic systems. *Brain Research, 222,* 335–349.

Fink, J. S., & Smith, G. P. (1980). Mesolimbic and mesocortical dopaminergic neurons are necessary for normal exploratory behavior in rats. *Neuroscience Letters, 17,* 61–65.

Fink, M. (1984). Theories of the antidepressant efficacy of convulsive therapy (ECT). In R. M. Post & J. C. Ballenger (Eds.), *Neurobiology of mood disorders* (pp. 721–730). Baltimore: Williams & Wilkins.

Fishman, R., Feigenbaum, J., Yanaiz, J., & Klawans, H. (1983). The relative importance of dopamine and norepinephrine in mediating locomotor activity. *Progress in Neurobiology, 20,* 55–58.

Floeter, M. K., & Greenough, W. T. (1979). Cerebellar plasticity: Modification of Purkinje cell structure by different rearing in monkeys. *Science, 206,* 227–229.

Flowers, K., & Robertson, C. (1985). The effect of Parkinson's disease on the ability to maintain mental set. *Journal of Neurology, Neurosurgery and Psychiatry, 48,* 517–529.

Fonberg, E. (1986). Amygdala, emotions, motivation, and depressive states. In E. Plutchik & H. Kellerman (Eds.), *Emotion: Theory, research, and experience: Vol. 3. Biological foundations of emotion* (pp. 301–331). New York: Academic Press.

Foote, S. L., Bloom, F. E., & Aston-Jones, G. (1983). Nucleus locus ceruleus: New evidence of anatomical and physiological specificity. *Physiological Reviews, 63,* 844–914.

Fowles, D. C. (1987). Application of a behavioral theory of motivation to the concepts of anxiety and impulsivity. *Journal of Research in Personality, 21,* 417–435.

Freeman, B. J., & Ray, O. S. (1972). Strain, sex, and environmental effects on appetitively and aversively motivated learning tasks. *Developmental Psychobiology, 5,* 101–109.

Friedman, H. R., Janas, J. D., & Goldman-Rakic, P. S. (1990). Enhancement of metabolicactivity in the diencephalon of monkeys performing working memory tasks: A 2-deoxyglucose study in behaving rhesus monkeys. *Journal of Cognitive Neuroscience, 2,* 18–31.

Funahashi, S., Bruce, C. J., & Goldman-Rakic, P. S. (1989). Mnemonic coding of visual space in the monkey's dorsolateral prefrontal cortex. *Journal of Neurophysiology, 61,* 331–349.

Fuster, J. M. (1973). Unit activity in prefrontal cortex during delayed-response performance: Neuronal correlates of transient memory. *Journal of Neurophysiology, 36,* 61–78.

Fuster, J. M. (1980). *The prefrontal cortex.* New York: Raven.

Fuster, J. M. (1989). *The prefrontal cortext* (2nd ed.). New York: Raven.

Gaffori, O., & LeMoal, M. (1979). Disruption of maternal behavior and appearance of cannibalism after ventral mesencephalic tegmentum lesions. *Physiology Behavior, 23,* 317–343.

Gallagher, M., Kapp, B. S., Pascoe, J. P., & Rapp, P. R. (1981). A neuropharmacology of amygdala systems which contribute to learning and memory. In Y. Ben-Ari (Ed.), *The amygdaloid complex* (pp. 175–184). Elsevier: Amsterdam.

Gallistel, C. R., Shizgal, P., & Yeomans, J. S. (1981). A portrait of the substrate for self-stimulation. *Psychological Review, 88*, 228–273.

Gaspar, P., Berger, B., Febvret, A., Vigny, A., & Henry, J. P. (1989). Catecholamine innervation of the human cerebral cortex as revealed by comparative immunohistochemistry of tyrosine hydroxylase and dopamine-beta-hydroxylase. *Journal of Comparative Neurology, 279*, 249–271.

Glazer, W. M., Charney, D. S., & Heninger, G. R. (1987). Noradrenergic function in schizophrenia. *Archives of General Psychiatry, 44*, 898–904.

Glennon, R. A. (1990). Serotonin receptors: Clinical implications. *Neuroscience and Biobehavioral Reviews, 14*, 35–47.

Goldberg, G. (1985). Supplementary motor area structure and function: Review and hypotheses. *The Behavioral and Brain Sciences, 8*, 567–616.

Goldman-Rakic, P. S. (1987). Circuitry of the prefrontal cortex and the regulation of behavior by representational memory. In *Handbook of Physiology* (Vol. 5, pp. 373–417). Washington, DC: American Physiological Society.

Goldman-Rakic, P. S. (1988). Topography of cognition: Parallel distributed networks in primate association cortex. *Annual Review of Neuroscience, 11*, 137–156.

Goldman-Rakic, P. S. (1990). Cellular and circuit basis of working memory in prefrontal cortex of nonhuman primates. In H. B. M. Uylings, C. G. Van Eden, J. P. C. De Bruin, M. A. Corner, & M. G. P. Feenstra (Eds.), *Progress in Brain Research, 85*, 325–336.

Goodman, W. K., Price, L. P., Delgado, P. L., Palumbo, J., Krystal, J. H., Nagy, L. M., Rasmussen, S. A., Heninger, G. R., & Charney, D. S. (1990). Specificity of serotonin reuptake inhibitors in the treatment of obsessive-compulsive disorder. *Archives of General Psychiatry, 47*, 577–585.

Gorman, J. M., Askanazi, J., Liebowitz, M. R., Fyer, A. J., Stein, J. S., Kinnery, J. M., & Klein, D. F. (1984). Response to hyperventilation in a group of patients with panic disorder. *American Journal of Psychiatry, 141*, 857–861.

Gorman, J. M., Cohen, B. S., Liebowitz, M. R., Fyer, A. J., Ross, D., Davies, S. O., & Klein, D. F. (1986). Blood gas changes and hpophosphatemia in lactate-induced panic. *Archives of General Psychiatry, 43*, 1067–1071.

Gorman, J. M., & Papp, L. A. (1989). Respiratory physiology of panic. In J. C. Ballenger (Ed.), *Neurobiology of Panic Disorder* (pp. 187–204). New York: Wiley-Liss.

Grant, S. J., Huang, Y. H., & Redmond, D. E. Jr. (1980). Benzodiazepines regulate single unit activity in the locus coeruleus. *Life Science, 27*, 2231–2236.

Grant, S. J., & Redmond, D. E. Jr. (1984). Neuronal activity of the locus coeruleus in awake *Macaca arctoides*. *Experimental Neurology, 84*, 701–708.

Gray, J. A. (1973). Causal theories of personality and how to test them. In J. R. Royce (Ed.), *Multivariate analysis and psychological theory* (pp. 409–463). New York: Academic Press.

Gray, J. A. (1982). *The neuropsychology of anxiety*. New York: Oxford University Press.

Graybiel, A. (1990). Neurotransmitters and neuromodulators in the basal ganglia. *Trends in Neuroscience, 13,* 244–254.

Green, E. J., Greenough, W. T., & Schlumpf, B. E. (1983). Effects of complex or isolated environments on cortical dendrites of middle-aged rats. *Brain Research, 264,* 233–240.

Greenough, W. T., & Black, J. E. (in press). Induction of brain structure by experience: Substrates for cognitive development. In M. R. Gunnar & C. A. Nelson (Eds.), *Minnesota Symposia on Child Psychology* (Vol. 24). Minneapolis: University of Minnesota Press.

Greenough, W. T., Black, J. E., & Wallace, C. S. (1987). Experience and brain development. *Child Development, 58,* 539–559.

Greenough, W. T., Fulcher, J. K., Yuwiler, A., & Geller, E. (1970). Enriched rearing and chronic electroshock: Effects on brain and behavior in mice. *Physiology and Behavior, 5,* 371–373.

Greenough, W. T., & Volkmar, F. R. (1973). Pattern of dendritic branching in rat occipital cortex after rearing in complex environments. *Experimental Neurology, 40,* 491–504.

Greenough, W. T., Volkmar, F. R., & Juraska, J. M. (1973). Effects of rearing complexity on dendritic branching in frontolateral and temporal cortex of the rat. *Experimental Neurology, 41,* 371–378.

Greenough, W. T., West, R. W., & DeVoogd, T. J. (1978). Subsynaptic plate perforations: Changes with age and experience in the rat. *Science, 202,* 1096–1098.

Greenough, W. T., Wood, W. E., & Madden, T. C. (1972). Possible memory storage differences among mice reared in environments varying in complexity. *Behavioral Biology, 7,* 717–722.

Greenough, W. T., Yuwiler, A., & Dollinger, M. (1973). Effects of post-trial eserine administration on learning in "enriched" and "impoverished" reared rats. *Behavioral Biology, 8,* 261–272.

Haber, S. N. (1986). Neurotransmitters in the human and nonhuman primate basal ganglia. *Human Neurobiology, 5,* 159–168.

Hange, A., Thoresen, M., & Wallace, L. (1980). Changes in cerebral blood flow during hyperventilation and CO_2 rebreathing in humans by a bidirectional, pulsed ultrasound doppler velocity meter. *Acta Physiologica Scandinavica, 110,* 167–173.

Hassler, R., & Dieckman, G. (1973). Relief of obsessive–compulsive disorders phobias and tics by sterotactic coagulation on the rostral intralaminar and medial thalamic nuclei. In L. V. Laiitinen & K. V. Livingston (Eds.), *Surgical approaches in psychiatry* (pp. 206–212). Baltimore: University Park Press.

Hebb, D. O. (1949). *The organization of behavior.* New York: Wiley.

Heinsimer, J. A., Davies, A. O., Dowens, R. W., Levine, M. A., Spiegel, A. M., Drezner, M. K., De Lean, A., Wreggett, K. A., Caron, M. G., & Lefkowitz, R. J. (1983). Impaired formation of β-adrenergic receptor-nucleotide regulatory protein complexes in pseudohypoparathyroidism. *Journal of Clinical Investigation, 21,* 1335–1343.

Heninger, G. R., Charney, D. S., & Price, L. H. (1988). Alpha$_2$-adrenergic receptor function in depression: The plasma MHPG, behavioral, and cardiovascular responses to yohimbine. *Archives of General Psychiatry, 45,* 718–726.

Herzog, A. G., & Van Hoesen, G. W. (1976). Temporal neocortical afferent connections to the amygdala in the rhesus monkey. *Brain Research, 115,* 57–69.

Hewlett, W. A., Agras, W. S., & Berman, S. (1989). Fenfluramine stimulation of hormone release in obsessive compulsive disorder. *Society for Neuroscience Abstracts, 15,* 1122.

Higley, J., Mehlman, P., Taub, D., Higley, S., Suomi, S., Linnoila, M., & Vickers, J. (1992). Cerebrospinal fluid monoamine and adrenal correlates of aggression in free-ranging rhesus monkeys. *Archives of General Psychiatry, 49,* 436–441.

Hill, R. T. (1970). Facilitation of conditioned reinforcement as a mechanism of psychomotorstimulants. In E. Costa & S. Garattini (Eds.), *Amphetamines and related compounds* (pp. 781–795). New York: Raven.

Hollander, E., Fay, M., Cohen, B., Campeas, R., Gorman, J. M., & Liebowitz, M. R. (1988). Serotenergic and noradrenergic sensitivity in obsessive compulsive disorder: Behavioral findings. *American Journal of Psychiatry, 145,* 1015–1017.

Hollander, E., DeCaria, C., Cooper, T., & Liebowitz, M. R. (1989). Neuroendocrine sensitivity in obsessive–compulsive disorder. *Biological Psychiatry, 25,* 5A.

Hollander, E., DeCaria, C., Fay, M., & Liebowitz, M. R. (1989). Repeat m-CPP challenge during fluoxetine treatment in obsessive–compulsive disorder: Behavioral and neuroendocrine responses. *Biological Psychiatry, 25,* 8A.

Hollander, D., Decaria, C. M., Nitescu, A., Gully, R., Sckow, R. F., Cooper, T. B., Gorman, J. M., Klein, D. F., & Liebowitz, M. R. (1992). Serotenergic function in obsessive–compulsive disorder: Behavioral and neuroendocrine responses to oral m-chlorophenypiperazin and fenfluramine in patients and healthy volunteers. *Archives of General Psychiatry, 49,* 21–28.

Hollander, E., Schiffman, E., Cohen, B., Rivera-Stein, M. A., Rosen, W. R., Gorman, J. M., Fyer, A. J., Papp, L., & Liebowitz, M. R. (1990). Signs of central nervous system dysfunction in obsessive–compulsive disorder. *Archives of General Psychiatry, 47,* 27–32.

Horowitz, M. (1975). Intrusive and repetitive thoughts after experimental stress. *Archives of General Psychiatry, 32,* 1457–1463.

Hoyer, D. (1988). Functional correlates of 5-HT$_1$ recognition sites. *Journal of Receptor Research, 8,* 59–81.

Huang, Y. H., Redmond, D. E., Jr., & Snyder, D. R. (1976). Loss of fear following bilateral lesions in the locus coeruleus in the *Macaca arctoides. Neuroscience Abstract, 2,* 573.

Huttenlocher, P. R. (1990). Morphometric study of human cerebral cortex development. *Neuropsychologia, 28,* 517–527.

Insel, T. J., Zohar, J., Benkelfat, C., & Murphy, D. L. (1990). Serotonin in obsessions, compulsions, and the control of aggressive impulses. *Annals of the New York Academy of Sciences, 600,* 574–586.

Insel, T. R., Mueller, E. A., Alterman, I., Linnoila, M., & Murphy, D. L. (1985). Obsessive–compulsive disorder and serotonin: Is there a connection? *Biological Psychiatry, 20,* 1174–1189.

Insel, T. R., Mueller, E. A., Gillin, J. C., Siever, L. J., & Murphy, D. L. (1984).

Biological markers in obsessive–compulsive and affective disorders. *Journal of Psychiatry Research, 18,* 407–423.

Iversen, S. D. (1978). Brain dopamine systems and behavior. In L. Iversen, S. Iversen, and S. Snyder (Eds.), *Handbook of psychopharmacology* (Vol. 8, pp. 333–384). New York: Plenum.

Iversen, S. D., & Mishkin, M. (1970). Perseverative interference in monkeys following selective lesions of the inferior prefrontal convexity. *Experimental Brain Research, 11,* 376–386.

Jacobs, B. L. (1986). Single unit activity of the locus coeruleus neurons in behavior animals. *Progress in Neurobiology, 27,* 83–194.

Jimerson, D. C., & Post, R. M. (1984). Psychomotor stimulants and dopamine agonists in depression. In R. M. Post & J. C. Ballenger (Eds.), *Neurobiology of mood disorders* (pp. 619–628). Baltimore: Williams & Wilkins.

Jones, E. G., & Powell, T. P. S. (1970). An anatomical study of converging sensory pathways within the cerebral cortex of the monkey. *Brain, 93,* 793–820.

Juraska, J. M., Fitch, J., Henderson, C., & Rivers, N. (1985). Sex differences in the dendritic branching of dentate granule cells following differential housing experience. *Brain Research, 333,* 73–80.

Juraska, J. M., Fitch, P., & Washburne, D. L. (1989). The dendritic morphology of pyramidal neurons in the rat hippocampal CA3 area: II. Effects of gender and experience. *Brain Research, 479,* 115–119.

Juraska, J. M., Greenough, W. T., Elliott, C., Mack, K. J., & Berkowitz, R. (1980). Plasticity in adult rat visual cortex: An examination of several cell populations after differential housing. *Behavioral and Neural Biology, 29,* 157–167.

Kahn, R. S., Asnis, G. M., Wetzler, S., & Van Praag, H. (1988). Neuroendocrine evidence for serotonin receptor hypersensitivity in panic disorder. *Psychopharmacology, 96,* 360–364.

Kehr, W. (1981). 3-Methoxytyramine and normetanephrine as indicators of dopamine and noradrenaline release in mouse brain *in vivo. Journal of Neural Transmission, 50,* 165–178.

Kelly, P. (1978). Drug-induced behavior. In S. D. Iversen, L. L., Iversen, & S. Snyder (Eds.), *Handbook of psychopharmacology* (Vol. 8, pp. 295–331). New York: Plenum.

Kemp, J. M., & Powell, T. P. S. (1970). The cortico-striate projections in the monkey. *Brain, 93,* 525–546.

Kennealy, J. A., McLellan, J. E., London, R. G., & McLaurin, R. L. (1980). Hyperventilation-induced cerebral hypoxia. *American Journal of Respiratory Disorders, 122,* 407–411.

Killackey, H. P. (1990). Neocortical expansion: An attempt toward relating phylogeny and ontogeny. *Journal of Cognitive Neuroscience, 2,* 1–17.

Kling, A. S. (1986). The anatomy of aggression and affiliation. In E. Plutchik & H. Kellerman (Eds.), *Emotion: Theory, research, and experience: Vol. 3. Biological foundations of emotion* (pp. 237–263). New York: Academic Press.

Ko, G. N., Elsworth, J. D., Roth, R. H., Rifkin, G. B., Leigh, H., & Redmond, D. E. Jr. (1983). Panic-induced elevation of plasma MHPG levels in phobic-anxious patients: Effects of clonidine and imipramine. *Archives of General Psychiatry, 40,* 425–430.

Kolbilka, B. (1992). Adrenergic receptors as models for G protein-coupled receptors. *Annual Review of Neuroscience, 15,* 87–114.

Konorski, J. (1967). *Integrative activity of the brain: An interdisciplinary approach.* Chicago: University of Chicago Press.

Koob, G. F., & Bloom, F. E. (1988). Cellular and molecular mechanisms for drug dependence. *Science, 242,* 715–723.

Kopin, I. J., Eisenhofer, G., & Goldstein, D. (1986). Sympathoadrenal medullary system and stress. In Chrousos, G. P., Loriaux, L., & Gold, P. W. (Eds.), *Mechanisms of physical and emotional stress* (pp. 11–23). New York: Plenum.

Kosslyn, S. M. (1988). Aspects of a cognitive neuroscience of mental imagery. *Science, 240,* 1621–1626.

Kravitz, E. A. (1988). Hormonal control of behavior. *Science, 241,* 1775–1781.

Kruesi, M., Hibbs, E., Zahn, T., Keysor, C., Hamburger, S., Bartko, J., & Rappoport, J. (1992). A 2-year prospective study of children and adolescents with disruptive behavior disorders. *Archives of General Psychiatry, 49,* 429–435.

Kubota, K., & Niki, H. (1971). Prefrontal cortical unit activity and delayed alternation performance in monkeys. *Journal of Neurophysiology, 34,* 337–347.

Laplane, D., Bulac, M., Widlocher, D., & Dubois, B. (1984). Pure psychic akinesia with bilateral lesions of the basal ganglia. *Journal of Neurology, Neurosurgery, and Psychiatry, 47,* 377–385.

Lauder, J. M., & Krebs, H. (1986). Do neurotransmitters, neurohumors, and hormones specify critical periods? In W. T. Greenough & J. Juraska (Eds.), *Developmental Neuropsychobiology* (pp. 120–174). New York: Academic Press.

LeDoux, J. E. (1987). Emotion. In *Handbook of physiology* (Vol. 5, pp. 419–459). Washington, DC: American Physiological Society.

Lefkowitz, R. J., Caron, M. G., & Stiles, G. L. (1984). Mechanisms of membrane–receptor regulation: Biochemical, physiological, and clinical insights derived from studies of the adrenergic receptors. *New England Journal of Medicine, 310,* 1570–1579.

Lefkowitz, R. J., Stadel, J. M., & Caron, M. G. (1983). Adenylate cyclase-coupled beta-adrenergic receptors: Structure and mechanisms of activation and desensitization. *Annual Review of Biochemistry, 52,* 159–186.

Levi, L. (1975). *Emotions: Their parameters and measurement.* New York: Raven.

Levitt, P., Rakic, P., & Goldman-Rakic, P. (1984a). Region-specific distribution of catecholamine afferents in primate cerebral cortex: A fluorescence histochemial analysis. *Journal of Comparative Neurology, 227,* 23–36.

Levitt, P., Rakic, P., & Goldman-Rakic, P. (1984b). Comparative assessment of monoamine afferents in mammalian cerebral cortex. In H. H. Jasper & N. van Gelder (Eds.), *Monoamine innervation of the cerebral cortex* (pp. 41–59). New York: Liss.

Lewis, D. A., Campbell, M. J., Foote, S. L., & Morrison, J. H. (1986). The monoaminergic innervation of primate neocortex. *Human Neurobiology, 5,* 181–188.

Lewis, D. A., Campbell, M. J., Foote, S. L., & Morrison, J. H. (1987). The distribution of tyrosine hydroxylase immunoreactive fibers in primate neocortex is widespread but regionally specific. *Journal of Neuroscience, 7,* 279–290.

Lewis, D. A., Foote, S. L., Goldstein, M., & Morrison, J. H. (1988). The dopaminergic innervation of monkey prefrontal cortex: A tyrosine hydroxylase immunohistochemical study. *Brain Research, 449,* 225–243.

Liang, K. C., Juler, R. G., & McGaugh, J. L. (1986). Modulating effects of posttraining epinephrine on memory: Involvement of the amygdala noradrenergic system. *Brain Research, 368,* 125–133.

Liang, K. C., McGaugh, J. L., & Yao, Y.-H. (1990). Involvement of amygdala pathways in the influence of post-training intra-amygdala norepinephrine and peripheral epinephrene on memory storage. *Brain Research, 508,* 225–233.

Lidberg, L., Tuck, J., & Asberg, M. (1985). Homicide, suicide, and CSF-5-HIAA. *Acta Psychiatrica Scandinavica, 71,* 230–236.

Lidow, M. S., Goldman-Rakic, P. S., Rakic, P., & Innis, R. B. (1989). Dopamine D2 receptors in the cerebral cortex: Distribution and pharmacological characterization with [3H]raclopride. *Proceedings of the National Academy of Science, 86,* 6412–6416.

Liebowitz, M. R., Gorman, J. M., Fyer, A. J., Levitt, M. M., Dillon, D., Levy, P., Appleby, I., Anderson, S., Palij, M., Davies, S. O., & Klein, D. F. (1985). Lactate provocation of panic attacks: II. Biochemical and physiological findings. *Archives of General Psychiatry, 42,* 709–719.

Limberger, N., Späth, L., & Starke, K. (1986). A search for receptors modulating the release of g-[^{3}H[aminobutyric acid in rabbit caudate nucleus slices. *Journal of Neurochemistry, 46,* 1109–1117.

Linnoila, M., Virkkunen, M., & Scheinin, M. (1983). Low cerebrospinal fluid 5-HIAA concentration differentiates impulsive from nonimpulsive violent behavior. *Life Sciences, 33,* 2609–2614.

Livingston, K. E., & Escobar, A. (1971). Anatomical bias of the limbic systems concept. *Archives of Neurology, 24,* 17–21.

Louilot, A., Taghzouti, K., Deminiere, J. M., Simon, H., & Le Moal, M. (1987). Dopamine and behavior: Functional and theoretical considerations. In M. Sandler (Ed.), *Neurotransmitter interactions in the basal ganglia* (pp. 193–204). New York: Raven.

Luciana, M., Depue, R. A., Arbisi, P., & Leon, A. (1992). Facilitation of working memory in humans by a D-2 dopamine receptor agonist. *Journal of Cognitive Neuroscience, 4,* 58–68.

Lum, L. C. (1976). The syndrome of chronic hyperventilation. In O. W. Hill (Ed.), *Modern trends in psychosomatic medicine* (Vol. 3, pp. 17–35). London: Buttersworth.

Luxenberg, J. S., Swedo, S. E., Flament, M. F., Friedland, R. P., Rapoport, J., & Rapoport, S. I. (1988). Neuroanatomical abnormalities in obsessive–compulsive disorder detected with quantitative x-ray computed tomography. *American Journal of Psychiatry, 145,* 1089–1093.

Lyness, W. H., Friedle, N. M., & Moore, K. E. (1979). Destruction of dopaminergic nerve terminals in nucleus accumbens: Effect on d-amphetamine self-administration. *Pharmacology, Biochemistry, and Behavior, 11,* 553–556.

MacLean, P. D. (1969). The hypothalamus and emotional behavior. In W.

Haymaker, E. Anderson, & W. J. H. Nauta (Eds.), *The hypothalamus* (pp. 42–65). Springfield, IL: Thomas.

MacLean, P. D. (1970). The triune concept of the brain and behavior. In F. O. Schmitt (Ed.), *The neurosciences second study program* (pp. 141–175). New York: Rockerfeller University Press.

MacLean, P. D. (1975). Sensory and perceptive factors in emotional functions of the triune brain. In L. Levi (Ed.), *Emotions: Their parameters and measurement* (pp. 71–92). New York: Raven.

MacLean, P. D. (1986). Ictal symptoms relating to the nature of affects and their cerebral substrate. In E. Plutchik & H. Kellerman (Eds.), *Emotion: Theory, research, and experience: Vol. 3: Biological foundations of emotion* (pp. 61–90). New York: Academic Press.

MacLean, P. D. (1990). *The triune brain in evolution: Role in paleocerebral functions.* New York: Plenum.

Malakhova, O. E., Popovkin, E. M., & Gudina, I. G. (1989). Efferent connections of various parts of the orbitofrontal cortex with the thalamic structures of the cat. *Neuroscience and Behavioral Physiology, 19,* 507–515.

Mandell, A. J., Knapp, S., Ehlers, C., & Russo, P. V. (1984). The stability of constrained randomness: Lithium prophylaxis at several neurobiological levels. In R. M. Post & J. C. Ballenger (Eds.), *Neurobiology of mood disorders* (pp. 744–776). Baltimore: Williams & Wilkins.

Mann, J., Stanley, M., & McBride, A. (1986). Increased serotonin-2 and beta-adrenergic receptor binding in the frontal cortices of suicide victims. *Archives of General Psychiatry, 43,* 954–959.

Marczynski, T. J. (1986). A model of brain function. In W. C. McCallum, R. Zappoli, & F. Denoth (Eds.), *Cerebral psychophysiology: Studies in event-related potentials* [Special issue]. *Electroencephalography and Clinical Neurophysiology, 38,* 351–367.

Marks, I. (1987). *Fears, phobias, and rituals: Panic, anxiety and their disorders.* New York: Oxford University Press.

Mason, S. T. (1981). Noradrenaline in the brain: Progress in theories of behavioral function. *Progress in Neurobiology,16,* 263–303.

Mason, S. T. (1984). *Catecholamines and Behavior.* New York: Cambridge University Press.

Mattson, M. P. (1988). Neurotransmitters in the regulation of neuronal cytoarchitecture. *Brain Research Reviews, 13,* 179–212.

Mattson, M. P., Dou, P., & Kater, S. B. (1988). Outgrowth-regulating actions of glutamate in isolated hippocampal pyramidal neurons. *Journal of Neuroscience, 8,* 2087–2100.

McGaugh, J. L., Introini-Collison, I. & Nagahara, A. (1988). Memory enhancing effects of postraining naloxone: Involvement of β-noradrenergic influences in the amygdaloid complex. *Brain Reseach, 446,* 37–49.

Meltzer, H., & Lowy, M. (1987). The serotonin hypothesis of depression. In H. Meltzer (Ed.), *Psychopharmacology: The third generation of progress* (pp. 513–526). New York: Raven Press.

Mesulam, M.-M. (1984). A cortical network for directed attention and unilateral neglect. In A. Ardila & F. Ostrosky-Solis (Eds.), *The right hemisphere* (pp. 61–96). New York: Gordon & Breach.

Mesulam, M.-M. (1990). Large-scale neurocognitive networks and distributed processing for attention, language, and memory. *Annals of Neurology, 28,* 597–613.

Mesulam, M.-M., & Mufson, E. J. (1982a). Insula of the old world monkey: Part I. Architectonics in the insulo-orbito-temporal component of the para-limbic brain. *Journal of Comparative Neurology, 212,* 1–22.

Mesulam, M.-M., & Mufson, E. J. (1982b). Insula of the old world monkey: Part III. Efferent cortical output and comments on function. *Journal of Comparative Neurology, 212,* 38–52.

Mesulam, M.-M., & Mufson, E. J. (1984). Neural inputs into the nucleus basalis of the substantia innominata (CH4) in the rhesus monkey. *Brain, 107,* 253–274.

Milner, B. (1963). Effects of different lesions on card sorting. *Archives of Neurology, 9,* 90–100.

Milner, B. (1964). Some effects of frontal lobectomy in man. In J. M. Warren & K. Akert (Eds.), *The frontal granular cortex and behavior* (pp. 313–334). New York: McGraw-Hill.

Milner, B. (1971). Interhemispheric differences and psychological processes in man. *British Medical Bulletin, 27,* 272–277.

Mindus, P., Bergstrom, K., Levandar, S. E., Noren, G., Hindmarsh, T. & Thuomas, K.-A. (1987). Magnetic resonance images related to clinical outcome after psychosurgical intervention in severe anxiety disorder. *Journal of Neurology, Neurosurgery and Psychiatry, 50,* 1288–1293.

Mishkin, M. (1982). A memory system in the monkey. *Philosophical Transactions of the Royal Society, B298,* 85–95.

Mogenson, G. J., Jones, D. L., & Yim, C. Y. (1980). From motivation to action: Functional interface between the limbic system and the motor system. *Progress in Neurobiology, 14,* 69–97.

Mogenson, G. J., Takigawa, M., Robertson, A., & Wu, M. (1979). Self-stimulation of the nucleus accumbens and ventral tegmental area of Tsai attenuated by microinjections of spiroperidol into the nucleus accumbens. *Brain Research, 171,* 247–259.

Monroe, S. M. (1992). Psychosocial factors in anxiety and depression. In J. Maser & C. R. Cloninger (Eds.), *Comorbidity in anxiety and mood disorders.* Washington, DC: American Psychiatric Press, Inc.

Monroe, S. M., & Depue, R. A. (1992). Life stress and depression. In J. Becker & A. Kleinman (Eds.), *Affective disorders: Theory and research. Vol. 1. Psychosocial aspects.* New York: Erlbaum.

Montigny, C. de, Chaput, Y., Blier, P. (1990). Modification of serotenergic neuron properties by long-term treatment with serotonin reuptake blockers. *Journal of Clinical Psychiatry, 51* (Suppl. B), 4–8.

Moore, R. Y., & Bloom, F. E. (1978). Central catecholamine neuron systems: Anatomy and physiology of the dopamine systems. *Annual Review of Neuroscience, 1,* 129–169.

Morgan, M. J. (1973). Effects of post-weanling environment on learning in the rat. *Animal Behaviour, 21,* 4429–4442.

Morrison, J. H., Foote, S. L., Molliver, M. E., Bloom, F. E., & Lidov, G. W. (1982). Noradrenergic and serotonergic fibers innervate complementary layers in monkey visual cortex: An immunohistochemical study. *Proceedings of the National Academy of Sciences USA, 79,* 2401–2405.

Murphy, D. L, Zohar, J., Benkelfat, C., Pato, M. T., Pigott, T. A., & Insel, T. R. (1989). Obsessive–compulsive disorder as a 5–HT subsystem-related behavioural disorder. *British Journal of Psychiatry, 155*(Suppl. 8), 15–24.

Nauta, W. J. H. (1964). Some efferent connections of the prefrontal cortex in the monkey. In J. M. Warren & K. Akert (Eds.), *The frontal granular cortex and behavior (pp. 397–409). New York: McGraw-Hill.*

Nauta, W. J. H. (1971). The problem of the frontal lobe: A reinterpretation. *Journal of Psychiatric Research, 8,* 167–187.

Nauta, W. J. H. (1986). Circuitous connections linking cerebral cortex, limbic system, and corpus striatum. In B. K. Doane & K. E. Livingston (Eds.), *The limbic system: Functional organization and clinical disorderss* (pp. 43–54). New York: Raven Press.

Nauta, W. J. H. & Domesick, V. B. (1981). Ramifications of the limbic system. In S. Matthysse (Ed.), *Psychiatry and the biology of the human brain* (pp. 165–188). Amsterdam: Elsevier North Holland.

Nee L., Caine, E., Polinsky, R., Eldridge, R., & Ebert, M. (1980). Gilles de la Tourette syndrome: Clinical and family studies of 50 cases. *Annals of Neurology, 7,* 41–49.

Niki, H. (1974a). Differential activity of prefrontal units during right and left delayed response trials. *Brain Research, 70,* 346–349.

Niki, H. (1974b). Prefrontal unit activity during delayed alternation in the monkey: I. Relation to direction of response. *Brain Research, 68,* 185–196.

Niki, H. (1974c). Prefrontal unit activity during delayed alternation in the monkey: I. Relation to absolute versus relative direction of response. *Brain Research, 68,* 197–204.

Nordahl, T. E., Benkelfat, C., Semple, W. E., Gross, M., King, A. C., & Cohen, R. M. (1989). Cerebral glucose metabolic rates in obsessive compulsive disorder. *Neuropsychopharmacology, 2,* 23–28.

Nutt, D. J. (1986). Increased central α_2-adrenoceptor sensitivity in panic disorder. *Psychopharmacology, 90,* 268–269.

Nutt, D. J. (1989). Altered central α_2-adrenoceptor sensitivity in panic disorder. *Archives of General Psychiatry, 46,* 165–169.

Oades, R. D. (1985). The role of noradrenaline in tuning and dopamine in switching between signals in the CNS. *Neuroscience and Biobehavioral Reviews, 9,* 261–282.

Oades, R. D., & Halliday, G. M. (1987). Ventral tegmental (A10) system: Neurobiology: 1. Anatomy and connectivity. *Brain Research Reviews, 12,* 117–165.

Oades, R. D., Rea, M., & Taghzouti, K. (1984). Modulation of selective processes in learning by neocortical and limbic dopamine: Studies of behavioral strategies. In B. E. Will, P. Schmitt, & J. C. Dalrymple-Alford (Eds.), *Brain plasticity, learning, and memory* (pp. 241–251). New York: Plenum.

Oades, R. D., Taghzouti, K., Simon, H., & LeMoal, M. (1985). Dopamine-sensitive alteration and collateral behaviour in a Y-maze: Effects of d-amphetamine and haloperidol. *Psychopharmacology, 85,* 123–128.

Oades, R. D., Taghzouti, K., Rivet, J.-M., Simon, H., & Le Moal, M. (1986).

Locomotor activity in relation to dopamine and noradrenaline in the nucleus accumbens, septal and frontal areas: A 6-hydroxydopamine study. *Neuropsychobiology, 16,* 37–43.

O'Kusky, J., & Colonnier, M. (1982). Postnatal changes in the number of neurons and synapses in the visual cortex (A17) of the macaque monkey. *Journal of Comparative Neurology, 210,* 291–296.

Olton, D. S., Becker, J. T., & Handelmann, G. E. (1979). Hippocampus, space, and memory. *Behavioral and Brain Sciences, 2,* 313–365.

Panksepp, J. (1986). The anatomy of emotions. In E. Plutchik & H. Kellerman (Eds.), Emotion: Theory, research, and experience: Vol. 3: Biological foundations of emotion (pp. 91–124). New York: Academic Press.

Papez, J. W. (1937). A proposed mechanism of emotion. *Archives of Neurology and Psychiatry, 79,* 217–224.

Parkinson, L., & Rachman, S.(1981)Intrusive thoughts: The effects of an uncontrived stress. *Advances in Behaviour Research and Therapy, 3,* 111–118.

Pascoe, J., & Kapp, B. S. (1985). Electrophysiological characteristics of amygdaloid central nucleus neurons during pavlovian fear conditioning in the rabbit. *Behavioral Brain Research, 16,* 117–133.

Pauls, D., Towbin, K, Leckman, J., Zahner, G., & Cohen, D. (1986). Gilles de la Tourette's syndrome and obsessive–compulsive disorder: Evidence supporting an etiological relationsihp. *Archives of General Psychiatry 43,* 1180–1182.

Pazos, A., Probst, A., & Palacios, J.M. (1987a). Serotonin receptors in the human brain: III. Autoradiographic mapping of serotonin-1 receptors. *Neuroscience, 21,* 97–122.

Pazos, A., Probst, A. & Palacios, J. M. (1987b). Serotonin receptors in the human brain: IV. Autoradiographic mapping of serotonin-2 receptors. *Neuroscience, 21,* 123–130.

Penney, J. B., & Young, A. B. (1983). Speculations on the functional anatomy of basal ganglia disorders. *Annual Review of Neuroscience, 6,* 73–94.

Pickar, D., Cowdry, R. W., Zis, A. P., Cohen, R. M., & Murphy, D. L. (1984). Mania and hypomania during antidepressant pharmacotherapy: Clinical and research implications. In R. M. Post & J. C. Ballenger (Eds.), *Neurobiology of mood disorders* (pp. 836–845). Baltimor: Williams & Wilkins.

Piggot, T. A., Pato, M. T., Bernstein, S. E., Grover, G. N., Hill, J. L., Tolliver, B., & Murphy, D. L. (1990). Controlled comparisons of clomipramine and fluoxetine in the treatment of obsessive–compulsive disorder. *Archives of General Psychiatry, 47,* 926–932.

Piggot, T. A., Zohar, J., Hill, J. L., Bernstein, S. E. ,Grover, G. N., Zohar-Kadouch, R. C., & Murphy, D. L. (1991). Metergoline blocks the behavioral and neuroendocrine effects of orally administered m-chlorophenylpiperazine in patients with obsessive–compulsive disorder. *Biological Psychiatry, 29,* 418–426.

Pitman, R., Green, R., Jenike, M. & Mesulam, M. (1987). Clinical comparison of Tourette's disorder and obsessive–compulsive disorder. *American Journal of Psychiatry, 144,* 1166–1171.

Ploog, D. (1986). Biological foundations of the vocal expressions of emotions. In E. Plutchik & H. Kellerman (Eds.), *Emotion: Theory, research, and experience:*

Vol. 3. Biological Foundations of emotion (pp. 173–197). New York: Academic Press.

Plutchik, E., & Kellerman, H. (1986). *Emotion: Theory, research, and experience: Vol. 3. Biological foundations of emotion.* New York: Academic Press.

Plutchik, R. (1980). *Emotion: A psychoevolutionary synthesis.* New York: Harper & Row.

Porrino, L. J. (1987). Cerebral metabolic changes associated with activation of reward systems. In J. Engel & L. Oreland (Eds.), *Brain reward systems and abuse* (pp. 51–60). New York: Raven.

Porrino, L. J., Crane, A. M., & Goldman-Rakic, P. S. (1981). Direct and indirect pathways from the amygdala to the frontal lobe in rhesus monkeys. *Journal of Comparative Neurology, 198,* 121–136.

Porrino, L. J., & Goldman-Rakic, P. S. (1982). Brain stem innervation of prefrontal and anterior cingulate cortex in the rhesus monkey revealed by retrograde transport of HRP. *Journal of Comparative Neurology, 205,* 63–76.

Posner, M. I., Petersen, S. E., Fox, P. T., & Raichle, M. E. (1988). Localization of cognitive operations in the human brain. *Science, 240,* 1627–1631.

Post, R. M. (1980). Biochemical theories of mania. In R. H. Belmaker & H. M. van Praag (Eds.), *Mania: An evolving concept* (pp. 217–267). New York: Spectrum.

Post, R. M., & Uhde, T. W. (1982). Biological relationships between mania and melancholia. *L'Encephale, 8,* 213–228.

Pysh, J. J., & Weiss, M. (1979). Exercise during development induces an increase in Purkinje cell dendritic tree size. *Science, 206,* 230–232.

Rachman, S. J., & Hodgson, R. J. (1980). *Obsessions and compulsions.* Englewood Cliffs, NJ: Prentice Hall.

Rakic, P., Bourgeois, J.-P., Eckenhoff, M. F., Zecevic, M., & Goldman-Rakic, P. S. (1986). Concurrent overproduction of synapses in diverse regions of primate cerebral cortex. *Science, 232,* 232–234.

Rapoport, M. H., Risch, S. C., Gillin, J. C., Golshan, S., & Janowsky, D. S.(1989). Blunted growth hormone response to peripheral infusion of human growth hormone releasing factor in patients with panic disorder. *American Journal of Psychiatry, 146,* 92–95.

Rasmussen, K., Morilak, D. A., & Jacobs, B. L. (1986). Single unit actibity of locus coeruleus neurons in the freely moving cat: I. During naturalistic behaviors and in response to simple and complex stimuli. *Brain Research, 371,* 324–334.

Rasmussen, S. A., Goodman, W. K., & Woods, S. W. (1987). Effects of yohimbine in obsessive compulsive disorder. *Psychopharmacology, 93,* 308–373.

Raymond, J. R., Hnatowich, M., Lefkowitz, R. J., Caron, M. G. (1990). Adrenergic receptors: Models for regulation of signal transduction processes. *Hypertension, 15,* 119–131.

Reader, T. A., Ferron, A., Descarries, L., & Jasper, H. H. (1979). Modulatory role for biogenic amines in the cerebral cortex. *Brain Research, 160,* 217–229.

Redmond, D. E. Jr., & Huang, Y. H. (1979). New evidence for a locus coeruleus-norepinephrine connection with anxiety. *Life Sciences, 25,* 2149–2162.

Redmond, D. E. Jr., Huang, Y. H., & Snyder, D. R. (1972). Behavioral changes following lesions of the locus coeruleus in the monkey. *Neuroscience Abstracts, 1,* 472.

Reiner, P. B. (1986). Correlational analysis of central noradrenergic neuronal activity and sympathetic tone in behaving cats. *Brain Research, 378,* 86–96.

Ricardo, J. A., & Koh, E. T. (1978). Anatomical evidence of direct projections from the nucleus of the solitary tract to the hypothalamus, amygdala, and other forebrain structures in the rat. *Brain Research, 153,* 1–26.

Risch, S. J., & Janowsky, D. S. (1984). Cholinergic–adrenergic balance in affective illness. In R. M. Post & J. C. Ballenger (Eds.), *Neurobiology of Mood Disorders* (pp. 652–663). Baltimore: Williams & Wilkins.

Robbins, T. W. (1975). The potentiation of conditioned reinforcement by psychomotor stimulant drugs: A test of Hill's hypothesis. *Psychopharmacology, 45,* 103–114.

Robbins T. W., & Everitt B. J. (1982). Functional studies of the central catecholamines. *International Review Neurobiology, 23,* 245–261.

Roberts, D. C. S., Corcoran, M. E., & Fibiger, H. C. (1977). On the role of the ascending catecholaminergic systems in intravenous self-administration of cocaine. *Pharmacology, Biochemistry, and Behavior, 6,* 615–620.

Roberts, D. C. S., Koob, G. F., Klonoff, P., & Fibiger, H. C. (1980). Extinction and recovery of cocaine self-administration following 6-hydroxydopamine lesions of the nucleus accumbens. *Pharmacology, Biochemistry, and Behavior, 12,* 781–787.

Roberts, D. C. S., & Zito, K. A. (1987). Interpretation of lesion effects on stimulant self-administration. In M. A. Bozarth (Ed.), *Methods of assessing the reinforcing properties of abused drugs* (pp. 119–132). New York: Springer-Verlag.

Robertson, A. (1989). Multiple reward systems and the prefrontal cortex. *Neuroscience and Biobehavioral Reviews, 13,* 163–170.

Roitblat, S. (1987). *Introduction to comparative cognition.* New York: Freeman Press.

Rolls, E. T. (1986). Neural systems involved in emotion in primates. In E. Plutchik & H. Kellerman (Eds.), *Emotion: Theory, research, and experience: Vol 3. Biological foundations of emotion (pp. 125–143).* New York: Academic Press.

Rolls, E. T. (1989). Information processing in the taste system of primates. *Journal of Experimental Biology, 146,* 141–164.

Rolls, E. T. (in press). Spatial memory, episodic memory, and neuronal network functions in the hippocampus. In L. Squire (Ed.), *The biology of memory, symposia Hoechst.* Frankfurt: Hoechst, AG.

Rolls, E. T., Thorpe, S. J., & Maddison, J. (1983). Responses of striatal neurons in the behaving monkey. 1. Head of the caudate nucleus. *Behavior Brain Research, 7,* 179–210.

Rolls, E. T., & Willisms, G. V. (1987). Sensory and movement-related neuronal activity in different regions of the primate striatum. In J. S. Schneider & T. I. Lidsky (Eds.), *Basal ganglia and behavior: Sensory aspects of motor functioning* (pp. 37–59). Toronto: Hans Huber.

Rosenkilde, C. E. (1979). Functional heterogeneity of the prefrontal cortex in the monkey: A review. *Behavioral and Neural Biology, 25,* 301–345.

Rosenzweig, M. R., & Bennett, E. L. (1978). Experiential influences on brain anatomy and brain chemistry in rodents. In G. Gottlieb (Ed.), *Studies on the development of behavior and the nervous system: Vol. 4. Early influences* (pp. 289–330). New York: Academic Press.

Roth, B. L., Hamblin, M., & Ciaranello, R. D. (1990). Regulation of 5-HT$_2$ and 5-HT$_{1c}$ serotonin receptor levels: Metholody and mechanisms. *Neuropsychopharmacology, 3,* 427–433.

Roy, A., Adinoff, B., & Linnoila, M. (1988). Acting out hostility in normal volunteers: Negative correlation with CSF 5-HIAA levels. *Psychiatry Research, 24,* 187–194.

Roy, A., DeLong, J., & Linnoila, M. (1989). Cerebrospinal fluid monoamine metabolite and suicidal behavior in depressed patients: A 5-year follow-up study. *Archives of General Psychiatry, 46,* 609–612.

Roy, A., Karoum, F., & Pollack, S. (1992). Marked reduction in indexes of dopamine metabolism among patients with depression who attempt suicide. *Archives of General Psychiatry, 49,* 447–450.

Roy, A., Pickar, D., & Linnoila, M. (1985). Cerebrospinal fluid monoamine and monoamine metabolite concentrations in melancholia. *Psychiatry Research, 15,* 281–292.

Russchen, F. T., Amaral, D. G., & Price, J. L. (1985). The afferent connections of the substantia innominata in the monkey. *Journal of Comparative Neurology, 242,* 1–27.

Rylander, G. (1979). Stereotactic radiosurgery in anxiety and obsessive–compulsive states: Psychiatric aspects. In E. R. Hitchock, H. R. Ballantine, & B. A. Neyerson (Eds.), *Modern concepts in psychiatric surgery* (pp. 235–240). Amsterdam: Elsevier North Holland Biomedical.

Salkovskis, P. M. (1985). Obsessional–compulsive problems: A cognitive behavioural analysis. *Behaviour Research and Therapy, 23,* 571–583.

Sanders-Bush, E. (1990). Adaptive regulation of central serotonin receptors linked to phosphoinsitide hydrolysis. *Neuropsychopharmacology, 3,* 411–416.

Sawaguchi, T., & Goldman-Rakic, P. S. (1991). D1 dopamine receptors in prefrontal cortex: Involvement in working memory. *Science, 251,* 947–950. Sawaguchi, T., Matsumura, M., & Kubota, K. (1988). Dopamine enhances the neuronal activity related to a spatial short-term meory task in the primate prefrontal cortex. *Neuroscience Research, 5,* 465–473.

Sawaguchi, T., Matsumura, M., & Kubota, K. (1990a). Catecholamine effects on neuronal activity related to a delayed response task in monkey prefrontal cortex. *Journal of Neurophysiology, 63,* 1385–1400.

Sawaguchi, T., Matsumura, M., & Kubota, K. (1990b). Effects of dopamine antagonists on neuronal activity related to a delayed response task in monkey prefrontal cortex. *Journal of Neurophysiology, 63,* 1401–1412.

Schneider, J. S.(1987). Basal ganglia-motor influences: Role of sensory gating. In J. S. Schneider & T. I. Lidsky (Eds.), *Basal ganglia and behavior: Sensory aspects of motor functioning* (pp. 103–122). Toronto: Hans Huber.

Schneirla, T. (1959). An evolutionary and developmental theory of biphasic processes underlying approach and withdrawal. In M. Jones (Ed.), *Nebraska symposium on motivation* (pp. 27–58). Nebraska: University of Nebraska Press.

Scoville, W. B., & Bettis D. B. (1977). Results of orbital undercutting today: a personal series. In W. H. Sweet, S. Obrador, & J. Martin-Rodriguez, J. (Eds.), *neurosurgical treatment in psychiatry, pain and epilepsy* (pp. 189–197). Baltimore: University Press.

Secunda, S. K., Swann, A., Katz, M. M., Koslow, S. H., Croughan, J., Chang, S. (1987). Diagnosis and treatment of mixed mania. *American Journal of Psychiatry, 144,* 96–98.

Seeger, T. F., Porrino, L. J., Esposito, R. U., Crane, A. M., Sullivan, T. L., & Pert, A. (1984). Amphetamine effects on intracranial self-stimulation as assessed by the quantitative 2-deoxyglucose method. *Society for Neuroscience Abstracts, 10,* 307.

Segal, M., & Bloom, F. E. (1976a). The action of norepinephrine in the rat hippocampus: III. Hippocampal cellular responses to locus coeruleus stimulation in the awake rat. *Brain Research, 107,* 499–511.

Segal, M., & Bloom, F. E. (1976b). The action of norepinephrine in the rat hippocampus: IV. The effects of locus coeruleus stimulation on the evoked hippocampal unit activity. *Brain Research, 107,* 513–525.

Seigel, J. (1987). Striatal and limbic modulating influences: A search for target sites. In J. S. Schneider & T. I. Lidsky (Eds.), *Basal ganglia and behavior: Sensory aspects of motor functioning* (pp. 183–196). Toronto: Hans Huber.

Selemon, L. D., & Goldman-Rakic, P. S. (1985). Longitudinal topography and interdigitation of corticostriatal projections in the rhesus monkey. *The Journal of Neuroscience, 3,* 776–794.

Siever, L. J., Uhde, T. W., & Silberman, E. K. (1982). Growth hormone response to clonodine as a probe of noradrenergic receptor responsiveness in affective disorder patients and controls. *Psychiatry Research, 6,* 171–183.

Silverstone, T. (1985). Dopamine in manic depressive illness. *Journal of Affective Disorders, 8,* 225–231.

Simon, H., Scatton, B., & Le Moal, M. (1980). Dopaminergic A10 neurons are involved in cognitive functions. *Nature, 288,* 150–151.

Sirevaag, A. M., & Greenough, W. T. (1985). Differential rearing effects on rat visual cortex synapses: II. Synaptic morphometry. *Developmental Brain Research, 19,* 215–226.

Sitiram, N., Gillin, C., & Bunney, W. E. (1984). Cholinergic and catecholaminergic receptor sensitivity in affective illness: Strategy and theory. In R. M. Post & J. C. Ballenger (Eds.), *Neurobiology of mood disorders* (pp. 629–651). Baltimore: Williams & Wilkins.

Soubrie, P. (1986). Reconciling the role of central serotonin neurons in human and animal behavior. *The Behavioral and Brain Sciences, 9,* 319–364.

Spoont, M. (in press). Modulation of behavior by serotonin. *Psychological Bulletin.*

Spyraki, C., & Fibiger, H. C. (1981). Behavioural evidence for supersensitivity of postsynaptic dopamine receptors in the mesolimbic system after chronic administration of desipramine. *European Journal of Pharmacology, 74,* 195–206.

Stanley, M. A., Bowers, T. C., Swann, A. C. & Taylor, D. J. (1991) Treatment of trichotillomania with fluoxetine. *Journal of Clinical Psychiatry, 52,* 282.

Stanley, M., & Mann, J. (1986). Serotonin and sertonergic receptors in suicide. *Annals of the New York Academy of Sciences, 487,* 122–127.

Starr, M. D., & Mineka, S. (1977). Determinants of fear over the course of avoidance learning. *Learning and Motivation, 8,* 332–350.

Stewart, J., de Wit, H., & Eikelboom, R. (1984). Role of unconditioned and conditioned drug effects in the self-administration of opiates and stimulants. *Psychological Review, 91,* 51–268.

Stiles, G. L., Stadel, J. M., De Lean, A., & Lefkowitz, R. J. (1981). Hypothyroidism modulates beta adrenergic receptor–adenylate cyclase interactions in rat reticulocytes. *Journal of Clinical Investigation, 68,* 1450–1455.

Struss, D. T., & Benson, D. F. (1986). *The frontal lobes.* New York: Raven Press.

Sumal, K. K., Blessing, W. W., Joh, T. H., Reiss, D. J. & Pickel, V. M. (1982). Ultrastructural evidence that vagal afferents terminate on catecholaminergic neurons in the nucleus tractus solitarius. *Society of Neuroscience Abstracts, 8,* 429.

Sutherland, G., Newman, B. & Rachman, S. (1982). Experimental investigations of the relations between mood and intrusive unwanted cognitions. *British Journal of Medical Psychology, 55,* 127–138.

Sved, A. F., Baker, H. A., & Reis, D. J. (1984). Dopamine synthesis in inbred mouse strains which differ in numbers of dopamine neurons. *Brain Research, 303,* 261–266.

Sved, A. F., Baker, H. A., & Reis, D. J. (1985). Number of dopamine neurons predicts prolactin levels in two inbred mouse strains. *Experientia, 41,* 644–646.

Svensson, T. H. (1987). Peripheral, autonomic regulation of locus coeruleus neoradrenergic neurons in brain: Putative implications for psychiatry and psychopharmacology. *Psychopharmacology, 92,* 1–7.

Swedo, S. E., Leonard, H. L., Krueski, M. J., Rettew, D. C., Listwak, S. J., Berrettini, W., Stipetic, M., Hamburger, S., Gold, P. W., Potter, W. Z., * Rapoport, J. L. (1992). Cerebrospinal fluid neurochemistry in children and adolescents with obsessive–compulsive disorder. *Archives of General Psychiatry, 49,* 29–36.

Swedo, S. E., Leonard, H. L., Rapoport, J. L., Lenane, M. C., Goldberger, E. L., & Cheslow, D. L. (1989). A double-blind comparison of clomipramine and desipramine in the treatment of trichotillomania (hair pulling). *New England Journal of Medicine, 321,* 497–501.

Swedo, S. E., Rapoport, J. L., & Cheslow, D. L. (1989). High prevalence of obsessive–compulsive symptoms in patients with Sydenham's chorea. *American Journal of Psychiatry, 146,* 246–249

Taghzouti, K., LeMoal, M., & Simon, H. (1985). Enhanced frustrative nonreward effect following 6-OHDA lesions of the lateral septum in the rat. *Behav. Neurosci., 99,* 1066–1073.

Taghzouti, K., Louilot, A., Herman, J. P., LeMoal, M., & Simon, H. (1985). Alternation behavior, spatial discrimination, and reversal disturbances following 6-hydroxydopamine lesions in the nucleus accumbens of the rat. *Behav Neural Biol, 44,* 354–363.

Taghzouti, K., Simon, H., & LeMoal, M. (1986). Disturbances in exploratory behavior and functional recovery in the Y and radial mazes following dopamine depletion of the lateral septum. *Behav Neural Biol, 45,* 48–56.

Taghzouti, K., Simon, H., Louilot, A., Herman, J. P., & LeMoal, M. (1985). Behavioral study after 6-hydroxydopamine lesions of the nucleus accumbens. *Brain Research, 344,* 9–20.

Taghzouti, K., Simon, H., Tazi, A., Dantzer, R., & LeMoal, M. (1985). The effect of 6-OHDA lesions of the lateral septum on schedule-induced polydipsia. *Behavioral Brain Res, 15,* 1–8.

Tellegen, A. (1985). Structures of mood and personality and their relevance to assessing anxiety, with an emphasis on self-report. In A. H. Tuma & J. D. Maser (Eds.), *Anxiety and the anxiety disorders* (pp. 681–706). Hillsdale, NJ: Erlbaum.

Tellegen, A., & Walker, N. G. (1992). Exploring personality through test construction: Development of the multidimensional personality questionnaire. In S. R. Briggs & J. M. Cheek (Eds.), *Personality measures: Development and evaluation* (Vol. 1, pp. 80–110). Greenwich, CT: JAI.

Thoren, P., Asberg, M., Bertilsson, L., Mellstrom, B., Sjoqvist, F., & Traskman, L. (1980). Clomipramine treatment of obsessive–compulsive disorder: II. Biochemical aspects. *Archives of General Psychiatry, 37,* 1289–1294.

Thoren, P., Asberg, M., Cronhom, B., Jornstedt, L. & Traskman, L., (1980). Clomipramine treatment of obsessive–compulsive disorder, a controlled trial. *Archives of General Psychiatry, 37,* 1281–1285.

Thorpe, S. J., Rolls, E. T., & Maddison, S. (1983). Neuronal activity in the orbitofrontal cortex of the behaving monkey. *Experimental Brain Research, 49,* 93–115.

Tork, I. (1990). Anatomy of the serotenergic system. *Annals of the New York Acadamy of Science, 600,* 9–31.

Traskman, L., Asberg, M., & Bertilsson, L. (1981). Monoamine metabolites in CSF and suicidal behavior. *Archives of General Psychiatry, 38,* 631–636.

Traskman, L., Asberg, M., & Bertilsson, L. (1984). CSF monoamine metabolites of depressed patients during illness and after recovery. *Acta Psychiatrica Scandinavica, 69,* 333–342.

Tsuda, A., & Tanaka, M. (1985). Differential changes in noradrenaline turnover in specific regions of rat brain produced by controllable and uncontrollable shocks. *Behavioral Neuroscience, 99,* 802–817.

Tsuda, A., Tanaka, M., Yoshishige, I., Tsujimaru, S., Ushijima, I., & Nagasaki, N. (1986). Effects of preshcok experience on enhancement of rat brain noradrenergic turnover induced by psychologcial stress. *Pharmacology Biochemistry & Behavior, 24,* 115–119.

Tuomista, J., & Mannisto, P. (1985). Neurotranmitter regulation of anterior pituitary hormones. *Pharmacology Review, 37,* 249–332.

Turner, A. M., & Greenough, W. T. (1983). Synapses per neuron and synaptic dimensions in occipital cortex of rats reared in complex, social, or isolation housing. *Acta Stereologica, 2*(Suppl. 1), 239–244.

Turner, A. M., & Greenough, W. T. (1985). Differential rearing effects on rat visual cortex synapses: I. Synaptic and neuronal density and synapses per neuron. *Brain Research, 329,* 195–203.

Turner, B. H., Mishkin, M., & Knapp, M. (1980). Organization of the amygdalopetal projections from modality-specific cortical association areas in the monkey. *Journal of Comparative Neurology, 191,* 515–543.

Turner, S. M., Jacob, R. G., Beidel, D. C., & Himmelhoch, J. (1985). Fluoxetine treatment of obsessive–compulsive disorder. *Journal of Clinical Psychopharmacology, 5,* 207–212.

Uhde, T. W., Boulenger, J.-P., Post, R. M., Siever, L. J., Vittone, B. J., Jimerson, D. C., Roy-Byrne, P. P. (1984). Fear and anxiety: Relationship to noradrenergic function. *Psychopathology, 17*(Suppl. 3), 8–23.

Uhde, T. W., Siever, L. J., Post, R. M., Jimerson, D., Boulenger, J.-P. & Buschsbaum, M. (1982). The relationship of plasma-free MHPG to anxiety and psychophysical pain in normal volunteers. *Psychopharmacological Bulletin, 18,* 129–132.

Uhde, T. W., Vittone, B. J., Siever, L. J., Kaye, W. H., & Post, R. M. (1986). Blunted growth hormone response in panic disorder patients. *Biological Psychiatry, 21,* 1081–1085.

Uylings, H. B. M., Kuypers, K., & Veltman, W. A. M. (1978). Envrionmental influences on neocortex in later life. In M. A. Corner, R. E. Baker, N. E. van de Poll, D. F. Swabb, & H. B. M. Uylings (Eds.), *Maturation of the nervous system: Progress in brain research* (Vol. 48, pp. 261–274). Amsterdam: Elsevier.

Valzelli, L. (1981). *Psychobiology of aggression and violence.* New York: Raven Press.

van De Kar, L.D., Lorens, S. A., Urban J. H., and Bethea, C. L. (1989). Effect of selective serotonin (5-HT) agonists and 5-HT2 antagonist on prolactin secretion. *Neuropharmacology, 28,* 293–305.

van Hoesen, G. W., Pandya, D. N., & Butters, N. (1975). Some connections of the entorhinal (area 28) and perirhinal (area 35) cortices of the rhesus monkey: II. Frontal lobe afferents. *Brain Research, 95,* 25–38.

van Hoesen, G. W., Yeterian, E. H. & Lavizzo-Mourey, R. (1981). Widespread corticostriate projections from temporalcortex of the rhesus monkey. *Journal of Comparative Neurology, 199,* 205–219.

van Praag, H. (1984). Studies in the mechanism of action of serotonin precursors in depression. *Psychopharmacology Bulletin, 20,* 599–602.

van Praag, H. (1986). (Auto)aggression and CSF 5-HIAA in depression and schizophrenia. *Psychopharmacology Bulletin, 22,* 669–673.

Virkkunen, M., Nuutila, A., & Goodwin, F. (1987). Cerebrospinal fluid monoamine metabolite events in male arsonists. *Archives of General Psychiatry, 44,* 241–247.

Watanabe, T., & Niki, H. (1985). Hippocampal unit activity and delayed response in the monkey. Brain Research, 325, 241–254.

Watkins, J. C., & Evans, R. H. (1981). Excitatory amino acid neurotransmitters. *Annual Review of Pharmacology and Toxicology, 21,* 165–204.

Watson, D., & Tellegen, A. (1985). Toward a consensual structure of mood. *Psychological Bulletin, 92,* 426–457.

Weilburg, J. B., Mesulam, M-M., Weintraub, S., Buonanno, F., Jenile, M., & Stakes, J. W. (1989). Focal striatal abnormalities in a patient with obsessive–compulsive disorder. *Archives of Neurology, 46,* 233–235.

West, R. W., & Greenough, W. T. (1972). Effect of environmental complexity of cortical synapses of rats: Preliminary results. *Behavioral Biology, 7,* 279–284.

Whitlock, D. G., & Nauta, W. J. H. (1956). Subcortical projections from the temporal neocortex in *Macaca mulatta. Journal of Comparative Neurology, 106,* 183–212.

Wise, R. A. (1978). Catecholamine theories of reward: A critical review. *Brain Research, 152,* 215–247.

Wise, R. A. (1982). Neuroleptics and operant behavior: The anhedonia hypothesis. *Behavioral and Brain Sciences, 5,* 39–53.

Wong, D. T., & Bymaster, F. P. (1980). Subsensitivity of serotonin receptors after long term treatment of rats with fluoxetine. *Research Communications in Chemical Pathological Pharmacology, 32,* 41–51.

Wood, K. (1985). The neurochemistry of mania. *Journal of Affective Disorders, 8,* 215–223.

Woods, S. W., Charney, D. S., McPherson, C. A., Gradman, A. H., & Heninger, G. R. (1987). Situational panic attacks: Behavioral, physiological, and biochemical characterization. *Archives of General Psychiatry, 44,* 365–375.

Yakovlev, P. I. (1948). Motility, behavior, and the brain. *Journal of Nervous and Mental Diseases, 107,* 313–335.

Yakovlev, P. I. (1959). Pathoarchitectonic studies of cerebral malformation. 3. Arrhinencephalies (holotelencephalies). *Journal of Neuropathology and Experimental Neurology, 18,* 22–55.

Yeterian, E. H., & Van Hoesen, G. W. (1978). Cortico-striate projections in the rhesus monkey: The organization of certain cortico-caudate connections. *Brain Research, 139,* 43–63.

Zohar, J., Insel, T. R., Zohar-Kadouch, R. C., Hill, J. L., & Murphy, D. L. (1988). Serotenergic responsivity in obsessive–compulsive disorder: Effects of chronic clomipramine treatment. *Archives of General Psychiatry, 45,* 167–172.

Zohar, J., Mueller, E.A., Insel, T. R., Zohar-Kadouch, R.C., & Murphy, D.L. (1987). Serotenergic responsivity in obsessive–compulsive disorder: A comparison of patients and healthy controls. *Archives of General Psychiatry, 44,* 946–951.

Zuckerman, M. (1983). *Biological bases of sensation seeking, impulsivity, and anxiety.* Hillsdale, NJ: Erlbaum.

6

The Causes
of Functional Psychosis

PAUL BEBBINGTON

CATHERINE WALSH

ROBIN MURRAY

Schizophrenic and manic–depressive disorders are conventionally grouped together as "functional psychoses." The term *functional* is a continuing reflection that the etiology of these conditions has been hard to identify. Thus, Jaspers (1963, p. 460) stated, "We give the term 'functional' to those psychic changes for which no physical cause can be found and where at present there is in the somatic sphere no real ground for supposing that such causes exist, and where such a supposition can only rest on the postulate that there must be physical causes for all psychic changes."

The attempt to discover physical substrates for conditions that are defined symptomatically, and are almost certainly etiologically quite diverse, has not been easy. Nevertheless, progress has been made, and a number of brain abnormalities at the neuroimaging and neuropathological level have been identified, particularly in schizophrenia. Likewise, there is now much more evidence concerning the genetic contribution to both schizophrenia and manic depression, although this comes more consistently from genetic epidemiological studies than from molecular genetics. Similarly, there is now evidence that the effects of aberrant genes may be mimicked by the operation of environmental factors and for the role of the physical environment in the causation of certain functional psychoses.

Theories of the etiology of psychosis that relate to the genetic or physical environment posit causes that are neither necessary nor sufficient for the emergence of psychosis. Nevertheless, it is generally assumed that, one way or another, a biological predisposition is a necessary precondition. In other words, something more particular than the general biological endowment of human beings is required before an individual is capable of developing the features characteristic of psychosis. Most workers in the field feel this is a reasonable working hypothesis, albeit unprovable. In this chapter, therefore, we will first review the evidence that there exists a biological predisposition to schizophrenia and manic depression and then proceed to discuss the more controversial role of social factors.

GENETICS

A substantial body of evidence now implicates genetic factors in the etiology of schizophrenia and manic depression.

Schizophrenia

Early investigators recognized a tendency for schizophrenia to cluster within families and observed that the risk to relatives correlated with genetic proximity (e.g., Rudin, 1916). Adoption studies, demonstrating higher rates of schizophrenia in the biological as opposed to the adoptive relatives of schizophrenic adoptees, indicated that this familial aggregation reflected genetic vulnerability and not the influence of intrafamilial environment (Heston, 1966; Kety, Rosenthal, Wender, Schulsinger, & Jacobson, 1978). Further support derived from twin studies showing concordance rates for schizophrenia among identical or monozygotic (MZ) twins of 35–58%, in contrast to rates of 12–27% for fraternal or dizygotic (DZ) twin pairs (Gottesman & Shields, 1982). The absence of 100% concordance in MZ twins can be explained in two ways. First, it is possible that the well cotwins represent unexpressed genotypes and that the clinical manifestation of schizophrenia requires an interaction between genetic and environmental cofactors (Gottesman & Bertelsen, 1989). Second, a proportion of schizophrenia may be of nongenetic origin (Murray, Lewis, & Reveley, 1985).

Some interesting findings have recently emerged from family studies. First, it appears that morbid risk of schizophrenia is significantly higher among the relatives of probands who develop schizophrenia before the age of 21 (Sham et al., 1992). This is, of course, very compatible with the idea that early-onset cases are especially likely to inherit a gene or genes that cause neurodevelopmental abnormality. Secondly, several studies (Bellodi et al., 1986; Goldstein, Tsuang, & Farmer, 1989; Sham et al., 1992) have reported that the relatives of female probands have a much higher risk of schizophrenia than the relatives of male probands. Similarly, concordance rates for monozygotic twins are higher for female than for male pairs (Kringlen & Cramer, 1989). These findings suggest that genetic factors are more important, on average, in female than male schizophrenics.

Schizophrenia is not inherited as a simple Mendelian disorder. There are a number of published pedigrees (e.g., Kennedy et al., 1988) in which genetic transmission appears to follow autosomal dominant patterns, but this is the exception rather than the rule, and epidemiological studies suggest that schizophrenia is unlikely to be caused by a single major gene (McGue, Gottesman, & Rao, 1986). Alternative possibilities include the involvement of a small number of major genes (oligogenic model) or the additive effect of many minor genes together with environmental factors (polygenic multifactorial model) (McGuffin, Farmer, & Gottsman, 1987).

Affective Psychosis

The morbid risk of bipolar illness in the first degree relatives of bipolar probands is approximately 8%, and that for unipolar illness is over 11% (McGuffin & Katz, 1986); by comparison, the lifetime risk in the general population for bipolar illness is less than 1% and for severe unipolar illness about 3%. Twin studies show that concordance rates for affective disorder in MZ twins are up to five times greater than in DZ twins (Bertelsen, Harvald, & Hauge, 1977); this disparity is even greater when only bipolar probands are considered. Once again, adoption studies show that this is due to a genetic effect rather than to the family culture (Mendelwicz & Rainer, 1977). The available evidence suggests that bipolar affective illness is under greater genetic control than schizophrenia, and that it lies at the more severe end of a continuum of liability, with unipolar depression of the neurotic type at the other; thus, genetic factors predominate in bipolar illness and environmental factors in nonendogenous unipolar disorder. However, the exact mode of transmission remains obscure (O'Rourke, McGuffin, & Reich, 1983).

MOLECULAR GENETICS

Until recently, the detailed study of psychotic disorders at a molecular level was hampered by a lack of suitable genetic markers. Genetic markers are stable biological traits that can be reliably measured, have simple Mendelian modes of inheritance, and are polymorphic (i.e., exist in many forms). By knowing the chromosomal location for a marker trait, the inheritance of a particular chromosomal region can be traced through families. In early studies of psychoses, blood groupings (ABO, Rh factor) and human leukocyte antigen types (HLA) were commonly employed as genetic markers (McGuffin, Festenstein, & Murray, 1983; Andrew, Watt, Gillespie, & Chapel, 1987). However, these classic markers cover only a fraction of the entire genome and are therefore limited in the information they supply (McGuffin, 1988).

The development of recombinant DNA technology led to the identification of a new type of genetic marker. These are sequences of DNA that occur throughout the genome, vary between individuals, and are inherited as simple Mendelian traits. Employing these markers enables locating a disease gene without knowing anything of the gene itself or of the pathopsysiological process. This approach, known as *reverse genetics*, has been spectacularly successful in many disorders, for example, familial Alzheimer's disease (St. George-Hyslop et al., 1987).

The first step in the process of reverse genetics is to collect families in which several members are affected with the disorder (multiplex families). Having defined the disease phenotype, the position of a putative disease gene must be specified. In some instances, there may be obvious candidate genes. In the case of psychosis, candidate genes might include those involved in the monoamine pathways, such as the dopamine receptor genes or genes encoding enzymes like tyrosine hydroxylase. Alternatively, the finding of chromosomal anomalies cosegregating with the disorder might highlight particular chromosomal regions worthy of study (e.g., chromosome 5 in schizophrenia; see next section). In the absence of such clues, the remaining strategy to locate a disease gene involves using a series of anonymous DNA markers on each chromosome to exclude each region systematically.

The next step is to examine DNA markers from the specified region in a series of multiply affected families. If the inheritance of a particular marker allele appears to cosegregate with the illness, it may be that the disease gene and marker allele are linked (linkage occurs when two loci on the same chromosome are situated so close to each other that alleles at these loci are not inherited independently). Alternatively, this cosegregation may simply be a chance happening. In order to establish which is most likely, a statistical analysis, the LOD score method, is applied (see Ott, 1985). LOD scores of 3 or more have traditionally been taken to indicate a high chance of linkage (the possibility of the observed findings having arisen by chance is 1,000:1); LOD scores below –2 signify no linkage, and anything in between is equivocal.

To date, linkage studies in psychosis have focused on chromosome 5, chromosome 11, and the sex chromosomes.

Chromosome 5

In 1988, a report suggested the possible involvement of the long arm of chromosome 5 in schizophrenia (Bassett, McGillivray, Jones, & Pantzar,

1988). A family had been identified in which an uncle and a nephew, both suffering from schizophrenia, were noted to have similar facial dysmorphologies. Cytogenetic testing revealed that both men possessed a trisomic segment of part of chromosome 5. Subsequently, Sherrington and his colleagues (1988) examined the segregation of chromosome 5 markers in two English and five Icelandic pedigrees and found evidence of linkage that, depending on phenotypic definition and specification of genetic parameters, generated LOD scores ranging from 2.45 to greater than 7.

The possibility that a schizophrenia gene had been found generated considerable excitement that was soon tempered by a number of negative reports (Kennedy et al., 1988; McGuffin et al., 1990; St. Clair et al., 1989), and to date no study has replicated the finding of positive linkage to chromosome 5.

There has been much speculation regarding the inconsistency of these studies (Lander, 1988). The most frequently proposed explanation has been genetic heterogeneity, with suggestions that Sherrington and colleagues (1988) may have detected a rare genetic form of schizophrenic psychosis in a genetic isolate. Recent data indicate that this is unlikely (McGuffin et al., 1990). Furthermore, Sherrington's group subsequently found evidence against linkage when using more informative markers in an extended pedigree set (Mankoo et al., 1991). It can be concluded that there is no linkage between chromosome 5 and schizophrenia.

Chromosome 11

The dopamine hypothesis of schizophrenia has evolved largely from the understanding that the efficacy of neuroleptic drugs relates to the degree of dopamine receptor blockade they induce. Consequently, any genes involved in the control of dopamine neurotransmission or dopamine receptor function become candidate genes for schizophrenia. In 1989, the gene encoding the dopamine D2 receptor gene (DRD2) was mapped to chromosome 11q (Grandy et al., 1989). Further interest in this region was fueled by a number of reports of families in which balanced translocations involving the long arm of chromosome 11 appeared to cosegregate with psychotic disorders (Holland & Gosden 1990; Smith et al., 1989; St. Clair et al., 1990).

However, using a marker linked to the DRD2 locus, Moises and colleagues (1991) reported no linkage (LOD score, −2.23) to schizophrenia in a large Swedish pedigree. Similarly, a study examining 12 different polymorphic markers from the 11q region excluded most of it as the location of a gene of major effect for schizophrenia (Gill et al., 1993).

The story has been somewhat similar for manic depression. In 1987, Egeland and associates reported linkage between manic depression and

two markers on the short arm of chromosome 11, the Harvey-ras onco-
gene and the insulin gene, in a large branch of the Old Order Amish in
Pennsylvania. The result could not, however, be replicated in other
North American pedigrees (Detera-Wadleigh et al., 1987), Icelandic
families (Hodgkinson et al., 1987), or an Irish family (Gill, McKeown, &
Humphries, 1988). This could have been a consequence of heterogeneity,
but recently doubt has been cast on the original Amish results. Indeed,
reanalysis of the Amish pedigree data after inclusion of further branches
of the family, and allowing for changes in diagnosis in two individuals,
reduced the final LOD score to below the level generally considered to be
statistically significant (Kelsoe et al., 1989).

Sex Chromosomes

The possible linkage of X chromosome markers to manic depression has
aroused interest for two decades. Evidence was originally derived from
studies using classical X-linked markers such as color blindness
(Mendlewicz, Fleiss, & Fieve, 1972) and glucose-6-phosphate dehydro-
genase (Mendlewicz, Linkowski, & Wilmotte, 1980). In the most systematic of such studies, Baron and colleagues (1987) found linkage between
these two markers and bipolar illness in several Israeli families, whereas
Mendlewicz and associates (1987) found linkage between the illness and
the factor IX gene, which is known to be on the X chromosome. Gill,
Castle, and Duggan (1992) also identified a pedigree in which affective
illness and Christmas disease (caused by factor IX deficiency) appeared to
cosegregate. Having said this, evidence of father-to-son transmission,
coupled with a number of negative linkage reports (e.g., Berrettini et al.,
1990), suggest that an X-linked form of manic depression can only be
present in a subset of patients.

There has been no strong evidence to suggest that X-linked inheritance is operating in schizophrenia, but it is well recognized that gender
may affect the expression of this disorder (Castle & Murray, 1991;
Lewine, 1988). Furthermore, it is known that sex chromosomal anomalies are more common in psychotic populations, and that related individuals with schizophrenia are more likely to be of the same sex. Such
observations could be explained if a gene for schizophrenia were situated
in the pseudoautosomal region of the sex chromosomes (Crow, 1988).
This region is a segment at the distal ends of the X and Y chromosomes in
which there is sequence homology and in which a single obligatory
crossover occurs during male meiosis. Depending on its exact location, a
gene situated within this region can be inherited either in an autosomal or
in a sex-linked manner (hence pseudoautosomal).

Crow (1988) proposed that a schizophrenia gene might be pseudoautosomal and tested this hypothesis with an affected sib-pair technique

(Collinge et al., 1991). The sib-pair method predicts that affected siblings are more likely to share alleles at a putative disease locus than would be expected by chance. Having examined a number of pseudoautosomal markers in 83 sibling pairs, Collinge and his colleagues found that schizophrenic siblings shared alleles more frequently than would be expected at a marker that maps to the distal pseudoautosomal region ($p <$ .05). However, because of the restricted sample size, this could only indicate a trend in the direction of positive linkage.

Future Directions

In summary, although much valuable information has come from classic genetic studies, molecular studies in psychosis have been less successful. This is not entirely surprising, considering the many obstacles facing psychiatric geneticists. Phenotypic definition depends on identification of groups of symptoms that, without biological markers, are of unknown validity. In addition, both schizophrenia and affective psychosis are likely to be genetically heterogeneous, and other factors such as variable age of onset, incomplete penetrance, and variable expression may also confuse the picture. However, similar problems have been defeated in other complex genetic disorders (e.g., diabetes), and research aimed at more clearly defining the phenotype and the development of biological markers to act as middle phenotypes (*endophenotypes*) are likely to facilitate this in psychosis.

STRUCTURAL BRAIN ABNORMALITIES

Neuroimaging

Molecular genetics promises much hope for the future, but the introduction of computerized tomography (CT) scanning in the 1970s has already brought substantial advances in understanding psychosis. This technique provided a noninvasive method of examining the brain *in vivo* and supplied quantitative evidence of structural brain changes in a proportion of schizophrenic cases. More recently, magnetic resonance imaging (MRI) has brought the ability to visualize smaller structures.

The first CT scanning study demonstrated that schizophrenic patients had larger cerebral ventricles compared with age-matched controls, a finding previously suggested by air encephalography (Johnstone, Crow, Frith, Husband, & Kreel, 1976). The observation that these changes occurred in both treated and untreated subjects indicated that the abnormalities were not merely a secondary effect of medication or ECT. Furthermore, it was found that the magnitude of ventriculomegaly correlated with the degree of cognitive impairment, an index of disease severity.

Similar studies followed, each confirming that cortical sulcal widening and ventriculomegaly were to be found in a subgroup of schizophrenic subjects (e.g., Andreasen, Olsen, Dennert, & Smith, 1982; Owens et al., 1985; Weinberger, Torrey, Neophytides, & Wyatt, 1979); the small number of negative reports can be questioned on methodological grounds (Raz & Raz, 1990). Positive correlations were also reported between structural brain changes and a number of premorbid, clinical, and outcome variables. Thus, CT abnormalities have been shown to be more common in males than in females with schizophrenia, and tend to be associated with negative symptoms, poor premorbid social and educational adjustment, poor treatment response, and a chronic deteriorating course (Castle & Murray, 1991).

Initially, the detection of concomitant brain abnormalities was thought to indicate that an underlying and progressive neurodegenerative process was operating in schizophrenia. However, it gradually became apparent that these lesions were not necessarily progressive; although greater degrees of ventriculomegaly were associated with more severe illness, ventricular size did not predict illness duration. Indeed, marked changes could be detected in a proportion of young patients shortly after the first onset of psychosis (Turner, Toone, & Brett-Jones, 1986). These findings, coupled with follow-up studies that failed to demonstrate evidence of progressive changes (e.g., Illowsky, Julliano, Bigelow, & Weinberger, 1988; Vita, Sacchetti, Valvassori, & Cazzullo, 1988), suggested that the observed abnormalities indicated static brain lesions antedating the onset of florid illness.

MRI studies have reaffirmed these observations and, in addition, shown a reduction in the volume of temporal lobe structures and of the hippocampus in particular (Bogerts et al., 1990; Johnstone et al., 1989; Suddath, Christison, Torrey, Casanova, & Weinberger, 1990). Some investigators have reported that these changes may be more prominent in the left temporal lobe (Johnstone et al., 1989). As we shall now see, the implication of the temporal lobe is of particular interest in view of recent neuropathological data.

Neuropathology

The brains of schizophrenic patients show a decrease in weight, estimated at 6% by Brown and associates (1986). Bogerts, Meertz, and Schonfeldt-Bausch (1985) showed a greater decrease (20–30%) in the volume of the limbic temporal lobe (amygdala, hippocampus, parahippocampal gyrus), a finding that is consistent not only with the neuroimaging studies but also with the evidence of particular enlargement of the temporal horn of the lateral ventricles (Brown et al., 1986).

Two groups (Falkai & Bogerts, 1986; Jeste & Lohr, 1989) found decreased cell counts in the hippocampus. Gliosis is the usual glial cell reaction to neuronal inflammation or damage, and its absence in most schizophrenic subjects (Roberts, 1991) suggests an abnormality of development rather than degeneration.

The hippocampus is formed by young neurons migrating from the ventricular surface, a process in which they are guided by the radial glia. If the neuronal migration is disrupted in the fetus, abnormally positioned cells result. Kovelman and Scheibel (1984) reported disarray of the normally regimented ranks of pyramidal neurons in the CA1/CA2 regions of the hippocampus in schizophrenia. A subsequent study from the same group failed to find a statistically significant difference in neuronal disorganization between schizophrenic subjects and controls, but did report greater disarray among those with a more severe psychosis. Jacob and Beckman (1986) noted that in the brains of some adults with schizophrenia, particularly those with early onset, groups of prealpha neurones normally located in the superficial layers of the parahippocampal gyrus are displaced deep to their expected position. This finding was replicated by Falkai, Bogerts, and Rozumek, (1988). Some defect in control of embryonal cell migration is an appealing explanation.

A large proportion of all cells generated in the developing nervous system die by the time it is mature. This process of selective neuronal death eliminates early errors of connection, and several authors have suggested that it might be abnormal in schizophrenia. Benes, Davidson, and Bird (1986) showed that, in schizophrenia, neuronal density is lower in certain layers of the cerebral cortex and suggest that this could have arisen from "an accelerated process of neuronal drop out early in life, perhaps related to a perinatal insult". A compensatory process could result in the persistence of immature patterns of cells and their connections into adult life. Indeeed, Deakin and colleagues (1989) attributed the abnormally dense glutaminergic innervation of the orbital cortex, which they found in schizophrenia to "an arrest or failure of the process by which transient callosal connections are normally eliminated during development."

THE EARLY PHYSICAL ENVIRONMENT

What causes these structural abnormalities? They could result from an abnormality in the genetic specification of early brain development (Jones & Murray, 1991). However, lack of 100% concordance for psychosis in MZ twin pairs indicates that genes alone cannot be responsible for the entire liability to schizophrenia; environmental factors must operate in at least some cases. In fact, there is considerable evidence of influence from the physical environment on risk of schizophrenia. For example, environmental agents are implicated by CT and MRI studies of discordant MZ twins in which brain changes are most apparent in the affected members (Reveley, Clifford, Reveley, & Murray, 1982; Suddath et al., 1990).

The most investigated finding relating to physical insult in schizophrenia is an association with obstetric complications (OCs). Most, but not all, studies have shown an increase in prenatal and perinatal difficulties in the birth histories of schizophrenic patients (Lewis & Murray, 1987; McNeil & Kaij, 1978). In addition, it has been reported that patients with a history of OCs are more likely to show evidence of ventricular enlargement (Owen, Lewis, & Murray, 1988), suggesting that OCs might directly cause structural brain changes and predispose to later schizophrenia (Murray, Lewis, Owen, & Foerster, 1988). Reports that enlarged ventricles were more likely to occur in the absence of family history supported this view and prompted suggestions that schizophrenia be divided on etiological grounds into "familial" and "sporadic" types (Murray, Lewis, & Reveley, 1985). However, more recent studies have failed to confirm the negative correlation with family history, and it now appears that genetic predisposition and environmental insult may frequently operate in unison. An alternative view regarding the role of OCs is that they are secondary phenomena that arise as a consequence of preexisting abnormality in the fetus and that this abnormality could be acquired or be the result of genetic factors (Goodman, 1989).

Evidence that people who develop schizophrenia are more likely to have been born in the late winter or early spring months has led to suggestions that exposure to some seasonal element, possibly an infective agent, might interfere with fetal brain development. In 1988, Mendick, Machon, Huttenen, and Bonet reported indirect evidence for an association between exposure to the influenza virus during the second trimester of fetal life and subsequent development of schizophrenia in adult life. A similar epidemiological study has recently demonstrated an increase in the incidence of schizophrenia among individuals who would have been in their fifth or sixth month of fetal life at the time of the Asian flu epidemic in England and Wales (O'Callaghan, Sham, Takei, Glover, & Murray, 1991). More importantly, two studies, in Denmark and England over four and two decades, respectively, have shown a consistent relationship between influenza epidemics and subsequent increased births of schizophrenics (Barr, Mendick, & Munk-Jorgensen, 1990; Takei, Sham, O'Callaghan, Glover, & Murray, 1992). The early physical environment has been much less frequently investigated in affective psychosis. Foerster, Lewis, Owen, and Murray (1991) reported that OCs are less common in the histories of those with affective psychosis than of those with schizophrenia. Paradoxically, however, Done and colleagues (1991) reported that perinatal complications increased the risk of later affective psychosis but not schizophrenia. Similar inconsistencies have arisen in relation to season of birth, with most studies reporting no seasonal effect on birth in affective psychosis but a few claiming a late winter/spring excess (Hare, 1975).

CONGENITAL AND ADULT-ONSET PSYCHOSES

It will be apparent to the reader that several lines of evidence now suggest that at least a proportion of cases of schizophrenia result from an abnormality of brain development during fetal or neonatal life (Murray & Lewis, 1987; Weinberger, 1987). Neuroimaging studies demonstrate that a significant percentage of sufferers have evidence of quantitative brain abnormalities and that these appear to be static lesions antedating clinical symptoms. The neuropathology found in the brain supports these data and, in addition, indicates that the brain changes are more likely to represent a failure of development rather than degeneration. Schizophrenic patients also show an excess of minor physical anomalies, for example, furrowed tongue, malformed ears, and curved fingers (Green, Satz, Gaier, Ganzell, & Kharabi, 1989). These minor defects are known to represent abnormalities in ectodermal development and have been associated with developmental disorders and early environmental insult. It has been suggested they may reflect simultaneous events occurring in the CNS—also of ectodermal origin—further supporting suggestions of an early brain lesion in schizophrenia (Jones & Murray, 1991).

Why, then, do positive symptoms not appear until late adolescence and early adult life? The most likely explanation is that the congenital cytoarchitectural abnormalities remain largely dormant until some maturational process brings them to light. Myelination of axons is one possibility, as Benes (1989) has shown strikingly increased myelination of the subicular and presubicular regions during late adolescence. She notes that these structures have a strategic location within the corticolimbic circuitry of the brain and asks whether myelination of one or two linkages in this circuitry could in some way permit a preexisting, but latent, defect to become manifest.

Recent data suggest that genetic factors may be more important in females with schizophrenia (Sham et al., 1992) and that obstetric hazards are more likely to be relevant in young male patients who show previous evidence of neurodevelopmental impairment, as measured by poor premorbid social, educational, and occupational adjustment (Castle &

Murray, 1991). Whether this anomalous development is secondary to environmental insult, aberrant gene function, or a combination of the two is not clear. However, the role of genetic and early environmental components need not be mutually exclusive, and it is possible that environmental agents (such as the influenza virus) may interact with genetic forces, as, for example, in conditions like leprosy and tuberculosis that develop in genetically susceptible individuals.

There is much less evidence to implicate neurodevelopmental abnormality in affective psychosis. Whereas preschizophrenic children frequently manifest poor cognitive and social function, this is unusual in those who later develop affective psychosis (Foerster et al., 1991). Similarly, when structural brain abnormalities are found in affective psychosis, they appear more frequently to be degenerative rather than developmental in origin (Sacchetti et al., 1990). Many people with acute schizophrenia also fail to show childhood abnormalities or structural brain changes. These facts together with their relatively good outcome led Murray, Callaghan, Castle, and Lewis (1992) to suggest that acute schizophrenia should be classified together with affective psychoses as the "adult-onset psychoses" in contrast to severe neurodevelopmental schizophrenia, which they regard as a "congenital psychosis." These authors further postulate that social factors may be of particular importance in precipitating the former type.

SOCIAL FACTORS

Big Social Theories

Could social factors not only precipitate but also cause psychosis? Following the Second World War, a number of attempts were made to provide etiological theories that discounted the role of biological influences. These "big" social theories were all concerned to explain the emergence of schizophrenia, although many of the cases that form the basis of the research would fit dubiously into current categories. These theories were all essentially cognitive. Early experience was said to result in ways of perceiving and therefore of interacting with the social world that corresponded to the observed symptoms of schizophrenia. All were couched in terms of parental and family behavior: schizophrenia was held to be the result of the families' "double-bind" communication (Bateson, Jackson, Hally, & Weakland, (1956), or of a "fragmented" or "amorphous" parental style of communication (Wynne & Singer, 1963, 1965). Lidz, Cornelison, Fleck, and Terry (1957) claimed that such parents showed "schism" or "skew" in their marriages, together with narcissistic egocentricity. Finally, Laing and Esterson (1964) held that schizophrenia was an understandable response to pressures in the family and in society at large.

These theories live on, after their scientific death, in a rather surprising way. Many psychiatrists seem to adhere, uncritically and subliminally, to the underlying ideas. This is despite the effective debunking carried out nearly two decades ago by Hirsch and Leff (1975). These authors' review of the experimental evidence for these theories concluded that oddities of parents were not marked, and almost certainly not the cause of the condition. There was some support for a few rather modest relationships, such as an increase in conflict and disharmony between the parents of schizophrenic patients, and in maternal concern and protectiveness. These seemed equally likely to be ordinary responses to illness in their offspring. Hirsch and Leff (1975) also attempted to replicate the findings of Wynne and Singer (1963, 1965) concerning abnormal parental communication. Despite being trained by the original authors, they were unable to repeat their findings.

The real problem with these theories is that causal direction is impossible to establish from retrospective studies. Straightforward prospective studies are impossibly expensive to pursue, as most subjects, laboriously followed up, will never develop schizophrenia. Some researchers have used the less costly approach of following up families with children who may be at high risk of developing schizophrenia (e.g., Goldstein, 1985; Venables, 1977), but such studies usually have high dropout rates, and may sometimes outlive the research workers.

Doane, West, Goldstein, Rodnick, and Jones (1981; Goldstein, 1987) reported one such study. They adopted the strategy of following up adolescents attending a psychiatric outpatient department for disturbed behavior, on the grounds that this group would be more at risk of developing schizophrenia. After a 15-year follow-up, only four of the adolescents actually developed definite schizophrenia, but others had evidence of more broadly defined schizophrenic spectrum disorders. These conditions were associated with a measure of family atmosphere and parental abnormalities of communication and affective style, all identified 15 years previously. The study reveals all the difficulties of the high risk strategy. First, few of the followed-up subjects have developed narrowly defined schizophrenia. Second, the causal direction remains almost as ambiguous as in the retrospective studies. In other words, it is possible that the more disturbed adolescents drew extreme reactions from their parents, and happened also to be those who went on to develop schizophrenia.

The Finnish adoption study places the big theories in what might be their proper perspective (Tienari et al., 1987). As might be expected under a genetic model, these workers found an excessive rate of schizophrenia in the adopted offspring of schizophrenic mothers. However, these cases all occurred in the 47% of adoptive families who were rated as severely disturbed, suggesting the possibility of genetic–environmental interactions. The early studies of the family context of schizophrenia combined imaginativeness with scientific naivete. With hindsight, it is possible to see that their imaginativeness did, at least, have the effect of obtaining acceptance for a social dimension to schizophrenia, thus opening the door for more refined hypotheses. Unfortunately, they also seem to have been responsible for the continuing tendency of some professionals to blame parents for the patient's state. The proponents of the modern social theories of schizophrenia have traded imagination for modesty, and may be the better for it. They propose that social influences operate, with factors at other levels, to determine the timing of breakdown. These theories rely on the concept of psychosocial stress, measured in terms of life events and expressed emotion. They are thus in line with the widely held clinical opinion that people with psychosis are, despite the social withdrawal seen in some cases, very responsive to their social environment.

Life Events and Psychosis

It has long been known that acute florid symptoms may reappear in patients subject to excessive pressure in rehabilitation programs, or discharged before they are ready (Drake & Sederer, 1986; Goldberg, Schooler, Hogarty, & Roper, 1977; Stevens, 1973; Wing, Bennett, & Denham, 1964). This reinforces the belief that social pressure may be important in shaping the symptoms of psychosis. Evidence from specific life events studies would be expected to confirm this. Although we have probably now reached the stage where we can say this with confidence, some questions remain unanswered.

A number of different strategies have been employed. In a few cases, researchers have identified an event common to a large group of subjects to see whether breakdown is more likely in the immediate aftermath of the event in question. Where randomly occurring life events are dated accurately over a sufficient period, within-case comparisons may reveal a significant peaking of events before onset. This provides at least prima facie evidence for an association. Another strategy is to use control groups, so that the rate of life events before the onset of psychosis can be compared with the rate of life events in an ordinary population. However, it is not clear what the appropriate control group would be for patients who, in any case, tend to be rather withdrawn and may therefore avoid social situations likely to engender life events. Finally, there are studies in which subjects known to have psychosis are followed at regular intervals; it is then possible to relate a relapse to the occurrence of events in the preceding period. Each strategy has its strengths and weaknesses, but between them we have fairly good direct evidence of a relationship between events and psychosis.

Steinberg and Durell (1968), in a study of the first type, observed recruits entering military service. They showed very high rates of admissions for schizophrenia in the first year after enlistment in comparison with the second, and this excess of admissions was even more notable in the first month. The finding did not appear to arise because of a greater likelihood of enlistment among people already showing signs of schizophrenia, nor did it seem to be an artifact of recognition. The soldiers who developed schizophrenia might have done so in any case, but the timing is suggestive, at least, of a precipitating effect of enlistment.

The first direct study of life events and schizophrenia was that of Brown and Birley (1968). Their chosen sample had experienced a mixture of first onsets and relapses of various types. Life events were rated through a semistructured interview. They found a significant excess of events of various degrees of impact compared with controls, limited to the specific period before onset. Controls were not ideal, being drawn from the employees of local firms. If anything, however, the inappropriateness of the control group may have worked against the hypothesis under test, in that people in employment probably have more opportunity to experience life events. Until recently, subsequent studies gave inconsistent results, and it was hard to come to any consensus because they were all open to criticisms of various sorts: less than appropriate control groups, small numbers, poor methods of establishing and dating life event histories, diagnostic idiosyncrasies, and combinations of these (Al Khani, Bebbington, Watson, & House, 1986; Canton & Fraccon, 1985; Chung, Langeluddecke, & Tennant, 1986; Jacobs & Myers, 1976; Malzacher, Merz, & Ebnother, 1981).

The large WHO collaborative study of life events and schizophrenia had the advantage of including over 400 patients, but was limited by the lack of a control group (Day et al., 1987). Again, a number of criticisms can be made of this study, but in all centers events seemed to cluster in the 3-week period before onset and perhaps, to a lesser extent, in the 3-week period before that. When all types of events were considered together, these findings were significant in six of nine centers, and the nonsignificance of similar trends in the remaining three centres probably arose because of small numbers or a low event rate.

Several studies have assessed life events over a period in patients who have recovered from a known episode of schizophrenia (S. Hirsch, personal communication, Oct. 26, 1992; Malla, Cortese, Shaw, & Ginsberg, 1990; Michaux, Gansereit, McCabe, & Kurland, 1967; Ventura, Nuechterlein, Lukoff, & Hardisty, 1989). In general, these studies have found that there are more events in the period preceding that in which relapse occurred than in any other similar period in the relapsing patients and in any equivalent period in those who did not. Results from the study by Ventura, Nuechterlein, Hardisty, and Gitlin (1992) are shown in Figure 6.1. These authors found an effect of life events restricted to those on medication, with the implication that medication raises the threshold to social adversity in established cases.

These prospective studies thus add to the evidence for a causal role of life events, although the subjects are inevitably restricted to those who have had at least one previous episode of illness.

There are fewer studies of life events in mania, and most of those use relatively crude measures of assessment (Ambelas, 1979; Ambelas, 1987; Dunner, Patrick, & Fieve, 1979; Glassner & Haldipur, 1983; Kennedy, Thompson, Stancer, Roy, & Persad, 1983; Sclare & Creed, 1990). With the exception of the last named study, the results are, nevertheless, again suggestive of an association. In line with the research literature on schizophrenia, the events preceding episodes of mania are reported to occur in close proximity to onset. It is possible that events are more associated with first than subsequent episodes of mania (e.g., Ambelas, 1987; Sclare & Creed, 1990). Some authors have suggested a similar pattern in schizophrenia (Al Khani et al., 1986). The suggestion that life events are more likely to be involved in first breakdowns is an interesting one. It implies that afterwards patients are somehow sensitized, such that breakdown

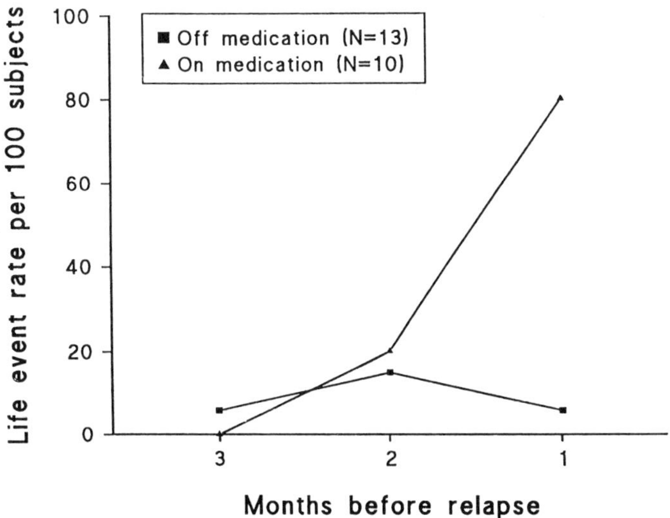

FIGURE 6.1. Life events before relapse in schizophrenia. From "Life events and schizophrenic relapse after medication withdrawal: A prospective study" by J. Ventura, K. H. Nuechterlein, J. P. Hardisty, and M. Gitlin, 1992, *British Journal of Psychiatry.* Copyright 1992 by the Royal College of Psychiatrists. Reprinted by permission.

does not require the same degree of stress. If true, this itself requires explanation, in either social or biological ways.

There have been very few studies of the role of life events in depressive psychosis. Such conditions are sometimes regarded as the extreme end of a continuum from mild depression onward. There are grounds from studies of less severe depressions to suggest that life events have a role at the psychotic end of the spectrum. For example, a number of authors have addressed the issue of whether life events are more likely before depressions with a neurotic rather than an endogenous symptom picture (Bebbington, Tennant, & Hurry, 1981; Bebbington et al., 1988; Benjaminsen, 1981; Brown & Harris, 1978; Brugha & Conroy, 1985; Hudgens, Morrison, & Barchka, 1967; Katschnig, 1984; Katschnig, Pakesh, & Egger-Zeidner, 1986; Katschnig et al., 1981, Leff, Roach, & Bunney, 1970; Nelson & Charney 1980; Paykel, Rao, & Taylor, 1984; Roy, Breier, Doran, & Pickar, 1985; Thompson & Hendrie, 1972; Zimmerman, Coryell, Pfohl, & Stangel, 1986). Some of these studies do support a reduced association of adversity with an endogenous symptom picture, many do not. They invariably involve dividing the cases of depression into a limited number of categories. This raises the possibility that the choice of criteria for making this division will influence the findings. However, Katschnig et al. (1986) divided their case series according to several different sets of criteria. In no case were they able to demonstrate that depressions with an endogenous symptom picture were less likely to be precipitated by life events than depressions with neurotic symptoms only. The conclusion must therefore be that, although events may be less implicated in the precipitation of severe than mild depression, this difference is slight.

Our most recent investigation, the Camberwell Collaborative Psychosis Study, has provided data that we feel clarifies the role of life events (Bebbington et al., 1993). *Psychosis* was defined broadly in this study, and we thus included cases of schizophrenic, manic, and depressive psychoses. Life events were much commoner in the 3-month period before onset of each of these conditions than in general population controls. These findings were statistically very significant. There was virtually no difference between the different types of psychosis: All seemed equally likely to be precipitated by events. The study used stringent methods of evaluation and analysis, and we think that weight can be placed on its findings. However, we did not find a marked peak of events in immediate proximity to onset. Rather, the increased event rate started several months before and increased gradually as the time of onset was approached. This implies that events can influence the onset of psychosis over a longer interval than has previously been thought. Our results are summarized in Figure 6.2. Two further studies of life events and schizophrenia will be published in the fairly near future (B. P. Dohrenwend, personal commu-

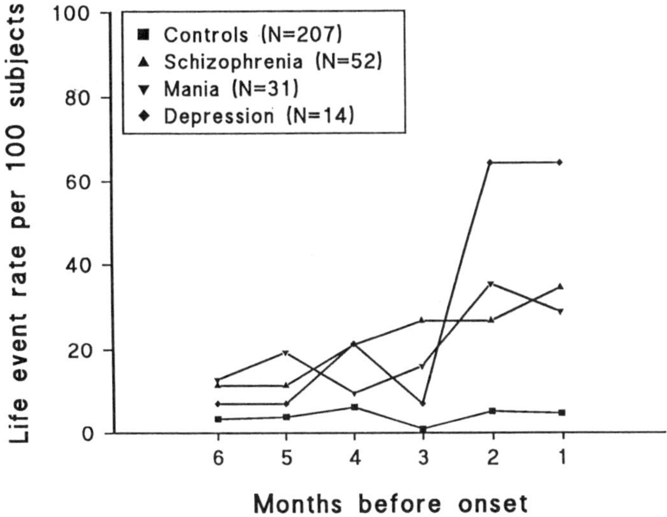

FIGURE 6.2. Life events before relapse in psychosis. From "Life events and psychosis: Initial results from the Camberwell Collaborative Psychosis Study" by P. E. Bebbington, S. Wilkins, P. Jones, A. Foerster, R. Murray, B. Toone, and S. Lewis, 1993, *British Journal of Psychiatry*. Copyright 1993 by the Royal College of Psychiatrists. Reprinted by permission.

nication, June 16, 1991; S. Hirsch, personal communication, Oct. 26, 1992).

Expressed Emotion as a Source of Stress

Expressed Emotion (EE) is now a long-established concept and has been reviewed at length elsewhere (Kuipers & Bebbington, 1988, 1990; Vaughn, 1989). The vast majority of studies have shown that the EE measure is predictive of relapse in schizophrenia (see review in Kuipers & Bebbington, 1990). The measure in based on the Camberwell Family Interview (CFI – Brown and Rutter, 1966; Rutter and Brown, 1966). The interview is taped and ratings are subsequently made of the number of critical comments made by relatives, their overall hostility and their emotional over-involvement. These ratings are used to construct a composite score of EE. The ability to reduce relapse rates by interventions that change the EE ratings of relatives with whom patients live, suggests that the behaviour of relatives reflected in the EE measure may have a genuine causal role (Bebbington & Kuipers, 1992).

It has always been assumed, not unreasonably, that the home environment characterized by high EE represents a form of psychosocial stress. There is now considerable evidence from psychophysiological studies to support this idea. Patients seem to be physiologically aroused in the presence of high EE relatives but not of low EE relatives (Sturgeon, Turpin, Kuipers, Berkowitz, & Leff, 1984; Tarrier, Barrowclough, Porceddu, & Watts, 1988; Tarrier, Vaughn, Lader, & Leff, 1979). Indeed Tarrier and Barrowclough (1987) demonstrated a differential physiological effect in a man living with one high and one low EE parent, depending on which was present. The arousal provoked by critical relatives seems to be nonspecific and has been observed in nonschizophrenic disturbed adolescents (Valone, Goldstein, & Morton, 1984).

Another key issue concerning EE is what the measure indicates about family relationships (Kuipers, 1979). Relatives who make frequent critical comments when interviewed alone behave similarly in the presence of the patient, although they are more restrained in the second setting (Rutter & Brown, 1966). EE is strongly correlated with negative affective style rated during direct interaction between family members (Miklowitz, Goldstein, Falloon, & Doane, 1984; Micklowitz et al., 1989; Strachan, 1986). Hubschmid and Zemp (1989) have shown that high EE relatives engender a more negative emotional climate, a more conflict-prone home structure, and more rigid patterns of interaction. Kuipers, Sturgeon, Berkowitz, and Leff (1983) studied direct interaction between relatives and patients and found that high-EE relatives talked longer and were poorer listeners than low-EE relatives. Highly critical relatives appear to provide an unpredictable home environment (MacCarthy, Hemsley, Schrank-Fernandez, Kuipers, & Katz, 1986). Another sequential analysis of interactions, this between couples where one partner was depressed, found that high-EE couples had a varied but largely negative style of interaction, whereas their low-EE counterparts appeared to provide a continuous positive exchange (Hooley & Hahlweg, 1986). Although relatives can in no way be blamed for what they cannot help, these findings suggest a number of ways in which their behavior may contribute to a stressful environment for people prone to psychosis.

Most work on expressed emotion has concerned patients suffering from schizophrenia, but two studies of bipolar and schizoaffective disorder suggest that patients with these disorders are also prone to break down in the face of a family environment that includes high-EE relatives (Miklowitz, Goldstein, Nuechterlein, Snyder, & Mintz, 1988; Priebe, Wildgrube, & Müller-Oerlinghausen, 1989).

Leff and his colleagues (Leff, Kuipers, Berkowitz, Vaughn, & Sturgeon, 1983) have incorporated the effects of psychosocial stress into an overall model of relapse in schizophrenia. They concluded from data available to them that patients unprotected by medication may relapse in response either to a life event or to living with high EE relatives, but that patients taking medication required exposure to both factors before they would relapse. In this model, medication operates generally to raise the threshold for the psychosocial provocation of relapse, suggesting that life events and expressed emotion might perhaps operate through a common mechanism.

Social Influences on the Negative Symptoms of Schizophrenia

Evidence for an important environmental influence on the negative symptoms of schizophrenia has long been established. This is of particular significance, as such symptoms are relatively resistant to modification by psychopharmacological means (Crow, 1989). Belknap (1956), Dunham and Weinberg (1960), and, perhaps most famously, Goffman (1961) propounded with force the view that large and environmentally impoverished mental institutions had a damaging effect on long-term inmates. They were able to do this because the association between the institutional environment and the impaired social behavior of many of those accommodated in institutions was quite obvious.

However, they did not consider the possibility that individuals handicapped by the chronic effects of severe psychiatric illness might themselves contribute to their own environment. This is apparent from the work of Wing and Freudenberg (1961), who arranged for nurses to provide extra social stimulation for long-term schizophrenic patients. The patients slowly improved, but when the stimulation was withdrawn they deteriorated again. Improvement was thus conditional upon the continuous provision of stimulation from an external source, and without it the patients would themselves create an environment of impoverishment.

The results of this experiment led Wing and his colleagues to mount a further study (Wing and Brown, 1970). Three area mental hospitals were selected on the basis that they provided demonstrably different environments for the patients they housed. A sample of female residents with long-standing schizophrenia was studied in each hospital. Measures of the social environment encountered in the hospitals confirmed differences between them in terms of the range of the patients' personal possessions, the attitudes of the nurses toward them, the amount of contact with the community outside, the restrictiveness of ward regimes, and the amount of time the patients spent doing nothing. It was hypothesized that these characteristics would be associated with equivalent clinical differences between the patient samples. This was corroborated by the results, which showed in particular that an impoverished and restricted ward environment was associated with prominent negative symptoms.

This cross-sectional association does not guarantee causal direction, but the three groups were followed up over an 8-year period. Externally induced improvements in the social environment were associated with improvements in the patients, and they were independent of medication policies. Although negative symptoms rarely disappeared entirely, the degree of improvement was clinically significant. These effects of the social environment have now been confirmed by other studies located outside large institutions (Hewitt, Ryan, & Wing, 1975; Tidmarsh & Wood, 1972).

Although the Three Hospitals Study is a classic of careful investigation that had a major impact on the management of long-term mental illness, no attempt to replicate it has been made until very recently (Curson, Pantellis, Ward, & Barnes, 1992). These authors examined the relationship between social and clinical poverty in long-stay patients with schizophrenia at a fourth British hospital. The patients were less than 60 years of age and had been resident for more than 2 years. All had a DSM-III diagnosis of schizophrenia. Assessments were made with the same instruments as in the Wing and Brown (1970) study. Levels of disability seemed comparable in the two studies.

In the earlier study, the time the patients spent doing nothing was a particularly important predictor of negative symptoms. Despite the fact that the nurse–patient ratio was 2.5 times greater in the later study, the patients spent almost 2 hours *more* doing nothing than in the least stimulating of the three hospitals in the earlier study. Overall, there was a relationship between environmental understimulation and negative symptoms, but the relationship was much weaker than that obtained by Wing and Brown (1970). However, this may reflect a constriction in the variability of the environment rather than unsatisfactory replication: The patients in this study were very much a residual group. The authors also found that there was a relationship between an impoverished social environment and *florid* symptoms. The definitive results of this study are awaited with interest.

As a result of these studies, there is little doubt that, although social disablement in schizophrenia to some extent represents an intrinsic part of the disease process, it responds considerably to enlightened clinical intervention.

CONCLUSIONS

Jaspers (1963) was clear about the way disease categories in psychiatry should be used to establish potential causes, but pessimistic about the progress that had been made at the time he was writing. The intervening years have seen an enormous volume of research into the functional psychoses, and the underlying postulate of a somatic cause has now been well corroborated at a number of levels.

Evidence of a genetic component in both schizophrenia and bipolar affective disorder has existed for many years, the lodestar of biological researchers when their bright hopes were revealed as will-o'-the-wisps. To the evidence from genetic epidemiology, we can now add the powerful modern techniques of molecular genetics. With the exception of the location of genes associated with bipolar disorder on the X chromosome, their specific claims have so far proved false, but it seems likely that they will eventually present us with the genetic basis of these disorders.

Apart from genetics, biological studies have tended to focus on schizophrenia. This has had the good effect of confirming definite anatomical abnormalities in this condition, through a range of imaging and neuropathological techniques. These cannot be attributed to medication, nor do they appear to be progressive. Taking the studies as a whole, it is possible to speculate that the term *schizophrenia* may cover separate conditions with either a predominantly genetic basis or a neurodevelopmental one, and to adduce evidence from a range of sources in support of this idea. The neurodevelopmental version is commoner in males and explains a number of features of male schizophrenia.

The disadvantage of this concentration on schizophrenia is that affective psychoses have been relatively neglected. Such evidence as there is suggests that bipolar disorder does not show the established anatomical and pathological changes seen in schizophrenia, nor is there corroborative epidemiological evidence that the disorder is much affected by agents in the physical environment. However, the strength of the genetic contribution is particularly striking in bipolar disorder, so this is not entirely surprising.

One of the major purposes of etiological research is to confirm that the clinical categories on which it is based are indeed useful. Until more studies of bipolar disorder have been completed, we cannot be sure that the distinction between it and schizophrenia can be validated in etiological terms. The preliminary evidence suggests that it can, but we must wait and see.

Our knowledge of the influence of social circumstances on these conditions also shows gaps and inconsistencies. However, the general conclusion must be that people suffering from either schizophrenia or bipolar disorder are indeed sensitive to the social environment in ways that may adversely affect the clinical course of their disorder. As far as can be seen, this sensitivity does not differentiate between the conditions, but there is no requirement that it should while biological factors look, as they do, a better bet.

It is perfectly possible that meaningful subcategories of the two major types of functional psychoses exist. One interesting proposition is that a sensitivity to social factors may assist the process of subdivision, for instance, into the "adult onset" and "congenital" psychoses proposed by Murray and his colleagues (1992). In any case, there is a strong argument for conducting studies in which variables at the biological and social levels are examined together, in terms of both their interaction with each other and their combined impact on clinical features. This was the approach adopted in both the Camberwell Collaborative Depression Study (Bebbington et al., 1988) and the Camberwell Collaborative Psychosis Study (Jones et al., 1993), some results of which have been adumbrated in the current chapter.

REFERENCES

Al Khani, M. A. F., Bebbington, P. E., Watson, J. P., & House, F. (1986). Life events and schizophrenia: A Saudi Arabian study. *British Journal of Psychiatry, 148,* 12–22

Ambelas, A. (1979). Psychologically stressful events in the precipitation of manic episodes. *British Journal of Psychiatry, 135,* 15–21.

Ambelas, A. (1987). Life events and mania: A special relationship? *British Journal of Psychiatry, 150,* 235–240.

Andreasen, N. C., Olsen S. A., Dennert J. W., Smith M. R. (1982). Ventricular enlargement in schizophrenia: Relationship to positive and negative symptoms. *American Journal of Psychiatry, 139,* 297–302

Andrew, B., Watt, D. C., Gillespie, C., Chapel, H. (1987). A family study of genetic linkage in schizophrenia. *Psychological Medicine 17,* 363–370

Baron, M., Risch, N., Hamburger, R., Mandel, B., Kushner, S., Newman, M., Drumer, D., Belmaker, R. H. (1987). Genetic linkage between X-chromosome markers and bipolar affective illness. *Nature, 326,* 289–291

Barr, C. E., Mendick, S. A., & Munk-Jorgensen, P. (1990) Exposure to influenza epidemics during gestation and adult schizophrenia: a 40-year study. *Archives of General Psychiatry, 47,* 869–874.

Bassett, A. S., McGillivray, B. C., Jones, B. D., & Pantzar, J. T. (198 8). Partial trisomy chromosome 5 cosegregating with schizophrenia. *Lancet, 1,* 799–801

Bateson, G., Jackson, D. D., Hally, J., & Weakland, J. H. (1956). Towards a theory of schizophrenia. *Behavioural Science, 1,* 251–64.

Bebbington, P. E., Brugha, T. MacCarthy, B., Potter, J., Sturt, E., Wykes, T., Katz, R., & McGuffin, P. (1988). The Camberwell Collaborative Depression Study: I. Depressed probands: Adversity and the form of depression. *British Journal of Psychiatry, 152,* 754–765.

Bebbington, P. E., & Kuipers, L. (1992). Social causation of schizophrenia. In D. Bhugra & J. P. Leff (Eds.), *Principles of Social Psychiatry* (pp. 82–98). Oxford: Blackwells.

Bebbington, P. E., Tennant, C., & Hurry, J. (1981). Adversity and the nature of psychiatric disorder in the community. *Journal of Affective Disorders, 3,* 345–366.

Bebbington, P. E., Wilkins, S., Jones, P., Foerster, A., Murray, R. M., Toone B., & Lewis, S. (1993). Life events and psychosis: Initial results from the Camberwell Collaborative Psychosis Study. *British Journal of Psychiatry, 162,* 72–79.

Belknap, I. (1956). *Human problems of a state mental hospital,* New York: McGraw-Hill.

Bellodi, L., Bussoleni, C., Scorza-Smeraldi, R., Grassi, G., Zacchetti, & L., Smeraldi, E. (1986). Family study of schizophrenia: Exploratory analysis for relevant factors. *Schizophrenia Bulletin, 12,* 120–128.

Benes, F. M. (1989). Myelination of cortical–hippocampal relays during late adolescence. *Schizophrenia Bulletin, 15,* 585–593.

Benes, F. M., Davidson, J., Bird, & E. D. (1986). Quantitative cytoarchitectural studies of the cerebral cortex of schizophrenics. *Archives of General Psychiatry, 43,* 31–35.

Benjaminsen, S. (1981). Primary non-endogenous depression and features attributed to reactive depression. *Journal of Affective Disorders, 3,* 245–259.

Berrettini, W. H., Goldin, L. R., Gelernter, J., Gejman, P. V., Gershon, E. S., & Detera-Wadleigh, S. (1990). X-chromosome markers and manic–depressive illness: Rejection of linkage to Xq28 in nine bipolar pedigrees. *Archives of General Psychiatry, 47,* 366–373.

Bertelsen, A., Harvald, B., & Hauge, M. (1977). A Danish twin study of manic–depressive disorders. *British Journal of Psychiatry, 130,* 330–351.

Bogerts, B., Ashtari, M., Degreef, G., Alvir, J., Bilder, R., & Lieberman, J. (1990). Reduced temporal limbic structure volumes on magnetic resonance images in first episode schizophrenia. *Psychiatry Research, Neuroimaging, 35,* 1–13 .

Bogerts, B., Meertz, E., & Schonfeldt-Bausch, R. (1985). Basal ganglia and limbic system pathology in schizophrenia: A morphometric study of brain volume and shrinkage. *Archives of General Psychiatry, 42,* 784–791.

Brown, G. W., & Birley, J. L. T. (1968). Crises and life changes and the onset of schizophrenia. *Journal of Health and Social Behaviour, 9,* 203–214.

Brown, G. W., & Harris, T. (1978). *Social origins of depression.* London, Tavistock.

Brown, G. W., & Rutter, M. L. (1966). The measurement of family activities and relationships. *Human Relations, 19,* 241–263.

Brown, R., Colter, N., Corsellis, J. A. N., Crow, T. J., Frith, C. D., Jagoe, R., Johnstone, E. C., & Marsh, L. (1986). Post-mortem evidence of structural brain changes in schizophrenia. *Archives of General Psychiatry, 42,* 36–42.

Brugha, T., & Conroy, R. (1985). Categories of depression: Reported life events in a controlled design. *British Journal of Psychiatry, 147,* 641–646.

Canton, G., & Fraccon, I. G. (1985). Life events and schizophrenia: A replication. *Acta Psychiatrica Scandinavica, 71,* 211–216.

Castle, D. J., & Murray, R. M. (1991). The neurodevelopmental basis of sex differences in schizophrenia. *Psychological Medicine, 21,* 565–575.

Chung, R. K., Langeluddecke, P., & Tennant, C. (1986). Threatening life events in the onset of schizophrenia, schizophreniform psychosis and hypomania. *British Journal of Psychiatry, 148,* 680–686.

Collinge, J. S., DeLisi, L. E., Boccio, A. Johnstone, E. C., Lane, A., Larkin, C.,

Leach, M., Lofthouse, R., Owen, F., Poulter, M., Shah, T., Walsh, C., & Crow, T. J. (1991). Evidence for a pseudoautosomal locus for schizophrenia using the method of affected sibling pairs. *British Journal of Psychiatry, 158,* 624–629.

Crow, T. J. (1988). Sex chromosomes and psychosis: The case for a pseudoautosomal locus. *British Journal of Psychiatry, 149,* 419–429.

Crow, T. J. (1989). A current view of the Type II syndrome: Age of onset, intellectual impairment and the meaning of structural changes in the brain. *British Journal of Psychiatry, 155*(Suppl. 7), 10–14.

Curson, D. A., Pantellis, C., Ward, J., & Barnes, T. R. E. (1992). Institutionalization and schizophrenia 30 years on: Clinical poverty and the social environment in three British mental hospitals in 1960 compared with a fourth in 1990. *British Journal of Psychiatry, 160,* 230–241.

Day, R., Neilsen, J. A., Korten, A., Ernberg, G., Dube, K. C., Gebhart, J., Jablensky, A., Leon, C., Marsella, A., Olatawura, M., Sartorius, N., Stromgren, E., Takahashi, R., Wig, N., & Wynne, L. C. (1987). Stressful life events preceding the acute onset of schizophrenia: A cross-national study from the World Health Organization. *Culture, Medicine and Psychiatry, 11,* 123–206.

Deakin, J. F. W., Slater, P., Simpson, M. D. C., Gilchrist, A. C., Skan, W. J., Royston, M. C., Reynolds, G. P., & Cross, A. J. (1989). Frontal cortical and and left temporal glutmatergic dysfunction in schizophrenia. *Journal of Neurochemistry, 52,* 1781–1786.

Detera-Wadleigh, S. D., Berrettini, W. H., Goldin, L. R., Boorman, D., Anderson, S. B., & Gershon, E. S. (1987) Close linkage of C-Harvey-ras-1 and the insulin gene to affective disorder is ruled out in three North American pedigrees. *Nature, 325,* 806–808.

Doane, J. A., West, K. L., Goldstein, M. J., Rodnick, E. H., & Jones, J. E. (1981). Parental communication deviance and affective style: Predictors of subsequent schizophrenia spectrum disorders in vulnerable adolescents. *Archives of General Psychiatry, 38,* 679–685.

Done, J. D., Johnstone, E. C., Frith, C. D., Golding, J., Sheperd, P. M., & Crow, T. J. (1991). Complications of pregnancy and delivery in relation to psychosis in adult life: Data from the British Perinatal Portality Study. *British Medical Journal, 302,* 1576–1580.

Drake, R. E., & Sederer, L. I. (1986). The adverse effects of intensive treatment of chronic schizophrenia. *Comprehensive Psychiatry, 27,* 313–326.

Dunham, H. W., & Weinberg, S. K. (1960). *Culture of the state mental hospital.* Detroit: Wayne State University Press.

Dunner, D. L., Patrick, V., & Fieve, R. R . (1979). Life events at the onset of bipolar affective illness. *American Journal of Psychiatry, 136,* 508–511.

Egeland, J. A., Gerahard, D. S., Pauls, D., Sussex, J. N., Kidd, K. K., Allen, C. R., Hostetter, A. M., & Housman, D. E. (1987). Bipolar affective disorders linked to DNA markers on chromosome 11. *Nature, 325,* 783–787.

Falki, P., & Bogerts, B. (1986). Cell loss in the hippocampus of schizohrenics. *European Archives of Psychiatry and Neurological Science, 236,* 154–161.

Falki, P., Bogerts, B., Rozumek, M. (1988). Limbic pathology in schizophrenia. The entorhinal region: a morphometric study. *Biological Psychiatry, 24,* 515–521.

Foerster, A., Lewis, S. W., Owen, M. J., & Murray, R. M. (1991). Low birth weight and a family history of schizophrenia predict poor premorbid functioning in psychosis. *Schizophrenia Research, 5*, 13–20.

Gill, M., Castle, D., & Duggan, C. (1992). Cosegregation of Christmas disease and major affective disorder in a pedigree. *British Journal of Psychiatry, 160*, 112–114.

Gill, M., McGuffin, P., Parfitt, E., Mant, R., Asherson, P., Collier, D., Vallada, H., Powell, J., Shaikh, S., Taylor, C., Sargeant, M., Clements, A., Nanko, S., Takazawa, N., Llewellyn, D., Williams, J., Whatley, S., Murray, R., & Owen M. (1993). A linkage study of schizophrenia with DNA markers from the long arm of chromosome 11. *Psychological Medicine, 23*, 27–44.

Gill, M., McKeown, P., & Humpries, P. (1988). Linkage analysis of manic depression in a large Irish pedigree using -ras-1 and INS DNA markers. *Journal of Medical Genetics, 24*, 634–635.

Glassner, B., & Haldipur, C. V. (1983). Life events and early and late onset of bipolar disorder. *American Journal of Psychiatry, 140*, 215–217.

Goffman, E. (1961). *Asylums*. New York: Anchor Books.

Goldberg, S. C., Schooler, N. R., Hogarty, G. E., & Roper, M. (1977). Prediction of relapse in schizophrenic outpatients treated by drug and sociotherapy. *Archives of General Psychiatry, 34*, 171–184.

Goldstein, J. M., Tsuang, M. T., & Farrone, S. V. (1989). Gender and schizophrenia: Implications for understanding the heterogeneity of the illness. *Psychiatry Research, 28*, 243–253.

Goldstein, M. (1985). Family factors that antedate the onset of schizophrenia and related disorders: The results of a 15 year prospective longitudinal study. *Acta Psychiatrica Scandinavica, 71*(Suppl. 319), 7–18.

Goldstein, M. (1987). The UCLA high-risk project. *Schizophrenia Bulletin, 13*, 505–514.

Goodman, R. (1989). Are complications of pregnancy and birth causes of schizophrenia? *Developmental Medicine and Child Neurology, 30*, 391–406.

Gottesman, I. I., & Bertelsen, A. (1989). Confirming unexpressed genotypes for schizophrenia. *Archives of General Psychiatry, 46*, 867–872.

Gottesman, I. I., & Shields, J. (1982). *Schizophrenia, the epigenetic puzzle*. Cambridge: Cambridge University Press.

Grandy, D. K., Litt, M., Allen, L., Bunzow, J. R., Marchionni, M., Makam, H., Reed, l., Magenis, R. E., & Civelli, O. (1989). The human dopamine receptor gene is located on chromosome 11 at q22–q23 and identifies a Taq1 RFLP. *American Journal of Human Genetics, 45*, 778–785.

Green, M. F., Satz, P., Gaier, J., Ganzell, S., & Kharabi, F. (1989). Minor physical anomalies in schizophrenia. *Schizophrenia Bulletin 15*, 91–100.

Hare, E. H. (1975). Manic-depressive psychosis and season of birth. *Acta Psychiatrica Scandinavica. 52*, 69.

Heston, L. L. (1966). Psychiatric disorders in foster home reared children of schizophrenic mothers. *British Journal of Psychiatry, 112*, 819–825.

Hewitt, S., Ryan, P., & Wing, J. K. (1975). living without the mental hospitals. *Journal of Social Policy, 4*, 391–404.

Hirsch, S. R., & Leff, J. P. (1975). *Abnormalities in the Parents of Schizophrenics*. Maudsley Monograph No. 22. Oxford: Oxford University Press.

Hodgkinson, S., Sherrington, R., Gurling, H., Marchbanks, R., Reeders, S.,

Mallet, J., McInnis, M., Petursson, H., & Brynjolfsson, J. (1987). Molecular genetic evidence for heterogeneity in manic depression. *Nature, 325,* 805–806.

Holland, A., & Gosden, C. (1990). A balanced chromosomal translocation partially co-segregating with psychotic illness in a family. *Psychiatric Research, 32,* 1–8.

Hooley, J. M., & Hahlweg, K. (1986). The marriages and interaction patterns of depressed patients and their spouses: Comparison of high and low EE dyads. In M. J. Goldstein, I. Hand, & K. Hahlweg (Eds.), *Treatment of Schizophrenia: Family Assessment and Intervention.* Berlin: Springer.

Hubschmid, T., & Zemp, M. (1989). Interactions in high- and low-EE families. *Social Psychiatry and Psychiatric Epidemiology, 24,* 113–119.

Hudgens, R. W., Morrison, J. R., & Barchka, R. (1967). Life events and onset of primary affective disorders. A study of 40 hospitalised patients and 40 controls. *Archives of General Psychiatry, 16,* 134–145.

Illowsky, B. P., Julliano, D. M., Bigelow, L. B., & Weinberger, D. R. (1988) Stability of CT scan findings in schizophrnia: results of an 8 year follow-up. *Journal of Neurology, Neurosurgery and Psychiatry, 51,* 209–213.

Jacob, H., & Beckman, H. (1984). Prenatal developmental disturbance in the limbic allocortex in schizophrenics. *Journal of Neural Transmission, 65,* 303–326.

Jacobs, S., & Myers, J. (1976). Recent life events and acute schizophrenic psychosis: A controlled study. *Journal of Nervous and Mental Disease, 162,* 75–87.

Jaspers, K. (1963). *General psychopathology* (7th ed., J. Hoenig & M. W. Hamilton, Trans.). Manchester, England: Manchester University Press.

Jeste, D. V., & Lohr, J. B. (1989). Hippocampal pathologic findings in schizophrenia: A morphometric study. *Archives of General Psychiatry, 46,* 1019–1024.

Johnstone, E. C., Crow, T. J., Frith, C. D., Husband, J., & Kreel, L. (1976). Cerebral ventricular size and cognitive impairment in chronic schizophrenia. *Lancet, 2,* 924–926.

Johnstone, E. C., Owens, D. G. C., Crow, T. J., Frith, C. D., Alexandropolis, K., Bydder, G. M., & Colter, N. (1989). Temporal lobe structure as determined by nuclear magnetic resonance in schizophrenia and bipolar affective disorder. *Journal of Neurology, Neurosurgery and Psychiatry, 52,* 736–741.

Jones, P., Bebbington, P. E., Foerster, A., Lewis, S., Murray, R. M., Russell. A., Sham, P., Toone B., & Wilkins, S. (1993). Poor scholastic achievement and pre-psychotic social decline are specific to schizophrenia: results from the Camberwell Collaborative Psychosis Study. *British Journal of Psychiatry, 162,* 65–71.

Jones, P., & Murray, R. M. (1991). The genetics of schizophrenia is the genetics of neurodevelopment. *British Journal of Psychiatry, 158,* 615–623.

Katschnig, H. (1984). Commentary to Paul Bebbington. Inferring causes: Some constraints in the social psychiatry of depressive disorders. *Integrative Psychiatry, 2,* 77–79.

Katschnig, H., Brandl-Nebehay, A., Fuchs-Robetin, G., Seelig, P., Eichberger, G., Strobl, R., & Sint, P. P. (1981). *Lebensverandernde Ereignisse, psychoziale Dispositionen und depressive Verstimmungzustande.* Vienna: Abteilung für Sozialpsychiatrie und Dokumentation, Psychiatrische Universitätsklinik.

Katschnig, H., Pakesh, G., & Egger-Zeidner, E. (1986). Life stress and subtypes of depression. In H. Katschnig (Ed.), *Life Events and Psychiatric Disorders: Controversial Issues,* Cambridge: Cambridge University Press.

Kelsoe, J. R., Ginns, E. I., Egeland, J. A., Gerhard, D. S., Goldstein, A. M., Bale, S. J., Pauls, D. L., Long, R. T., Kidd, K. K., Conte, G., Housman, D. E., & Paul, S. M. (1989). Re-evaluation of the linkage relationship between chromosome 11p loci and the gene for bipolar affective disorder in the Old Order Amish. *Nature, 324,* 238–243.

Kennedy, J. L., Giuffra, L. A., Moises, H. W., Cavalli-Sforza, L. L., Pakstsis, A. J., Kidd, J. R., Castiglione, C. M., Sjogren, B., Wetterberg, L., & Kidd K. (1988). Evidence against linkage to markers on chromosome 5 in a northern Swedish pedigree. *Nature, 336,* 167–169.

Kennedy, S., Thompson, R., Stancer, H. C., Roy, A., & Persad, E. (1983). Life events precipitating mania. *British Journal of Psychiatry, 142,* 398–403.

Kety, S. S., Rosenthal, D., Wender, P. H., Schulsinger, F., & Jacobson, B. (1978). The biologic and adoptive families of individuals who became schizophrenic: prevalence of mental illness and other characteristics. In L. C. Wynne, R. L. Cromwell, & S. Mathysse (Eds.), *The nature of schizophrenia: New approaches to research and treatment.* New York: Wiley.

Kovelman, J. A., & Scheibel, A. B. (1984). A neurohistological correlate of schizphrenia. *Biological Psychiatry, 19,* 1601–1602 .

Kringlen, E., & Cramer, G. (1989). Offspring of monozygotic twins discordant for schizophrenia. *Archives of General Psychiatry, 46,* 873–877.

Kuipers, L. (1979). Expressed emotion: A review. *British Journal of Social and Clinical Psychology, 18,* 237–243.

Kuipers, L., & Bebbington, P. E. (1988). Expressed emotion research in schizophrenia: theoretical and clinical implications. *Psychological Medicine, 18,* 893–910.

Kuipers, L., & Bebbington, P. E. (1990). *Working in partnership: Clinicians and carers in the management of longstanding mental illness.* Oxford: Heinemann Medical.

Kuipers, L., Sturgeon, D., Berkowitz, R., & Leff, J. P. (1983). Characteristics of expressed emotion: Its relationship to speech and looking in schizophrenic patients and their relatives. *British Journal of Clinical Psychology, 22,* 257–264.

Laing, R. D., & Esterson, A. (1964). *Sanity, madness and the family.* Harmondsworth, England: Penguin.

Lander E. (1988). Splitting schizophrenia. *Nature, 336,* 105–106.

Leff, J. P., Kuipers, L., Berkowitz, R., Vaughn, C. E., & Sturgeon, D. (1983). Life events, relatives' Expressed Emotion and maintenance neuroleptics in schizophrenic relapse. *Psychological Medicine, 13,* 799–806.

Leff, M. H., Roach, J. F., & Bunney, W. E. (1970). Environmental factors preceding the onsets of severe depressions. *Psychiatry, 33,* 293–311.

Lewine, R. (1988). Gender and Schizophrenia. In M. T. Tsuang & J. C. Simpson (Eds.), *Handbook of Schizophrenia* (Vol. 3, pp. 379–397). Amsterdam: Elsevier

Lewis, S. W., & Murray, R. M. (1987). Obstetric complications, neurodevelopmental deviance and schizophrenia. *Journal of Psychiatric Research, 21,* 413–421.

Lidz, T., Cornelison, A. R., Fleck, S., & Terry, D. (1957). The intrafamilial environment of the schizophrenic patient. *Psychiatry, 20,* 329–342.

MacCarthy, B., Hemsley, D., Schrank-Fernandez, C., Kuipers, L., & Katz, R. (1986). Unpredictability as a correlate of expressed emotion in the relatives of schizophrenics. *British Journal of Psychiatry, 148,* 727–730.

Malla, A. K., Cortese, L., Shaw, T. S., & Ginsberg, B. (1990). Life events amd relapse in schizophrenia: A one year prospective study. *Social Psychiatry and Psychiatric Epidemiology, 25,* 221–224.

Malzacher, M., Merz, J., & Ebnother, D. (1981). Einschneidende Lebensereignisse im Vorfeld akuter schizophrener Episoden: Erstmals erkrankte Patienten im Vergleich mit einer Normalstichprobe. *Archiv fur Psychiatrie und Nervenkrankheiten, 230,* 227–242.

Mankoo, B., Sherrington, R., Brynjolfsson, J., Kalsi, G., Petursson, H., Sigmundsson, T., Read, T., Murphy, P., Curtis, D., Melmer, G., & Gurling, H. (1991). New microsatellite polymorphisms provide a highly polymorphic map of chromosome 5 bands q11.2–q13.3 for linkage analysis of Icelandic and English families affected by schizophrenia [Abstract] *Psychiatric Genetics, 2,* 17.

McCreadie, R., Wilson, A., & Burton, L. (1983). The Scottish Survey of "new chronic" inpatients. *British Journal of Psychiatry, 143,* 564–571.

McGue, M., Gottesman, I. I., Rao, D. C. (1986). The analysis of schizophrenia family data. *Behavioural Genetics, 16,* 75–87.

McGuffin, P. (1988). Major genes for major affective disorder. *British Journal of Psychiatry, 153* 591–596.

McGuffin, P., Farmer, A., Gottesman, I. I. (1987). Is there really a split in schizophrenia? *British Journal of Psychiatry, 150,* 581–592.

McGuffin, P., Festenstein W., Murray R. M. (1983). A family study of HLA antigens and other genetic markers in schizophrenia. *Psychological Medicine, 13,* 31–43.

McGuffin, P., & Katz, R. (1986). Nature, nurture and affective disorder. In J. W. Deakin (Ed.), *The biology of affective disorders.* London: Royal College of Psychiatrists, Gaskell Press.

McGuffin, P., Sargeant, M., Hett, G., Tidmarsh, S., Whatley, S., & Marchbanks, R. M. (1990). Exclusion of a schizophrenia susceptibility gene from the chromosome 5q11–13 region: New data and a reanalysis of previous reports. *American Journal of Human Genetics, 47,* 524–535.

McNeil, R. F., & Kaij, L. (1978). Obstetric factors in the development of schizophrenia. In L. C. Wynne, R. L. Cromwell, & S. Matthysse (Eds.), *The Nature of Schizophrenia.* New York: Wiley.

Mendick, S. A., Machon, R. A., Huttenen, M. O., & Bonet, D. (1988). Adult schizophrenia following prenatal exposure to an influenza epidemic. *Archives of General Psychiatry, 45,* 188–192.

Mendelwicz, J., Fleiss, J. L., & Fieve, R. R. (1972). Evidence for X-linkage in the transmission of manic–depressive illness. *Journal of the American Medical Association, 222,* 1624–1627.

Mendlewicz, J., Linkowski, P., & Wilmotte, J. (1980). Linkage between glucose-6-phosphate dehydrodgenase deficiency and manic–depressive psychosis. *British Journal of Psychiatry, 137,* 337–342.

Mendlewicz, J., & Rainer, J. D. (1977). Adoption study supporting genetic transmission in manic–depressive illness. *Nature, 268,* 327–329.

Mendlewicz, J., Simon, P., Sevy, S., Charon, F., Brocas, H., Legros, S., & Vassart, G. (1987). Polymorphic DNA marker on X chromosome and manic depression. *Lancet, 1,* 1230–1232.

Michaux, W., Gansereit, K., McCabe, O., & Kurland, A. (1967). The psychopathology and measurement of environmental stress. *Community Mental Health Journal, 3,* 358–371.

Miklowitz, D. J., Goldstein, M. J., Doane, J. A., Nuechterlein, K. H., Strachan, A. M., Snyder, K. S., & Magana-Amato, A. (1989). Is expressed emotion an index of a transactional process: I. Parent's affective style. *Family Process, 28,* 153–167.

Miklowitz, D. J., Goldstein, M. J., Falloon, R. H., & Doane, J. A. (1984). Interactional correlates of expressed emotion in the families of schizophrenics. *British Journal of Psychiatry, 144,* 482–487.

Miklowitz, D. J., Goldstein, M. J., Nuechterlein, K. H., Snyder, K. S., & Mintz, J. (1988). Family factors and the course of bipolar affective disorder. *Archives of General Psychiatry, 45,* 225–231.

Moises, H. W., Gelernter, J., Giuffra, L., Zarcone, V., Wetterberg, L., Civelli, O., Kidd, K. K., & Cavalli-Sforza, L. (1991). No linkage between D2 dopamine receptor gene region and schizophrenia. *Archives of General Psychiatry, 48,* 643–647.

Murray, R. M., Callaghan, E., Castle, D., & Lewis, S. W. (in press). A neurodevelopmental approach to the classification of schizophrenia. *Schizophrenia Bulletin.*

Murray, R. M., & Lewis, S. W. (1987). Is schizophrenia a neurodevelopmental disorder? *British Medical Journal, 295,* 681–682.

Murray, R. M., Lewis, S. W., & Reveley, A. M. (1985). Towards an aetiological classification of schizophrenia. *Lancet, 1,* 1023–1026.

Murray, R. M., Lewis, S. W., Owen, M. J., & Foerster, A. (1988). The neurodevelopmental origins of dementia praecox. In P. McGuffin & P. Bebbington (Eds.), *Schizophrenia: The major issues.* London: Heinmann.

Nelson, C. J., & Charney, D. S. (1980). Primary affective disorder criteria and the endogenous–reactive distinction. *Archives of General Psychiatry, 37,* 787–793.

O'Callaghan, E., Sham, P., Takei, N., Glover, G., & Murray, R. (1991). Schizophrenia after prenatal exposure to 1957 A2 influenza epidemic. *Lancet, 337,* 1248–1249.

O'Rourke, D. H., McGuffin, P., & Reich, T. (1983). Genetic analysis of manic–depressive illness. *American Journal of Physical Anthropology, 62,* 51–59.

Ott, J. (1985) *Analysis of human genetic linkage.* Baltimore: Johns Hopkins University Press.

Owen, M. J., Lewis, S. W., Murray, R. M. (1988). Obstetric complications and cerebral abnormalities in schizophrenia. *Psychological Medicine, 18,* 331–340.

Owens, D. G. C., Johnstone, E. C., Crow, T. J., Frith, C. D., Jagoe, V. R., & Kreel, L. (1985). Lateral ventricular size in schizophrenia: Relationship to the disease process and its clinical limitations. *Psychological Medicine, 15,* 27–41.

Paykel, E. S., Rao, B. M., & Taylor, C. N. (1984). Life stress and symptom pattern in out-patient depression. *Psychological Medicine, 14*, 559–568.

Priebe, S., Wildgrube, C., & Müller-Oerlinghausen, D. (1989). Lithum prophylaxis and expressed emotion. *British Journal of Psychiatry, 154*, 396–399.

Raz, S., & Raz, N. (1990). Structural brain abnormalities in the major psychoses: A quantitative review of the evidence from computerised imaging. *Psychological Bulletin, 108*, 93–108.

Reveley, A. M., Clifford, C. A., Reveley, M. A., & Murray, R. M. (1982). Cerebral ventricular size in twins discordant for schizophrenia. *Lancet, 1*, 540–541.

Roberts, G. W. (1991). Schizophrenia: A neuropathological perspective. *British Journal of Psychiatry, 158*, 8–17.

Roy, A., Breier, A., Doran, A. R., & Pickar, D. (1985). Life events and depression: Relation to subtypes. *Journal of Affective Disorders, 9*, 143 –148.

Rudin E. (1916). *Zur Vererbung und Neuenstehung der Dementia Praecox.* Berlin: Springer-Verlag.

Rutter, M. L., & Brown, G. W. (1966). The reliability and validity of measures of family life and relationships in families containing a psychiatric patient. *Social Psychiatry, 1*, 38–53.

Sacchetti, E., Vita, A., Calezeroni, A., Conte, G., Pallastio, F., Terzi, A., Valvassori, G., Invernizzi, G., & Cazzullo, C. L. (1990) Neuromorphological correlates of mood disorders. In C. L. Cazzullo, E. Sacchetti, G. Conte, G. Invernizzi, & A. Vita (Eds.), *Plasticity and Morphology of the Central Nervous System.* Lancaster, England: Kluwer Academic Publications.

Sclare, P., & Creed, F. (1990). Life events and the onset of mania. *British Journal of Psychiatry, 156*, 508–514.

Sham, P., Bebbington, P., Jones, P., Russell, A., Gilvarry, K., Wilkins, S., Lewis, S., Toone, B., & Murray, R. M. (1992). *The Camberwell functional psychosis family study: 2. Age at onset, gender, and familial morbidity in schizophrenia.* Manuscript submitted for publication.

Sherrington, R., Brynjolfsson, J., Petursson, H., Potter, M., Dudleston, K., Barraclough, B., Wasmuth, J., Dobbs, M., & Gurling, H. (1988). Localisation of a susceptibility locus for schizophrenia on chromosome 5. *Nature, 336*, 164–167.

Smith, M., Wasmuth, J., McPherson, J. D., Wagner, C., Grandy, D., Civelli, O., Potkin, S., & Litt, M. (1989). Cosegregation of an 11q22–9p22 translocation with affective disorder: proximity of the dopamine D2 receptor gene relative to the translocation breakpoint. *American Journal of Human Genetics 45*, A220 .

St. Clair, D., Blackwood, D., Muir, W., Baillie, D., Hubbard, A., Wright, A., & Evans, H. J. (1989). No linkage of chromosome 5q11–13 markers to schizophrenia in Scottish families. *Nature, 339*, 305–309.

St. Clair, D., Blackwood, D., Muir, W., Carothers, A., Walker, M., Spowart, G., Godsen, C., & Evans, H. J. (1990). Association within a family of a balanced autosomal translocation with major mental illness. *Lancet, 336*, 13–16.

St. George-Hyslop, P. H., Tanzi, R. E., Polinsky, R. J., Haines, J. L., Nee, L., Watkins P. C., Myers, R. H., Feldman, R. G., Pollen, D., Drachman, D.,

Growdon, J., Bruni, A., Fonci, J. -F., Salmon, D., Frommelt, P., Amaducci, L., Sorbi, S., Piacentini, S., Stewart, G. D., Hobbs, W. J., Conneally, M., & Gusealla, J. F. (1987) The genetic defect causing Alzheimer's disease maps on chromosome 21. *Science, 235*, 885–889.

Steinberg, H., & Durell, J. (1968). A stressful situation as a precipitant of schizophrenic symptoms: An epidemiological study. *British Journal of Psychiatry, 114*, 1097–1105.

Stevens, B. C. (1973). Evaluation of rehabilitation for psychotic patients in the community. *Acta Psychiatrica Scandinavica, 46*, 136–140.

Strachan, A. M. (1986). Family intervention for the rehabilitation of schizophrenia. *Schizophrenia Bulletin, 12*, 678–698.

Sturgeon, D., Turpin, D., Kuipers, L., Berkowitz, R., & Leff, J. (1984). Psychophysiological responses of schizophrenic patients to high and low expressed emotion relatives: a follow-up study. *British Journal of Psychiatry, 145*, 62–69.

Suddath, R. L., Christison, G. W., Torrey, E. F., Casanova, M. F., & Weinberger, D. R. (1990). Anatomical abnormalities in the brains of monozygotic twins discordant for schizophrenia. *New England Journal of Medicine, 322*, 789–794.

Takei, N., Sham, P. C., O'Callaghan, E., Glover, G., & Murray, R. M. (1992). *Early risk factors in schizophrenia: Season and place of birth.* Manuscript submitted for publication.

Tarrier, N., & Barrowclough, C. (1987). A longitudinal psychophysiological assessment of a schizophrenic patient in relation to the expressed emotion of his relatives. *Behavioural Psychotherapy, 15*, 45–57.

Tarrier, N., Barrowclough, C., Porceddu, K., & Watts, S. (1988). The assessment of psychophysiological reactivity to the expressed emotion of the relatives of schizophrenic patients. *British Journal of Psychiatry, 153*, 618–624.

Tarrier, N., Vaughn, C. E., Lader, M. H. and Leff, J. P. (1979). Bodily reactions to people and events in schizophrenics. *Archives of General Psychiatry, 36*, 311–315.

Thompson, K. C., & Hendrie, H. C. (1972). Environmental stress in primary depressive illness. *Archives of General Psychiatry, 26*, 130–132.

Tidmarsh, D., & Wood, S. (1972). Psychiatric aspects of destitution. In J. K. Wing & A. M. Hailey (Eds.), *Evaluating a community psychiatric service,* London: Oxford University Press.

Tienari, P., Sorri, A., Lahti, I., Naarala, M., Wahlberg, K.-E., Moring, J., Pohjola, J., & Wynne, L. C. (1987). Genetic and psychosocial factors in schizophrenia: The Finnish adoptive family study. *Schizophrenia Bulletin, 13*, 477–484.

Turner, S. W., Toone, B. K., Brett-Jones, J. R. (1986). Computed tomographic scan changes in early schizophrenia: Preliminary findings. *Psychological Medicine, 16*, 219–226.

Valone, K., Goldstein, M. G., & Morton, J. P. (1984). Parental expressed emotion and psychophysiological reactivity in an adolescent sample at risk for schizophrenic spectrum disorders. *Journal of Abnormal Psychology, 93*, 448–457.

Vaughn, C. E. (1989). Annotation: Expressed emotion in family relationships. *Journal of Child Psychology, 30*, 13–22.

Venables, P. (1977). Psychophysiological high risk strategy with Mauritian children: Methodological issues. Paper presented at the Psychophysiological Conference, London.

Ventura, J., Nuechterlein, K. H., Lukoff, D., & Hardisty, J. P. (1989). A prospective study of stressful life events and schizophrenic relapse. *Journal of Abnormal Psychology, 98*, 407–411.

Ventura, J., Nuechterlein, K. H., Hardisty, J. P., & Gitlin, M. (1992). Life events and schizophrenic relapse after withdrawal of medication: A prospective study. *British Journal of Psychiatry, 161*, 615–620.

Vita, A., Sacchetti, I., Valvassori, G., & Cazzullo, C. L. (1988). Brain morphology in schizophrenia: A 2- to 5-year CT scan follow-up study. *Acta Psychiatrica Scandinavica, 78*, 618–621.

Weinberger, D. R. (1987). Implications of normal brain development for the pathogenisis of schizophrenia. *Archives of General Psychiatry, 44*, 660–669.

Weinberger, D. R., Torrey, E. F., Neophytides, A. N., & Wyatt, R. J. (1979). Lateral ventricular enlargement in chronic schizophrenia. *Archives of General Psychiatry, 36*, 735–739.

Wing, J. K., Bennett, D. H., & Denham, J. (1964). *The industrial rehabilitation of long stay schizophrenic patients* (Medical Research Council Memo No. 42). London: HMSO.

Wing, J. K., & Bransby, E. R. (1970). *Psychiatric case registers* (DHSS Statistical Report Series No. 8). London: HMSO.

Wing, J. K., & Brown, G. W. (1970). *Institutionalism and schizophrenia: A comparative study of three mental hospitals 1960–68.* Cambridge: Cambridge University Press.

Wing, J. K., & Freudenberg, R. K. (1961). The response of serverely ill chronic schizophrenic patients to social stimulation. *American Journal of Psychiatry, 118*, 311–322.

Wynne, L. C., & Singer, M. (1963). Thought disorder and family relations of schizophrenics. I. *Archives of General Psychiatry, 9*, 191–206.

Wynne, L. C., & Singer, M. (1965). Thought disorder and family relations of schizophrenics. II. *Archives of General Psychiatry, 12*, 187–212.

Zimmerman, M., Coryell, W., Pfohl, B., & Stangel, D. (1986). The validity of four definitions of endogenous depression: II. Clinical, demographic, familial and psychosocial correlates. *Archives of General Psychiatry, 43*, 234–244.

7

Children at Risk
for Psychopathology

IAN H. GOTLIB

WILLIAM R. AVISON

Over the past two decades, researchers and clinicians have devoted increasing attention to the identification of factors that may place children at elevated risk for manifesting deviant or disordered behavior, either during childhood or later, during adolescence or adulthood. In this context, investigators have examined the influence of genetic, environmental, and situational factors on behaviors ranging from autism, depression, and hyperactivity in childhood; to conduct disorder, juvenile delinquency, and Type A behavior in adolescence; to schizophrenia, alcoholism, depression, criminality, and personality disorder in adulthood. Given the extraordinary diversity both in the types of risk factors and in the nature of the outcomes examined in these investigations, it is clear that a comprehensive review and discussion of all of these areas of study are well beyond the scope of a single chapter.

Consequently, in determining the focus and breadth of this chapter, we made a number of decisions regarding the range of risk factors and outcomes to be examined. With respect to risk factors, an obvious distinction can be made between genetic influences and environmental factors. Given the emphasis developmental psychopathologists place on the importance of environmental factors and socialization experiences, and particularly on experiences within the family environment (cf. Cummings & Cicchetti, 1990; Masten & Garmezy, 1985), we focus in this chapter on risk factors that fall within this domain. As Loeber (1990) notes, there have been definitional difficulties surrounding the term *risk factors*. Consistent with Loeber's use, we define *risk* as exposure to factors that increase the probability of manifesting deviant behavior. In the context of the family environment, therefore, we examine the effects of children's exposure to social disadvantage, disrupted family structures, dysfunctional family processes, and various forms of parental psychopathology.

With respect to outcome, investigators have considered children to be at risk for demonstrating disturbed or deviant behavior either during their childhood or later, when they reach adolescence or adulthood. A distinction can be drawn, therefore, between those outcomes that involve the relatively proximal expression of psychopathology in childhood and those that involve more distal manifestations of disturbance in adolescence or adulthood. Because investigation of the long-term consequences of exposure to risk factors requires the use of stringent, prospective, longitudinal designs, there are very few methodologically sound studies in this area. Indeed, most of the investigations assessing long-term consequences of early exposure to various risk factors use retrospective case-control designs, which are often characterized by methodological shortcomings (cf. Barnett & Gotlib, 1988). Thus we focus our discussion in this chapter on those outcomes involving deviant behavior in childhood. Nevertheless, we do point out when results from methodologically sound studies of early risk factors for adult psychopathology are consistent with findings of investigations of risk factors for disturbance in childhood.

Finally, we should note that in the vast majority of investigations of the impact of specific risk factors for childhood psychopathology, child functioning has been measured in one of two ways: with structured clinical interviews that yield clinical psychiatric diagnoses (e.g., Kiddie Schedule for Affective Disorders and Schizophrenia, Diagnostic Interview for Children and Adolescents) or with measures of relatively undifferentiated symptoms of emotional distress (e.g., Child Behavior Checklist, Child Depression Inventory). Although there is obviously some overlap between continuous measures of distress and categorical assessments of clinical diagnoses, each type of outcome variable has unique advantages and disadvantages (see Kessler & Magee [in press], and Mirowsky [in press] for more detailed discussions of this issue). Consequently, we shall note throughout this chapter when we are discussing categorical or continuous outcome measures.

We begin this chapter by examining the impact of social disadvantage, particularly low socioeconomic status and poverty, on the mental health of children. We continue this discussion by examining aspects of the family structure that may represent risk factors for child psychopathology. In this context, we review studies assessing the impact of parental divorce, single-parent families, and early parental loss on child mental health. We then turn to an examination of the effects on children's psychosocial functioning of specific types of parental disturbance. In this section we review studies assessing the impact of parental depression, schizophrenia, and alcoholism. Following this extended discussion of the effects of various risk factors on child psychopathology, we examine a number of common processes that might mediate this impact. Finally, we conclude the chapter with a presentation of outstanding issues and recommendations for future work in this area.

FAMILY MILIEU AND CHILD PSYCHOPATHOLOGY

There is substantial agreement among psychologists, sociologists, and psychiatrists that the family environment plays a critical role in the development of mental health problems among children. Indeed, almost every perspective on developmental psychopathology attributes considerable importance to the ways in which family contexts affect the lives of children. Moreover, a central theme of virtually all sociological and psychological theories of socialization asserts the prominence of family factors in influencing children's behavior.

At the same time, however, it has become increasingly apparent that the family environment cannot be described adequately in terms of any single attribute. Instead, it appears that a more accurate characterization of the family milieu requires consideration of two related, yet theoretically distinct, dimensions: the socioeconomic circumstances of the family and the structure of the family.

A distinctive contribution of sociologists to the study of children's mental health has been to draw attention to the impact of *social disadvantage* as a risk factor for the manifestations of psychopathology in childhood. These disadvantaged socioeconomic circumstances are most frequently indexed by measures such as family incomes that fall below "poverty lines," families that receive welfare benefits, and families that live in subsidized housing. In contrast, *family structure* refers to the composition of the family unit. In this regard, researchers have been especially interested in comparing children from two-parent families with offspring from single-parent families. These comparisons have often been further elaborated by distinguishing among separated or divorced single-parent families, families in which one parent has died, and families headed by never-married mothers.

Social Disadvantage and Child Psychopathology

Scope of the Problem

There is ample evidence that a significant number of children in North America live in poverty. Barancik (1989) estimates that the proportion of children in poverty in the United States increased from 15.1% to 19.6% between 1974 and 1988, an increase of approximately 2.5 million children. Moreover, Duncan and Rodgers (1991) have recently argued that the proportion of children living in persistent (as opposed to sporadic) poverty and the proportion of children whose families depend on social assistance have also increased over time. In Canada, with a population of almost 27 million, it is estimated that approximately 1.5 million adults are unemployed and that 1 million children live in poverty.

Child Psychopathology

Over the last three decades, several major studies of children's mental health have been conducted to assess the relation between social disadvantage and child psychopathology. A number of investigators have addressed the broad question of whether there is an association between socioeconomic disadvantage and such negative outcomes in children as poor school performance, emotional disturbance, and elevated rates of juvenile delinquency. The results of these studies clearly indicate that such a link does exist (Loeber & Stouthamer-Loeber, 1986; Rutter & Madge, 1976). Increasingly, however, researchers have recognized the need to specify more explicitly those aspects of disadvantage that are most highly correlated with children's psychopathology.

Several studies have focused on parental social class as the measure of families' economic circumstances. The conclusions of these investigations concerning the importance of social class as a risk factor have been equivocal. Whereas some early studies reported correlations between social class and emotional and behavioral problems in children (Langner, McCarthy, Gersten, Simcha-Fagan, & Eisenberg, 1979), these associations were modest at best. Moreover, other investigations have found no relation between social class and children's mental health problems (e.g., Campbell & Redfening, 1979; Leslie, 1974). More recent investigations suggest that the class–disorder correlation may be stronger for children's externalizing problems, such as conduct disorders and attention deficit disorder, than it is for internalizing disorders, such as separation anxiety or depression (Velez, Johnson, & Cohen, 1989).

Results from some of the classic studies of children's mental health suggest that rates of emotional and behavioral problems are significantly higher only among children from the most severely disadvantaged circumstances. In the Manhattan Survey of Psychiatric Impairment in Urban Children, for example, Langner and his associates (e.g., Langner et al., 1974) randomly sampled 1,000 welfare families and 1,034 nonwelfare families. In each family the investigators surveyed one randomly selected child between the ages of 6 and 18 years. They reported that welfare children were almost twice as likely as nonwelfare children to have "marked" or "severe" impairment ratings (23.1% versus 13.5%). Moreover, when income was controlled, rates of impairment were significantly higher for children from low-income welfare families than for children from low-income nonwelfare families (Langner 1979).

In their study of children on the Isle of Wight, Rutter and his associates (e.g., Rutter, Cox, Tupling, Berger, & Yule, 1975) screened all 10- and 11-year-old children by means of interviews with parents and teachers. In the second stage of the study, informants were interviewed again and the children themselves underwent psychiatric interviews. The investigators' initial results revealed no social class differences in rates of emotional or behavioral problems among these children (Rutter, Tizard, & Whitmore, 1970). In a parallel study, a large sample of children from an inner-city borough of London was also screened for disorders and problem behaviors. Rutter (1973) reported significantly higher rates of disorder among these inner-city children than in the children from the Isle of Wight. Thus, whereas family social class per se did not appear to correlate strongly with children's mental health problems, other measures of more pervasive and severe social disadvantages did.

Perhaps the most comprehensive investigation of the association between social disadvantage and children's mental health has been conducted by Offord and his colleagues (e.g., Offord, Boyle, Szatmari, et al., 1987). The Ontario Child Health Study (OCHS) is a survey of almost 2,700 4- to 16-year-old children in the province of Ontario, Canada. In this study, Offord and his colleagues investigated the risk and protective factors associated with hyperactivity, conduct disorder, emotional disorder, and somatization as indexed by the Survey Diagnostic Instrument, a checklist substantially similar to the Child Behavior Checklist.

In a systematic fashion, Offord and his associates have been able to examine the relations among various measures of disadvantage and children's mental health problems. Offord, Boyle, and Racine (1989) reported that children from families with very low incomes were significantly more likely to suffer from at least one of the four disorders assessed in this study. However, when analyses were computed separately for each diagnosis and controlled for the source of symptom reporting (i.e., parent, child, or teacher reports), the researchers found no consistent effects of low income on the presence of specific disorders.

Offord and associates (1989) offer an alternative explanation for the absence of consistent effects of low income on specific diagnoses. They suggest that variations in case ascertainment by informant (parent, teacher, or child) indicate that the context in which symptomatic behavior occurs is important. Moreover, they contend that correlates of disorder vary by informant. They conclude:

> If child features associated with disorder vary by informant, there is a risk of attenuating or masking these associations when informant assessments are combined. This would occur, for example, if economic disadvantage was

strongly associated strongly with teacher assessments of childhood externalizing problems, as in this study. In such instances, the method used to combine information from different informants could have important effects on inferences made about associated features of disorder. Invariably, these inferences would be biased to a greater or lesser extent by the rules developed for combining information. (Offord et al., 1989, p. 860)

Offord and colleagues (1989) speculate on the reasons for these results. They suggest that case ascertainment is influenced by a number of factors. Perhaps the most important is the apparent lack of agreement among parents, teachers, and children themselves in reporting symptoms. The researchers argue that this reflects the extent to which the identification of children's mental health problems is influenced both by informants' perceptions and by their social contexts.

Although this interpretation is reasonable, the absence of any stable pattern of associations between low income and specific diagnoses may be an artifact of the statistical procedures employed or the relatively small proportions of cases meeting diagnostic criteria. Offord and associates (1989) employ a dichotomous dummy variable as an indicator of the presence or absence of low income (defined as family income less than $10,000 in 1982). Given the relatively low prevalence of any specific diagnosis (seldom more than 10%) and of low income, it seems unlikely that significant associations between these two variables with restricted variances could be expected. However, when the dependent variable is specified as "any diagnosis," prevalence increases to almost 17% for girls and more than 19% for boys. With substantially greater variation in the dependent variable, the probability of observing a significant association with low income may increase.

Despite the equivocal evidence from the OCHS on the effects of low income on children's disorders, a much stronger case can be made for the significance of family welfare status on children's mental health. Offord, Boyle, and Jones (1987) found that the presence of any psychiatric disorder was significantly higher among children whose families are on welfare. This association between welfare status and disorder persisted even when age, sex, income levels, and the presence of family dysfunction were held constant. Furthermore, the importance of this risk factor was most pronounced for conduct disorders (Offord & Boyle, 1988) and attention deficit disorder with hyperactivity (Szatmari, Offord, & Boyle, 1989).

What can we conclude, then, about the impact of socioeconomic disadvantage on children's mental health? Whereas parental social class and low family income appear to exert modest effects on the prevalence of children's disorders, their independent impact may not be as substantial as one might have anticipated. There is some indication, however, that as these economic difficulties aggregate, the risk to the child increases as well. Moreover, there is little doubt that children whose families are on welfare are at considerably elevated risk of mental health problems. Although the explanation for this pattern is not clear, Offord, Boyle, and Jones (1987) speculate that being on welfare may signify the accumulation of a number of other risk factors that create a family environment that is not conducive to the positive mental health of children. This formulation is consistent with what Rutter and Madge (1976) have described as "inter-generational cycles of disadvantage," in which mothers on welfare or social assistance tend to be very young, poorly educated, and from more economically disadvantaged backgrounds. In turn, their children experience similar circumstances, which significantly increase their risk of emotional and behavioral disorders. In this sense, then, when troubles cluster together, the prognosis for children's psychopathology is not encouraging.

Family Structure and Child Psychopathology

Scope of the Problem

There has been a substantial increase in the number of children living in single-parent families in North America in the last 30 years. In the United States, the proportion of children under age 18 living with one parent increased from from 13% in 1970 to more than 25% by 1984. This change has been due largely to increasing rates of marital separation and divorce and to an increase in the proportion of never-married single parents. For example, the percentage of female-headed households in the United States increased from 9.3% in 1960 to 15.9% in 1984 while the divorce rate during the same period rose from 0.9% to 5.2% of all married women aged 15 and older (Giele, 1988). More recently, Bumpass and Sweet (1989) estimate that 44% of all children in the United States will live in a single-parent family before age 16. In Canada, approximately 12.9% of all families in 1987 were headed by single parents, as opposed to 9.4% in 1971; more than 80% of these families were female-headed.

These significant demographic patterns of increased separations and divorces, together with increasing rates of birth outside marriage, have attracted attention because these families are far more likely to have younger, dependent children who require more care and exact demands from their single parents. At the same time, it is evident that a substantial proportion of single-parent families suffer from significant socioeconomic disadvantage (Holden & Smock, 1991; McQuillan, 1990). Moreover, it is likely that a large number of children in single-parent families have witnessed parental conflict or discord that has resulted in separation or divorce. Finally, in a small but significant proportion of single-parent families, the death of a parent will have resulted in a traumatic experience for all family members and a concomitant change in the structure of the family that requires considerable adjustment. For all these reasons, single-parent families have often been conceptualized as family environments that may contribute to child psychopathology. In the following sections, we consider the effects of exposure to separation and divorce, unmarried mothers, and death of a parent as risk factors for psychopathology in childhood.

Separation/Divorce and Child Psychopathology

Less than a decade ago, studies of divorce were surprisingly rare. Indeed, Garmezy (1986) recently noted that

> with such a powerful psychosocial problem now evident, one would have expected an outpouring of research aimed at gaining an understanding of the impact of divorce on children. Unfortunately, this is not the case. It is encouraging to note, however, that the neglect has been tempered by two research programs, one strongly clinical (Wallerstein, 1983; Wallerstein & Kelly, 1975, 1980), and the other strongly experimental/observational (Hetherington, Cox, & Cox, 1979a, 1979b, 1982). (p. 311)

Hetherington and her colleagues conducted a 2-year study of 48 white, middle-class, divorcing families with a preschool child and a matched sample of intact families. They describe the stresses associated with divorce and how mothers and fathers cope with such problems. As well, Hetherington and associates comment on problems in parenting associated with divorce and document some of the behavioral problems experienced by children in these families. Families in this study experienced a period of extreme disequilibrium during the first year following the divorce. During this initial phase of family disruption, deficits in the children's behavior were noted both at home and in school (Hetherington et al., 1979a, 1979b). This pattern of initial disruption was followed, however, by a tendency for parents to reestablish patterns of childcare and for the family to regain stability.

In the second set of studies, Wallerstein and Kelly (1975, 1980) conducted a series of clinical interviews with 60 families at the time of parental separation, at 1 year after separation, and at 4 years afterward. These interviews were augmented by observations of the children, by school records, and by information obtained from the children's teachers. Their findings are consistent with those reported by Hetherington and colleagues (1982). Emotional strains during the first year of separation hampered parenting abilities and were associated with problems in the children's adjustment.

Since these landmark studies, the number of investigations of children in single-parent families has grown dramatically. These more recent analyses have enriched our understanding of problems encountered in single-parent families. Kurdek and associates (e.g., Kurdek & Berg, 1983; Kurdek, Blisk, & Seisky, 1981) conducted interviews and administered questionnaires to 74 single, divorced, custodial parents (60 mothers and 14 fathers) and to their 132 children, ranging in age from 5 to 19. Two years later, they were able to reinterview a small subsample of 24 parents and children. Kurdek and his colleagues describe how the adjustment of children to divorce varies over time. With passage of time after parental divorce, children continued to regard the event negatively; there was some indication, however, that children became increasingly better adjusted to their circumstances. The researchers also indicate that adjustment appeared to be better among older children.

Guidubaldi, Cleminshaw, Perry, Nastasi, and Lightel (1986) designed the National Associate of School Psychologists–Kent State University Impact of Divorce Project to examine the effects of divorce on children. They conducted a longitudinal study of 341 children from divorced families and 358 from intact families; data were collected from children and parents. Two years later, they reinterviewed 123 children whose families' marital situation had not changed. They report that children of divorce suffer from a variety of deficits, including social, behavioral, and mental health problems. This study indicates that children of divorce experience significantly more academic, social, and physical health problems than do children from intact families and that there are important variations by the age and sex of the child. Guidubaldi and associates (1986) also found that females from divorced families performed similarly to females from intact families as these children move through elementary school grades. In contrast, with progression through school, boys from divorced families exhibited considerably more problematic behaviors than did boys from intact families.

Guidubaldi and colleagues (1986) also explored the impact of various aspects of the home environment across different sex and age groups. For example, the quality of same-sex parent–child relationships were found to be crucially important predictors of good adjustment. As well, parental satisfaction with their own parenting behavior was found to be a more important predictor of adjustment among boys than among girls. Interestingly, there is evidence that permissive parenting practices may be associated with more positive outcomes for girls but more negative outcomes among boys. These interactions with the child's gender are important specifications that clearly warrant greater consideration in future research.

In the National Survey of Children, Peterson and Zill (1986) interviewed 2,301 children aged 12 to 16. Over 4 years, a small subsample had experienced parental separation and divorce. This group and those whose parents were already separated or divorced at the first interview have been examined in detail by Peterson and Zill. They reported that levels of conflict and disruption in intact and divorced families have important effects on children's behaviors. Peterson and Zill concluded that the maintenance of good parent–child relationships, even in the face of marital discord and disruption, contributes dramatically toward better adjustment among children.

Furstenberg and Cherlin (1991) have also presented a comprehensive account of the consequences of divorce for children. They document how separation and divorce place mothers and their children in economically distressed circumstances with potentially dysfunctional consequences for children. In addition, they argue that children in divorced families are likely to experience high levels of uncertainty that continue even if their mothers remarry. Furstenberg and Cherlin conclude that children's reactions to separation and divorce are very much influenced by the quality of the custodial parent's functioning.

We have conducted interviews with 518 single-parent mothers, of whom 379 were either separated or divorced at the time of interview, and a comparison sample of 502 married mothers (Avison, Gotlib, Rae-Grant, Speechley, & Turner, 1992). Based on the mothers' reports on the Child Behavior Checklist (CBCL), we found that children in separated or divorced families scored significantly higher on both the internalizing and externalizing dimensions of the CBCL than did children in two-parent families. Furthermore, children from separated or divorced homes were more than twice as likely as children from intact families to have externalizing and internalizing scores that exceeded the clinical threshold.

Investigators in the United Kingdom have reported similar patterns. In this regard, Michael Rutter has made a number of significant contributions to our understanding of childhood behavioral problems associated with parental separation and divorce. In his earlier work, Rutter (1971) reported that parent–child separation as a result of marital discord was associated with elevated rates of conduct disorders. However, this association was modified considerably by the existence of a strong relationship between the child and at least one parent. These observations led Rutter to conclude in later work (e.g., Rutter, 1985a, 1985b) that parental separation or divorce per se may not be as critical as the existence of parental discord or family conflict and the nature of parent–child relationships. We shall return to this point in greater detail in a later section of this chapter.

In addition to these large-scale investigations, several other studies of children in separated and divorced families have been conducted over the last few years. Perhaps the most comprehensive review of this body of literature on family structure and children's well-being is that presented by Amato and Keith (1991). They review 92 studies that compared children from divorced single-parent families with children living in two-parent families. They examine contrasts between these two groups on a number of outcome variables, including measures of psychological adjustment (depression, anxiety, or happiness), social adjustment (loneliness, popularity, or cooperativeness), self-concept (self-esteem, perceived competence, or internal locus of control), and misconduct (aggression, misbehavior, or delinquency). Amato and Keith's meta-analyses are instructive insofar as they find that the effects of divorce on children's behaviors are rather modest. On average, children from divorced families scored 0.23 standard deviations higher on misconduct measures than did children from two-parent families. Average effect sizes for psychological adjustment, self-concept, and social adjustment were even smaller. They hasten to point out, however, that there is substantial variability in this effect size from study to study. In general, Amato and Keith reported that the estimated effect of divorce on children's outcomes declines when research designs employed large, random samples and when multiple-indicator measures of misconduct were used.

Criminologists have been interested in the effects of family structure on juvenile delinquency. Because many self-report measures of delinquency contain indicators of conduct disorder, research in this area may be relevant to our concerns here. Wells and Rankin (1991) present a comprehensive review of more than 50 studies on this topic. They conclude that the relationship between broken homes and delinquency is modest. Their meta-analysis reveals that a reliable estimate of the correlation (as expressed by a phi coefficient) between family structure and delinquency is between .05 and .15. Perhaps their most important conclusion, however, is that the effect of "broken homes" on delinquency is most pronounced for status offenses (misconduct that is noncriminal) and drug use, and the smallest coefficients are for violent delinquency.

It appears, therefore, that the effects of parental separation or divorce on children's psychopathology may not be as substantial as was previously thought. Furthermore, both Amato and Keith (1991) and Wells and Rankin (1991) reported that the significance of family structure for delinquency has declined over time. How do we interpret these findings? One possibility is that the selection factors that contribute to separation or divorce are less important today than they were several years ago. In the past, divorce may have occurred only in the face of extreme family conflict, spouse abuse, or spousal pathology. Thus, children from single-parent families in the past may have been exposed to much more severe stress than they are today.

Another possibility is that the stigma of coming from a single-parent home was greater in previous decades than it is today. In the past, children from single-parent families may have encountered more difficulty in integrating with their schoolmates, or they may have experienced some significant labeling by their teachers. Today, children from separated or divorced families are no longer rare in any classroom, and there are few expectations that they will differ significantly from other children.

Unmarried Mothers and Child Psychopathology

A substantial body of literature documents the socioeconomic difficulties experienced by unwed mothers and their children. At least two aspects of this circumstance require comment. First, numerous studies argue that unwed mothers tend to be very young, poorly educated, and from more economically disadvantaged backgrounds (cf. Rutter & Madge, 1976). Furstenberg and Brooks-Gunn (1986) have argued that early pregnancy represents a major obstacle to further education. Thus, the unwed mother is likely to possess few resources for coping with her situation. This condition leads to a second aspect of socioeconomic disadvantage. Lacking such resources, these young women experience considerable deprivation and report numerous difficulties in finding employment, meeting financial needs, and arranging for suitable living accommodations. Furstenberg and Brooks-Gunn find that such problems frequently result in unmarried mothers residing in disadvantaged neighborhoods where informal and formal support networks are less well developed and where services are less available.

In turn, these disadvantages contribute to a family environment that places children at elevated risk of mental health problems. By virtue of their young age, low education, poor socioeconomic circumstance, and single status, we would expect unmarried mothers to be at significantly increased risk for depression (Lewinsohn, Hoberman, & Rosenbaum, 1988). When this status is exacerbated by frequent perceptions of isolation, role strains associated with being the prime income provider and child caregiver, and a lack of emotional and instrumental support, elevated levels of distress are common consequences (cf. Guttentag, Salasin, & Belle, 1980; Ross & Sawhill, 1975).

Few studies have examined socioemotional development among children of unmarried mothers. Those investigations that have attempted to address this issue have usually focused on teenage mothers, most of whom are unmarried at the time of the child's birth. These studies find clear evidence of elevated levels of behavior disorders and lower levels of social competence among these children. In addition, there is some indication that these children's problems increase in frequency and magnitude as they reach adolescence (Furstenberg, Brooks-Gunn, & Morgan, 1987). Finally, in our own comparative study of 518 single-parent mothers and 502 married mothers and their children, we interviewed 115 mothers who had never been married (Avison et al., 1992). We found that children of the unmarried mothers were significantly more likely to score above the clinical cutpoints on both the externalizing and internalizing dimensions of the Child Behavior Checklist than were children whose mothers were currently married.

Death of a Parent and Child Psychopathology

Despite the widespread view that the loss of a parent through death is likely to be a severely traumatizing event to children, relatively little empirical research has addressed this issue. Indeed, the major interest in this area has been in evaluating the impact of parental loss on subsequent adult psychiatric disorder. The conclusions generated from these investigations, however, have been equivocal. Whereas some researchers have reported that loss of a parent in childhood is associated with depression in adulthood (e.g., Pfohl, Stangl, & Tsuang, 1983), other investigators have not been able to replicate these findings (e.g., Munro, 1966; see Brewin, Andrews, & Gotlib [in press] and Gotlib & Hammen [1992] for more detailed discussions of this literature).

Less attention has been paid to the effects of early parental loss on emotional disorders in children. Perhaps the most influential work on the impact of parental loss on children's psychological well-being is Bowlby's (1973) seminal work on the ways in which childhood attachments and losses are associated with subsequent clinical depression and anxiety. Bowlby and Parkes (1979) argue that bereavement must be considered in a family context and suggest that family relationships before the loss may condition the effect upon the child. As well, the loss of a parent usually marks the loss of a constellation of roles and responsibilities within the family. The resulting redistribution of these responsibilities may place additional strains upon the child and therefore may have direct consequences for the child's well-being. Alternatively, the surviving parent may experience role burdens that manifest themselves in problems in parenting that, in turn, have deleterious effects on children. In a similar vein, Rutter (1981) has underscored the need to understand early maternal loss in the context of the family situation. Indeed, he focuses his examination of this topic on the social circumstances within the family that precede, accompany, and follow the loss of a parent.

In his review of bereavement in childhood, Garmezy (1983) notes that most studies on this topic are characterized by serious methodological flaws. Even among more sophisticated studies, the results have been somewhat contradictory, with some reporting widespread emotional problems among bereaved children (e.g., Forman, 1974) and others suggesting that children adjust reasonably well to such losses after a relatively short period (e.g., Van Eerdewegh, Bieri, Parilla, & Clayton, 1982). Rutter (1966) has observed that breakdown among children after bereavement is probably more strongly related to situations that follow the parent's death, presumably to factors associated with the redefinition of family roles and responsibilities. Garmezy (1983) concludes that there is need for additional studies that compare children of divorce with those who have been bereaved. He argues further for studies that examine outcomes among children over a longer follow-up period. Finally, Garmezy suggests that, in examining children's adjustment to the loss of a parent, investigators must also consider such factors as child age and gender, parent gender, the "suddenness" as opposed to the gradual onset of the loss, and the nature of the relationship that existed between the affected child and the deceased parent.

These recommendations are echoed by other investigators. For example, Berlinsky and Biller (1982) and Norris and Murrell (1987) contend that parental death should not be conceptualized as a single stressor but as a series of stressful experiences occurring before and after the death. Other factors that require consideration include breakdowns in the continuity of the child's life after the loss of a parent (Reese, 1982), the nature of the child's existing social network (Silverman & Worden, 1992), and the ways in which the surviving parent interacts with the child. Finally, Silverman and Worden (1992) note that the study of bereaved children suffers from a number of design flaws that must be corrected in future research. Many studies base their conclusions on small samples of children who are in psychiatric treatment. Still others obtain information about bereaved children from their mothers and often fail to survey other potential informants, including their teachers and the bereaved children themselves.

In summary, our knowledge of the sequelae of parental loss on children is incomplete. Although there is good reason to believe that most children adjust to such parental loss, we have little insight into those factors that hinder such adaptation. Wallerstein (1983) has drawn parallels between divorce and bereavement and, while noting that there are differences between the two experiences, has suggested that they are both stressful experiences whose impact on child and parent could be examined within a similar conceptual framework. Similarly, Rutter (1966); Brown, Harris, and Bifulco (1986); and Garmezy (1986) have all called for research on parental loss that takes into consideration variability in stressors, vulnerability factors, and other environmental factors that are presumed to operate within the family.

PARENTAL PSYCHIATRIC DISTURBANCE AND CHILD PSYCHOPATHOLOGY

In this section we examine the association between parental psychiatric disturbance and psychopathology in children. A growing literature is documenting the effects of specific parental psychiatric diagnoses on the functioning of their children. The importance of parental psychopathology in this regard is reflected in Goldstein's (1988) statement that "the best risk marker for most mental disorders is still the rather crude index of being an offspring of a parent with that disorder" (p. 285). Although, as we shall see, there is not an isomorphic relation between parent and child psychiatric diagnoses, most investigators continue to examine the impact of specific parental psychiatric disorders on child functioning. The most extensive literatures assess the effects of parental depression, schizophrenia, and alcoholism on the psychosocial functioning of children. We now examine each of these three bodies of literature in turn.

Children of Depressed Parents

Scope of the Problem

Of all the psychiatric disorders, depression is by far the most common. Each year, more than 100 million people worldwide develop clinically recognizable depression, an incidence 10 times greater than that of schizophrenia. Furthermore, the World Health Organization believes that this number is likely to increase (Sartorius, 1979). During the course of a lifetime, it is estimated that between 8% and 18% of the general population will experience at least one clinically significant episode of depression (Karno et al., 1987) and that approximately twice as many women as men will be affected by depression (Frank, Carpenter, & Kupfer, 1988; Robins et al., 1984).

The term *depression* has a number of meanings, covering a wide range of emotional states that range in severity from normal, everyday moods of sadness, to psychotic episodes with increased risk of suicide. To receive a clinical psychiatric diagnosis of major depression according to the current diagnostic system in North America, the third revised edition of the *Diagnostic and Statistical Manual of Mental Disorders* (DSM-III-R) (American Psychiatric Association, 1987), an individual must have experienced one or more major depressive episodes. In a major depressive episode, the individual exhibits, over at least a 2-week period, depressed mood or a loss of interest or pleasure in almost all daily activities, as well as a number of other symptoms of depression, such as weight loss or gain, loss of appetite, sleep disturbance, psychomotor agitation or retardation, fatigue, feelings of guilt or worthlessness, and concentration difficulties.

The study of the children of depressed parents is an important area of investigation for a number of reasons. Given the prevalence of depression in the population, it seems clear that a significant number of children grow up in homes where at least one parent is depressed. Moreover, epidemiological studies consistently indicate that a greater proportion of women than men are diagnosed as depressed, and that women who are raising children and who are not employed outside the home are particularly vulnerable to depression (Gotlib, Whiffen, Mount, Milne, & Cordy, 1989). Other researchers have reported that depressed women find it difficult to be warm and consistent mothers, derive less satisfaction from being mothers, and feel inadequate in this role (Bromet & Cornely, 1984). Indeed, the disturbed relationship between a depressed mother and her child may be one key means by which a vulnerability to depression in adulthood is transmitted (cf. Goodman, 1992; Lee & Gotlib, 1991b). Similarly, Carlson and Strober (1983) have postulated that the roots of adult bipolar disorders lie in childhood or early adolescence and that the deprivations experienced as a consequence of being raised by a depressed parent may augment whatever genetic risk may be present. Interestingly, several studies have that found currently depressed adults report having experienced difficult early family environments and problems in their relationships with their parents (e.g., Gotlib, Mount, Cordy, & Whiffen, 1988; Parker, 1981) and, further, that early adverse experiences might predict the onset of depression in adulthood (Gotlib, Whiffen, Wallace, & Mount, 1991). Given these findings and formulations, it is not surprising that accumulating evidence suggests that the children of depressed parents are at increased risk for a variety of psychological and social difficulties (Beardslee, Bemporad, Keller, & Klerman, 1983; Gotlib & Lee, 1990).

Child Functioning

The growing importance of this area of research is underscored by the number of recent reviews of studies of the offspring of depressed parents (e.g., Gelfand & Teti, 1990; Goodman, 1992; Gotlib & Lee, 1990; Hammen, 1991). The consensus of these reviews is that there are relatively few large-scale, methodologically sound investigations of the children of depressed parents, and that much of the existing information must be derived from studies in which depressed parents and their children were included as comparison groups in high-risk studies of children of schizophrenic parents, a point to which we shall return in the next section of this chapter. Unfortunately, many studies in this area are limited by other methodological shortcomings. For example, some of the early studies failed to separate unipolar and bipolar depressed groups, and many studies compared depressed subjects only with normals. Other studies included only mildly depressed subjects, or confounded mild and severe depression in the same sample. Finally, only a few of the studies provided longitudinal follow-ups of children's functioning to evaluate the long-term status of children's adjustment.

Despite these methodological and conceptual limitations, the results of investigations of the functioning of the offspring of depressed parents are remarkably consistent. In several early investigations, researchers interviewed depressed mothers about the functioning of their children. Investigators using this design found that depressed mothers reported various psychological and physical problems in their children and viewed their children's behaviors more negatively than did nondepressed women (e.g., Forehand, Wells, McMahon, Griest, & Rogers, 1982; Webster-Stratton & Hammond, 1988). Depressed mothers also reported more depressed and anxious mood in their children, greater suicidal ideation, more physical problems, and more difficulties in school (Billings & Moos, 1983; Weissman et al., 1984). Moreover, in a 1-year follow-up assessment, Billings and Moos (1986) compared the children of remitted and nonremitted depressed parents to nondepressed controls. Interestingly, despite the abatement of their own depressive symptoms, parents in the remitted group continued to report more dysfunction in their children than did the control parents; as expected, the nonremitted depressed group reported the highest incidence of dysfunction in their children.

In a similar study, Weissman and colleagues (1984) interviewed 133 mildly and severely depressed parents and 82 normal community controls about their children's adjustment. According to the parents' reports, 34% of the children of the depressed parents had psychiatric symptoms or had received psychological treatment, compared with only 16% of the children of the controls. Furthermore, 24% of the children of the depressed parents were diagnosable by DSM-III criteria, compared with only 8% of the control children, and 25% of the depressives' children had received treatment for emotional problems, compared with 9% of the controls. Differences between the two groups of children were also noted for the use of psychotropic medication and the incidence of problems in school (e.g., school failures, repeating a grade). Finally, the Weissman group found that children with both parents depressed were at greater risk for a diagnosis of a psychiatric disorder than were children with one depressed parent. On the basis of these findings, Weissman and associates (1984) concluded that children of depressed parents are at increased risk for psychological symptoms, treatment for emotional problems, school problems, suicidal behavior, and multiple DSM-III diagnoses.

Although the results of these studies indicate that children of depressed parents function more poorly than do children of nondepressed parents, it is important to bear in mind that these early findings were based on parental reports rather than on direct observations of the children. Because depressed parents' reports may be biased by a tendency to see both their parenting and their children's behavior in a negative light (cf. Rickard, Forehand, Wells, Griest, & McMahon, 1981; but see also

Conrad & Hammen, 1989), a more rigorous research strategy would require that the functioning of children of depressed parents be assessed directly.

A recent cohort of observational investigations has incorporated these design considerations to provide specific information both about the functioning of children of depressed parents and about the quality of the relationship between depressed mothers and their offspring. Whiffen and Gotlib (1989), for example, have conducted observational studies with one of the youngest samples of children of depressed mothers. They examined the 2-month-old infants of women who had been diagnosed with an episode of clinically significant depression shortly following childbirth (i.e., postpartum depression). Whiffen and Gotlib not only observed and rated the infants while they interacted with their mothers but also administered the Bayley Scales of Infant Development to the infants. The results of this study indicated that infants of the depressed mothers were rated as less happy, tenser, and more easily fatigued during the interaction than were the infants of the nondepressed women. The infants of the depressed women also scored significantly lower on the Bayley scales.

Field and her colleagues (e.g., Field, 1984; Field et al., 1985) examined the interactions of subclinically depressed and nondepressed mothers and their infants. Compared to the infants of the nonsymptomatic women, the infants of the depressed mothers were rated as drowsier, more passive, or fussier, and as less relaxed or content. Finally, findings from other studies suggest that the infants of depressed mothers may be temperamentally difficult. Cutrona and Troutman (1986) and Whiffen (1988) found depressive symptomatology in mothers to be correlated with their reports of infant crying and unsoothability. Considered collectively, these results indicate that the presence of depression in mothers in the period following childbirth represents a significant risk factor for infants.

A number of investigations have examined the psychosocial functioning of older children of depressed mothers. In general, the results of these investigations indicate that children of depressed parents demonstrate poorer functioning than do children of nondepressed parents. For example, Radke-Yarrow, Cummings, Kuczynski, and Chapman (1985) observed 2- and 3-year-old children interacting with their mothers, who had either unipolar or bipolar depression. These investigators found that more children of women with affective disorders, particularly bipolar depression, displayed insecure attachment to their mothers, an important indicator of child adjustment. Using essentially the same sample, Zahn-Waxler and her colleagues (e.g., Zahn-Waxler, Cummings, McKnew, & Radke-Yarrow, 1984) reported that the 2-year-old children of the bipolar parents exhibited more impairments in affect regulation, altruism, and aggressive and affiliative interactions than did children of normal parents. Finally, Ghodsian, Zayicek, and Wolkind (1984) reported that depressed mothers rated their 2-year-old children as having a greater number of behavior problems than did nondepressed mothers, and that this pattern continued to be evident when the children were between 3 and 4 years of age. These findings clearly suggest that impairments are evident in the children of depressed parents from an early age.

In a study of older school-age children, Welner, Welner, McCrary, and Leonard (1977) compared children of depressed parents with offspring of nondepressed controls. Both mothers and children were seen in interviews covering such areas as physical problems, academic performance, conduct problems, and other symptoms of psychopathology. Welner and associates, reported that the children of the depressed parents had more depressed mood, death wishes, frequent fighting, unexplained headaches, loss of interest in usual activities, hypochondriacal concerns, crying for no apparent reason, and disturbed classroom behavior. In fact, the eight children in the study who were diagnosed as depressed by Welner's criteria (five or more depressive symptoms) all had at least one depressed parent.

In a subsequent study, Hirsch, Moos, and Reischl (1985) interviewed a group of adolescent children of unipolar depressed parents and found that these adolescents reported more symptoms than did a sample of offspring of nondepressed parents. Similar results were also reported by Turner, Beidel, and Costello (1987) in a study of children of dysthymic parents, and by Cytryn, McKnew, Bartko, Lamour, and Hamovitt (1982) and by Decina and associates (1983) in samples of offspring of bipolar depressed parents. In fact, in these latter three investigations of the functioning of children of bipolar parents, at least 30% (and more often more than 50%) of the children received a psychiatric diagnosis on the basis of a direct clinical interview.

In an intriguing study, Hops and colleagues (1987) conducted home observations of clinically depressed women and their families found that children of mothers who were depressed and maritally distressed emitted significantly more "irritated" affect (nonverbal behavior suggesting that they were angry) than did children in the normal or depressed-only families. Interestingly, analyses revealed that the women's displays of dysphoric affect and behavior were effective in suppressing aggressive behavior in both their spouses and their children; however, they also resulted in a suppression of caring behavior.

A number of investigators have demonstrated that a remarkably high proportion of children of depressed parents meet diagnostic criteria for psychiatric disorder. In independent studies, Beardslee, Schultz, and Selman (1987) and Klein, Clark, Dansky, and Margolis (1988) administered structured diagnostic interviews to adolescent offspring of depressed parents. These investigators found that between 40% and 77% of these children met criteria for a diagnosis of past or current psychiatric disturbance, compared with a rate of 2–14% in children of nondepressed parents. Hammen and associates (1987) obtained even higher rates in a more extensive investigation, but also reported that group differences were attenuated when psychosocial stresses were covaried. Moreover, as Goodman (1992) notes, symptoms of psychiatric disorder in children of depressed parents have been noted across the age range from infancy to adolescence.

Finally, in a recent investigation in our own laboratory (Lee & Gotlib, 1989a, 1989b, 1991a), we examined the psychological adjustment of four groups of school-age children: children of depressed psychiatric patient mothers, children of nondepressed psychiatric patient mothers; children of nondepressed medical patient mothers, and children of community mothers. Child functioning was assessed both by a clinical interview with the child and by maternal ratings. Children were interviewed using the Child Assessment Schedule (CAS) (Hodges, Kline, Stern, Cytryn, & McKnew, 1982), a semistructured protocol designed for the clinical assessment of children 7 years and older. The CAS assesses fears and anxieties, worries and concerns, self-image, mood disturbance, physical complaints, and conduct problems. All mothers also completed the CBCL, on which behavior problems are rated in terms of aptness in describing the child's behavior over the previous 6 months.

The results of this study revealed that the children of depressed mothers had more severe psychiatric symptoms on the CAS and poorer overall adjustment on the Global Assessment Scale for Children than did the children of nondepressed mothers. Using the mean ratings on the CAS presented by Hodges and associates (1982), the children of the depressed mothers functioned at a level comparable to a group of behaviorally disordered outpatient children. The children of depressed mothers were also rated by their mothers as having a greater number of both internalizing and externalizing problems than were the children of the nondepressed control mothers; indeed, two thirds of the children of the depressed mothers were placed in the clinical range on the CBCL (greater than the 90th percentile), an incidence three times greater than that observed in the nondepressed controls. Interestingly, the children of depressed mothers typically did not differ from the children of nondepressed psychiatric-patient mothers, suggesting that the effects of maternal depression on child dysfunction may be nonspecific.

In a 10-month follow-up assessment conducted on this sample of children, Lee and Gotlib (1991a) reported that despite a significant reduction in the mothers' depressive symptomatology, the formerly depressed women continued to describe their children as having a higher number of internalizing and externalizing problems than did the nondepressed controls. Finally, interviewer ratings on the CAS indicated that children of both the depressed and the nondepressed psychiatric-patient mothers were rated as having a greater number of mood symptoms and somatic complaints than were children of the community mothers. Thus, children of both depressed and nondepressed mothers demonstrated problematic adjustment, even when their mothers were no longer overtly symptomatic, indicating that there may be a substantial lag between alleviation of maternal symptomatology and improvement in child functioning. These findings not only corroborate Billings and Moos's (1986) observations that remitted depressed parents continue to report adjustment difficulties in their children but further replicate these results with ratings by clinicians.

In sum, there is little question that depression in a parent affects the functioning of children and significantly increases their risk of developing a psychiatric disorder and/or emotional difficulties. Moreover, this pattern of results has been found in assessments utilizing parental reports, child self-reports, and teacher, peer, and clinician ratings. Combining results across studies, it appears that 30% to 50% of the children of depressed parents (compared with less than 20% of unselected children) experience diagnosable psychiatric disorder, both affective diagnoses and attention deficits/conduct disturbance. Furthermore, the nature and severity of problems found in children of depressed parents appear to be similar to those observed among offspring of schizophrenics. Indeed, some investigators have posited that difficulties in child functioning may be due not to depression or schizophrenia per se, but rather to global parental psychopathology (e.g., Fisher & Jones, 1980; Kokes, Harder, Fisher, & Strauss, 1980). Despite this formulation, however, research to date has not fully examined the specificity to depression of observed child adjustment difficulties. It is unclear, for example, whether child problems are associated only with parental psychological disorders or whether they are related to parental disturbance in general, including physical disorders. In the following section, we examine the psychosocial functioning of children of schizophrenic parents.

Children of Schizophrenic Parents

Scope of the Problem

Schizophrenia is a severe psychiatric disorder characterized by gross distortions of reality, social withdrawal, and perceptual, cognitive, and affective disorganization. A clinical definition of schizophrenia is beyond the scope of this chapter. Generally, however, schizophrenic individuals may exhibit multiple psychiatric symptoms, such as delusions (false beliefs), hallucinations (false perceptions), incoherent speech, disturbed motor functioning, and flat or inappropriate affect. Furthermore, DSM-III-R lists several subtypes of schizophrenia, including catatonic, disorganized, paranoid, undifferentiated, and residual.

After mood disorders, schizophrenia is the most frequently diagnosed psychiatric disorder. Eaton, Ritter, and Brown (1990) reviewed 34 studies that attempted to estimate either lifetime or point prevalence rates of schizophrenia from samples of 2,500 or more. These epidemiological surveys from several different countries indicate that the point prevalence of schizophrenia ranges from 0.6 to 7.4 per 1,000, whereas estimates of lifetime prevalence fall between 0.9 and 9.5 per 1,000. Perhaps the best estimates of the prevalence of schizophrenia in the United States have been generated from the NIMH Epidemiologic Catchment Area (ECA) program. On the basis of data collected from three large cities, Robins and associates (1984) report lifetime prevalence rates of schizophrenic and schizophreniform disorders between 1.1% and 2.0%. They also conclude that females are at somewhat greater risk of schizophrenia than are males. Six-month prevalence rates were estimated to be between 0.6% and 1.1%.

Child Functioning

For some time, researchers have been aware of clear patterns of familial aggregation of schizophrenia. For example, whereas lifetime risk for schizophrenia is between 0.9% and 0.95% for the general population, this number can rise to more than 10% for relatives of schizophrenics (cf. Willerman & Cohen, 1990). Indeed, Gottesman and Shields (1982) have estimated that children with a schizophrenic parent have a morbid risk of 12% of becoming schizophrenic themselves. Although it is widely accepted that genetic factors play a significant role in the transmission of schizophrenia, there has also been a consistent focus on the family environment of the schizophrenic. In fact, as early as 1948, Fromm-Reichmann coined the term *schizophrenogenic* mother to describe mothers of schizophrenics who were overprotecting but distant. Fromm-Reichmann postulated that this mothering style was a critical factor in the development of schizophrenia. These patterns of familial aggregation, coupled with an early focus on the family environment, led investigators to identify groups of young children with a schizophrenic parent and to follow them longitudinally in order to chart the emergence of symptoms of the disorder.

Early studies in this area (e.g., Mednick & Schulsinger, 1984) assessed children of schizophrenic parents on a number of constitutional and physiological variables, psychological tasks, and inventories and then compared these children with offspring of normal parents. Not surprisingly, the results of these investigations indicated that children of schizophrenic parents performed less well on these tasks and inventories than did the children of normal parents. However, because these initial studies did not include psychiatric control groups (i.e., children of parents exhibiting other types of psychiatric symptomatology), it was not possible to examine the specificity of obtained deficits to schizophrenia or to make statements concerning early or causal factors unique to the development of this disorder. It is possible, for example, that the difficulties manifested by the offspring of schizophrenics were a function of global psychopathology rather than deficits specific to schizophrenia per se.

As more investigations in this area were initiated, the inclusion of psychiatric control groups became more common. Many studies included control groups composed of children of a heterogeneous group of psychiatric patients with a variety of diagnoses (cf. McNeil and Kaij, 1980). As we noted earlier, however, other investigators used psychiatric control groups composed exclusively of depressed patients. Among the most notable of these investigations are the Stony Brook High Risk Project (e.g., Emery, Weintraub, & Neale, 1982), the Massachusetts Mental Health Center Project (e.g., Cohler, Gallant, & Grunebaum, 1977), the Rochester Longitudinal Study (e.g., Sameroff, Seifer, & Zax, 1982), and the University of Rochester Child and Family Study (e.g., Fisher & Jones, 1980). It is apparent from the results of these projects that children of schizophrenic parents demonstrate clear and consistent deficits in their social and cognitive functioning.

In the Stony Brook High Risk Project, school-age children of schizophrenic mothers were compared on a number of indices with children of mothers who were not psychiatric patients. In addition, in order to assess the specificity of any deficits observed in the offspring of the schizophrenic mothers, this project also included a group of children of unipolar and bipolar depressed mothers. Interestingly, in virtually every report from this project, both children of schizophrenic parents and children of depressed parents were significantly different from their nonpsychiatric counterparts, although few differences were found between these two clinical groups. For example, using peer ratings of adjustment, Weintraub, Prinz, and Neale (1975) found that both school-age children of psychotic depressed and schizophrenic mothers were significantlly more impaired in their social adjustment than were children of well mothers, although they did not differ significantly from each other. In a second report, Weintraub, Liebert, and Neale (1978) examined the teacher ratings of these three groups of children on the 11-factor Devereux Elementary School Behavior Rating Scale. They found that teachers rated both the children of schizophrenics and the children of depressives higher than the controls on the factors of classroom disturbance, disrespect–defiance, comprehension, and need for closeness to teacher.

A similar pattern of results was reported by Winters, Stone, Weintraub, and Neale (1981) and by Harvey, Winters, Weintraub, and Neale (1981), who examined the performance of these children on cognitive and attentional tasks. Reliable differences were consistently found between children of schizophrenics and controls. The offspring of the depressed parents, and particularly unipolar depressed parents, were also more deviant than controls but were indistinguishable from the children of schizophrenics on general measures of attentional distractibility (see also Nuechterlein, Phipps-Yonas, Driscoll, & Garmezy [1990] for similar findings concerning attentional vigilance obtained in an independent sample of children). Interestingly, Harvey and associates (1981) reported that significant differences between the children of depressed and schizophrenic parents emerged when they ventured beyond a global assessment of the children's overall performance and examined more specifically finer-grained aspects of their attentional task. It may be necessary for researchers to emulate this procedure of developing more refined measures of attention and behavior in order to examine subtle differences between various psychopathological groups that appear similar on global measures of performance.

In general, these reports from the Stony Brook High Risk Project suggest that children of schizophrenic parents are at high risk for maladjustment, as are children of depressed parents. Other high-risk investigations of the offspring of schizophrenic parents have also documented difficulties in these children. In the Massachusetts Mental Health Center Project, Cohler and his associates examined the young children of schizophrenic, psychotically depressed, and normal mothers over a period of about 10 years. In one of the earliest reports from this project, Gamer, Gallant, Grunebaum, and Cohler (1977) assessed the cognitive functioning of these children when they were approximately 3 years old. Children of psychotically ill parents were found to perform worse than children of well parents on a complex task (the Embedded Figures Test) but not on the Peabody Vocabulary Test, a relatively straightforward task. Interestingly, as was the case in the findings reported from the Stony Brook Project, no differences were found between children of schizophrenics and children of depressed mothers. On the basis of these results, the Gamer group suggested that living with a mother who is generally mentally disordered may adversely influence the cognitive development of young children.

Similar results were reported by Cohler and associates (1977), who examined the relationships of these children with their mothers. The sick mothers, regardless of whether they were schizophrenic or depressed, were less likely to develop interactive relationships with their child and had greater difficulty separating their own needs from the needs of their children.

The pattern emerging from this early report of Cohler's group suggests that very young children of both schizophrenic and depressed mothers show impaired cognitive functioning and more maladaptive interactive behavior, relative to children of well mothers. These accounts are consistent with the reports of the Stony Brook Project, indicating that children of schizophrenic or depressed parents appear to function at a lower level than do children of nonpsychiatric patients. This pattern of findings persisted as the children from the Massachusetts project grew older and were assessed at 5 years of age (e.g., Cohler et al., 1977) and at 8 to 12 years of age (e.g., Grunebaum, Cohler, Kaufman, & Gallant, 1978). The children of schizophrenic parents continued to demonstrate deficits not only on measures of intellectual functioning and sustained and selective attention but with respect to home and school adjustment as well.

Finally, in the University of Rochester Child and Family Study, Fisher and his colleagues examined the associations between parental psychopathology and behavioral competence in a sample of children whose parents had previously been hospitalized for a psychiatric disorder. Family interaction studies indicated an association between parental communication deviance and nonacknowledgment and child problem solving (Fisher & Jones, 1980). The impact of parental psychopathology was noted to be particularly important in mother–patient cases, and severity of disturbance appeared more important than specific disturbance (Kokes et al., 1980). Regardless of diagnosis, parental depression, incongruous affect, and, most importantly, withdrawal were associated with poor child adjustment. Moreover, the degree of recovery attained following hospitalization appeared to be more critical in predicting child outcome than was the diagnosis or intensity of an acute episode. Thus, the long-term impairment of a parent was the most important determinant of child functioning, and the emotional availability of the parent to the child appears to play a crucial role in successful child adjustment to parental schizophrenia.

Considered collectively, the results of these projects indicate that children of schizophrenic parents are at considerable risk not only for psychopathology, but for cognitive and social impairment as well. In many cases, children of schizophrenic parents were indistinguishable from offspring of depressed parents, although children in both groups generally demonstrated higher levels of psychopathology than did children of nonpsychiatric controls. In the final section focusing on the effects of parental disturbance, we examine the functioning of children of alcoholic parents.

Children of Alcoholic Parents

Scope of the Problem

Alcohol-related damage involves interference with individuals' social, psychological, economic, or physical functioning. Such damage can result from *alcohol abuse,* defined as relatively isolated events of drinking, or from *alcoholism,* defined as a dependence on alcohol that seriously interferes with life adjustment (President's Commission on Mental Health, 1978). There is no commonly accepted distinct line that unequivocally separates alcohol use from abuse or alcoholism. Nevertheless, there is evidence that the greater one's level of consumption, the greater one's risk of developing alcohol-related damage, either in episodic or chronic fashion (Schmidt & Popham, 1975).

Recent investigations have used standardized interviews to estimate the incidence and prevalence of alcohol use disorders, according to DSM-III criteria. In Canada, it has been estimated that 5–10% of adult drinkers are addicted to alcohol and/or experience damage in the form of alcohol-related disabilities (Expert Committee on Alcohol Statistics, 1981). A further 10% can be termed *hazardous drinkers,* in the sense that their level of consumption puts them at elevated risk of developing alcohol-related damage. In their review of 12 surveys on the prevalence of alcoholism in the United States, Warheit and Auth (1985) conclude that 12–33% of males and 2–5% of females drink heavily. These estimates have been confirmed by the recent Epidemiologic Catchment Area (ECA) studies in the United States. Using the Diagnostic Interview Schedule in a multisite survey, for example, Helzer, Canino, Bland, Newman, and Yeh (1988) estimate the average lifetime prevalence of alcoholism to be approximately 14%. Finally, the number of children under the age of 20 who reside with an alcoholic parent has been estimated to be as high as 28 million (Booz-Allen & Hamilton, 1974). Without question, therefore, if parental alcoholism is a demonstrable risk factor for child psychopathology, a large portion of the child population is at risk.

Child Functioning

There is little doubt that children of alcoholic parents are at elevated risk for alcoholism in adulthood (cf. Kubicka, Kozeny, & Roth, 1990; Sher, 1991). Although less is known about the impact of parental alcoholism on younger children, the incidence of psychiatric problems in this population has been a concern of clinicians for some time. Early studies of this issue produced mixed results. For example, Haberman (1966) compared children of alcoholics to offspring of a sample of medical patients and to a community sample. Maternal reports indicated that the children of alcoholics had a greater frequency of temper tantrums, fighting, and school trouble than did the other two groups of children. In contrast, Chafetz, Blane, and Hill (1971) reported that children of alcoholic parents were not overrepresented in a review of records of children attending a child psychiatry clinic. They did find, however, that the numbers of illnesses and accidents, school problems, and police contacts were higher for these children. Kanmeier (1971) found similar results in her comparison of adolescents from families with and without alcohol problems: Although there were no differences in measures of maladjusted behavior, adolescents from alcoholic families were more often absent from school, and their parents had less stable marriages.

The results of more recent studies continue to be equivocal, particularly with respect to alcohol and substance abuse among children of alcoholic parents. For instance, whereas Merikangas, Weissman, Prusoff, Pauls, and Leckman (1985) reported that adolescent children of alcoholic parents were at elevated risk for both alcohol and drug use, Knop, Teasdale, Schulsinger, and Goodwin (1985) and Pandina and Johnson (1989) failed to replicate this finding, and Johnson, Leonard, and Jacob (1989) reported differences between children of alcoholics and children of nonalcoholics with respect to drug use, but not with respect to alcohol consumption. In a large study of college students, Sher, Walitzer, Wood, and Brent (1991) found that children of alcoholic parents, compared with children of controls, reported more problems with alcohol consumption and substance abuse, higher levels of behavioral undercontrol and neuroticism, and greater psychiatric distress. They also evidenced lower academic achievement. In terms of psychiatric diagnoses, children of alcoholic parents received alcohol diagnoses and diagnoses of major depression and anxiety more frequently than did children of nonalcoholic parents.

West and Prinz (1987) recently presented a comprehensive review of more recent studies (those published between 1975 and 1985) on the prevalence of psychopathology among children of alcoholics. They organized their review according to specific classifications of children's emotional and behavioral problems. In addition, they distinguished between, on one hand, those studies that sampled alcoholic and nonalcoholic parents and then assessed children's psychopathology and, on the other hand, those studies that assessed parental alcoholism among samples of children with and without indications of child psychopathology. West and Prinz concluded that these studies find only a weak association between parental alcoholism and child hyperactivity and conduct disorder. There are, however, a number of interpretational problems associated with this conclusion. West and Prinz observe that the association may be stronger for boys than for girls; moreover, few studies distinguished between aggressive behavior and hyperactivity. Furthermore, these results may be confounded by prenatal exposure to alcohol because of maternal drinking and the possibility that Attention–Deficit Disorder with Hyperactivity and alcoholism may be genetically linked. Accordingly, it is difficult to assert unequivocally that environmental factors associated with alcoholism in the family are causally implicated in this particular type of child psychopathology.

As West and Prinz (1987) note, several investigators have reported an association between parental alcoholism and delinquent and deviant behavior in their offspring. Children of alcoholics appear to have elevated rates of truancy, more contacts with police, more substance abuse, and a greater likelihood of dropping out of school. Chassin, Rogosch, and Barrera (1991) recently reported that children of alcoholic parents demonstrated drug and alcohol problems and also elevated externalizing behavior. Despite these risks, however, it is imperative to remain cognizant of the fact that not all children of alcoholics experience difficulties. Parental alcoholism, therefore, should not be considered to be inevitably associated with poor child adjustment.

Finally, with respect to internalizing childhood symptoms such as anxiety and depression, there is consistent evidence that parental problems with alcohol constitute a significant risk factor for young children. Moos and Billings (1982), for example, reported higher levels of anxiety and depression among children of alcoholic parents than among those with nonalcoholic parents. Offspring from alcoholic families have also been found to exhibit higher levels of internalizing behavior and lower levels of self-esteem and sense of control (cf. Chassin et al., 1991). Again, however, we should point out that much of this research is flawed methodologically: Measures are often not standardized and designs do not eliminate the confounding influences of other potential explanatory factors.

West and Prinz (1987) succinctly summarize the state of research on the consequences of parental alcoholism for children:

> The findings taken as a whole support the contention that parental alcoholism is associated with a heightened incidence of child symptomatology. . . . Nevertheless . . . neither all nor a major portion of the population of children from alcoholic homes are inevitably doomed to psychological disorder. This limiting conclusion derives from the relatively low magnitude of effects typically reported by investigators in this area. That is, they found significant group differences, but considerable overlap still existed in the distributions for children of alcoholic and nonalcoholic parents. Furthermore, the observed pattern of association may have been inflated by a heavy reliance on single measures of child outcome (particularly parental rating scales) and by the lack of confirmation of actual diagnoses of child psychological disorders. That childhood psychological disorder was not pervasive underscores the need to study individual differences in this population of children and to uncover specific factors that lead to positive outcomes. (pp. 214–215)

In summary, the studies reviewed examining the functioning of the offspring of depressed, schizophrenic, and alcoholic parents suggest that these children are at risk for developing a variety of emotional problems.

Clearly, as we noted earlier, there is not an isomorphic relation between parental diagnosis and child functioning. Thus, for example, children of depressed parents have been found not only to exhibit higher rates of depression than do offspring of nondepressed controls but also to demonstrate higher levels of conduct disorder, global psychiatric symptoms, and multiple psychiatric diagnoses. Similarly, children of alcoholic parents have been found not only to be at elevated risk for alcohol and drug use but further to receive diagnoses of major depression and anxiety. Finally, it is important to note that there are common problems exhibited by children in all three groups, as well as by children from disadvantaged family environments. These problems include difficulties at school, temper tantrums, headaches, problematic social functioning, and emotional disorder. The lack of diagnostic specificity in the impact of parental psychopathology on children's psychosocial adjustment, juxtaposed with the adverse effects of social disadvantage and problematic family structures reviewed earlier in this chapter, suggests that there are common factors or processes that may mediate the effects of these environmental variables on child functioning. In the following section of this chapter we consider two such factors: exposure to marital and/or family discord and emotional unavailability of the parents.

COMMON PROCESSES

There is little question from our preceding review that a number of seemingly diverse aspects of the family environment place children at elevated risk for demonstrating psychopathology. More specifically, we have seen that children's exposure to such factors as socioeconomic disadvantage, parental loss or absence, parental divorce, and parental psychopathology in the form of depression, schizophrenia, and substance abuse increases the likelihood that the children themselves will exhibit symptoms of psychopathology. In this section we examine two processes through which exposure to these factors might increase children's risk for psychopathology: exposure to marital and/or family discord and emotional unavailability of the parents.

Marital/Family Discord

The results of several diverse investigations attest to the strong link between marital/family discord and the factors that we have suggested place children at elevated risk for psychopathology. For example, some of the most compelling evidence of the effects of economic loss on marital relationships has been presented by Elder and his associates (e.g., Elder & Caspi, 1988). Elder's studies of Depression-era families clearly indicate that economic difficulties increase marital tensions in most families, especially those that were most vulnerable prior to the economic hardship. Similar findings have been reported by Conger and colleagues (1990) in their research on families whose lives have been affected by the farm crises of the 1980s.

Other investigators have examined the effects of job loss and economic stress on family functioning (e.g., Voydanoff, 1990). The results of these studies converge to indicate that socioeconomic hardships or disadvantages increase marital conflict, reduce marital satisfaction, and impair family interaction patterns. Liem and Liem (1990) have developed an analytic model that specifies the linkages between economic hardship (in the form of unemployment) and disruptions in family functioning. They have also presented strong evidence in support of this model from their longitudinal survey of couples (e.g., Liem & Liem, 1988). These reports clearly indicate that unemployment and social disadvantage have negative consequences for a number of different dimensions of marital and family functioning.

It goes without saying that there is also a strong link between marital/family discord and divorce. In addition, a number of studies have also demonstrated a consistent association between marital or family discord and parental psychopathology. For example, Sager, Gundlach, and Kremer (1968) estimated that 50% of all patients who seek psychotherapy do so because of marital problems. More specifically, with respect to depression, investigators have found not only that depressed persons report higher levels of marital distress and discord than do their nondepressed counterparts (e.g., Crowther, 1985; Ruscher & Gotlib, 1988) but further that the interactions of depressed persons with their spouses are significantly more negative than are the marital interactions of nondepressed couples (e.g., Biglan et al., 1985; Gotlib & Whiffen, 1989). Schless, Schwartz, Goetz, and Mendels (1974) demonstrated that depressed persons remain vulnerable to marriage-related stresses after they recover from their depressive episode. Indeed, Merikangas (1984) reported that the divorce rate in depressed patients 2 years after discharge is nine times that of the general population (see Gotlib & Hooley [1988] for a detailed review of this literature). Furthermore, because one of the most common reactions to divorce is depression (Bloom, Asher, & White, 1978), there is likely to be considerable overlap between the populations of divorced/discordant and depressed parents. Finally, Emery and associates (1982) suggested that the association between parental depression and children's disturbed behavior is largely accounted for by concomitant marital discord.

Although the literature examining the association of marital distress with alcoholism and schizophrenia is smaller than that focusing on depression, the results of studies in these areas indicate that the marriages of alcoholic and schizophrenic persons are characterized by tension and discord. O'Farrell and Birchler (1987) demonstrated that marital discord and dissatisfaction were a function of periods of intoxication and sobriety in families with an alcoholic spouse. These reports were corroborated by direct observations of the negative marital interactions of alcoholics (e.g., Billings, Kessler, Gomberg, & Weiner, 1979; Jacob & Krahn, 1988). Indeed, West and Prinz (1987) suggested that marital conflict might be an important link between parental alcoholism and child dysfunction, and Offord, Allen, and Abrams (1978) postulated that the elevated rates of delinquency among children of alcoholics may be due to the higher rates of marital conflict and divorce in these families. Finally, Hooley, Richters, Weintraub, and Neale (1987) reported that the marriages of schizophrenic persons, and particularly schizophrenics with predominantly negative symptoms (cf. Andreasen, 1982), were characterized by elevated marital distress. Therefore, given these documented associations between marital/family discord and disrupted family structures, on one hand, and between discord and parental psychopathology on the other, it is possible that the adverse effects of these factors are mediated by children's exposure to the concomitant marital or family discord.

The association between marital discord and children's psychopathology was first observed in samples of children receiving clinical treatment (e.g., Johnson & Lobitz, 1974; Oltmanns, Broderick, & O'Leary, 1977). These studies seemed to indicate that discordant parents led their children to exhibit problematic behavior by serving as poor role models (i.e., demonstrating aggressive behavior themselves) or by providing inconsistent discipline. Emery (1982), however, noted that it might also be the case that emotionally or behaviorally troubled children create stress in the family that results in parental discord. Moreover, the results of a number of studies suggest that reports by maritally discordant parents of their children's mental health problems are influenced by the parents' negative perceptions; their assessments of their children's adjustment may not be entirely accurate (e.g., Bond & McMahon, 1984; Emery & O'Leary, 1982).

Recent work in this area has emphasized the distinction between overt marital discord or conflict, on the one hand, and marital dissatisfaction on the other (cf. Grych & Fincham, 1990). The importance of this distinction is underscored by such findings as those reported by Rutter and colleagues (1974) and Hetherington and associates (1982), who found that overt marital conflict or hostility was more strongly associated with child problems than was marital dissatisfaction. Studies that have explicitly examined the impact of overt marital conflict on children's adjustment have documented high rates of conduct disorder (Jouriles, Murphy,

& O'Leary, 1989), aggression (Johnston, Gonzalez, & Campbell, 1987), depression (Peterson & Zill, 1986), anxiety (Wierson, Forehand, & McCombs, 1988), and school-related difficulties (Wierson et al., 1988).

Grych and Fincham (1990), in a review of studies of marital conflict and children's adjustment, concluded that 15 of 19 relevant studies support the existence of an association between parental discord and children's psychopathology. Moreover, marital conflict appeared to be a stronger predictor of children's adjustment than marital status (e.g., divorced, separated). Interestingly, this finding is consistent with Emery's (1982) and Kurdek and Sinclair's (1988) formulations that the negative impact of divorce on children may have less to do with the separation of family members than with the extent of family conflict that precedes, accompanies, or follows separation and divorce. Indeed, a number of researchers have reported explicitly that parental conflict in divorced families is associated with adjustment difficulties among children and adolescents (e.g., Krantz, Clark, Pruyn, & Usher, 1985; Shaw & Emery, 1987).

Perhaps the most compelling support for the importance of family discord as a critical determinant of children's adjustment is contained in Amato and Keith's (1991) meta-analysis described earlier. They review these studies to assess support for three different explanations for elevated levels of psychopathology among children of divorced families: the parental absence perspective, the economic disadvantage explanation, and the family discord perspective. Amato and Keith conclude:

> In contrast to the modest support for the [other] perspectives, the family conflict explanation was strongly supported. The hypothesis that children in intact families marked by high levels of interparental conflict reveal problems comparable to those of children in divorced families was confirmed. In fact, children in divorced families appear to have a higher level of well-being than do children in high-conflict intact families. (p. 40)

Parental Emotional Unavailability

The second process that may mediate children's elevated risk for psychopathology involves the degree to which parents are emotionally available to respond to their children's needs. There is consistent evidence that the nature and quality of children's interactions with their parents affect their school performance, social competence, and interpersonal behaviors (cf. Amato, 1989; Dornbusch, 1989). There is also a large body of literature indicating that the quality of parent–child interactions has a significant, direct effect on children's self-concept, sense of efficacy, and ego development (cf. Avison & McAlpine, 1992). Analyses of interactions of parents and their adolescents, for example, indicate that families that are characterized by sensitivity and individuality promote environments that facilitate the development of high self-esteem and a clear self-identity in the adolescents (e.g., Walker & Greene, 1986).

The results of investigations examining more explicitly the effects of poor parent–child involvement and inadequate parental supervision indicate an association between dysfunctional parenting behaviors and child psychopathology. For example, in their review of more than 30 studies, Loeber and Stouthamer-Loeber (1986) report strong support for the proposition that parental unavailability to, or insularity from, their children is a significant predictor of children's misconduct and delinquency. Similarly, Patterson and Stouthamer-Loeber (1984) have presented striking evidence concerning the impact of coercive parent–child relationships on children's antisocial behaviors. Finally, several studies have documented the strong relations between parental neglect and children's maladjustment, especially conduct problems and delinquency (e.g., McCord, 1983).

It is clear, therefore, that there is a significant association between dysfunctional parenting (typically characterized by emotional unavailability) and difficulties in children's mental health. In this context, it is important to note that the results of a number of investigations suggest that there are also consistent links between dysfunctional parenting and many of the factors we have considered earlier that place children at risk for psychopathology. In particular, as we shall discuss later, empirical studies have documented an association between parental emotional unavailability and parental psychopathology.

The majority of investigations that have explicitly examined the parenting styles and behaviors of individuals exhibiting some form of psychopathology have focused on the disorder of depression. Early studies of the parenting behaviors of depressed mothers relied on the women's self-reports. Compared with nondepressed women, depressed women in these studies reported being less involved, less affectionate, and more emotionally distant with their children (e.g., McLean, 1976). More recent investigations that have examined more directly the behaviors of depressed mothers in interactions with their children corroborate these results. Livingood, Daen, and Smith (1983), for example, found that depressed mothers gazed less often at their infants than did nondepressed women, reflecting withdrawal and a consequent interference with the development of mutual visual regard and a strong attachment bond. Similar findings of the decreased responsivity of depressed mothers to their infants have also been reported by Bettes (1988) and by Field, Healy, Goldstein, and Guthertz (1990).

These studies clearly indicate that depression interferes with the responsiveness of mothers toward their infants. Other investigators have replicated these findings with older children. Breznitz and Sherman

(1987), for example, observed 2- and 3-year-old children interacting with their depressed mothers. These investigators reported that depressed mothers and their children spoke less to each other and more slowly than did nondepressed control mothers and their offspring. Similarly, Goodman and Brumley (1990) reported that depressed mothers were significantly less responsive and involved with their children than were normal control mothers. Cohler and colleagues (1977) reported that the depressed mothers they studied were less likely than nondepressed controls to develop an interactive relationship with their children. Mills, Puckering, Pound, and Cox (1985) found that depressed women were less responsive in their interactions with their children than were nondepressed women. Finally, Weissman and associates (1987) reported that interactions between depressed mothers and their children were characterized by lack of interest and low involvement on the part of the mother and, further, that depressed mothers exhibited decreasing levels of involvement as their children grew older.

A number of researchers have reported strikingly similar findings in examining the parenting styles of individuals exhibiting other forms of psychopathology. For example, Jacob, Ritchey, Cvitkovic, and Blane (1981) videotaped the interactions of alcoholic and nonalcoholic families, and found that alcoholic fathers were less instrumental and directive than were their nonalcoholic counterparts; they also displayed less leadership. Similar to the pattern of results seen for families with a depressed parent, these findings suggest that alcoholism in fathers is related to lack of involvement with children. Corroborating these results, Steinglass (1981) and Moos and Billings (1982) reported that members of families in which an alcoholic is currently drinking tend to function more independently of each other and to be less cohesive and responsive than are members of nonalcoholic families. These studies highlight the association between drinking and lack of family involvement and suggest that one mechanism by which parental alcoholism may be associated with child problems is through a tendency for the parent to be relatively unavailable or unresponsive to the child. As Lee and Gotlib (1991b) speculate, alcoholic parents may often be physically absent from the home because of the time spent drinking outside the home, because of being hospitalized for treatment of alcoholism or other illnesses, or because the nonalcoholic parent has requested that the spouse leave the home for a period of time. Alternatively, an alcoholic spouse may be physically present in the home, but uninvolved in parenting and caretaking responsibilities.

Finally, several investigators have examined the interactions of families in which a parent has been diagnosed with schizophrenia. Fisher and Jones (1980) reported an association between parental communication deviance and nonacknowledgment and child problem-solving ability, and Kokes and associates (1980) found that incongruous affect and withdrawal in the parents were associated with poor child adjustment. More recently, Miklowitz and Stackman (1992) reviewed the literature concerned with the construct of "communication deviance" in schizophrenia and noted that parental communication deviance, which includes nonresponsivity, was the strongest individual predictor of the likelihood that the children would develop a schizophrenic disorder at a 15-year follow-up. It appears, therefore, that parental emotional unavailability plays a critical role in children's successful adjustment in the face of parental psychopathology and, in particular, in response to parental depression, alcoholism, and schizophrenia.

CONCLUSIONS

In this chapter we have examined several environmental factors that have been implicated in increasing children's risk for psychopathology. Specifically, we have explored the effects of children's exposure to social disadvantage, disrupted family structures, dysfunctional family processes, and parental depression, alcoholism, and schizophrenia. Certainly, these factors are diverse. Nevertheless, it is clear from our review that they all have been found to increase the probability that exposed children will demonstrate some form of psychosocial dysfunction. There does not appear to be an isomorphic relation between risk factor and outcome. Thus, as we noted earlier, children of depressed parents exhibit not only elevated rates of depression but in addition high levels of conduct disorder and multiple psychiatric diagnoses. Similar findings have been reported for children of alcoholic and schizophrenic parents. Indeed, it is clear that children in all three of these groups, as well as children from disadvantaged family environments, share common adjustment difficulties, which include difficulties at school, physical illness, social dysfunction, and emotional disorder.

In attempting to explain this apparent commonality of outcomes, we suggested that the effects of the diverse risk factors examined in this chapter might be mediated by two higher-level constructs: marital conflict/distress and parental emotional unavailability. We reviewed evidence indicating both that these two constructs can affect children's psychosocial functioning and that virtually all of the risk factors examined in this chapter may be linked with these two constructs. It is also important at this point to emphasize that, although we examined each of the various risk factors separately in this chapter, in fact they rarely occur independently. For example, there is high comorbidity or cooccurrence among the three forms of parental psychopathology we examined in this chapter (cf. Gotlib & Cane, 1989; Knights & Hirsch, 1981; Schuckit, 1983). Moreover, a number of studies have demonstrated that this comorbidity substantially increases the risk of psychopathology among the children of disturbed parents. For example, several investigators have reported higher rates of delinquency and truancy among children whose alcoholic parents also suffer from symptoms of other mental illnesses (e.g., Offord et al., 1978).

In addition to psychiatric comorbidity, other types of risk factors also tend to cooccur. For example, the families of alcoholics have been found to be more violent than nonalcoholic families, and children in these families may be exposed to abuse. For example, in a study of 11 families in which one parent was in treatment for alcoholism, Wilson and Orford (1978) found evidence of violence toward the children in four families, with consequent anxiety and tension. Similarly, West and Prinz (1987) observed that several types of stressors occur at elevated rates in alcoholic families, including family conflict and divorce, parental psychopathology, substance abuse, parental criminality, physical abuse and neglect, perinatal birth complications, and poverty. Indeed, children who are exposed to four or more risk factors have been found to exhibit greater psychopathology than do children with fewer risk factors (Werner, 1989). It will be important in future research that investigators attempt to examine the relative contributions of these factors to increasing children's risk for psychopathology.

In closing, we would like to underscore the importance of examining factors that increase children's risk for psychopathology. In this chapter we have focused on the adverse impact of disrupted family structures and parental psychopathology. It is clear from our review that much work remains to be done. In particular, although there is considerable overlap among populations of socioeconomically disadvantaged families and families experiencing parental psychopathology, simple dichotomous characterizations of these families are unlikely to capture adequately the features that are most critical in contributing to children's mental health problems. Distinctions between socially disadvantaged versus more fortunate families, families with a depressed parent versus intact families without major parental psychopathology, or discordant versus maritally satisfied parents are simply too coarse to provide us with powerful predictions about children's well-being. In addition, we know relatively little about children's psychosocial resources that may protect them from the negative consequences of experiencing multiple risk factors. The literature strongly suggests characteristics in children reflecting invulnerability, resilience, or competence (e.g., Garmezy, 1983; Werner, 1984) that buffer the adverse effects of parental psychopathology, but this area is clearly underexplored. As we begin to consider these factors in combination with one another and to learn more about how they affect children's functioning, we will begin to gain a better understanding of how we might reduce children's risk for psychopathology.

ACKNOWLEDGMENTS

Preparation of this chapter was facilitated by an Ontario Mental Health Foundation Senior Research Fellowship to Ian H. Gotlib and by Grants 6606-3465-51, 6606-4262-66, and 6606-4193-MH-L from Health and Welfare Canada.

REFERENCES

Amato, P. R. (1989). Family processes and the competence of adolescents and primary school children. *Journal of Youth and Adolescence, 18,* 39–53.

Amato, P. R., & Keith, B. (1991). Parental divorce and the well-being of children: A meta-analysis. *Psychological Bulletin, 110,* 26–46.

American Psychiatric Association. (1987). *Diagnostic and statistical manual of mental disorders* (3rd ed., rev.). Washington, DC: American Psychiatric Association.

Andreasen, N. C. (1982). Negative symptoms in schizophrenia: Definition and reliability. *Archives of General Psychiatry, 39,* 784–788.

Avison, W. R., Gotlib, I. H., Rae Grant, N. I., Speechley, K. N., & Turner, R. J. (1992, April). *Single-parent mothers and their children: Social, economic, and health issues.* Paper presented at Prevention Congress V, Healthy and Supportive Communities: The Promise of Change, London, Ontario, Canada.

Avison, W. R., & McAlpine, D. D. (1992). Gender differences in symptoms of depression among adolescents. *Journal of Health and Social Behavior, 33,* 77–96.

Barancik, S. (1989). *Poverty tables.* Washington, DC: Center on Budget and Policy Priorities.

Barnett, P. A., & Gotlib, I. H. (1988). Psychosocial functioning and depression: Distinguishing among antecedents, concomitants, and consequences. *Psychological Bulletin, 104,* 97–106.

Beardslee, W. R., Bemporad, J., Keller, M. B., & Klerman, G. L. (1983). Children of parents with major affective disorder: A review. American Journal of Psychiatry, 140, 825–832.

Beardslee, W. R., Schultz, L. H., & Selman, R. L. (1987). Level of social–cognitive development, adaptive functioning, and DSM-III diagnoses in adolescent offspring of parents with affective disorders: Implications for the development of the capacity for mutuality. *Developmental Psychology, 23,* 807–815.

Berlinsky, E. B., & Biller, H. B. (1982). *Parental death and psychological development.* Lexington, MA: D. C. Heath.

Bettes, B. A. (1988). Maternal depression and motherese: Temporal and intonational features. *Child Development, 59,* 1089–1096.

Biglan, A., Hops, H., Sherman, L., Friedman, L. S., Arthur, J., & Osteen, V. (1985). Problem-solving interactions of depressed women and their husbands. *Behavior Therapy, 16,* 431–451.

Billings, A. G., Kessler, M., Gomberg, C. A., & Weiner, S. (1979). Marital conflict resolution of alcoholic and nonalcoholic couples during drinking and nondrinking sessions. *Journal of Studies on Alcohol, 40,* 183–195.

Billings, A. G., & Moos, R. M. (1983). Comparisons of children of depressed and nondepressed parents: A social–environmental perspective. *Journal of Abnormal Child Psychology, 11,* 463–486.

Billings, A. G., & Moos, R. H. (1986). Children of parents with unipolar depression: A controlled one year follow-up. *Journal of Abnormal Child Psychology, 14,* 149–166.

Bloom, B. L., Asher, S. J., & White, S. W. (1978). Marital disruption as a stressor: A review and analysis. *Psychological Bulletin, 85,* 867–894.

Bond, C. R., & McMahon, R. J. (1984). Relationships between marital distress and child behavior problems, maternal adjustment, maternal personality, and maternal parenting behavior. *Journal of Abnormal Psychology, 93,* 348–351.

Booz-Allen & Hamilton. (1974). *An assessment of the needs of and resourses for children of alcoholic parents* (Report No. PB-241-119). Springfield, VA: National Technical Information Service.

Bowlby, J. (1973). *Attachment and loss: Vol. 2. Separation.* New York: Basic Books.

Bowlby, J., & Parkes, C. M. (1979). Separation and loss within the family. In E. J. Anthony & C. Koupernik (Eds.), *The child in his family* (pp. 197–216). Huntington, NY: Krieger.

Brewin, C. R., Andrews, B., & Gotlib, I. H. (in press). Psychopathology and early experience. *Psychological Bulletin.*

Breznitz, Z., & Sherman, T. (1987). Speech patterning of natural discourse of well and depressed mothers and their young children. *Child Development, 58,* 395–400.

Bromet, E. J., & Cornely, P. J. (1984). Correlates of depression in mothers of young children. *Journal of the American Academy of Child Psychiatry, 23,* 335–342.

Brown, G. W., Harris, T. O., & Bifulco, A. (1986). Long-term effects of early loss of parent. In M. Rutter, C. E. Izard, & P. B. Read (Eds.), *Depression in young people: Developmental and clinical perspectives* (pp. 251–296). New York: Guilford Press.

Bumpass, L. L., & Sweet, L. L. (1989). Children's experience in single-parent families: Implications of cohabitation and marital transitions. *Family Planning Perspectives, 6,* 256–260.

Campbell, E., & Redfening, D. L. (1979). Relationship among environmental and demographic variables and teacher-rated hyperactivity. *Journal of Abnormal Child Psychology, 7,* 77–81.

Carlson, G. A., & Strober, M. (1983). Affective disorders in adolescence. In D. P. Cantwell & G. A. Carlson (Eds.), *Affective disorders in childhood and adolescence: An update* (pp. 85–96). New York: Spectrum.

Chafetz, M. E., Blane, H. T., & Hill, M. J. (1971). Children of alcoholics: Observations in a child guidance clinic. *Quarterly Journal of Studies on Alcohol, 32,* 687–698.

Chassin, L., Rogosch, F., & Barrera, M. (1991). Substance use and symptomatology among adolescent children of alcoholics. *Journal of Abnormal Psychology, 100,* 449–463.

Cohler, B. J., Gallant, D. H., & Grunebaum, H. U. (1977). Disturbance of attention among schizophrenic, depressed and well mothers and their five-year-old children. *Journal of Child Psychology and Psychiatry, 18,* 115–136.

Conger, R.D., Elder, G.H. Jr., Lorenz, F.O., Conger, K.J., Simons, R.L., Whitbeck, L.B., Huck, S., & Melby, J. N. (1990). Linking economic hardship to marital quality and instability. *Journal of Marriage and the Family, 52,* 643–656.

Conrad, M., & Hammen, C. (1989). Role of maternal depression in perceptions of child maladjustment. *Journal of Consulting and Clinical Psychology, 57,* 663–667.

Crowther, J. H. (1985). The relationship between depression and marital maladjustment: A descriptive study. *Journal of Nervous and Mental Disease, 173,* 227–231.

Cummings, E. M., & Cicchetti, D. (1990). Attachment, depression, and the transmission of depression. In M. T. Greenberg, D. Cicchetti, & E. M. Cummings (Eds.), *Attachment during the preschool years.* Chicago: University of Chicago Press.

Cutrona, C. E., & Troutman, B. R. (1986). Social support, infant temperament, and parenting self-efficacy: A mediational model of postpartum depression. *Child Development, 57,* 1507–1518.

Cytryn, L., McKnew, D. H., Bartko, J. J., Lamour, M., & Hamovitt, J. (1982). Offspring of patients with affective disorders: II. *Journal of the American Academy of Child Psychiatry, 21,* 389–391.

Decina, P., Kestenbaum, C. J., Farber, S., Kron, L., Gargan, M., Sackeim, H. A., & Fieve, R. R. (1983). Clinical and psychological assessment of children of bipolar probands. *American Journal of Psychiatry, 140,* 548–553.

Dornbusch, S. M. (1989). The sociology of adolescence. *Annual Review of Sociology, 15,* 233–259).

Duncan, G. J., & Rodgers, W. (1991). Has children's poverty become more persistent? *American Sociological Review, 56,* 538–550.

Eaton, W. W., Ritter, C., & Brown, D. (1990). Psychiatric epidemiology and psychiatric sociology: Influences on the recognition of bizarre behaviors as social problems. In J. R. Greenley (Ed.), *Research in community and mental health* (Vol. 6, pp. 41–68). Greenwich, CT: JAI Press.

Elder, G. H. Jr., Caspi, A. (1988). Human development and social change: An emerging perspective of the life course. In N. Bolger, A. Caspi, G. Downey, & M. Moorehouse (Eds.), *Persons in context: Developmental processes* (pp. 77–113). Cambridge: Cambridge University Press.

Emery, R., & O'Leary, K. D. (1982). Children's perceptions of marital discord and behavior problems of boys and girls. *Journal of Abnormal Child Psychology, 10,* 11–24.

Emery, R., Weintraub, S., & Neale, J. M. (1982). Effects of marital discord on the children of schizophrenic, affectively disordered, and normal parents. *Journal of Abnormal Child Psychology, 10,* 215–228.

Emery, R. E. (1982). Interparental conflict and the children of discord and divorce. *Psychological Bulletin, 92,* 310–330.

Expert Committee on Alcohol Statistics. (1981). Special report on alcohol statistics. Ottawa: Health and Welfare Canada.

Field, T., Healy, B., Goldstein, S., & Guthertz, M. (1990). Behavior-state matching and synchrony in mother–infant interactions of nondepressed versus depressed dyads. *Developmental Psychology, 26,* 7–14.

Field, T., Sandberg, D., Garcia, R., Vega-Lahr, N., Goldstein, S., & Guy, L.

(1985). Pregnancy problems, postpartum depression and early mother–infant interactions. *Developmental Psychology, 21,* 1152–1156.

Field, T. M. (1984). Early interactions between infants and their postpartum depressed mothers. *Infant Behavior and Development, 7,* 517–522.

Fisher, L., & Jones, J. E. (1980). Child competence and psychiatric risk. II. Areas of relationship between child and family functioning. *Journal of Nervous and Mental Disease, 168,* 332–342.

Forehand, R., Wells, K., McMahon, R., Griest, D., & Rogers, T. (1982). Maternal perception of maladjustment in the clinic-referred children: An extension of earlier research. *Journal of Behavioral Assessment, 4,* 145–151.

Forman, E. (1974). *A child's parent dies: Studies in childhood bereavement.* New Haven: Yale University Press.

Frank, E., Carpenter, L. L., & Kupfer, D. J. (1988). Sex differences in recurrent depression: Are there any that are significant? *American Journal of Psychiatry, 145,* 41–45.

Fromm-Reichmann, F. (1948). Notes on the development of treatment of schizophrenics by psychoanalytic therapy. *Psychiatry, 11,* 263–273.

Furstenburg, F. F., & Brooks-Gunn, J. (1986). Teenage childbearing: Causes, consequences, and remedies. In L. H. Aiken & D. Mechanic (Eds.), *Applications of social science to clinical medicine and health policy* (pp. 307–334). New Brunswick, NJ: Rutgers University Press.

Furstenberg, F. F., Brooks-Gunn, J., & Morgan, S. P. (1987). *Adolescent mothers in later life.* New York: Cambridge University Press.

Furstenberg, F. F., & Cherlin, A. J. (1991). *Divided families: What happens to children when parents part.* Cambridge, MA: Harvard University Press.

Gamer, E., Gallant, D., Grunebaum, H., & Cohler, B. J. (1977). Children of psychotic mothers. *Archives of General Psychiatry, 34,* 592–597.

Garmezy, N. (1983). Stressors of childhood. In N. Garmezy & M. Rutter (Eds.), *Stress, coping, and development in children* (pp. 43–84). New York: McGraw-Hill.

Garmezy, N. (1986). Developmental aspects of children's responses to the stress of separation and loss. In M. Rutter, C. E. Izard, & P. B. Read (Eds.), *Depression in young people: Developmental and clinical perspectives* (pp. 297–324). New York: Guilford Press.

Gelfand, D. M., & Teti, D. M. (1990). The effects of maternal depression on children. *Clinical Psychology Review, 10,* 320–354.

Ghodsian, M., Zayicek, E., & Wolkind, S. (1984). A longitudinal study of maternal depression and child behavior problems. *Journal of Child Psychology and Psychiatry, 25,* 91–109.

Giele, J. Z. (1988). Gender and sex roles. In N. J. Smelser (Ed.), *Handbook of sociology.* Newbury Park, CA: Sage.

Goldstein, M. J. (1988). The family and psychopathology. *Annual Review of Psychology, 39,* 283–299.

Goodman, S. H. (1992). Understanding the effects of depressed mothers on their children. In E. F. Walker, B. A. Cornblatt, & R. H. Dworkin (Eds.), *Progress in experimental personality and psychopathology research* (Vol. 15, pp. 47–109). New York: Springer.

Goodman, S. H., & Brumley, H. E. (1990). Schizophrenic and depressed mothers: Relational deficits in parenting. *Developmental Psychology, 26,* 31–39.

Gotlib, I. H., & Cane, D. B. (1989). Self-report assessment of depression and anxiety. In P. C. Kendall & D. Watson (Eds.), *Anxiety and depression: Distinctive and overlapping features* (pp. 131–169). Orlando, FL: Academic Press.

Gotlib, I. H., & Hammen, C. L. (1992). *Psychological aspects of depression: Toward a cognitive–interpersonal integration.* Chichester, England: Wiley.

Gotlib, I. H., & Hooley, J. M. (1988). Depression and marital distress: Current status and future directions. In S. Duck (Ed.), *Handbook of personal relationships* (pp. 543–570). Chichester, England: Wiley.

Gotlib, I. H., & Lee, C. M. (1990). Children of depressed mothers: A review and directions for future research. In C. D. McCann & N. S. Endler (Eds.), *Depression: New directions in theory, research, and practice* (pp. 187–208). Toronto: Wall & Thompson.

Gotlib, I. H., Mount, J. H., Cordy, N. I., & Whiffen, V. E. (1988). Depressed mood and perceptions of early parenting: A longitudinal investigation. *British Journal of Psychiatry, 152,* 24–27.

Gotlib, I. H., & Whiffen, V. E. (1989). Depression and marital functioning: An examination of specificity and gender differences. *Journal of Abnormal Psychology, 98,* 23–30.cos c7g5 ts

Gotlib, I. H. , Whiffen, V. E., Mount, J. H., Milne, K. , & Cordy, N. I. (1989). Prevalence rates and demographic characteristics associated with depression in pregnancy and the postpartum. *Journal of Consulting and Clinical Psychology, 57,* 269–274.

Gotlib, I. H., Whiffen, V. E., Wallace, P. M., & Mount, J. H. (1991). A prospective investigation of postpartum depression: Factors involved in onset and recovery. *Journal of Abnormal Psychology, 100,* 122–132.

Gottesman, I. I., & Shields, J. (1982). Schizophrenia: The epigenetic puzzle. Cambridge: Cambridge University Press.

Grunebaum, H., Cohler, B., Kaufman, D., & Gallant, D. (1978). Children of depressed and schizophrenic mothers. *Child Psychiatry and Human Development, 8,* 219–228.

Grych, J. H., & Fincham, F. D. (1990). Marital conflict and children's adjustment: A cognitive–contextual framework. *Psychological Bulletin, 108,* 267–290.

Guidubaldi, J., Cleminshaw, H. K., Perry, J. D., Nastasi, B. K., & Lightel, J. (1986). The role of selected family environment factors in children's post-divorce adjustment. Family Relations, 35, 141–151.

Guttentag, M., Salasin, S., & Belle, D. (1980). *The mental health of women.* New York: Academic Press.

Haberman, P. W. (1966). Childhood symptoms in children of alcoholics and comparison group parents. *Journal of Marriage and the Family, 28,* 152–154.

Hammen, C. (1991). *Depression runs in families: The social context of risk and resilience in children of depressed mothers.* New York: Springer-Verlag.

Hammen, C., Gordon, D., Burge, D., Adrian, C., Jaenicke, C., & Hiroto, D. (1987). Maternal affective disorders, illness, and stress: Risk for children's psychopathology. *American Journal of Psychiatry, 144,* 736–741.

Harvey, P., Winters, K., Weintraub, S., & Neale, J. M. (1981). Distractibility in children vulnerable to psychopathology. *Journal of Abnormal Psychology, 90,* 298–304.

Helzer, J. E., Canino, G. J., Bland, R. C., Newman, S., & Yeh, E. (1988). Alcoholism: A cross-national comparison of population surveys with the Diagnostic Interview Schedule. In R. M. Rose & J. Barrett (Eds.), *Alcoholism: Origins and outcomes* (pp. 31–47). New York: Raven Press.

Hetherington, M. E., Cox, M. E., & Cox, R. (1979a). Family interaction and the social emotional and cognitive development of children following divorce. In V. Vaughn & T. Brazelton (Eds.), *The family: Setting priorities* (pp. 71–87). New York: Science and Medicine.

Hetherington, M. E., Cox, M. E., & Cox, R. (1979b). Play and social interaction in children following divorce. *Journal of Social Issues, 35,* 26–49.

Hetherington, M. E., Cox, M. E., & Cox, R. (1982). Effects of divorce on parents and children. In M. Lamb (Ed.), *Non-traditional families* (pp. 233–288). Hillsdale, N.J.: Erlbaum

Hirsch, B. J., Moos, R. H., & Reischl, T. M. (1985). Psychosocial adjustment of adolescent children of a depressed, arthritic, or normal parent. *Journal of Abnormal Psychology, 94,* 154–164.

Hodges, K., Kline, J., Stern, L., Cytryn, L., & McKnew, D. (1982). The development of a child assessment interview for research and clinical use. *Journal of Abnormal Child Psychology, 10,* 173–189.

Holden, K. C., & Smock, P. M. (1991). The economic costs of marital dissolution: Why do women bear a disproportionate cost? *Annual Review of Sociology, 17,* 51–78.

Hooley, J. M., Richters, J. E., Weintraub, S., & Neale, J. M. (1987). Psychopathology and marital distress: The positive side of positive symptoms. *Journal of Abnormal Psychology, 96,* 27–33.

Hops, H., Biglan, A., Sherman, L., Arthur, J., Friedman, L., & Osteen, V. (1987). Home observations of family interactions of depressed women. *Journal of Consulting and Clinical Psychology, 55,* 341–346.

Jacob, T., & Krahn, G. L. (1988). Marital interactions of alcoholic couples: Comparison with depressed and nondistressed couples. *Journal of Consulting and Clinical Psychology, 56,* 73–79.

Jacob, T., Ritchey, D., Cvitkovic, J. F., & Blane, H. T. (1981). Communication styles of alcoholic and nonalcoholic families when drinking and not drinking. *Journal of Studies on Alcohol, 42,* 466–482.

Johnson, S., Leonard, K., & Jacob, T. (1989). Drinking, drinking styles, and drug use in children of alcoholics, depressives, and controls. *Journal of Studies on Alcohol, 50,* 427–432.

Johnson, S. M., & Lobitz, G. K. (1974). The personal and marital adjustment of parents as related to observed child deviance and parenting behaviors. *Journal of Abnormal Child Psychology, 2,* 193–207.

Johnston, J. R., Gonzalez, R., & Campbell, L. E. G. (1987). Ongoing post-divorce conflict and child disturbance. *Journal of Abnormal Child Psychology, 15,* 493–509.

Jouriles, E. N., Murphy, C. M., & O'Leary, K. D. (1989). Interspousal aggression, marital discord, and child problems. *Journal of Abnormal Child Psychology, 57,* 453–455.

Kanmeier, M. L. (1971). Adolescents from families with and without alcohol problems. *Quarterly Journal of Studies on Alcohol, 32,* 364–372.

Karno, M., Hough, R. L., Burnam, M. A., Escobar, J. I., Timbers, D. M., Santana, F., & Boyd, J. H. (1987). Lifetime prevalence of specific psychiatric disorders among Mexican Americans and non-Hispanic whites in Los Angeles. *Archives of General Psychiatry, 44,* 695–701.

Kessler, R. C., & Magee, W. J. (in press). The disaggregation of vulnerability to depression as a function of the determinants of onset and recurrence. In W. R. Avison & I. H. Gotlib (Eds.), *Stress and mental health: Contemporary issues and prospects for the future.* New York: Plenum Press.

Klein, D. N., Clark, D. C., Dansky, L., & Margolis, E. T. (1988). Dysthymia in the offspring of parents with primary unipolar affective disorder. *Journal of Abnormal Psychology, 97,* 265–274.

Knights, A., & Hirsch, S. R. (1981). "Revealed" depression and drug treatment of schizophrenia. *Archives of General Psychiatry, 38,* 806–811.

Knop, J., Teasdale, T., Schulsinger, F., & Goodwin, D. (1985). A prospective study of young men at high risk for alcoholism: School behavior and achievement. *Journal of Studies on Alcohol, 46,* 273–278.

Kokes, R. F., Harder, D. W., Fisher, L., & Strauss, J. S. (1980). Child competence and psychiatric risk. V. Sex of patient parent and dimensions of psychopathology. *Journal of Nervous and Mental Disease, 168,* 348–352.

Krantz, S. E., Clark, J., Pruyn, J. P., & Usher, M. (1985). Cognition and adjustment among children of separated or divorced parents. *Cognitive Therapy and Research, 9,* 1–77.

Kubicka, L., Kozeny, J., & Roth, Z. (1990). Alcohol abuse and its psychosocial correlates in sons of alcoholics as young men and in the general population of young men in Prague. *Journal of Studies on Alcohol, 51,* 49–58.

Kurdek, L. A., & Berg, B. (1983). Correlates of children's adjustment to their parents' divorces. In L. A. Kurdek (Ed.), *Children and divorce* (pp. 47–60). San Francisco: Jossey-Bass.

Kurdek, L. A., Blisk, D., & Seisky, A. E. (1981). Correlates of children's long-term adjustment to their parents' divorce. *Development Psychology, 17,* 565–579.

Kurdek, L. A., & Sinclair, R. J. (1988). Adjustment of young adolecents in two-parent nuclear, stepfather, and mother custody families. *Journal of Consulting and Clinical Psychology, 56,* 91–96.

Langner, T. S., Gersten, J. C., Greene, E. L., Eisenberg, J. G., Herson, J. H., & McCarthy, E. (1974). Treatment of psychological disorders among urban children. *Journal of Consulting and Clinical Psychology, 42,* 170–179.

Langner, T. S., McCarthy, E. D., Gersten, J. C., Simcha-Fagan, O., & Eisenberg, J. G. (1979). Factors in children's behavior and mental health over time: The Family Research Project. In R. G. Simmons (Ed.), *Research in community and mental health* (Vol. 1., pp, 127–181). Greenwich, CT: JAI Press.

Lee, C. M., & Gotlib, I. H. (1989a). Clinical status and emotional adjustment of children of depressed mothers. *American Journal of Psychiatry, 146,* 478–483.

Lee, C. M., & Gotlib, I. H. (1989b). Maternal depression and child adjustment: A longitudinal analysis. *Journal of Abnormal Psychology, 98,* 78–85.

Lee, C. M., & Gotlib, I. H. (1991a). Adjustment of children of depressed mothers: A ten-month follow-up. *Journal of Abnormal Psychology, 100,* 473–477.

Lee, C. M., & Gotlib, I. H. (1991b). Family disruption, parental availability, and child adjustment: An integrative review. In R. J. Prinz (Ed.), *Advances in the behavioral assessment of children and families* (Vo. 5., pp. 166–199). London: Jessica Kingsley.

Leslie, S. A. (1974). Psychiatric disorder in the young adolescents of an industrial town. *British Journal of Psychiatry, 125,* 113–124.

Lewinsohn, P. M., Hoberman, H. M., & Rosenbaum, M. (1988). A prospective study of risk factors for unipolar depression. *Journal of Abnormal Psychology, 97,* 251–264.

Liem, J. H., & Liem, G. R. (1988). Understanding the individual and family effects of unemployment. In J. Eckenrode & S. Gore (Eds.), *Stress between work and family* (pp. 175–204). New York: Plenum Press.

Liem, R., & Liem, J. H. (1990). The psychological effects of unemployment on workers and their families. *Journal of Social Issues, 44,* 87–106.

Livingood, A. B., Daen, P., & Smith, B. D. (1983). The depressed mother as a source of stimulation for her infant. *Journal of Clinical Psychology, 39,* 369–375.

Loeber, R. (1990). Development and risk factors of juvenile antisocial behavior and delinquency. *Clinical Psychology Review, 10,* 1–14.

Loeber, R., & Stouthamer-Loeber, M. (1986). Family factors as correlates and predictors of delinquency. In M. Tonry & N. Morris (Eds.), *Crime and justice: An annual review of research* (Vol. 7, pp. 29–149). Chicago: University of Chicago Press.

Masten, A. S., & Garmezy, N. (1985). Risk, vulnerability, and protective factors in developmental psychopathology. In B. B. Lahey & A. E. Kazdin (Eds.), *Advances in clinical child psychology* (Vol. 8, pp. 1–52). New York: Plenum Press.

McCord, J. (1983). A forty year perspective on effects of child abuse and neglect. *Child Abuse and Neglect, 7,* 265–270.

McLean, P. D. (1976). Parental depression: Incompatible with effective parenting. In E. J. Mash, C. Handy, & L. A. Hammerlynck (Eds.), *Behavior modification approaches to parenting* (pp. 209–220). New York: Brunner/ Mazel.

McNeil, T. F., & Kaij, L. (1980, February). *Offspring of women with nonorganic psychosis: Progress report.* Paper presented at the Risk Research Consortium Plenary Conference, San Juan.

McQuillan, K. (1990). Family change and family income in Ontario. In L. C. Johnson & D. Barnhorst (Eds.), *Children, families and public policy in the 90s* (pp. 153–174). Toronto: Thompson Educational.

Mednick, S. A., & Schulsinger, F. (1968). Some premorbid characteristics related to breakdown in children with schizophrenic mothers. In D. Rosenthal & S. S. Kety (Eds.), *The transmission of schizophrenia.* Oxford, England: Pergamon Press.

Merikangas, K., Weissman, M., Prusoff, B., Pauls, D., & Leckman, J. (1985). Depressives with secondary alcoholism: Psychiatric disorders in offspring. *Journal of Studies on Alcohol, 46,* 199–204.

Merikangas, K. R. (1984). Divorce and assortative mating among depressed patients. *American Journal of Psychiatry, 141,* 74–76.

Miklowitz, D. J., & Stackman, D. (1992). Communication deviance in families of schizophrenic and other psychiatric patients: Current state of the construct. In E. F. Walker, B. A. Cornblatt, & R. H. Dworkin (Eds.), *Progress in experimental personality and psychopathology research* (Vol. 15, pp. 1–46). New York: Springer.

Mills, M., Puckering, C., Pound, A., & Cox, A. (1985). What is it about depressed mothers that influences their children's functioning? In J. E. Stevenson (Ed.), *Recent research in developmental psychopathology* (pp. 11–17). Oxford, England: Pergamon Press.

Mirowsky, J. (in press). The advantages of indexes over diagnoses in scientific assessment. In W. R. Avison & I. H. Gotlib (Eds.), *Stress and mental health: Contemporary issues and prospects for the future.* New York: Plenum Press.

Moos, R., & Billings, A. (1982). Children of alcoholics during the recovery process: Alcoholic and matched control families. *Addictive Behaviors, 7,* 155–163.

Munro, A. (1966). Parental deprivation in depressive patients. *British Journal of Psychiatry, 112,* 443–457.

Norris, F. H., & Murrell, S. A. (1987). Older adult family stress and adaptation before and after bereavement. *Journal of Gerontology, 42,* 606–612.

Nuechterlein, K. H., Phipps-Yonas, S., Driscoll, R., & Garmezy, N. (1990). Vulnerability factors in children at risk: Anomalies in attentional functioning and social behavior. In J. Rolf, A. S. Masten, D. Cicchetti, K. H. Nuechterlein, & S. Weintraub (Eds.), *Risk and protective factors in the development of psychopathology* (pp. 445–479). Cambridge, England: Cambridge University Press.

O'Farrell, T. J., & Birchler, G. R. (1987). Marital relationships of alcoholic, conflicted, and nonconflicted couples. *Journal of Marital and Family Therapy, 13,* 259–274.

Offord, D., Allen, N., & Abrams, N. (1978). Parental psychiatric illness, broken homes, and delinquency. *Journal of the American Academy of Child Psychiatry, 17,* 224–238.

Offord, D. R., & Boyle, M. H. (1988). The epidemiology of antisocial behavior in early adolescents, aged 12 to 14. In M. D. Levine & E. R. NcAnarney (Eds.), *Early adolescent transitions* (pp. 245–259). Lexington, MA: Lexington.

Offord, D. R., Boyle, M. H., & Jones, B. R. (1987). Psychiatric disorder and poor school performance among welfare children in Ontario. *Canadian Journal of Psychiatry, 32,* 518–525.

Offord, D. R., Boyle, M. H., & Racine, Y. (1989). Ontario Child Health Study: Correlates of disorder. *Journal of the American Academy of Child and Adolscent Psychiatry, 28,* 856–860.

Offord, D. R., Boyle, M. H., Szatmari, P., Rae-Grant, N. I., Links, P. S., Cadman, D. T., Byles, J. A., Crawford, J. W., Blum, H. M., Byrne, C., Thomas, H., & Woodward, C. A. (1987). Ontario Child Health Study. II. Six-month prevalence of disorder and rates of service utilization. *Archives of General Psychiatry, 44,* 832–836.

Oltmanns, T. F., Broderick, J. E., & O'Leary, K. D. (1977). Marital adjustment and the efficacy of behavior therapy with children. *Journal of Consulting and Clinical Psychology, 45,* 724–729.

Pandina, R. J., & Johnson, V. (1989). Familial drinking history as a predictor of alcohol and drug consumption among adolescent children. *Journal of Studies on Alcohol, 50,* 245–253.

Parker, G. (1981). Parental reports of depressives: An investigation of several explanations. *Journal of Affective Disorders, 3,* 131–140.

Patterson, G. R., & Stouthamer-Loeber, M. (1984). The correlation of family management practices and delinquency. *Child Development, 55,* 1299–1307.

Peterson, J. L., & Zill, N. (1986). Marital disruption, parent–child relationship and behavior problems in children. *Journal of Marriage and the Family, 48,* 295–307.

Pfohl, B., Stangl, D., & Tsuang, M. T. (1983). The association between early parental loss and diagnosis in the Iowa 500. *Archives of General Psychiatry, 40,* 965–967.

President's Commission on Mental Health. (1978). *Report to the President.* Washington, DC: U. S. Government Printing Office.

Radke-Yarrow, M., Cummings, M., Kuczynski, L., & Chapman, M. (1985). Patterns of attachment in two- and three-year olds in normal families and families with parental depression. *Child Development, 56,* 884–893.

Reese, M. F. (1982). Growing up: The impact of loss and change. In D. Belle (Ed.), *Lives in stress: Women and depression* (pp. 65–88). Beverly Hills, CA: Sage.

Rickard, K. M., Forehand, R., Atkeson, B. M., & Lopez, C. (1982). An examination of the relationship of marital satisfaction and divorce with parent–child interactions. *Journal of Clinical Child Psychology, 11,* 61–65.

Rickard, K. M., Forehand, R., Wells, K. C., Griest, D. L., & McMahon, R. J. (1981). Factors in the referral of children for behavioral treatment: A comparison of mothers of clinic-referred deviant, clinic-referred non-deviant, and non-clinic children. *Behaviour Research and Therapy, 19,* 201–205.

Robins, L. N., Helzer, J. E., Weissman, M. M., Orvaschel, H., Gruenberg, E., Burke, J. D., & Regier, D. A. (1984). Lifetime prevalence of specific psychiatric disorders in three sites. *Archives of General Psychiatry, 41,* 949–958.

Ross, H. L., & Sawhill, I. V. (1975). *Time of transition: The growth of families headed by women.* Washington, DC: Urban Institute.

Ruscher, S. M., & Gotlib, I. H. (1988). Marital interaction patterns of couples with and without a depressed partner. *Behavior Therapy, 19,* 455–470.

Rutter, M. (1966). *Children of sick parents: An environmental and psychiatric study.* Oxford: Oxford University Press.

Rutter, M. (1971). Parent–child separation: Psychological effects on the children. *Journal of Child Psychology and Psychiatry, 12,* 233–260.

Rutter, M. (1973). Why are London children so disturbed? *Proceedings of the Royal Society of Medicine, 66,* 1221–1225.

Rutter, M. (1981). Stress, coping, and development: Some issues and some questions. *Journal of Child Psychology and Psychiatry, 22,* 323–356.

Rutter, M. (1985a). Resilience in the face of adversity: Protective factors and resistance to psychiatric disorder. *British Journal of Psychiatry, 147,* 598–611.

Rutter, M. (1985b). Family and school influences on behavioral development. *Journal of Child Psychology and Psychiatry, 26,* 349–368.

Rutter, M., Cox, A., Tupling, C., Berger, M., & Yule, W. (1975). Attainment and adjustment in two geographic areas: I. *British Journal of Psychiatry, 126,* 493–509.

Rutter, M., & Madge, N. (1976). *Cycles of disadvantage.* London: Heinemann.

Rutter, M., Tizard, J., & Whitmore, K. (1970). *Education, health and behaviour.* London: Longmans.

Rutter, M., Yule, B., Quinton, D., Rowlands, O., Yule, W., & Berger, M. (1974). Attainment and adjustment in two geographic areas: III. Some factors accounting for area differnces. *British Journal of Psychiatry, 125,* 520–533.

Sager, C. J., Gundlach, R., & Kremer, M. (1968). The married in treatment. *Archives of General Psychiatry, 19,* 205–217.

Sameroff, A. J., Seifer, R., & Zax, M. (1982). Early development of children at risk for emotional disorder [Special issue]. *Monographs of the Society for Research in Child Development, 47*(7).

Sartorius, N. (1979). Research on affective psychoses within the framework of the WHO programme. In M. Schon & E. Stromgren (Eds.), *Origin, prevention and treatment of affective disorders* (pp. 207–213). London: Academic Press.

Schless, A. P., Schwartz, L., Goetz, C., & Mendels, J. (1974). How depressives view the significance of life events. *British Journal of Psychiatry, 125,* 406–410.

Schmidt, W., & Popham, R. E. (1975). Heavy alcohol consumption and physical health problems: A review of epidemiological evidence. *Drug and Alcohol Dependence, 1,* 27–50.

Schuckit, M. A. (1983). Alcoholism and other psychiatric disorders. *Hospital and Community Psychiatry, 34,* 1022–1027.

Shaw, D. S., & Emery, R. E. (1987). Parental conflict and other correlates of the adjustment of school-age children whose parents have separated. *Journal of Abnormal Child Psychology, 15,* 269–281.

Sher, K. J. (1991). *Children of alcoholics: A critical appraisal of theory and research.* Chicago: University of Chicago Press.

Sher, K. J., Walitzer, K. S., Wood, P. K., & Brent, E. E. (1991). Characteristics of children of alcoholics: Putative risk factors, substance use and abuse, and psychopathology. *Journal of Abnormal Psychology, 100,* 427–448.

Silverman, P. R., & Worden, J. W. (1992). Children's reactions in the early months after the death of a parent. *American Journal of Orthopsychiatry, 62,* 93–104.

Steinglass, P. (1981). The alcoholic family at home: Patterns of interaction in dry, wet, and transitional stages of alcoholism. *Archives of General Psychiatry, 38,* 578–584.

Szatmari, P., Offord, D. R., & Boyle, M. H. (1989). Ontario Child Health study: Prevalence of attention deficit disorder with hyperactivity. *Journal of Child Psychology and Psychiatry, 30,* 219–230.

Turner, S. M., Beidel, D. C., & Costello, A. (1987). Psychopathology in the offspring of anxiety disorder patients. *Journal of Consulting and Clinical Psychology, 55,* 229–235.

Van Eerdewegh, M. M., Beiri, M. D., Parilla, R. H., & Clayton, P. J. (1982). The bereaved child. *British Journal of Psychiatry, 140,* 23–29.

Velez, C. N., Johnson, J., & Cohen, P. (1989). A longitudinal analysis of selected risk factors for childhood psychopathology. *Journal of the American Academy of Child and Adolescent Psychiatry, 28,* 861–864.

Voydanoff, P. (1990). Economic stress and family relations. *Journal of Marriage and the Family, 52,* 1099–1115.

Walker, L. S., & Greene, J. W. (1986). The social context of adolescent of self-esteem. *Journal of Youth and Adolescence, 15,* 315–322.

Wallerstein, J. S. (1983). Children of divorce: Stress and development tasks. In N. Garmezy & M. Rutter (Eds.), *Stress, coping, and development in children* (pp. 265–302). New York: McGraw-Hill.

Wallerstein, J. S., & Kelly, J. B. (1975). The effects of parental divorce: Experiences of the pre-school child. *Journal of the American Academy of Child Psychiatry 14,* 600–616.

Wallerstein, J. S., & Kelly, J. B. (1980). *Surviving the breakup: How children and parents cope with divorce.* New York: Basic Books.

Warheit, G. J., & Auth, J. B. (1985). Epidemiology of alcohol abuse in adulthood. In J. O. Cavenar (Ed.), *Psychiatry* (Vol. 3, pp. 1–18). Philadelphia: J. P. Lippincott.

Webster-Stratton, C., & Hammond, M. (1988). Maternal depression and its relationship to life stress, perceptions of child behavior problems, parenting behaviors, and child conduct problems. *Journal of Abnormal Child Psychology, 16,* 299–315.

Weintraub, S., Liebert, D., & Neale, J. M. (1978). Teacher ratings of children vulnerable to psychopathology. In E. J. Anthony (Ed.), *The child and his family: Vol. 4. Vulnerable children* (pp. 335–346). New York: Wiley.

Weintraub, S., Prinz, R., & Neale, J. M. (1975). Peer evaluations of the competence of children vulnerable to psychopathology. *Journal of Abnormal Child Psychology, 6,* 461–473.

Weissman, M. M., Gammon, G. D., John, K., Merikangas, K. R., Warner, V., Prusoff, B. A., & Sholomskas, D. (1987). Children of depressed parents: Increased psychopathology and early onset of major depression. *Archives of General Psychology, 44,* 847–853.

Weissman, M. M., Prusoff, B. A., Gammon, G. D., Merikangas, K. R., Leckman, J. F., & Kidd, K. K. (1984). Psychopathology in the children (ages 6–18) of depressed and normal parents. *Journal of the American Academy of Child Psychiatry, 23,* 78–84.

Wells, L. E., & Rankin, J. H. (1991). Families and delinquency: A meta-analysis of the impact of broken homes. *Social Problems, 38,* 71–93.

Welner, Z., Welner, A., McCrary, M., & Leonard, M. A. (1977). Psychopathology in children of inpatients with depression: A controlled study. *Journal of Nervous and Mental Disease, 164,* 408–413.

Werner, E. E. (1984). Resilient children. *Young Children, 40,* 68–72.

Werner, E. E. (1989). High-risk children in young adulthood: A longitudinal study from birth to 32 years. *American Journal of Orthopsychiatry, 59,* 72–81.

West, O. M., & Prinz, R. J. (1987). Parental alcoholism and childhood psychopathology. *Psychological Bulletin, 102,* 204–218.

Whiffen, V. E. (1988). Vulnerability to postpartum depression: A prospective multivariate study. *Journal of Abnormal Psychology, 97,* 467–474.

Whiffen, V. E., & Gotlib, I. H. (1989). Infants of postpartum depressed mothers: Temperament and cognitive status. *Journal of Abnormal Psychology, 98,* 274–279.

Wierson, M., Forehand, R., & McCombs, A. (1988). The relationship of early adolescent functioning to parent-reported and adolescent-perceived interparental conflict. *Journal of Abnormal Child Psychology, 16,* 707–718.

Willerman, L., & Cohen, D. B. (1990). *Psychopathology.* New York: McGraw-Hill.

Wilson, C., & Orford, J. (1978). Children of alcoholics: Report of a preliminary study and comments on the literature. *Journal of Studies on Alcohol, 39,* 121–142.

Winters, K. C., Stone, A. A., Weintraub, S., & Neale, J. M. (1981). Cognitive and attentional deficits in children vulnerable to psychopathology. *Journal of Abnormal Child Psychology, 9,* 435–453.

Zahn-Waxler, C., Cummings, E. M., McKnew, D. H., & Radke-Yarrow, M. (1984). Altruism, aggression and social interactions in young children with a manic-depressive parent. *Child Development, 55,* 112–122.

8

Cognitive Causes
of Psychopathology

CHARLES G. COSTELLO

The word *cognition* usually refers to (1) the *processes* involved in receiving current information from the world around us, from our bodies, and from the information already stored in our brains—and thus embraces processes involved in attention, perception, learning, language, and memory—and to (2) the *processes* involved in our use of this information as we face the tasks of daily life—and thus embraces processes involved in problem solving, reasoning, believing, and judging. In many investigations of psychopathological disorders, however, it is cognitive *contents* (e.g., what is remembered) rather than cognitive *processes* (e.g., how the remembering is done) that have been studied. As shown later in the chapter, the measurement of cognitive contents rather than cognitive processes often makes it difficult to interpret research findings.

I am concerned in this chapter only with studies that have investigated whether certain cognitive processes or contents can cause a disorder. There is no question that cognitive processes such as attention and memory are impaired in some kinds of psychopathology. There are also biases in cognition that appear to be peculiar to some kinds of psychopathology, although they do not necessarily imply an impairment in cognitive processes. For instance, people with mood disorders appear to have a negative bias in their memory functioning such that unpleasant memories are more accessible to them than pleasant memories. I shall not be concerned with this research, which works within what Beck (1987) has called the cross-sectional model. He gives as an example, with respect to depression, the model that "asserts that negative content is an integral part of the depressive symptomatology and is as much a symptom as the affect of sadness or the behavioral impairments or deficiencies" (p. 7). Because I shall not cover cross-sectional studies, I shall not review the extensive literature on the cognitive dysfunction in those diagnosed as schizophrenic.

There is also good evidence that cognitive therapy is effective for some psychopathological conditions, particularly some of the mood disorders and some of the anxiety disorders, but I shall not review this research.

I shall then discuss the evidence for hypotheses that propose that cognitive processes and contents play a causal role in the occurrence of psychopathology. No one expects to find that some peculiarity in cognitive processes or contents is a necessary or sufficient cause of any kind of psychopathology. However, showing that some peculiarity in one or more of the cognitive processes or contents is significantly associated with a succeeding occurrence of psychopathology, with a worsening and persistence of psychopathology, or with a recurrence of psychopathology after recovery from an episode of illness will at least suggest the possibility that cognition has a causal role in some stage of the natural history of psychopathology.

I shall review the evidence for hypotheses that have been proposed as to how dysfunctional cognitive processes or contents may play a contributory causal role for mood disorders, anxiety disorders, conduct disorders, and substance use disorders.

There is some variability in how the term *psychopathology* is explicitly or implicitly used in the literature. A psychopathological condition, as the term is used in this chapter, is one that satisfies the criteria for a syndrome listed in a diagnostic system such as one of the editions of the *Diagnostic and Statistical Manual* (e.g., DSM-III, DSM-III-R [American Psychiatric Association, 1980, 1987]). I shall review only the research in which subjects have been identified as having a psychopathological disorder in this sense either on entry into the study or at some point in the course of the study. Some of the research on the cognitive hypotheses of psychopathology has measured psychopathology by using scores on a self-report instrument such as the Beck Depression Inventory (BDI) (Beck, Ward, Mendelson, Mock, & Erbaugh, 1961) or the Center for Epidemiological Studies Depression Scale (CES-D) (Radloff, 1977). If there were strong agreement between the identification of disturbances such as those in the BDI and the syndromes identified by systems such as the DSM-III-R, the research findings from investigations using such self-report instruments could be considered valid tests of the cognitive hypotheses, but the agreement is not strong (see Smith & Rhodewalt, 1991). A good review of the literature with respect to depression that is less restrictive than the present one in that it includes research using self-report measures can be found in Brewin (1985). Although I shall review only studies whose subjects have been diagnosed using a standardized diagnostic interview and associated diagnostic criteria, some of the data to be reviewed concerns changes in symptomatology as measured by self-report instruments such as the BDI.

With respect to mood disorders, another research area that I shall not review involves attempts to produce dysphoric moods by manipulating people's cognitions. If there were some good evidence that dysphoria at the intensity levels produced by such manipulations was the first stage at some point in the natural history of mood disorders, the data would be relevant to the concerns of this chapter, but there is no such evidence.

MOOD DISORDERS

The Beckian Hypothesis

This hypothesis states that people who are vulnerable to the onset, perseveration, and recurrence of mood disorders are those who have dysfunctional schemas that, when activated by, for instance, a stressful event or a mood disturbance, result in abnormalities in information processing, which in turn result in those people having negative views of themselves, their current experiences, and their future prospects.

The Seligmanian Hypothesis

This hypothesis states that people who are vulnerable to the onset, perseveration, and recurrence of some of the major symptoms of mood disorders (feelings of helplessness, loss of motivation, loss of self-esteem) possess some combination of the following beliefs: (1) that the negative events and circumstances of their lives are inevitable; (2) that they are personally responsible for their occurrence; (3) that their engendering of negative events and circumstances is due to enduring incapacities in their personalities; and (4) that these personal incapacities hinder their effectiveness in all aspects of their lives.

These hypotheses have been called the Beckian and the Seligmanian hypotheses rather than Beck's and Seligman's hypotheses because a number of writers have contributed to the elaborations of the hypotheses, and it is not always clear if Beck and Seligman endorse all components of the hypotheses or if they give more emphasis to some components than to others. For instance, the attributional reformulation of the learned helplessness hypothesis is often associated with the name of Abramson rather than Seligman because she was the senior author on the paper that first proposed the reformulation (Abramson, Seligman, & Teasdale, 1978). In relation to the Beckian hypothesis, Teasdale (1988) rather than Beck has emphasized the importance of abnormal cognitions in the worsening and perseveration rather than the onset of mood disorders.

Are Cognitions Involved in the Onset of Mood Disorders?

Cognitive measures did not predict onsets of depression in six studies: a community study (Lewinsohn, Steinmetz, Larson, & Franklin, 1981), three studies of postpartum depression (Gotlib, Whiffen, Wallace, & Mount, 1991; O'Hara, Neunaber, & Zekoski, 1984; O'Hara, Schlecte, Lewis, & Varner, 1991), a study of college students (Hammen, Marks, de Mayo, & Mayol, 1985), and a study of children at risk for depression (Hammen, Adrian, & Hiroto, 1988).

Positive results have been reported in five articles. Brown, Andrews, Harris, Adler, and Bridge (1986) in a 12-month follow-up of 303 working-class women found that 150 of the women had a severe life event or chronic difficulty. Thirty-three percent of those who had low self-esteem and experienced a life event or difficulty developed an onset of depression as against 13% of those who did not have low self-esteem. Level of self-esteem was not related to onset of depression in the 153 women who did not experience a severe life event or chronic difficulty. In further analyses of these data, reported in Brown, Bifulco, Veiel, and Andrews (1990) and in Brown, Bifulco, and Andrews (1990a), it was found that (1) with respect to the source of low self-esteem, negative interactions in current close relationships and early inadequate parenting were both significantly associated with low self-esteem; and (2) poor self-esteem in combination with negative interactions in current close relationships was significantly associated with both occurrence in a 12-month follow-up period of severe events arising out of chronic difficulties and severe events that were related to role conflicts, and lack of crisis support at the time of occurrence of the severe event.

In an analysis of some other data from this study, Andrews and Brewin (1990) found that six of the seven women who had been in a violent marital relationship and blamed their own character for the violence had an onset of depression during a 3-year study period when they were no longer in the relationship, compared with 12 of the 36 women who had experienced similar violence but had not blamed their character for the violence inflicted on them. However, a further analysis of the data for these women, which excluded six women who had not experienced a severe life event or major difficulty within the 3-year study period, suggests the possibility that the characterological blame variable was confounded with one of the life-stress variables. Among the 37 women with a stressor, all six with characterological self-blame were depressed in the study period compared with a third of the remaining 31 women; however, five of the six self-blaming women (83%) "were depressed as a result of problems in *subsequent* interpersonal relationships" (Andrews & Brewin, 1990, p. 764, original italics). Only 33% (4/12) of the women who did not blame themselves for the previous violence and who were depressed during the study period had problems in subsequent interpersonal relationships. Although the difference between these two percentages is not significant at the .05 level by Fisher's exact test, one would have to be very cautious about assigning a causal role in the development of depression to the cognitive variable of self-blame rather than to the problems in interpersonal relationships.

Miller, Kreitman, Ingham, and Sashidharan (1989) in a community study of women found that (1) women with low self-esteem who had made a previous psychiatric contact were at risk for onset of depression even in the absence of severe stress, and (2) women with low self-esteem with no previous psychiatric contact but with severe stress were at risk for depression.

Parry and Brewin (1988), using the Present State Examination (PSE), identified 27 cases of depression in a community sample of 193 working-class mothers with young children. They found that the depressed women who had *not* suffered a severely stressful event in the 12 months before the interview took greater responsibility for negative occurrences in their lives and had lower self-esteem than (1) the depressed women who had suffered such an event and (2) the nondepressed women whether or not they had suffered such an event. If the distinctive cognitive characteristics in relation to the attributions for negative events and perception of one's worth had occurred in both groups of depressed women—those who had and those who did not have an event—the hypothesis that these cognitive characteristics were simply a concomitant of depression would be just as plausible as the hypothesis that they were a cause of depression. Their occurrence only in the subgroup of depressed women who did not have an event does give some support to the causal hypothesis—as much support as one is likely to get in a cross-sectional study.

Hammen, Marks, Mayol, and deMayo (1985) classified their college students into *dependent* self-schematic individuals and *self-critical* schematic individuals on the basis of the recall of events that happened to them during the previous month. The students in the former group were hypothesized to experience negative interpersonal events as relatively more depressing than negative achievement events. The students in the latter group were hypothesized to show the opposite pattern. The psychiatric statuses of the students were monitored with the Schedule for Affective Disorders and Schizophrenia-Lifetime version (SADS-L) (Endicott & Spitzer, 1978) over a 4-month follow-up period. The occurrence of life events was also monitored over the same period. It was found that students with dependent self-schema were more likely to have an onset of depression according to the Research Diagnostic Criteria (RDC) (Spitzer, Endicott, & Robins, 1978) if they suffered a negative interpersonal event than if they suffered a negative achievement event.

Because of the difficulty of obtaining cognitive measures before the onset of depression, some researchers have examined the cognitions of individuals who have recovered from an episode of depression and argue that any evidence of cognitive abnormalities during remission would suggest that the abnormality is a stable characteristic of the individual. Some researchers have obtained evidence for such cognitive abnormalities after recovery from depression (Altman & Wittenborn, 1980; Cofer & Wittenborn, 1980; Eaves & Rush, 1984; Fennell & Campbell, 1984; Peselow, Robins, Block, Barouche, & Fieve, 1990), but many others have not found such evidence (Caine, 1970; Dobson & Shaw, 1987; Gotlib & Cane, 1987; Hamilton & Abramson, 1983; Hollon, Kendall, & Lumry, 1986; McCabe & Gotlib, 1990; Mayo, 1967; Miller & Norman, 1986; Reda, Carpiniello, Secchiaroli, & Blanco, 1985; Segal, Shaw, Vella, & Katz, 1992; Silverman, Silverman, & Eardley, 1984; Simons, Garfield, & Murphy, 1984; Wilkinson & Blackburn, 1981). More serious than the conflicting data is the questionable soundness of the argument. It is just as likely, as Lewinsohn and associates (1981) suggested, that any cognitive abnormalities detected after recovery from an episode of depression are simply residual effects of the depressive illness rather than an indication of some stable trait that existed before the illness occurred. Some evidence in support of this possibility was reported by Peselow and colleagues (1990). Then again, where no such abnormalities are detected they may have been removed by treatment.

A somewhat similar design to the one that examines patients in remission was used by Alloy, Lipman, and Abramson (1992). They found that among currently nondepressed individuals those who possessed a putative depressogenic attributional style, as assessed by the Attributional Style Questionnaire (ASQ) (Seligman, Abramson, Semmel, & von Baeyer, 1979), when compared with individuals who had a putative nondepressogenic attributional style, were more likely to have had major depressive episodes in the past, to have had more episodes, and to have had more severe episodes. The authors themselves noted, however, that it is not possible to distinguish with certainty between the hypotheses that increased rates of past depression among attributionally vulnerable individuals are due to the negative attributional style contributing to risk to past depression or due to past episodes of depression leading to a negative attributional style as a psychosocial "scar" or consequence of the depression.

In an interesting variation of the postrecovery design, Teasdale and Dent (1987) used music to induce a depressed mood in recovered-depressed and never-depressed people. While in the depressed mood, these individuals read a list of positive and negative trait adjectives indicating the adjectives that described them and those that did not. When asked to recall these adjectives in a later induced depressed mood, the recovered-depressed individuals recalled more negative adjectives than did the never-depressed individuals. In a similar study, Miranda and Persons (1988) found that individuals who reported a history of depression and high levels of momentary negative mood had more dysfunctional attitudes as measured by the Dysfunctional Attitude Scale than those with lower levels of momentary negative mood. Momentary mood did not have an effect on the dysfunctional attitudes scores of the never-depressed individuals. Despite the fact that the findings from these two studies and similar studies on mood (see, for instance, Nolen-Hoeksema, 1991) pique one's interest, they do not provide any clear evidence that abnormal cognitions are among the causes of the onset of mood disorders.

Are Cognitions Involved in the Maintenance of a Mood Disorder?

Gotlib and colleagues (1991) found no relationship between cognitions as measured by the Dysfunctional Attitudes Scale (DAS) (Weissman & Beck, 1978) during a woman's pregnancy and recovery from a depressive episode that had been experienced during pregnancy. However, some authors have claimed that evidence has been found for a significant relationship between cognitions and the course of a depressive episode.

A variety of cognitive measures have been used in these studies. For instance, Lewinsohn and associates (1981) investigated persistence of depression in a self-selected community sample of individuals 8 months after they had been diagnosed as having a mood disorder according to Research Diagnostic Criteria (RDC) (Spitzer et al., 1978). They found that, after control for initial severity of depression, those individuals who, at first testing, had low expectancy of positive outcomes (i.e., they responded in the negative to items such as "I will have periods of great happiness") and those who perceived that they had no control over their lives were more likely to still meet criteria for depression at the follow-up second testing 8 months later. However, as Teasdale (1988) has noted, there is a difficulty in interpreting these data. Agreeing with statements such as "I have little control over the things that happen to me" may indicate an objectively difficult life situation rather than a cognitive vulnerability.

In a study of individuals receiving treatment, Steinmetz, Lewinsohn, and Antonuccio (1983) found that a set of six variables (expected post-treatment Beck Depression Inventory [BDI] [Beck et al., 1961] scores, reading ability, age, social support from the family, concurrent treatment, and perceived mastery of the environment) was significantly related to outcome as determined by RDC 1 month after a psychoeducational group treatment. Unfortunately, the significance of each variable was not presented. However, the standard canonical discriminant function coefficients made available to me by Steinmetz (personal communication, 1990) were as follows: expected posttreatment BDI, $-.24190$; reading ability, .64983; age, .55516; social support from family, .09707; concurrent treatment, .41549; perceived mastery over the environment, $-.54767$. These coefficients indicate that the cognitive variable called *perceived mastery over the environment* was one of the important variables in the discrimination between the groups. Once again, however, Teasdale's (1988) cautionary comments concerning the possible confounding of cognitive and environmental factors must be kept in mind.

In Dent and Teasdale's (1988) study, 28 women identified in a community survey as meeting the RDC for a major or minor depressive episode or for intermittent depressive disorder were reassessed 5 months later. Two cognitive measures obtained at the first assessment correlated significantly with scores on the BDI obtained at the second assessment: repeated frequency of negative thoughts and the number of global trait words (e.g., *unloved, worthless*) endorsed as self-descriptive. However, only the second cognitive measure contributed significantly to the variance in the BDI scores on the second assessment after first assessment BDI scores were taken into account.

Brown, Bifulco, and Andrews (1990b) found that in a group of 40 women suffering from chronic depression 6 women who viewed themselves positively recovered during a 2-year follow-up period, whereas only 10 of the 34 women without such a positive view of themselves recovered. They did not find a significant association between the presence or absence of such a positive view of self and recovery in the 29 women who had an onset of depression in the period of the study.

Williams, Healy, Teasdale, White, and Paykel (1990) found that 6 (35%) of 16 patients with a major depressive disorder who also had high dysfunctional attitudes had not recovered 6 weeks after admission to hospital, whereas only 1 (6%) of 17 equally depressed patients with low dysfunctional attitudes had not recovered. There was a significant correlation between level of dysfunctional attitudes on admission and level of depression 6 weeks later, even after initial depression level and number of negative words the patients endorsed about themselves were taken into account. The dysfunctional attitudes were measured by the Dysfunctional Attitudes Questionnaire (DAQ) (Burns, 1980).

Although Gotlib and colleagues (1991) did not find a significant relationship between scores on the DAS and the course of depression, a number of studies that have used this measure of cognitions have reported positive findings. For instance, Simons, Murphy, Levine, and Wetzel (1986) followed up over a period of 1 year 44 patients of an original cohort of 70 patients, all of whom had a diagnosis of unipolar primary affective disorder as determined by the administration of the Diagnostic Interview Schedule (DIS) (Robins, Helzer, Croughan, & Ratcliff, 1981). The 44 patients who were followed up had responded to treatment of either cognitive therapy, pharmacotherapy, cognitive therapy plus active placebo, or cognitive therapy plus pharmacotherapy. Within the 1-year follow-up, 16 of the 44 patients had relapsed. Patients who had high scores on the DAS at the termination of treatment were significantly more likely to relapse, even after taking into account BDI scores at the termination of treatment.

Peselow and associates (1990) found that 112 patients with DSM-III major depression who responded to antidepressant drug treatment had significantly lower scores on the DAS before treatment than did the nonresponding patients.

The problem with studies using the DAQ and the DAS is that it is not at all clear that they are simply measuring cognitions. For instance, the questions in the DAQ ask respondents how much they agree with statements reflecting seven domains: needs for approval, love, achievement, perfectionism, entitlement, omnipotence, and autonomy. Two examples of the items in the questionnaire are: "My value as a person depends greatly on what others think of me" (need for approval) and "I should be able to please everybody" (need to be omnipotent). One may very well ask if these questions are clearly measuring cognitions. It may be that they are measuring needs that individuals report because the needs appear in consciousness as desires or because the individuals are aware of the needs from the observation of their behaviors.

A number of studies have investigated if risk of relapse in depression is increased when a life event of an interpersonal or achievement-related sort occurs that matches the predominant needs of an individual, that is, needs with respect to interpersonal relationships or in relation to achievements. Some of these studies have used the DAS to classify subjects in relation to their needs. Segal, Shaw, and Vella (1989) monitored every 2 months for a period of 6 months 26 remitted RDC unipolar depressed patients, 10 of whom were of a dependent personality type according to their DAS responses and 16 of whom were of a self-critical personality type. They found that for dependent subjects, if an interpersonal stressful life event occurred, there were significant increases in self-reported levels of depression and in clinical relapse. Self-critical subjects did not show a significant vulnerability to either interpersonal events or achievement events. The authors were careful not to make any claims that they had found evidence for cognitive vulnerability. They discussed their findings in terms of personality types and simply proposed that the personality type might be influential through the mediation of some cognitive process:

> In attempting to account for the congruency effect in the dependent group, one explanation which has been offered regarding a possible mechanism of action suggests that the experience of dysphoria following exposure to a subtype-congruent life event in predisposed individuals results from the activation of a cognitive/affective structure or schema . . . This structure may be comprised of negative or depressive elements and may begin to exert an increasingly intrusive influence on the patient's information processing, thereby making the conclusions or appraisals regarding those life events less amenable to experimental disconfirmation. (p. 397)

Segal and colleagues (1992) seem to have been less careful in their interpretation of data from a later study. In this study they monitored 59 remitted RDC depressed people over six occasions spaced 2 months apart. Thirty of these individuals relapsed during the 1-year follow-up. Those who were self-critical, as determined by the DAS, relapsed more often after experiences with achievement-related events than after the occurrence of interpersonal events. This significant effect was found after taking into account the number of prior episodes of depression. The title of the article refers to cognitive and life stress predictors of relapse, and the authors implied at two points in their article that with the DAS they had measured a cognitive variable. At other points in the article, however, they referred to the DAS as measuring personality styles, personality traits, character traits, motivations, and concerns related to needs. It is significant that the authors, commenting on the lack of agreement between studies measuring similar personality types with different measures, suggested that there might be more consistency if there was "a comparison of self-report with behavioral measures of these concerns and the retention of subjects who satisfied criteria derived from both assessment methods" (p. 32). If one were to do this, one would surely not be simply investigating the effects of a cognitive variable.

Another instrument that has been used to measure subjects' needs is the Sociotropy–Autonomy Scale (SAS; Beck, Epstein, Harrison, & Emery, 1983). Hammen, Ellicott, and Gitlin (1989) monitored every 2 to 4 weeks over a period of 6 to 24 months the symptoms of 27 patients with a DSM-III unipolar major depressive episode. The patients were also interviewed every 3 months to determine if life events had occurred in the

3 months since the last interview. They also completed, at the beginning of the study, the SAS. It was found that in the 3 months prior to the patient's worst symptom period there occurred significantly more life stress that matched the patient's vulnerability type than stress that did not match it. In a regression analysis, the interaction of autonomy needs and the occurrence of achievement events, but not the interaction of sociotropy needs and the occurrence of interpersonal events, predicted the severity of depressive symptoms. Although the authors described their study as one that investigated a cognitive–life stress integrative model, one might again wonder if the description is justified. Beck and colleagues (1983) describe their scale as measuring personality factors. The authors of the study themselves commented:

> Although we have suggested that it is the manner in which life events are appraised that makes them "depressing" or not, the present study does not directly test the mechanism by which events are associated with depression. We speculate that personal values and cognitions about self-worth determine the nature of interpretation of events, but it remains for future studies to clarify the cognitive processes likely to be involved. (p. 385)

One might add: "If indeed the crucial causal processes are of a cognitive sort."

Hammen, Ellicott, Gitlin, and Jamison (1989) monitored 22 unipolar and 25 bipolar DSM-III mood disordered patients every 2 to 4 weeks for a 6-month period. They found that, for unipolar patients, symptom exacerbations were significantly more likely to be preceded by life events that were congruent with the patient's personality type as measured by the SAS. Although they wrote that they used the SAS as "an indicator of 'meaning' attached to events in the achievement and interpersonal domains" (p. 155), implying that the variable investigated was a cognitive one, other comments in their article suggest some hesitancy. For instance, the first sentence of the discussion section reads: "Unipolar patients displayed specific vulnerability to stressful life events that matched their relative *motivation* for autonomous achievement or affiliation" (p. 158, italics added). Later in the section they commented:

> We have hypothesized that the sociotropy/autonomy distinction captures a construct of personal meaning about the self that is associated with having depressive cognitions when negative events occur. We might further speculate that a self-schema process accounts for the way in which information is appraised for its relevance to the self. . . . However, the present study provides no test of such a process, and the actual mechanism linking personal motives, appraisal of events and depression remains to be clarified. (p. 159)

Discussion

Although there is some evidence here and there that cognitions play a causal role in the natural history of mood disorders, there is considerable inconsistency in the findings and ambiguity in their interpretation. This inconsistency and ambiguity may be due to the inadequacy of the cognitive theories (Coyne & Gotlib, 1983, 1986; Hilton, 1990; Power, 1991; Power & Champion, 1986; Safran, Segal, Hill, & Whiffen, 1990; Segal, 1988), the poor conceptual status of the cognitive concepts (Peterson, 1991a, 1991b, with twelve commentaries), and problems in the designs of the research used to test the theories (Brewin, 1985; Costello, 1992; Kuiper, Olinger, & Martin, 1990; Power, 1990; Robins, 1988; Segal & Shaw, 1986, Williams, Watts, MacLeod, & Mathews, 1988).

The most serious problems seem to be:

1. The inadequate statistical power of many of the studies. Robins (1988) found that analyses involving psychiatric patients (the focus of the present review) had significantly lower power than those using other subjects such as undergraduate students. This was due to the categorizing of patients samples.

2. All of the research that has been done used concepts of psychopathology that are either too intricate or too isolated. *Major depressive episode,* as defined in DSM-III-R, is an example of a too intricate concept because it refers to a polythetic class, the members of which suffer from different combinations of a set of quite different symptoms such as dysphoria, anhedonia, sleep problems, and psychomotor retardation, which are probably functionally related in quite complex ways. Abramson and her colleagues (Abramson, Alloy, & Metalsky, 1990; Abramson, Metalsky, & Alloy, 1989) have attempted to deal with this problem by identifying a specific subtype of depression, which they have called *hopelessness* depression. They have stated that a necessary condition for the validity of their hopelessness theory of depression is that the hypothesized symptoms of hopelessness depression should be intercorrelated with one another and not as highly correlated with other symptoms of depression. However, eight of the list of nine symptoms of hopelessness depression they have presented are essentially the same as eight of the nine symptoms listed for a major depressive episode in DSM-III-R, so it is not clear just what is supposed to be distinctive about the symptoms of hopelessness depression.

Research on the cognitive variables associated with depressed mood is an example of research with a too isolated concept of psychopathology. If the goal of such research is to discover the cognitive causes of a mood disorder, it is unlikely that much progress will be made without including at least one other symptom and demonstrating the relationships with the cognitions and the two or more symptoms of the disorder.

3. With respect to research on the role played by cognitive schemas in psychopathology, there are a number of problems: (1) The reliance on self-reports in some of the research in which pathogenic schemas are assessed by measuring cognitions such as dysfunctional attitudes or the occurrence of automatic negative thoughts. In view of the complexity of the cognitive material that people are asked to report on, there is understandable doubt about the veracity of the reports (see Nisbett and Wilson [1977] for a discussion of problems concerning the veracity of verbal reports). Furthermore, some of the cognitive processes that cause psychopathological disorders may be out of awareness (see Clark [1988] and Hammen and Krantz [1985] for critical reviews of methods of cognitive assessment). (2) Beckian theories postulate that in order to demonstrate the role played by cognitive schemas in causing psychopathology the schema must be primed either by stimuli that occur naturally, such as stressful life events, or by stimuli presented in the laboratory, and this is overlooked by some researchers. (3) When the stimuli that are presented in the laboratory are chosen by the experimenter because in a general sense they are expected to evoke pathogenic schemas, they may not do so because the stimuli are not relevant to a particular individual's schemas. For instance, stimuli designed to evoke pathogenic schemas concerning achievement failure would not have much effect on an individual whose pathogenic schemata concern interpersonal relationships.

4. With respect to tests of Seligmanian attributional or explanatory style theories postulating that some of the cognitive causes of psychopathology can be found in the beliefs people hold concerning characteristics of the causes of stressful events, the problems are that (1) the construct validity of the concept of attributional style has not been well established; for instance, its distinctiveness from concepts such as neuroticism, negative affectivity, and pessimism is uncertain. (2) There is controversy over whether a composite measure of attributions such as those concerning the internality, stability, and globality of the putative cause of a event should be used in research rather than each component separately. If a composite measure was to be used, it is not yet known if it should be an additive or interactive composite. A related concern is that researchers appear to have ignored the specific predictions arising from the reformulated model of learned helplessness (Abramson, Seligman, & Teasdale, 1978) to the effect that attributions relating to the *stability* of the cause of an event affect the *persistence* of depression, attributions relating to *globality* affect the *pervasiveness* of depression, and attributions relating to *internality* affect an individual's level of *self-esteem*. (3) There is controversy over whether the perception of the controllability of the perceived cause of an event is subsumed under one or more of the attributions concerning the internal-

ity, stability, and globality of the cause. (4) The social context of the individual whose attributions are being assessed has been neglected. (5) It is unlikely that attributions about the causes of events are the only or even most important cognitive causes of psychopathology. Other contenders are judgements about the morality of events and one's ability to cope with the consequences of events.

ANXIETY DISORDERS

There are three theories concerning the causal role of cognitions in anxiety disorders: Clark's (1986) catastrophic misinterpretations theory, Chambless's cognitive theory of panic (Goldstein & Chambless, 1978; Chambless & Goldstein, 1988; Chambless, Beck, Gracely & Bibb, 1989), and Rachman's (1988) theory concerning the role of expectations in panic attacks.

The Clark and Chambless Theories

Clark (1986) has proposed that a panic occurs when a person catastrophically misinterprets the significance of some bodily sensation. He gave the following examples: "a healthy individual perceiving palpitations as evidence of impending heart attack; perceiving a slight feeling of breathlessness as evidence of impending sensation of breathing and consequent death; or perceiving a shaky feeling as evidence of impending loss of control and insanity" (Clark, 1986, p. 462).

Goldstein and Chambless (1978) proposed that panics are due to (1) a fear of body sensations associated with panic and (2) maladaptive thoughts about the consequences of becoming anxious. More recently (Chambless & Goldstein, 1988; Chambless, Beck, Gracely, & Bibb, 1989), the theory was modified to include the misinterpretation of cues that do not arise from anxiety, which has made the theory more similar to Clark's theory.

Clark (1988) has argued that the following findings support his theory:

1. Patients report the occurrence of catastrophic interpretations during panic attacks. Of course, this finding provides no support because there is no evidence that the catastrophic interpretations occur before the onset of panic. They could be concomitants or consequences of the panic.

2. Normal subjects, given the expectation that CO_2 inhalation would produce a state of relaxation, reported a pleasant experience. Those who were told that it would produce a mild aversive state had an unpleasant experience. Apart from the fact that the subjects' responses to

the demand characteristics of the situation might account for the findings, however, demonstrating that cognitive set can modify the affective response to induced bodily sensations would seem to have very little bearing on the problem of what causes panic attacks.

The findings reported by Rapee, Mattick, and Murrell (1986) look a little more promising. In their study, single inhalations of a 50% carbon dioxide and 50% oxygen gas mixture were administered to 16 subjects with spontaneous panic attacks and 16 social phobics who did not experience such attacks. Half of each of the panic and social phobic subjects were randomly allocated to an explanation condition in which all possible sensations resulting from the inhalation were described, and half were allocated to a no explanation condition. The panic attack subjects who were given no explanation reported a greater proportion of catastrophic cognitions, greater panic, and a greater similarity of the overall experience to naturally occurring panic attacks than the panic attack subjects who received an explanation. Both groups of social phobics reported similar effects of the inhalation regardless of the explanation given. The ameliorative effects of the cognitive manipulation does suggest that the panic that results from CO_2 inhalations is mediated by a cognitive mechanism. However, the study is far from providing any unequivocal evidence for the causal role of cognitions in the onset of a panic attack.

3. Cognitive therapy directed at the reduction of catastrophic misinterpretations of bodily sensations reduces the frequency of panic attacks. However, there does not appear to have been a test of the effectiveness of *pure* cognitive therapy. The therapy always includes other interventions such as training in respiratory control.

One of the most direct tests of Clark's theory has been reported by Rachman, Levitt, and Lopatka (1987). Their subjects have been panic disorder patients and university undergraduates whose answers to a Fear of Enclosed Spaces Questionnaire (FOESQ) (Rachman, 1993) indicated that they were claustrophobic. After each of a number of exposures to their feared situations (a closet for the claustrophobics and behavioral test walks for those with panic disorder), the subjects reported the bodily sensations and cognitions they had experienced in the situations. The self-reports of body sensations were obtained by means of the list of symptoms in the diagnostic criteria for panic disorder in the DSM-III 14-item checklist of body symptoms and a 10-item shortened version of the Agoraphobics Cognitions Questionnaire (Chambless, Caputo, Bright, & Gallagher, 1984).

Rachman and his colleagues reported a number of findings they considered to be consistent with Clark's theory:

1. They found that bodily sensations and fearful cognitions were endorsed more frequently on trials when the subjects experienced panics than on trials when no panics were experienced. However, it is not at all surprising that the subjects experienced more bodily sensations on panic trials because the experience of body sensations are predominant in diagnostic criteria for panic disorder. Fearful cognitions do not receive the same emphasis, but they are included, for instance, in DSM-III-R, where one of the criteria is "fear of dying, going crazy or doing something uncontrolled during an attack."

2. Rachman and colleagues (1987) wrote: "Clark's writing leads one to expect that there should be a meaningful, if not always rational, relationship between body symptoms and cognition; they should fit. The sensation of heart palpitations should be associated with the fear of cardiac illness, dizziness should be linked to the fear that one might lose control, etc." (p. 411). They found that, of the 140 correlations calculated between 14 body sensations and 10 cognitions, 7 (5%) were significant for the panic disorder patients and 17 (12%) for the claustrophobic subjects. The small proportion of significant correlations might not be a cause for concern because a conservative alpha level ($p < .001$) was adopted, and it was predicted in a general manner that only the sensations and cognitions that could be *meaningfully* linked (e.g., "palpitations" and "I am going to have a heart attack") would be significantly correlated. However, specific predictions were not made as to which sensations would be significantly correlated with which cognitions, and deciding which of the significant correlations reported by Rachman and his colleagues reflect meaningful links cannot be confidently done. For instance, the cognition "I am going to pass out" was significantly correlated with "choking," "faintness," and "depersonalization." The first two correlations would seem to be measures of the strength of meaningful links, but there would not seem to be any compelling reason to consider the link between "I am going to pass out" and "depersonalization" to be a meaningful link. The problem of which links could be considered meaningful needs to be addressed with a clearer understanding of what is meant by "meaningful links" and by an investigation of the reliability of classifying links as meaningful or not.

3. Two related findings were that (1) panics that were accompanied by fearful cognitions (cognitive panics) were also accompanied by more body sensations than were noncognitive panics, and (2) when combinations of two or three of the most common body sensations were selected and matched with each of the 10 cognitions, no panics were reported if the combination of sensations occurred without an associated cognition. Even if one could assume that the constructs "panic," "bodily sensations," and "cognitions" are being measured independently, the problem

still remains of what is causing what. Rachman and his colleagues clearly believe that fearful cognitions play a causal role:

> When they *were* associated with a panic cognition . . . [the] combination of [bodily sensation] symptoms ended in a panic in most instances. So, for example, the combination of breathlessness and dizziness plus a cognition (pass out, lose control, panic) ended in panic on 11 out of 13 occasions; but in all of the *no-panic* trials with this combination of [bodily sensation] symptoms there was no associated panic cognition." (Rachman et al., 1987, p. 418, original italics)

But there are many other causal pathways. For instance, the awareness of bodily sensations may increase the likelihood of fearful cognitions and the experience of panic without the cognitions playing a causal role.

There have been four other tests of the Clark and Chambless theories, those by Chambless and colleagues (1989); Pollard and Frank (1990); Street, Craske, and Barlow (1989); and Warren, Zgourides, and Englert (1990). The main purpose of these four studies was the same as that of the Rachman group (1987) study, namely, to examine the extent to which during periods when they were panicking (or fearful in the Warren et al. [1990] study) subjects would experience certain pairs of body sensations and cognitions. In all five studies, except the one by Street and colleagues (1989), where no predictions in this connection were made, it was specifically predicted that the subjects would experience combinations of body sensations and cognitions that could be considered meaningfully related.

There are three problems with these five studies:

1. The first is the ambiguity and indistinguishability of the "body sensations" and "cognitions" concepts. It is not clear what the measures of body sensations and cognitions used in the five studies are actually measuring. The body sensations measure includes items such as "dizziness," which would indeed appear to be a body sensation, and "fear of dying," which most people would probably not consider to be a body sensation, not, at least, in the same sense as dizziness. It is also not at all certain that the measures of body sensations and cognitions are measuring different variables. The Agoraphobics Cognitions Questionnaire (Chambless et al., 1984) includes items such as "I am going to pass out" and "I am going to suffocate." There is no obvious reason why these items should be cognitions rather than body sensations. Similarly, in Pollard and Frank's (1990) investigation, if individuals check the items "I will faint" on the cognitions list to indicate that it is an experience they have when they panic, and if they also check on the physical symptoms

list that the sensation of faintness occurs, can they really be said to be referring to two different phenomena, one of which causes the other? Is "nausea" in Pollard's physical symptoms list referring to a different experience than the experience referred to as "I am going to throw up" on the cognitions list?

Suspicion that the body sensations and cognition concepts in these studies are indistinguishable is increased when one examines the results of the Chambless and associates (1989) study. In a factor analysis of the items of the Agoraphobics Cognitions Questionnaire and Body Sensations Questionnaire (Chambless et al., 1984) that had been administered to 142 agoraphobic outpatients, they found that the semantically related descriptions of body sensations and cognitions loaded on the same factors. For instance, on Factor 1 the cognition "I am going to have a heart attack" had a high loading, as did the body sensations "heart palpitations" and "pressure in chest." On Factor 2 there was a high loading for the cognition "I am going to pass out" and the body sensation "dizziness." On Factor 3, the cognition "I am going to throw up" had a high loading, as did the body sensation "nausea." Similar results were found for samples of anxious outpatients without panic disorder and normal volunteers. Chambless and her colleagues interpret their findings as being supportive of theories that postulate that one cause of panic is the catastrophic misinterpretations of body sensations. However, a more plausible interpretation is that self-report items such as "I am going to throw up" and "nausea" simply denote the same experience.

2. Another problem is the uncertain meaning of "meaningful relationships." In none of the five studies being discussed has the meaning of a meaningful relationship between body sensations and cognitions been spelled out, and only two of the studies (Chambless et al., 1989; Pollard & Frank, 1990) have made predictions as to which pairs of body sensations and cognitions could be considered meaningfully linked and therefore would be significantly correlated.

Because the meaning of "meaningful relationships" has not been clearly defined and because the measurements of body sensations and cognitions are not clearly distinguishable, one might have predicted that the conceptual framework for the tests of the catastrophic misinterpretation theories would be loose enough to produce consistency in the findings of the five studies. However, there is a surprising lack of consistency. Not one pair of body sensations and cognitions resulted in significant correlations in all five studies, even when one takes into consideration obvious synonyms. For instance, the body sensation "shortness of breath" and the cognition "I will pass out" were significantly correlated in the Chambless group's (1989) study and in the Warren group's (1990) study, and the body sensation "difficulty in breathing" and the cognition "I will faint" were correlated in Pollard and Frank's (1990) study. But the body sensation "shortness of breath" and the cognition "I will pass out" were not significantly correlated in either the Rachman group's (1987) study or the Street group's (1989) study. For these particular body sensations and cognitions, then, the correlations were significant in only three of the five studies. But this hit rate might be considered good when one takes into account that only one other body sensation/cognition pair (i.e., the body sensation "faintness" and the cognition "I will pass out" or "I will faint") were significantly correlated in three of the five studies. Of the 84 pairs of body sensations and cognitions that were significantly correlated in one or another of the five studies, none was significant in all five or even four of the studies; as noted before, two pairs were significantly correlated in three studies, although not the same three studies; 17 pairs were significantly correlated in two studies, although not the same two studies; and 65 pairs in only one or other of the five studies.

3. The third problem is differences between Clark's theory and Chambless's theory. The lack of consistency in the findings of the five studies suggests that the conceptual frameworks of Clark's and Chambless's theories are too loose, that the differences between the two theories may be more crucial than they seem, and that the ways in which the theories were tested in the five studies may not be as comparable as they seem at first glance.

As noted previously, Chambless and colleagues (1989) considered their revised theory to be similar to Clark's (1986) theory because it recognizes the possibility that panic may be caused by the catastrophic misinterpretation of body sensations that are not associated with anxiety. However, whereas Clark simply proposes that panic occurs when the occurrence of certain body sensations is accompanied by catastrophic misinterpretations of those sensations, Chambless proposes that panic occurs when there is a *fear of* certain body sensations accompanied by catastrophic misinterpretations of the sensations. Therefore, the Chambless theory is a less pure cognitive theory than Clark's theory in that one component of their theory involves the affective concept of fear.

The five studies also differ in the degree to which they are pure tests of the cognitive causes of panic. The studies by the Rachman group (1987) and Pollard and Frank (1990) are purer in that their subjects were simply asked to indicate the extent to which, when they were panicking, certain body sensations and cognitions occurred. In the Chambless group's (1989) study and the Warren group's (1990) study, the subjects also simply had to indicate how often the cognitions occurred when they were panicking or anxious, but on the body sensations list they had to indicate how *frightened* they were by the body sensations when they were panicking or anxious. In the Street and associates (1989) study, affective variables appear to be introduced in relation to both body sensations and cognitions in that the subjects had to indicate how *frightened* they were by the body sensations and how *disturbed* they were by the cognitions.

This review of the tests of two cognitive theories of panic suggests that:

1. The theories are too loosely formulated, and the differences between them are not always appreciated. For instance, Chambless and colleagues (1989) wrote that one of the purposes of their investigation was to determine, whether, as predicted by Clark (1986), agoraphobics' self-reported fear of somatic symptoms would be reliably associated with logically related catastrophic cognitions; however, Clark's theory refers to the *occurrence* of body sensations and not to the *fear* of such sensations.

2. The construct and discriminant validity of the measures of body sensations and cognitions has not been established. The problem of the indistinguishability of the body sensations and cognitions when measured by self-reports may be overcome to some extent by the use of objective measurements of physiological responses.

3. There is no clear definition of *meaningful relationships* between body sensations and cognitions and no evidence that judges can reliably classify the relationships with respect to meaningfulness.

4. There is too great a reliance on correlational data. Because of the difficulties in arriving at any conclusions concerning causal processes on the basis of such data, priority should be given to experimental studies in which body sensations and cognitions are manipulated. Whether experimental or nonexperimental studies are conducted, measurements of body sensations and cognitions should be done concurrently with their occurrence rather than retrospectively.

5. Finally, there is a general issue that perhaps should be kept in mind: It is possible that some of the relationships between body sensations and cognitions will *not* be meaningful and that herein lies one of the causes of the psychopathological condition known as panic disorder. Pollard and Frank (1990) noted that in their study, "Despite the many physical symptoms associated with panic attacks, concern about psychological catastrophe (e.g. I will lose control and I will embarrass myself) appears to be a more usual feature of agoraphobic panic than does concern about medical or physical incapacitation" (p. 13). The links between body sensations and thoughts about what Pollard and Frank call psychological catastrophe may not always, or even usually, be meaningful. In the Rachman and associates (1987) study, significant correlations were found between thoughts of "losing control" and each of the following body sensations: palpitations, sweating, and flushes/chills. In the Street and colleagues (1989) study, significant correlations were found between

thoughts of screaming and each of the following body sensations: faintness, wobbly legs, sweating, and knots in stomach.

There might be advantages from the point of view of the researcher
if the cognitive aspects of panic involved meaningless rather than meaningful relationships between body sensations and cognitions. In the first
chapter of this book I discussed the problem of researching relationships
between concepts that are incontrovertibly related. Smedslund (1987) has
presented a similar argument noting that "Causal relationships, as traditionally conceived, can only exist between semantically unrelated entities" (p. 43). Significant correlations between semantically related statements such as the body sensation "faintness" and the cognition "I am
going to faint" do not enjoy much of a status as empirical findings because
the correlation is a logical consequence of their semantic relatedness and,
therefore, is knowable a priori. It may be argued that in the studies
reviewed there has been a remarkable absence of consistent significant
correlations between semantically related body sensations and cognitions. This may be a measurement problem and not of particular theoretical interest, although it may have important implications for the validity
of our measurement procedures. Smedslund (1984) described this situation as follows:

> A noncontingent proposition states under what conditions something must
> necessarily occur or be the case. This means that, if the expected outcome is
> obtained, one may surmise, but not know for certain, that the procedure was
> indeed efficient. On the other hand, if the expected outcome is *not* obtained,
> then one knows with certainty that the required conditions have not been
> established and, therefore, that the procedure was not efficient. . . . Noncon-
> tigent propositions offer unique advantages in the testing of psychological
> procedures. Indeed, it would seem that procedure-testing research should,
> whenever possible, rely on noncontingent propositions for maximal effi-
> ciency. (p. 245, original italics)

Alternatively, it may be that under certain conditions, such as having
a panic attack, things happen in a more illogical than logical manner.
Perhaps this has something to do with the puzzle that Seligman (1988) has
pointed out: If the cause of panic attacks is the catastrophic misinterpretation of bodily sensations, why is this cognitive habit not given up when
it is repeatedly disconfirmed in the experience of the panic-disordered
patient? The heart attacks, the passing out, the madness, the other catas-
trophes do not occur, and yet the cognitive habit persists.

Rachman's Hypothesis Concerning the Role
of Expectations

Rachman (1988) has hypothesized that unexpected panic attacks are more
likely than expected panic attacks to increase (1) subsequent intensity of

fear, (2) the probability of further panic attacks, (3) the intensity of further panic attacks, (4) the probability of avoidance behavior, (5) the level of tonic arousal, and (6) the development of conditioned psychophysiological responses.

There appears to be evidence only in relation to the first hypothesis concerning the relationship between unexpected panic attacks and the subsequent intensity of fear. One experiment, discussed in Rachman and Levitt (1985) and Rachman (1988), involved asking 13 claustrophobic undergraduate students to enter a small enclosed room on a number of trials and getting them to provide reports of their *expectations* of panic and fear *before* each trial. Reports of their *experiences* of panic and fear *during* each trial were also obtained. The findings indicate that whether or not a panic experienced on any trial had been expected had no significant effect on the amount of fear experienced on the following trial and that the occurrence of neither expected nor unexpected panics on any trial was followed by a significant increase in the fear experienced in the subsequent trial.

These findings indicate that, contrary to Rachman's hypothesis, expectations of panic in a specific situation and the confirmation or disconfirmation of those expectations do not play a causal role in an individual's subsequent experiences of fear in the same situation. However, the occurrence of unexpected panics, when compared with the occurrence of expected panics, resulted in a significantly greater increase in an individual's expectancies of future panic attacks. Similar results were found in studies of patients with panic disorder (Rachman, Lopatka, & Levitt, 1988; Street, Craske, & Barlow, 1989) and students with snake phobias (Rachman & Lopatka, 1986a, 1986b).

It might be expected that the increase in predictions of panic and fear that occurs after unexpected occurrences of panic and fear would increase avoidance behavior. There does not appear to have been a test of this specific hypothesis concerning the effects on avoidance behavior of the increased expectations of panic and fear following an unexpected panic attack or fear. However, Rachman and Lopatka (1986b) have presented evidence that inclinations toward avoidance, indicated by slower approaches to a feared snake and hesitations, increased after snake-phobic subjects had experienced on a previous trial more fear than they had predicted. No evidence was presented that these avoidancelike behaviors were mediated by increased expectations of fear.

Three studies have obtained evidence that the more one expects to panic or experience fear in a situation, the more one is likely to avoid it, but only one of these studies went beyond self-report data. Twenty-eight patients with panic disorder in a study reported by Craske, Rapee, and Barlow (1988) attempted to perform three behavioral tests that were self-rated as evoking low, moderate, and high degrees of fear/avoidance. There were 57 cases of task completion, 11 cases of escape (the patient entered the test situation but withdrew before the test was completed), and 15 cases of complete avoidance. They found that the greater the predicted probability of panic, the more likely the patient was to avoid or escape the test situation.

Warren, Zgourides, and Jones (1989), in a study of 33 anxiety-disordered patients, 57 patients with a variety of psychiatric disorders, and 60 normal subjects, found that the more individuals thought it was likely that something catastrophic would happen when they were anxious or panicking, as indicated by their responses to the Agoraphobics Cognitions Questionnaire (ACQ) (Chambless, Caputo, Bright, & Gallagher, 1984), the more likely it was that they avoided situations associated with anxiety or panic, as indicated by their responses to the Mobility Inventory for Agoraphobia (MI) (Chambless, Caputo, Jasin, Gracely, & Williams, 1985). Similarly, Telch, Brouillard, Telch, Agras, and Taylor (1989) found that patients diagnosed as having panic disorder with agoraphobia when compared with patients with panic disorder without avoidance anticipated more panic in a variety of situations.

It does seem that expectancies of panic and fear are a determinant of avoidance behavior. However, there is no clear evidence at present that expectancies or any other cognitions play a causal role in the onset of fear and panic.

CONDUCT PROBLEMS

A number of cross-sectional studies have found significant associations between IQ and conduct disorder (Berger, Yule, & Rutter, 1975; Farrington, 1978; Richman, Stevenson, & Graham, 1982; Rutter, Tizard, & Whitmore, 1970; West & Farrington, 1973), between IQ and aggression (Huesmann, Eron, Lefkowitz, & Walder, 1984; Kellam, Branch, Agrawal, & Ensminger, 1975; Lewis, Shanok, & Pincus, 1981), and between social–cognitive competence and conduct problems (Dodge, 1986; Freedman, Rosenthal, Donahoe, Schlundt, & McFall, 1978). Although these studies suggest the possibility of a causal role for cognition in the development of conduct problems, they provide no clear evidence for such a role.

One of these studies does not provide some indirect support for impaired cognitive functioning as a cause of conduct problems. Rutter and colleagues (1970) found that families of conduct-disordered children with reading retardation had lower rates of parental discord than families of conduct-disordered children without reading retardation. This suggests the possibility of at least two routes to conduct disorder: cognitive dysfunction and parental discord.

However, nonexperimental evidence with any persuasiveness can come only from longitudinal studies. In one such study, Schonfeld, Schaffer, O'Connor, and Portnoy (1988) analyzed data for 115 17-year-old black males, 30 of whom had a conduct disorder and for whom data on a number of variables were available at age 4 and age 7. They found that the young men with conduct disorders had, at age 7, significantly lower full-scale WISC IQs. However, in a path analysis of the data for the 30 subjects with conduct disorder and the 64 with no psychiatric disorder, the age 7 WISC IQ did not have a significant path coefficient relating it to a global assessment of psychiatric functioning (GAS) at age 17. The global assessments were described by the authors as giving an index of the severity of the conduct disorder. The full scale WAIS IQ at age 17 did have a significant path coefficient to GAS, and its predictive validity was equal to that of parent psychopathology and signs of aggression at age 7. Because the WAIS IQs at age 17 were measured at the same time as the GAS, one might question whether there was any convincing evidence of IQ level being among the causes of conduct disorder. The authors gave two arguments in favor of entertaining the possibility of such a causal relationship:

> We considered the possibility that we misspecified our path-analytic models. For example, adolescent psychopathology and WAIS IQ may influence each other bidirectionally, or some third factor may cause both WAIS IQ and GAS. In order to rule out these alternatives we examined the WAIS IQ and GAS residuals using LISREL procedures (Joreskog & Sorbom, 1981). In each analysis the residuals were uncorrelated, a result that is incompatible with those two possibilities (Kenny, 1979). (p. 1002)

> One final test was conducted to rule out the possibility that change in IQ from age 7 to 17 (either increase or decrease) rather than trait IQ affected psychiatric functioning. The least-squares regression analyses were repeated with an IQ change scores replacing full-scale IQ. The results of the analysis failed to reveal anything approaching an effect for IQ change. (p. 1002)

Some other data presented by the authors are not as supportive of the causal status of IQ. They found that whereas a subscale of acquired knowledge (based on the WAIS tests of Information, Vocabulary, and Arithmetic) showed a significant path coefficient to GAS, for a subscale of spatial ability (Block Design, Object Assembly, and Picture Completion) the path coefficient to GAS was not significant. The authors considered the acquired knowledge and spatial ability scales to reflect, respectively, acculturation (crystallized) and native (fluid) aspects of intelligence. Patterson's (1990) suggestion, when commenting on this study, that the impairment in acquired knowledge may have been a consequence of the conduct problems because the child's noncompliance and coercive style would have made it difficult to teach him academic subjects is as plausible as the Schonfeld and associates' (1988) hypothesis, which gives a causal role to the cognitive impairment.

Another longitudinal study was conducted by Huessman, Eron, and Yarmel (1987). They examined the correlations between IQ and aggression measured at age 8 and aggression and intellectual competence at age 30 for a variable number of men and women (from 63 to 335), depending on the measures used. They found that for males only three of the eight measures of aggression at age 30 were significantly correlated with IQ at age 8, and the correlations were small (age-8 IQ correlation with aggression measured by the MMPI scales $F + 4 + 9 = -.19$; with criminal justice convictions $r = -.15$; with seriousness of criminal act, $r = -.14$). Only one of the eight age 30 measures of aggression, punishment of child by subject, was significantly correlated ($r = .21$) with age-8 aggression for the female subjects, and it is noteworthy that the brighter young children were more likely to abuse their children when adults.

By contrast, aggression at age 8 was significantly correlated with all three measures of intellectual competence at age 30 for the male and female subjects (r's ranged from $-.20$ to $-.37$, $M = -.30$). Regression analyses indicated that the subject's change in intellectual functioning from age 8 to age 30 is partially predictable from the subject's age-8 aggression, but the subject's change in aggression from age 8 to age 30 is not at all predictable from the subject's age-8 IQ.

In summary there is no good evidence for the causal role of cognition in the development of conduct disorders.

SUBSTANCE USE DISORDERS

There has been a considerable amount of research on the relationships between alcohol expectancies—the beliefs that individuals hold about the effects of alcohol on their behavior, moods, and emotions—and the drinking of alcohol. There has also been a fair amount of cross-sectional research comparing expectancies of alcoholics, problem drinkers, and nonproblem drinkers concerning the effects of alcohol (see Leigh [1989] for a review). However, these studies do not provide any evidence that cognition plays a causal role in substance use disorders. Neither does research that indicates that the sons of male alcoholics have comparatively poor linguistic, abstraction, and problem-solving abilities and poor academic performance records (see review by Pihl, Peterson, & Finn, 1990).

A number of longitudinal studies have been done. In their 33-year follow-up of the 456 nondelinquent controls from the Gluecks' delinquency study, Vaillant and Milofsky (1982) found that 30% of 71 alcohol-dependent men had IQs lower than 90 at age 14 ± 2 compared with 28% of the men who were social drinkers, a nonsignificant difference.

Christiansen, Smith, Roehling, and Goldman (1989) reported data from a 1-year longitudinal investigation of 637 seventh- and eight-grade students. They found that expectancies concerning the effects of alcohol measured at Time 1 significantly predicted the likelihood of problem drinking having occurred by Time 2, a year later. However, alcohol expectancy was significantly correlated with alcohol consumption at Time 1, and there was no analysis of the relationship between Time 1 expectancies and Time 2 problem drinking after controlling for Time 1 alcohol consumption. Appropriate controls were made in a study by Stacy, Newcomb, and Bentler (1991). They found that cognitive motivation factors reflecting anticipated positive effects of using alcohol and marijuana, measured during adolescence ($M = 17.95$ years), predicted the use and abuse of these drugs 9 years later ($M = 26.95$ years), even after controlling for the effects of the frequency of drug use in adolescence and general social conformity in adolescence. The cognitive factors related to alcohol that were measured in adolescence predicted problems with drug use in adulthood, but the cognitive factors related to marijuana did not.

In the study reported by Hull, Young, and Jouriles (1986), investigating the role played by self-awareness in causing relapse, 35 males nearing completion of a detoxification program completed a self-consciousness inventory and a life event survey. When a life event that reflected the individual's successful or unsuccessful performance of a role had occurred during the previous 12 months, the subject rated the event on a seven-unit scale ranging from -3 (very negative impact on my life) to $+3$ (very positive impact on my life). When relapse was examined 3 months later, the correlation between the valence of self-relevant life events and relapse was significant for the 17 high-self-conscious subjects ($r = -.54$) but not for the 18 low-self-conscious subjects ($r = .09$). Similar results were obtained for the 6-months relapse data, with the respective correlations being $-.40$ and $.14$. However, a study reported by Chassin, Mann, and Sher (1988) did not find data in support of the causal role of self-awareness. In their study, 308 high school students, 49% of whom were male, were assessed at the beginning of the high school year in relation to level of self-awareness, perceived school achievement, and the occurrence of negative and positive self-relevant life events in the previous 12 months. Level of self-awareness either alone or in interaction with poor school achievement or the occurrence of negative life events did not predict symptomatic drinking, which was assessed at the end of the school year.

Researchers have not found any evidence that neuropsychological test performance measured at the time of treatment predicts posttreatment drinking status (Donovan, Kivilahan, & Walker, 1984; Eckardt et al., 1988; Parsons, Schaeffer, & Glenn, 1990).

In summary, there does not appear to be any evidence that those at risk for substance use disorders have any specific cognitive deficits or that they have particularly high levels of self-awareness. However, there is some evidence that expectancies concerning the effects of drugs play a causal role in the development of such disorders.

CONCLUSIONS

The notion that cognition may play a causal role in the development of psychopathology, although eminently sensible on an intuitive level, has not received much research support. The only exception seems to be the predictive validity of people's expectancies. It has been found that if people expect to be fearful in a situation they will avoid that situation, and the finding appears to be replicable. Unfortunately, it does not take us any closer to understanding the causes of fear and similar experiences such as anxiety and panic. A more interesting finding concerning expectancy is that if children and adolescents expect that alcohol and drugs will have positive effects on them they are more likely to develop substance use disorders as adults. However, the replicability of this finding has not been firmly established, and the possibility of confounding variables needs more attention.

In general, there is a lot of inconsistency in the findings of the research into the possible cognitive causes of psychopathology. However, that is not the most serious problem. More serious is the ambiguity of the findings. The ambiguity arises from the cognitive variables that have been investigated.

In some instances, the variables do not appear to be pure cognitive variables at all but are simply cognitive assessments of noncognitive variables such as environmental circumstances (e.g., the controllability of one's life), somatic conditions (e.g., the likelihood of fainting), or motivations (e.g., the extent to which one desires good interpersonal relationships.) Such reports, although they involve cognitive processes of some sort, cannot be described simply as cognitive variables. Should we measure the discrepancy between such reports and the actual circumstances being reported, our measure might be considered more cognitive in nature, but even here considerable ambiguity remains. A person's report is an action. Anything noteworthy about it may be due to something significant about that person's cognitions. Nevertheless, there are many other possible sources of the report, such as motivation, affect, and habit. So, for instance, a person's report about need for good interpersonal relationships may not jibe with observers' assessments of the need made on the basis of the person's behavior. The discrepant report may have its source not in the person's cognitive processes but in some motivation such as the desire to deceive the hearer.

The fundamental problem seems to be that psychopathologists have, for the most part, investigated cognitive contents rather than processes. If a case is to be made for cognitive causes of psychopathology, then one must demonstrate that people are more likely to develop psychopathological conditions if they show some peculiarity in cognitive processes, such as the way of perceiving or remembering things, and not simply in the things they perceive or remember.

One problem, then, with researching cognitive contents is that although cognitive processes may be involved in the measurement of the variable it is not cognitive per se. Another problem is that the cognitive content (e.g., self-appraisal) may be semantically linked with the psychopathological disorder (e.g., depression) being investigated. Beck (1984) is aware of this problem. Commenting on the inadvisability of the notion that such cognitions are a cause of depression, he wrote:

> This notion has always struck me as rather far-fetched, somewhat in the same class as an assertion that "delusions cause schizophrenia" . . . a far more satisfactory view of causality in depression would view this condition as the resultant of a variety of innate and environmental factors . . . cognitive phenomena such as the unmitigated negative self-references and expectancies are an integral part of depression; consequently, hardly capable of causing themselves. (p. 1113)

Segal and Shaw (1986), having presented this quotation from Beck, wrote: "Seen in this light the importance of cognition is not due to its hypothesized causal role, but rather to the fact that it allows access to the system of integrated dysfunctions which characterize the disorder and which are observable at both a molecular (biochemical changes) or molar (cognitive changes) level of analysis" (p. 672).

No one would disagree with Beck's statement that cognitive contents may be one way in which a psychopathological condition manifests itself, and many people would agree with the implication of Segal and Shaw's statement, namely, that the examination of cognitive contents may be one way of accessing the causes of disorder. If researchers wish to demonstrate that cognitions are themselves among the causes of psychopathology, however, then cognitive processes will have to be investigated. Furthermore, it would seem advisable to investigate the possible cognitive causes of specific symptoms of disorder and their interrelationships rather than attempt to discover the cognitive causes of complex, chameleon-like diagnoses.

REFERENCES

Abramson, L., Seligman, M., & Teasdale, J. (1978). Learned helplessness in humans: Critique and reformation. *Journal of Abnormal Psychology, 87,* 49–74.

Abramson, L. Y., Alloy, L. B., & Metalsky, G. I. (1990). Hopelessness depression: An empirical search for a theory-based subtype. In R. E. Ingram (Ed.), *Contemporary psychological approaches to depression* (pp. 37–58). New York: Plenum Press.

Abramson, L. Y., Metalsky, G. I., & Alloy, L. B. (1989). Hopelessness depression: A theory-based subtype of depression. *Psychological Review, 96,* 358–372.

Alloy, L. B., Lipman, A. J., & Abramson, L. Y. (1992). Attributional style as a vulnerability factor for depression: Validation by past history of mood disorders. *Cognitive Therapy and Research, 16,* 391–407.

Altman, J. H., & Wittenborn, J. R. (1980). Depression-prone personality in women. *Journal of Abnormal Psychology, 89,* 303–308.

American Psychiatric Association. (1980). *Diagnostic and statistical manual of mental disorders* (3rd ed.). Washington, DC: Author.

American Psychiatric Association. (1987). *Diagnostic and statistical manual of mental disorders* (3rd ed., rev.). Washington, DC: Author.

Andrews, B., & Brewin, C. R. (1990). Attributions of blame for marital violence: A study of antecedents and consequences. *Journal of Marriage and the Family, 52,* 757–767.

Beck, A. T. (1984). Cognition and therapy. *Archives of General Psychiatry, 411,* 1112–1114.

Beck, A. T. (1987). Cognitive models of depression. *Journal of Cognitive Psychotherapy, 1,* 5–37.

Beck, A. T., Epstein, N., Harrison, R., & Emery, G. (1983). *Development of the Sociotropy–Autonomy Scale: A measure of personality factors in psychopathology.* Unpublished manuscript, University of Pennsylvania, Philadelphia.

Beck, A. T., Ward, C. H., Mendelson, M., Mock, J., & Erbaugh, J. (1961). An inventory for measuring depression. *Archives of General Psychiatry, 4,* 561–571.

Berger, M., Yule, W., & Rutter, M. (1975). Attainment and adjustment in two geographical areas: II. The prevalence of specific reading retardation. *British Journal of Psychiatry, 126,* 510–519.

Brewin, C. R. (1985). Depression and causal attributions: What is their relation? *Psychological Bulletin, 98,* 297–309.

Brown, G. W., Andrews, B., Harris, T. O., Adler, Z., & Bridge, L. (1986). Social support, self-esteem and depression. *Psychological Medicine, 16,* 813–831.

Brown, G. W., Bifulco, A., & Andrews, B. (1990a). Self-esteem and depression: III. Aetiological issues. *Social Psychiatry and Psychiatric Epidemiology, 25,* 235–243.

Brown, G. W., Bifulco, A., & Andrews, B. (1990b). Self-esteem and depression: IV. Effect on course and recovery. *Social Psychiatry and Psychiatric Epidemiology, 25,* 244–249.

Brown, G. W., Bifulco, A., Veil, H. O. F., & Andrews, B. (1990). Self-esteem and depression: II. Social correlates of self-esteem. *Social Psychiatry and Psychiatric Epidemiology, 25,* 225–234.

Burns, D. D. (1980). *Feeling good: The new mood therapy.* New York: Signet.

Caine, T. M. (1970). Personality and illness. In P. Mittler (Ed.), *The psychological assessment of mental and physical handicap* (pp. 781–817). London: Methuen.

Chambless, D. L., Beck, A. T., Gracely, E. J., & Bibb, J. L. (1989). *The relationship of cognitions to fear of somatic symptoms: A test of the cognitive theory of panic.* Unpublished manuscript.

Chambless, D. L., Caputo, G. C., Bright, P., & Gallagher, R. (1984). Assessment of fear of fear in agoraphobics: The Body Sensations Questionnaire and the Agoraphobic Cognitions Questionnaire. *Journal of Consulting & Clinical Psychology, 52,* 1090–1097.

Chambless, D. L., Caputo, G. C., Jasin, S. E., Gracely, E. J., & Williams, C. (1985). The mobility inventory for agoraphobia. *Behaviour Research and Therapy, 23,* 35–44.

Chambless, D. L., & Goldstein, A. J. (1988). Fear of fear: A reply to Reiss. *Behavior Therapy, 19,* 85–88.

Chassiu, L., Mann, L. M., & Sher, K. J. (1988). Self-awareness theory, family history of alcoholism and adolescent alcohol involvement. *Journal of Abnormal Psychology, 97,* 206–217.

Christiansen, B. A., Smith, G. T., Roehling, P. V., & Goldman, M. S. (1989). Using alcohol expectancies to predict adolescent drinking behavior after one year. *Journal of Consulting and Clinical Psychology, 57,* 93–99.

Clark, D. A. (1988). The validity of measures of cognition: A review of the literature. *Cognitive Therapy and Research, 12,* 1–20.

Clark, D. M. (1986). A cognitive approach to panic. *Behaviour Research and Therapy, 24,* 461–470.

Clark, D. M. (1988). A cognitive model of panic attacks. In S. Rachman & J. D. Maser (Eds.), *Panic: Psychological perspective* (pp. 71–89). Hillsdale, NJ: Erlbaum.

Cofer, D. H., & Wittenborn, J. R. (1980). Personality characteristics of formerly depressed women. *Journal of Abnormal Psychology, 89,* 309–314.

Costello, C. G. (1992). Conceptual problems in current research on cognitive vulnerability to psychopathology. *Cognitive Therapy & Research, 16,* 379–390.

Coyne, J. C., & Gotlib, I. H. (1983). The role of cognition in depression: A critical appraisal. *Psychological Bulletin, 94,* 472–505.

Coyne, J. C., & Gotlib, I. H. (1986). Studying the role of cognition in depression: Well trodden paths and cul-de-sacs. *Cognitive Therapy and Research, 10,* 794–812.

Craske, M. G., Rapee, R. M., & Barlow, D. H. (1988). The significance of panic expectancy for individual patterns of avoidance. *Behavior Therapy, 19,* 577–592.

Dent, J., & Teasdale, J. D. (1988). Negative cognition and the persistence of depression. *Journal of Abnormal Psychology, 97,* 29–34.

Dobson, K. S., & Shaw, B. F. (1987). The specificity and stability of self-referential encoding in clinical depression. *Journal of Abnormal Psychology, 96,* 34–40.

Dodge, K. A. (1986). A social information processing model of social competence in children. In M. Perlmutter (Ed.), *Minnesota symposium on child psychology* (Vol. 18, pp. 77–125). Hillsdale, NJ: Erlbaum.

Donovan, D. M., Kivilahan, D. R., & Walker, R. D. (1984). Clinical limitations of neuropsychological testing in predicting treatment outcome among alcoholics. *Alcoholism: Clinical and Experimental Research, 5*, 470–475.

Eaves, G., & Rush, A. J. (1984). Cognitive patterns in symptomatic and remitted unipolar major depression. *Journal of Abnormal Psychology, 56*, 431–445.

Eckardt, M. J., Rawlings, R. R., Graubard, B. I., Fader, V., Martin, P. R., & Gottschalk, L. A. (1988). Neuropsychological performance and treatment outcome in male alcoholics. *Alcoholism: Clinical and Experimental Research, 12*, 88–93.

Endicott, J., & Spitzer, R. L. (1978). A diagnostic interview: The Schedule for Affective Disorders and Schizophrenia. *Archives of General Psychiatry, 35*, 837–844.

Farrington, D. P. (1978). The family backgrounds of aggressive youths. In L. A. Hersov, M. Berger, & D. Shaffer (Eds.), *Aggression and antisocial behaviour in childhood and adolescence* (pp. 73–93). Oxford: Pergamon Press.

Fennell, M. J. V., & Campbell, E. A. (1984). The Cognitions Questionnaire: Specific thinking errors in depression. *British Journal of Clinical Psychology, 23*, 81–92.

Freedman, B. J., Rosenthal, L., Donahoe, C. P. Jr., Schlundt, D. G., & McFall, R. M. (1978). A social–behavioral analysis of skill deficits in delinquent and non-delinquent adolescent boys. *Journal of Consulting and Clinical Psychology, 46*, 1448–1462.

Goldstein, A. J., & Chambless, D. L. (1978). A reanalysis of agoraphobia. *Behavior Therapy, 9*, 47–59.

Gotlib, I. H., & Cane, D. B. (1987). Construct accessibility and clinical depression: A longitudinal investigation. *Journal of Abnormal Psychology, 96*, 199–204.

Gotlib, I. H., Whiffen, V. E., Wallace, P. M., & Mount, J. H. (1991). A prospective investigation of postpartum depression: Factors involved in onset and recovery. *Journal of Abnormal Psychology, 100*, 122–132.

Hamilton, E. W., & Abramson, L. Y. (1983). Cognitive patterns and major depressive disorder: A longitudinal study in a hospital setting. *Journal of Abnormal Psychology, 92*, 173–184.

Hammen, C., Adrian, C., & Hiroto, D. (1988). A longitudinal test of the attributional vulnerability model in children at risk for depression. *British Journal of Clinical Psychology, 27*, 37–46.

Hammen, C., Ellicott, A., & Gitlin, M. (1989). Vulnerability to specific life events and prediction of course of disorder in unipolar depressed patients. *Canadian Journal of Behavioural Science, 21*, 377–388.

Hammen, C., Ellicott, A., Gitlin, M., & Jamison, K. R. (1989). Sociotropy/autonomy and vulnerability to specific life events in patients with unipolar depression and bipolar disorders. *Journal of Abnormal Psychology, 98*, 154–160.

Hammen, C., & Krantz, S. E. (1985). Measures of psychological processes in depression. In E. E. Beckham & W. R. Leber (Eds.), *Handbook of depression:*

Treatment assessment and research (pp. 408–444). Homewood, IL: Dorsey Press.

Hammen, C., Marks, T., de Mayo, R., & Mayol, A. (1985). Self-schemas and risk for depression: A prospective study. *Journal of Personality and Social Psychology, 49,* 1147–1159.

Hammen, C., Marks, T., Mayol, A., & de Mayo, R. (1985). Depressive self-schemas, life stress, and vulnerability to depression. *Journal of Abnormal Psychology, 94,* 308–319.

Hilton, D. J. (1990). Conversational processes and causal explanation. *Psychological Bulletin, 107,* 65–81.

Hollon, S. D., Kendall, P. C., & Lumry, A. (1986). Specificity of depressotypic cognitions in clinical depression. *Journal of Abnormal Psychology, 95,* 52–59.

Huesmann, L. R., Eron, L. D., Lefkowitz, M. M., & Walder, L. O. (1984). Stability of aggression over time and generations. *Developmental Psychology, 20,* 1120–1134.

Huesmann, L. R., Eron, L. D., & Yarmel, P. W. (1987). Intellectual functioning and aggression. *Journal of Personality and Social Psychology, 52,* 232–240.

Hull, J. G., Young, R. D., & Jouriles, E. (1986). Applications of the self-awareness model of alcohol consumption: Predicting patterns of use and abuse. *Journal of Personality and Social Psychology, 51,* 790–796.

Joreskog, K. G., & Sorbom, D. (1981). *LISREL V: User's guide.* Chicago: National Educational Resources.

Kellam, S. G., Branch, J. D., Agrawal, D. C., & Ensminger, M. E. (1975). *Mental health and going to school: The Woodlawn Program of Assessment, Early Intervention and Evaluation.* Chicago: University of Chicago Press.

Kenny, D. A. (1979). *Correlation and causality.* New York: Wiley.

Kuiper, N. A., Olinger, L. J., & Martin, R. A. (1990). Are cognitive approaches to depression useful? In C. D. McCann & N. S. Endler (Eds.), *Depression: New directions in theory, research, and practice* (pp. 53–75). Toronto: Wall & Emerson.

Leigh, B. C. (1989). In search of the seven dwarves: Issues of measurement and meaning in alcohol expectancy research. *Psychological Bulletin, 105,* 361–373.

Lewinsohn, P., Steinmetz, J., Larson, D., & Franklin, J. (1981). Depression-related cognitions: Antecedent or consequence? *Journal of Abnormal Psychology, 90,* 213–219.

Lewis, D. O., Shanok, S. S., & Pincus, J. N. (1981). The neuropsychiatric status of violent male delinquents. In D. O. Lewis (Ed.), *Vulnerabilities to delinquency* (pp. 67–88). New York: Spectrum.

McCabe, S. B., & Gotlib, I. H. (1990). *Attentional processing in clinically depressed subjects: A longitudinal investigation.* Unpublished manuscript, University of Western Ontario.

Mayo, P. R. (1967). Some psychological changes associated with improvement in depression. *British Journal of Social and Clinical Psychology, 6,* 63–68.

Miller, I. W., & Norman, W. H. (1986). Persistence of depressive cognitions within a subgroup of depressed inpatients. *Cognitive Therapy and Research, 10,* 211–225.

Miller, P. McC., Kreitman, N. B., Ingham, J. G., & Sashidharan, S. P. (1989).

Self-esteem, life stress and psychiatric disorder. *Journal of Affective Disorders, 17,* 65–75.

Miranda, J., & Persons, J. B. (1988). Dysfunctional attitudes are mood-state dependent. *Journal of Abnormal Psychology, 97,* 76–79.

Nisbett, R. E., & Wilson, T. D. (1977). Telling more than we can know: Verbal reports on mental processes. *Psychological Review, 84,* 231–259.

Nolen-Hoeksema, S. (1991). Responses to depression and their effects on the duration of depressive episodes. *Journal of Abnormal Psychology, 100,* 569–582.

O'Hara, M. W., Neunaber, D. J., & Zekoski, E. M. (1984). A prospective study of postpartum depression: Prevalence, course and predictive factors. *Journal of Abnormal Psychology, 93,* 158–171.

O'Hara, M. W., Schlecte, J. A., Lewis, D. A., & Varner, M. W. (1991). Controlled prospective study of postpartum mood disorders: Psychological, environmental and hormonal variables. *Journal of Abnormal Psychology, 100,* 63–73.

Parry, G., & Brewin, C. R. (1988). Cognitive style and depression: Symptom related, event-related or independent provoking factor? *British Journal of Clinical Psychology, 27,* 23–35.

Parsons, O. A., Schaeffer, K. W., & Glenn, S. W. (1990). Does neuropsychological test performance predict resumption of drinking in posttreatment alcoholics? *Addictive Behaviors, 15,* 297–307.

Patterson, G. R. (1990). Some comments about cognitions as causal variables. *American Psychologist, 45,* 984–985.

Peselow, E. D., Robins, C., Block, P., Barouche, F., & Fieve, R. R. (1990). Dysfunctional attitudes in depressed patients before and after clinical treatment and in normal control subjects. *American Journal of Psychiatry, 147,* 439–444.

Peterson, C. (1991a). The meaning and measurement of explanatory style. *Psychological Inquiry, 2,* 1–10.

Peterson, C. (1991b). Further thoughts on explanatory style. *Psychological Inquiry, 2,* 50–57.

Pihl, R. O., Peterson, J., & Finn, P. (1990). An heuristic model for the inherited predisposition to alcoholism. *Psychology of Addictive Behaviors, 4,* 12–25.

Pollard, C. A., & Frank, M. A. (1990). Catastrophic cognitions and physical sensations of panic attacks associated with agoraphobia. *Phobia Practice and Research Journal, 3,* 3–18.

Power, M. J. (1990). A prime time for emotion: Cognitive vulnerability and the emotional disorders. In K. J. Gilhooly, M. T. G. Keane, R. H. Logie, & G. Erdos (Eds.), *Lines of thinking* (Vol. 2, pp. 157–165). New York: Wiley.

Power, M. J. (1991). Cognitive science and behavioral psychotherapy: Where behaviour was, there shall cognition be? *Behavioural Psychotherapy, 19,* 20–41.

Power, M. J., & Champion, L. A. (1986). Cognitive approaches to depression: A theoretical critique. *British Journal of Clinical Psychology, 25,* 201–212.

Rachman, S. (1988). Panics and their consequences: A review and prospect. In S. Rachman & J. Maser (Eds.), *Panic: Psychological perspectives* (pp. 259–303). Hillsdale, NJ: Erlbaum.

Rachman, S. (1993). *The Fear of Enclosed Spaces Questionnaire.* Manuscript in preparation.

Rachman, S., & Levitt, K. (1985). Panics and their consequences. *Behaviour Research and Therapy, 23,* 585–600.

Rachman, S., Levitt, K., & Lopatka, C. (1987). Panic: The links between cognitions and bodily symptoms: I. *Behaviour Research and Therapy, 25,* 411–423.

Rachman, S., & Lopatka, C. (1986a). Match and mismatch in the prediction of fear: I. *Behaviour Research and Therapy, 24,* 387–393.

Rachman, S., & Lopatka, C. (1986b). Match and mismatch of fear in Gray's Theory: II. *Behaviour Research and Therapy, 24,* 395–401.

Rachman, S., Lopatka, C., & Levitt, K. (1988). Experimental analyses of panic: II. Panic patients. *Behaviour Research and Therapy, 26,* 33–40.

Radloff, L. S. (1977). The CES-D Scale: A self-report depression scale for research in the general population. *Applied Psychological Measurement, 1,* 385–401.

Rapee, R., Mattick, R., & Murrell, E. (1986). Cognitive mediation in the affective component of spontaneous panic attacks. *Journal of Behavior Therapy and Experimental Psychiatry, 17,* 245–253.

Reda, M. A., Carpiniello, B., Secchiaroli, L., & Blanco, S. (1985). Thinking, depression, and antidepressants: Modified and unmodified depressive beliefs during treatment with amitriptyline. *Cognitive Therapy and Research, 9,* 135–143.

Richman, N., Stevenson, J., & Graham, P. J. (1982). *Pre-school to school: A behavioural study.* London: Academic Press.

Robins, C. J. (1988). Attributions and depression: Why is the literature so inconsistent? *Journal of Personality and Social Psychology, 54,* 880–889.

Robins, L. N., Helzer, J. E., Croughan, J., & Ratcliff, K. S. (1981). National Institute of Mental Health Diagnostic Interview Schedule: Its history, characteristics and validity. *Archives of General Psychiatry, 38,* 381–389.

Rutter, M., Tizard, J., & Whitmore, K. (1970). *Education, health and behaviour.* London: Longman.

Safran, J. D., Segal, Z. V., Hill, C., & Whiffen, V. (1990). Refining strategies for research on self-representations in emotional disorders. *Cognitive Therapy and Research, 14,* 143–160.

Schonfeld, I. S., Shaffer, D., O'Connor, P., & Portnoy, S. (1988). Conduct disorder and cognitive functioning: Testing three causal hypotheses. *Child Development, 59,* 993–1007.

Segal, Z. V. (1988). Appraisal of the self-schema construct in cognitive models of depression. *Psychological Bulletin, 103,* 147–162.

Segal, Z. V., & Shaw, B. F. (1986). Cognition in depression: A reappraisal of Coyne and Gotlib's critique. *Cognitive Therapy and Research, 10,* 671–693.

Segal, Z. V., Shaw, B. F., & Vella, D. D. (1989). Life stress and depression: A test of the congruency hypothesis for life event content and depressive subtype. *Canadian Journal of Behavioural Science, 21,* 389–400.

Segal, Z. V., Shaw, B. F., Vella, D. D., & Katz, R. (1992). Cognitive and life stress predictors of relapse in remitted unipolar depressed patients: Test of the congruency hypothesis. *Journal of Abnormal Psychology, 101,* 26–36.

Seligman, M. E. P. (1988). Competing theories of panic. In S. Rachman & P. D. Maser (Eds.), *Panic: Psychological perspectives.* Hillsdale, NJ: Erlbaum.

Seligman, M. E. P., Abramson, L. Y., Semmel, A., & von Baeyer, C. (1979). Depressive attributional style. *Journal of Abnormal Psychology, 88,* 242–247.

Silverman, J. S., Silverman, J. A., & Eardley, D. A. (1984). Do maladaptive attitudes cause depression? *Archives of General Psychiatry, 41,* 28–30.

Simons, A. D., Garfield, S. L., & Murphy, G. E. (1984). The process of change in cognitive therapy and pharmacotherapy for depression: Changes in mood and cognition. *Archives of General Psychiatry, 41,* 45–51.

Simons, A. D., Murphy, G. E., Levine, J. L., & Wetzel, R. D. (1986). Cognitive therapy and pharmacotherapy for depression. *Archives of General Psychiatry, 43,* 43–48.

Smedslund, J. (1984). What is necessarily true in psychology? In J. R. Royce & L. P. Mos (Eds.), *Annals of theoretical psychology* (Vol. 2, pp. 241–272). New York: Plenum Press.

Smedslund, J. (1987). The epistemic status of inter-item correlations in Eysenck's Personality Questionnaire: The *a priori* versus the empirical in psychological data. *Scandinavian Journal of Psychology, 28,* 42–55.

Smith, T. W., & Rhodewalt, F. T. (1991). Methodological challenges at the social/clinical interface. In C. R. Snyder & D. R. Forsyth (Eds.), *Handbook of social and clinical psychology* (pp. 739–756). Elmsford, NY: Pergamon Press.

Spitzer, R. L., Endicott, J., & Robins, E. (1978). Research diagnostic criteria. *Archives of General Psychiatry, 34,* 773–782.

Stacy, A. W., Newcomb, M. D., & Bentler, P. M. (1991). Cognitive motivation and drug use: A 9-year longitudinal study. *Journal of Abnormal Psychology, 100,* 502–515.

Steinmetz, J. L., Lewinsohn, P. M., & Antonuccio, D. O. (1983). Prediction of individual outcome in a group intervention for depression. *Journal of Consulting and Clinical Psychology, 51,* 331–337.

Street, L. L., Craske, M. G., & Barlow, D. H. (1989). Sensations, cognitions and the perception of cues associated with expected and unexpected panic attacks. *Behaviour Research and Therapy, 27,* 189–198.

Teasdale, J. D. (1988). Cognitive vulnerability to persistent depression. *Cognition and Emotion, 2,* 247–274.

Teasdale, J. D., & Dent, J. (1987). Cognitive vulnerability to depression: An investigation of two hypotheses. *British Journal of Clinical Psychology, 26,* 113–126.

Telch, M. J., Brouillard, M., Telch, C. F., Agras, W. S., & Taylor, C. B. (1989). Role of cognitive appraisal in panic-related avoidance. *Behaviour Research and Therapy, 27,* 373–383.

Vaillant, G. E., & Milofsky, E. S. (1982). The etiology of alcoholism: A prospective viewpoint. *American Psychologist, 37,* 494–503.

Warren, R., Zgourides, G., & Englert, M. (1990). Relationship between catastrophic cognitions and body sensations in anxiety disordered, mixed diagnosis and normal subjects. *Behaviour Research and Therapy, 28,* 355–357.

Warren, R., Zgourides, G., & Jones, A. (1989). Cognitive bias and irrational belief as predictors of avoidance. *Behaviour Research and Therapy, 27,* 181–188.

Weissman, A. N., & Beck, A. T. (1978, November). *Development and validation of the dysfunctional attitude scale: A preliminary investigation.* Paper presented at the annual meeting of the American Educational Research Association, Toronto, Canada.

West, D. J., & Farrington, D. P. (1973). *Who becomes delinquent?* London: Heinemann.

Wilkinson, I. M., & Blackburn, I. M. (1981). Cognitive style in depressed and recovered depressed patients. *British Journal of Clinical Psychology, 20,* 283–292.

Williams, J. M. G., Healy, D., Teasdale, J. D., White, W., & Paykel, E. S. (1990). Dysfunctional attitudes and vulnerability to persistent depression. *Psychological Medicine, 20,* 375–381.

Williams, J. M. G., Watts, F. N., MacLeod, C., & Mathews, A. (1988). *Cognitive psychology and emotional disorders.* Chichester, England: Wiley.

III

THE COURSES
AND CONSEQUENCES
OF PSYCHOPATHOLOGY

9

Specific and Nonspecific Effects in Psychological Treatments

LISA GRENCAVAGE

RICHARD R. BOOTZIN

VARDA SHOHAM

Many different psychological interventions have been applied to the treatment of psychopathology. They include interpersonal psychotherapy, counseling, cognitive–behavioral therapy, family therapy, psychoeducational therapy, and group therapy, among others. Each of these broad categories includes a wide range of interventions that vary by orientation, goals of the intervention, and breadth of focus. Some interventions are highly focused (e.g., relaxation training), whereas others are broad and have a general goal, such as self-understanding (e.g., some forms of insight-oriented psychotherapy). Given the diversity of interventions and problem areas to which they can be applied, it is not possible in one chapter to review the literature for every intervention as applied to every problem with regard to specific and nonspecific effects. In this chapter we address general issues that apply to all interventions and illustrate those points by an examination of studies in two problems areas, insomnia and depression. We use the term *psychotherapy* to encompass the entire range of psychological interventions. Where appropriate, specific interventions are identified.

Clinical outcome research (e.g., Elkin et al., 1989; Frances, Sweeney, & Clarkin, 1985; Kazdin, 1986; Lambert, Shapiro, & Bergin, 1986;

Landman & Dawes, 1982; Luborsky, Singer, & Luborsky, 1975; Shapiro & Shapiro, 1982; Smith, Glass, & Miller, 1980; Stiles, Shapiro, & Elliott, 1986) has established that psychotherapy is generally effective. Although doing much to settle the question of general efficacy, this collective body of research does little to enlighten our understanding of how and why psychotherapy works.

How are we to account for psychotherapeutic success (and failure)? Are they due to specific or nonspecific factors? Specific factors are those particular therapeutic maneuvers espoused by a particular theoretical orientation as being necessary for the amelioration of a particular symptom or disorder. By definition, they are well-defined, theoretically derived, intentional actions or intervention strategies on the part of the therapist (Jones, Cumming, & Horowitz, 1988) that are unique to a specific brand of psychotherapy. The application of these techniques is believed to be causally responsible for client relief, with the explanation for this causal connection coming from the theory from which the techniques were derived (Butler & Strupp, 1986). For example, a specific factor in cognitive therapy is the alteration of a client's distorted cognitions to more adaptive ones. A specific factor in psychoanalysis is the resolution of unconscious conflicts through interpretation and the working through of the transference.

Nonspecific factors are those unspecified variables (Kazdin, 1979) that are common to all forms of effective psychotherapy. Elements of the client–therapist relationship (Frank, 1981; Hobbs, 1962; Kempler, 1980) have been most frequently referred to as nonspecific factors (Butler & Strupp, 1986; Grencavage & Norcross, 1990). Other variables that have been referred to in this way include client characteristics (Torrey, 1972), therapist qualities (Rosenzweig, 1936; Patterson, 1989), elements of the treatment structure (Frank, 1981; Hobbs, 1962; Mahrer, 1989; Torrey, 1972), and change processes or strategies (Davison, 1980; Goldfried, 1980; Prochaska, 1984; Torrey, 1972).

Much confusion surrounds the specific–nonspecific hypothesis in the literature. Kazdin (1979) points out that there is no clear and consistent meaning to the term *nonspecific treatment factors.* Grencavage & Norcross (1990), in their review of the literature, found 27 different terms used to describe nonspecific factors, including *common factors, common* [or *universal*] *elements/components,* and *effective principles,* as well as four extant coding schemes used to organize them, to which they added a fifth. Common factors posited to date have been "numerous and varied" (Patterson, 1989) in both composition and characterization (Karasu, 1986; Lambert, 1986). Furthermore, different authors have focused on different domains or levels of psychosocial treatment. Others have described nonspecific treatment factors primarily in terms of the healer–patient relationship (Butler & Strupp, 1986), the placebo effect (Shapiro & Morris, 1978), and even in such broad terms as "qualities inherent in any positive human relationship that felicitously affect an individual's expectations or morale" (Jones et al., 1988, p. 48).

Such a state of affairs is unfortunate. Before we can agree or disagree on a certain matter, we need to ensure that we are, in fact, discussing the same phenomenon (Norcross, 1987). It is difficult, if not impossible, to discuss, study, and apply the notion of specific and nonspecific treatment factors in the absence of accord over what it is we are discussing.

HISTORICAL DEVELOPMENT

Efforts to unravel the effects of psychotherapy by dividing it into specific and nonspecific components date back to the earliest psychotherapy research (Butler & Strupp, 1986; Rosenthal & Frank, 1956), as the field has long observed that disparate forms of psychotherapy share common elements or core features (Goldfried & Newman, 1986; Grencavage & Norcross, 1990; Thompson, 1987). As early as 1936, Rosenzweig, noting that all forms of psychotherapy have cures to their credit, invoked the famous dodo bird verdict from Alice in Wonderland, "Everybody has won and all must have prizes," to characterize psychotherapy outcome. As a possible explanation, he proposed common factors shared by all psychotherapies, such as psychological interpretation, the personality of the therapist, and catharsis.

Four years later, a meeting was held with the purpose of ascertaining areas of agreement among leading psychotherapy approaches (Watson, 1940). The assemblage, which included such leading figures as Alexandra Adler, Saul Rosenzweig, and Carl Rogers, concurred that behavior change, insight, support, psychological interpretation, certain therapist characteristics, and a good therapeutic relationship were common to successful psychotherapy approaches.

Perhaps the most vocal proponent of the nonspecific hypothesis through the decades has been Jerome Frank (1961, 1971, 1981), noted for his elaboration of the elements common to successful psychotherapies and folk traditions of healing. He argues that all psychotherapy clients suffer from a common "disorder"—demoralization, a chronic feeling of being overwhelmed and unable to cope effectively with problems—and that all successful psychotherapies work by helping clients to overcome it. He proposes that all therapies (and all healing endeavors) share (1) a client in distress, (2) a therapist who is perceived as an expert in dealing with the client's distress, (3) an acceptable explanation or "myth" provided by the therapist of the client's distress, and (4) some sort of healing ritual conducted by the therapist that serves to instill hope and positive expectation in the client. To Frank, the specific content of the therapist's technical interventions is important, not because any of the theoretical tenets represent the "correct" way to view the human psyche or the psychotherapeutic process, but because it helps to provide a shared belief system between the client and therapist as well as to give form to the prescribed rituals.

Along the lines of Frank's work, Torrey (1972) provides a fascinating analysis of modern-day psychotherapeutic endeavors by placing them in the context of age-old healing processes employed through the centuries. He equates contemporary mental health professionals with the witch doctors of more primitive cultures, outlining four elements common to our collective healing endeavors: personal qualities of the therapist; the use of rituals and techniques; client hope for improvement and confidence in the therapist, which he terms the *edifice complex,* describing it as "faith in the institution itself, the door at the end of the pilgrimage" (p. 49); and the naming of the client's problem, which he creatively called the *Rumpelstiltskin principle,* maintaining that the very act of naming the problem results in therapeutic benefit to the client.

More recently, the "common factors" approach (as it has come to be known) has been recognized as one of the three central thrusts of the psychotherapy integration movement (Arkowitz, 1989; Beitman, Goldfried, & Norcross, 1989; Norcross, 1986), along with theoretical integration, aimed at synthesizing diverse theoretical systems, and technical eclecticism, which incorporates a variety of therapeutic methods regardless of their theoretical derivation. This search for common factors across differing therapeutic schools has been described by some as one of the most significant trends in psychotherapy in the 1980s (Bergin, 1982; Gurman, 1980).

NONSPECIFIC FACTORS AND TREATMENT OUTCOME RESEARCH

Even before the notion of nonspecific factors operating across the various forms of psychotherapy had been considered, the search for specific factors operating within a particular form had been underway. In fact, arguments that a specific psychotherapy is effective because of specific components operating uniquely within it have been made as long as psychotherapy itself has been practiced. Practitioners of a particular brand of therapy have always been under pressure, at first primarily from practitioners of other schools of therapy, but now more from third-party reimbursement sources as well as the public, to demonstrate that what they are doing is more effective than what other practitioners are doing and why.

To many, the best way to demonstrate effectiveness is to show that the treatment surpasses the effectiveness of a placebo treatment (e.g., Prioleau, Murdock, & Brody, 1983). This has been the model successfully employed in drug evaluations. However, it is not really the effectiveness of the drug that is being evaluated, but rather its mechanism of action (Bootzin, 1985a). The assumption of the model is that the effect of a drug consists of two components, a specific physiological component and a nonspecific psychological component, whereas the effect of a placebo consists of only one, the nonspecific psychological component. Leaving aside the issue of whether this simple, dualistic model is an accurate portrayal of physiological mechanisms, it is not overall effectiveness that is being evaluated. Rather, it is the extent to which the *specific* physiological component adds significantly to the *nonspecific* psychological component.

In psychological treatment research, it is not relevant to partition the outcome into physiological and psychological components. Instead, placebo controls are used to distinguish the *specific* effects dictated by theory from the *nonspecific* effects associated with all therapy. For example, there is substantial evidence that systematic desensitization (SD) is an effective treatment of anxiety disorders (Kazdin & Wilson, 1978; Paul, 1969). Placebo control groups are used to evaluate not whether SD is effective, but whether its effectiveness is due to counterconditioning or to the ingredients common to SD and the placebo treatment (Bootzin & Lick, 1979).

A fundamental problem with the strategy of using placebo control groups in psychotherapy research is that placebos vary in effectiveness, depending on a variety of contextual factors. These factors include the credibility of the therapy rationale and instructions, the experiences during therapy implying improvement, subtle cues from the therapist, the context of the evaluation, and the apparent appropriateness of the treatment for the problem (Bootzin, 1985a). Placebos are not just an embodiment of "nonspecific" factors, but may vary in effectiveness because of the elicitation of active psychological change processes such as self-efficacy (Bandura, 1977).

Although the notion of nonspecific factors operating in the various psychotherapies does not necessarily preclude the operation of specific factors (and vice versa), these two approaches are often contrasted against each other as if they are mutually exclusive. It is entirely possible, perhaps even likely, that the nonspecifics operating across therapies do so in conjunction with the specific components of any one given therapy (Omer & London, 1989). The nonspecifics may be the necessary, but not sufficient, components of successful therapy, without which a given technique would be devoid of meaning and therefore ineffective.

Supporting evidence for this hypothesis has been reported by Alexander, Barton, Schiavo, and Parsons (1976), who, in a study of the behavioral treatment of delinquents and their families, found that therapist relationship skills (affect–behavior integration, warmth and humor, directiveness, and self-confidence) accounted for 60% of the variance of outcome. However, in an earlier study of a Rogerian approach, relationship skills alone were not effective in modifying the behavior of delinquent families (Parsons & Alexander, 1973). Thus, one nonspecific factor, relationship skills, appears to enhance the effectiveness of interventions rather than substitute for them.

The field has turned to research to help tease apart the quandary. Such research has typically focused on demonstrating mode-specific treatment effects through the use of comparative outcome studies (Kazdin, 1986; Pilkonis, Imber, Lewis, & Rubinsky, 1984), broadly defined as studies that compare two or more alternative treatments against each other. If specific factors are indeed the "active" ingredients of psychotherapy, then specific techniques employed in specific psychotherapies should result in specific treatment effects, or differential change across treatments, dependent upon the type of treatment offered. For example, cognitive therapy should result in clients being more rational and less dysfunctional in their thinking, whereas interpersonal therapy should result in more satisfying interpersonal relationships for those who participate in it. If such research fails to demonstrate specific treatment effects, or if all psychotherapies appear to have equal effectiveness rates, then it is often taken as de facto evidence in favor of the nonspecific hypothesis of treatment effectiveness.

Indeed, such has been the state of the field over the past few decades. To date, studies comparing different forms of psychotherapy have shown very few differences in outcome among the schools investigated (Bergin & Lambert, 1978; Sloan, Staples, Cristol, Yorkston, & Whipple, 1975; Luborsky et al., 1975; Smith & Glass, 1977; Smith et al., 1980). This paradox of lack of differential effectiveness in the face of technical diversity (Stiles et al., 1986) has led some to conclude that all psychotherapies are equivalent, and that it is the common, or nonspecific, elements, that are responsible for psychotherapeutic success (Cornsweet, 1983; Frank, 1981; O'Connell, 1983; Shapiro & Morris, 1978).

This "acceptance of the null hypothesis" (Butler & Strupp, 1986)—concluding that, because there have been no major discernible differences in outcome among the various psychotherapies found to date, they must therefore be equivalent—is, at the least, premature and, at the most, completely wrong. Other plausible explanations are possible for these findings (or lack of findings, as the case may be). The paucity of differential effects of treatments does not warrant the conclusion that nonspecific factors are responsible for the effect of psychotherapy. Specific interventions that are fundamentally different from each other may interact with nonspecific factors to produce the same overall results. The mechanisms through which they facilitate change (thus, their *specific* effects) may still be different from those of other specific interventions (Shoham-Salomon & Hannah, 1991).

The debate over which type of factors contributes more to psychotherapy outcome is diluted by the lack of *conceptual* clarity regarding the boundary definition of these factors. We would like to propose that part of the confusion in the field stems from the possibility that the specific–nonspecific dimension is orthogonal, rather than parallel, to the unique–common dimension.

Table 9.1 illustrates how orthogonal dimensions would interact. *Specific interventions* are therapist actions designed to improve client outcome (alleviate the symptom, relieve pain, solve problems, promote insight, etc.). *Common specific interventions* are outcome-oriented therapist actions shared by many therapeutic schools. An example is the therapist offering an alternative perspective from which the client can view his or her symptom, variously referred to as *reframing, interpretation, or cognitive restructuring,* depending on one's theoretical orientation. *Unique specific interventions* are therapist actions applied in one (or a few types of) therapy. Examples include systematic desensitization, paradoxical interventions, and empty–chair work.

Nonspecific interventions are therapist actions designed to promote a *process* that can serve as ground for the implementation of specific interventions. *Common nonspecific interventions* are therapist process-oriented actions shared by many therapeutic schools such as rapport building and joining. *Unique nonspecific interventions* are therapeutic messages conveyed by the setting and applied in one (or a few types of) therapy, such as a decision to invite family members to the session.

In this portrayal, the distinction between the common and unique emerges as less useful than the one between the specific and nonspecific. *Common* and *unique* are relative labels. Techniques and strategies that were once considered to be unique to a particular brand of therapy have often become a matter of common practice (e.g., some forms of brief therapy).

To complicate matters even further, the distinction between specific, outcome-oriented interventions and nonspecific, process-oriented interventions, although making more conceptual sense, is also problematic. Outcome- and process-oriented interventions serve as each other's context; each gets its meaning within the context of the other and is not independent (Shoham-Salomon, 1990). A relational message that pre-

TABLE 9.1. Specificity and Uniqueness of Therapeutic Interventions: Two Interacting Dimensions

	Common	Unique
Specific	Offer alternative view (reframing, interpretations)	An intervention (paradoxical)
Nonspecific	Rapport (empathy, emotional support)	Therapeutic setting (number of people in the room)

cedes a homework assignment is not equivalent to a relational message followed by an insight-oriented interpretation. The specific intervention lends meaning to its relational context.

A potentially useful distinction is the one between specific and nonspecific *factors* versus specific and nonspecific *effects.* Rather than focusing on the therapist's intentions (outcome versus process) while delivering the interventions, the focus shifts to the effects of the interventions on the client. Thus, the question becomes whether the therapeutic act (specific or nonspecific) achieves what it is purported to achieve. Does the therapist's specific intent to alter a client's distorted cognitions result in the client exhibiting more functional cognitions? Do such altered cognitions follow a therapy that does not specifically attempt to accomplish this? Do therapist's efforts at joining the client's system in fact result in better therapeutic relationships? Do better relationships serve as more fertile ground for interventions to achieve their specific effects (e.g., compliance with homework)? In the following section, we review empirical attempts at examining specific therapeutic effects in two problem areas, insomnia and depression.

EMPIRICAL EXAMINATION OF SPECIFIC THERAPEUTIC EFFECTS

Insomnia

We have selected insomnia for two reasons. First, there is a long tradition in this area of concern about nonspecific effects; second, there have been a number of comparative treatment studies, allowing for the identification of specific effects. We would expect there might be different profiles of results associated with different treatments.

A number of nonpharmacological treatments have been found to be effective for insomnia, including sleep hygiene information, stimulus-control instructions, sleep restriction, chronotherapy, bright light therapy, relaxation training, biofeedback, paradoxical intention, and cognitive therapy (see Bootzin & Perlis, 1992).

In many studies, nonspecific effects have been evaluated through the use of placebo control conditions and/or the use of a counterdemand control (Steinmark & Borkovec, 1974). In a counterdemand condition, patients are told not to expect therapeutic change for a specified number of weeks. Between-treatment comparisons are then assessed the week prior to the expected change. Using these control procedures, relaxation training, stimulus control instructions, and paradoxical intention have all been found to produce significantly more change than control conditions (Borkovec, 1982; Espie, Lindsay, Brooks, Hood, & Turvey, 1989; Lacks, Bertelson, Gans, & Kunkel, 1983).

Comparative studies of different treatments indicate considerable overlap in effectiveness. The treatments that have been most evaluated are relaxation training, stimulus-control instructions, and paradoxical intention. Of these treatments, stimulus-control instructions appears to have the edge in comparative studies (Bootzin, 1985b, Study 1; Espie, Lindsay et al., 1989; Lacks et al., 1983). Although some studies have found no difference between the treatments (Turner & Ascher, 1979, 1982), in no study has some other treatment been found to be more effective than stimulus-control instructions.

The elusive promise of specific treatment effects is that it should ultimately be possible to tailor a treatment to a problem, depending upon the causal factors for the individual. In insomnia, for example, one might expect that relaxation training would be more effective than stimulus-control instruction for someone who is tense and anxious, and that paradoxical intention would be most effective for reactant patients with presleep anticipatory anxiety. The evidence does not support this level of specificity. For example, in a large multitreatment study, relaxation training was less effective than stimulus-control instructions or paradoxical intention, even for anxious insomniacs (Espie, Brooks, & Lindsay, 1989). Each presumed casual mechanism must be tested and evaluated. There is no advantage to tailoring treatments if weak treatments are included and strong treatments are omitted.

Depression

There is evidence that psychotherapy and pharmacotherapy of depression result in differential treatment effects. Specifically, pharmacotherapy seems to have more rapid effects on the neurovegetative symptoms of depression, such as sleep and appetite disturbances, whereas psychotherapy results in more rapid improvement in social functioning (DiMascio et al., 1979; Weissman, Klerman, Prusoff, Sholomskas, & Padian, 1981) and self-concept and feelings of hopelessness (Rush, Beck, Kovacs, Weissenberger, & Hollon, 1982), although the latter findings were not confirmed by Simons, Garfield, and Murphy (1984).

Interestingly, when specific forms of psychotherapy are compared with each other in the treatment of depression, differential effects have not been as readily found. Zeiss, Lewinsohn, & Munoz (1979) investigated three theoretically and empirically derived outpatient approaches to the treatment of depression, each of which was targeted toward a specific depressive symptom. Treatment A focused on increasing the client's rate of mood-related pleasant activities; Treatment B on increasing assertiveness, positive social impact, and social interaction; and Treatment C on changing maladaptive cognitions. Depressed subjects were randomly assigned to one of the three treatment groups and randomly assigned to begin therapy immediately or after a 1-month waiting period. All groups underwent four assessment periods spaced 1 month apart, with the immediate treatment group having a pretest, posttest, 1-month follow-up, and 2-month follow-up, and the delayed treatment group a pretest, second pretest, posttest, and one-month follow-up. The purpose of the study was to examine the relative effects of the three treatment approaches, particularly in terms of the degree to which a particular therapy would result in specific changes in those behaviors targeted by it.

The results of this study indicate that all three treatment approaches were equally effective in alleviating depression and that their effects were nonspecific. That is, subjects were less depressed after treatment, but this improvement could not be attributed to any specific change in any target behavior because they did not improve differentially dependent on the type of treatment they received. The authors explain their results in terms of nonspecific treatment factors generally and Bandura's (1977) model of self-efficacy specifically.

Another interesting finding from this study was that the delayed treatment group exhibited much improvement in their depression levels on the second pretest, before they received any formal treatment. The authors noted, in retrospect, that the delayed treatment group had considerable contact with the project staff because of the extensive assessment procedures they were required to undergo; they hypothesized that this contact and activity may have resulted in the observed improvement via nonspecific treatment effects. (The authors noted, however, that in the absence of a traditional no-treatment, wait-list control group, it cannot be established that this improvement is anything more than a spontaneous remission effect.)

In another study designed to investigate differential treatment effects among psychological treatments for depression, Rehm, Kaslow, and Rabin (1987) developed three separate versions of Rehm's (1977, 1981) self-control therapy program for depression, a highly structured, group format therapy based on a model that conceptualizes depression as resulting from a series of specific deficits in self-management behavior. Of the three developed versions, one targets behavioral control by increasing specific categories of overt behavior, the second targets cognitive control through monitoring and altering evaluative self-statements and then contingently rewarding oneself with them, and the third targets both behavioral and cognitive control. No control conditions were employed. The purpose of this study was to evaluate the relative efficacy of these three therapy versions and to examine any interactions between specific subject characteristics and the therapy program.

Results of this study indicate that all three versions of the self-control therapy program were equally effective in reducing subject depression across self-report, interviewer, and clinician ratings. No significant differences were found between the three conditions on any of the outcome measures of depression and psychopathology. Additionally, there were no significant differences in the rate of subject improvement on self-control attitudes, beliefs, dysfunctional attitudes, or on any measures of the target behaviors, despite the therapies being developed specifically for this purpose and the use of a fairly large sample size ($n = 104$). The authors offer as potential explanations for their findings the possibility that these therapies are effective for reasons separate from the validity of their therapeutic rationales or that the positive findings are a result of features that the treatments share in common.

Finally, the National Institute of Mental Health's Treatment of Depression Collaborative Research Program, which compared two forms of psychotherapy (interpersonal and cognitive–behavioral) with a pharmacological treatment (imipramine) plus clinical management and a pill placebo plus clinical management, also found very little evidence for mode-specific treatment effects (Imber et al., 1990). All treatments, which have been shown to be precisely specified, appropriately applied, and discriminable, demonstrated significant symptom reduction with relatively few differences in general outcome (Elkin et al., 1989), in spite of the fact that outcome measures were selected on the basis of presumed sensitivity to the different treatments and the employment of a large sample size ($n = 250$). In their discussion of the results, Imber and associates (1990) note that the most parsimonious explanation of their findings is that core processes operating across the differing treatments are responsible for their effectiveness, noting that such "nonspecific factors" were present even in the pharmacotherapy treatment in its clinical management portion. However, they do not take this as the probable explanation. Instead, they point to limitations in the study's design, especially the selected assessment measures (which may have been too general and limited) and the time of their application (only at termination), as the likely reasons for their inability to find differential treatment effects.

What are we to conclude on the basis of this admittedly small body of empirical evidence for depression? The lack of differentiation of effects in psychological interventions could be due to a number a factors. First, it could be that common factors are the most important ingredients in the treatment of depression. However, other alternatives must be considered as well.

Second, it may be that it does not matter where one initially intervenes with depression in that depression may be influenced by any change in the system. Recent theories of depression have tended to be multicomponent, systems theories (e.g., Lewinsohn, Hoberman, Teri, & Hautzinger, 1985; Coyne, 1988), in which differential treatment effects might only be seen early in the process of change.

Third, an alternative possibility is that our current theories of depression and treatments derived from them are too broad. It may be that we need narrower theories and stronger treatments. Furthermore, more specific theories from which more focused treatments are derived may allow for better-differentiated hypotheses and more specific effects.

Finally, it may be that the existing studies were just methodologically limited. For example, Zeiss and colleagues (1979) used the same therapists to administer the three different therapy approaches investigated. Each therapist was conducting each therapy concurrently, treating one client in each of the conditions at any given phase of the study. No checks were made to determine the degree to which therapies were discriminable from each other. Thus, any conclusions based on this study must be treated with extreme caution.

It is not possible to choose among these alternatives from the existing evidence. Additional comparative studies in depression will be necessary to help sort out the alternative explanations. However, results from depression should not be taken as representative of results in other problem areas. An encouraging development in recent years has been the development of powerful treatments for specific problems.

Perhaps the best recent illustration of the development of powerful treatments has involved the treatment of panic disorder. A recent review (Michelson & Marchione, 1991) concluded that the treatment of choice for panic disorder without phobic avoidance is cognitive–behavioral therapy involving panic management, breathing retraining, exposure to interoceptive cues, and applied relaxation training. This treatment both reduces symptoms and maintains improvement, whereas pharmacological treatment reduces symptoms but has a high degree of relapse when medication is withdrawn. Nonspecific factors become a less plausible alternative explanation for the effectiveness of therapy when the treatment is highly effective and outperforms alternate interventions.

METHODOLOGICAL CONSIDERATIONS

As stated before, the specific–nonspecific hypotheses of therapeutic effectiveness are often pitted against each other. The debate, in fact, gets quite heated at times, as evidenced by the many critiques, predominantly against the nonspecific hypothesis, written to date (see, e.g., Butler & Strupp, 1986; Haaga, 1986; Jones et al., 1988; Mahrer, 1989; Messer, 1986; Messer & Winokur, 1980, 1981; Norcross, 1981; Wilson, 1982).

Critics (e.g., Jones et al., 1988; Strupp, 1983) have pointed out that the fact that psychotherapies share common elements and that the client–therapist relationship resembles other nonprofessional human relationships does not make all therapies equivalent to each other and especially not to any other human relationship. Psychotherapy is an interpersonal endeavor and does incorporate some "generic" or "common" procedures in order to help clients reach their goals. Nonetheless, there are specific aspects and operations unique to psychotherapy that set it apart from other means of human influence and helping endeavors.

In regard to the research methodology that has been popularly used thus far in efforts to delineate active therapeutic components, Jones and associates (1988) assert that treatment outcomes are not good criteria for deciding whether specific factors are operating in the psychotherapies. They argue that psychotherapy outcome cannot be precisely measured and cannot be readily compared between clients. Additionally, they note that in comparative studies, therapies are typically brief and sample sizes are small (usually 20 or fewer in a group). Thus, it is not surprising that differential treatment effects have not been readily apparent. Given the methodological limitations, such effects would need to be robust indeed (Kazdin, 1986).

Jones and colleagues (1988) point out that one of the crucial questions for our field remains the relationship of psychotherapy process and outcome and a methodology to adequately assess it. They state:

> One reason for the field's inability to identify strong and consistent corre-
> lations between specific aspects of process and treatment outcomes is that
> studies typically attempt to find simple, direct associations without consid-
> eration of the complex interaction of the multiple variables that constitute
> psychotherapy. What is needed is a method of sufficient complexity to
> adequately reflect the phenomenon it is attempting to assess, one that can tap
> configurations or patterns in process and that allows the discovery of
> associations or relations. (p. 49)

At a more fundamental level, Butler and Strupp (1986) argue that the specific–nonspecific hypothesis is itself a false dichotomy completely inappropriate to psychotherapy. Instead, they advocate a new paradigm to guide psychotherapy research that emphasizes the interpersonal context in which psychotherapy takes place, pointing out that specific techniques cannot be separated from the therapist–client context in which they are applied. They proclaim: "Psychotherapy research must move away from simplistic notions of 'active ingredients' and disembodied or decontextualized 'factors' and move toward the identification of fundamental principles of human interaction which underlie the interpersonal conditions essential for therapeutic change" (p. 38).

CONCLUSIONS

Taken to an extreme, the nonspecific hypothesis implies that the efforts invested in developing specific interventions capable of alleviating specific problems are wasted. It is our contention that the knowledge accumulated so far, sparse as it is, does not support such an implication. As Omer and London (1989) point out, nonspecific factors are manifested in therapy only when specific treatments are applied. Given the methodological problems entailed in therapy outcome designs, the "signal" seems inseparable from the "noise." A more fruitful route is to continue to develop specific, theory-derived treatments, along with alliance-promoting techniques, and to study their combined effects in the treatment of specific problems.

ACKNOWLEDGMENT

This work was supported by NIAA Grant R01AA08970.

REFERENCES

Alexander, J. F., Barton, C., Schiavo, R. S., & Parsons, B. V. (1976). Systems behavioral intervention with families of delinquents: Therapists' characteristics, family behavior, and outcome. *Journal of Consulting and Clinical Psychology, 44,* 656–664.

Arkowitz, H. (1989). The role of theory in psychotherapy integration. *Journal of Integrative and Eclectic Psychotherapy, 8,* 8–16.

Bandura, A. (1977). Self-efficacy: Toward a unifying theory of behavioral change. *Psychological Review, 84,* 191–215.

Beitman, B. D., Goldfried, M. R., & Norcross, J. C. (1989). The movement toward integrating the psychotherapies: An overview. *American Journal of Psychiatry, 146,* 138–147.

Bergin, A. E. (1982). *Comment on converging themes in psychotherapy.* New York: Springer.

Bergin, A. E., & Lambert, M. J. (1978). The evaluation of therapeutic outcomes. In S. Garfield & A. Bergin (Eds.), *Handbook of psychotherapy and behavior change* (pp. 139–189). New York: Wiley.

Bootzin, R. R. (1985a). The role of expectancy in behavior change. In L. White, B. Tursky, & G. E. Schwartz (Eds.), *Placebo: Theory, research, and mechanisms* (pp. 196–210). New York: Guilford Press.

Bootzin, R. R. (1985b). Evaluation of stimulus control instructions, progressive relaxation, and sleep hygiene as treatments for insomnia. In W. P. Koella, E. Ruther, & H. Schulz (Eds.), *Sleep '84* (pp. 142–144). Stuttgart: Gustav Fischer Verlag.

Bootzin, R. R., & Lick, J. R. (1979). Expectancies in therapy research: Interpretive artifact or mediating mechanism? *Journal of Consulting and Clinical Psychology, 47,* 852–855.

Bootzin, R. R., & Perlis, M. L. (1992). Nonpharmacologic treatments of insomnia. *Journal of Clinical Psychiatry, 53* (Suppl.), 37–41.

Borkovec, T. D. (1982). Insomnia. *Journal of Consulting and Clinical Psychology, 50,* 880–895.

Butler, S. F., & Strupp, H. H. (1986). Specific and nonspecific factors in psychotherapy: A problematic paradigm for psychotherapy research. *Psychotherapy, 23,* 30–40.

Cornsweet, C. (1983). Nonspecific factors and theoretical choice. *Psychotherapy: Theory, Research, and Practice, 20,* 307–313.

Coyne, J. C. (1988). Strategic therapy. In J. Clarkin, G. Haas, & I. Glick (Eds.), *Affective disorders and the family: Assessment and treatment* (pp. 89–113). New York: Basic Books.

Davison, G. C. (1980). Some views on effective principles of psychotherapy. *Cognitive Therapy and Research, 4,* 269–306.

DiMascio, A., Weissman, M. M., Prusoff, B. A., Neu, C., Zwilling, M., & Klerman, G. L. (1979). Differential symptom reduction by drugs and psychotherapy in acute depression. *Archives of General Psychiatry, 36,* 1450–1456.

Elkin, I., Shea, M. T., Watkins, J. T., Imber., S. D., Sotsky, S. M., Collins, J. F., Glass, D. R., Pilkonis, P. A., Leber, W. R., Docherty, J. P., Fiester, S. J., & Parloff, M. B. (1989). NIMH Treatment of Depression Collaborative Research Program: General effectiveness of treatments. *Archives of General Psychiatry, 46,* 971–983.

Espie, C. A., Brooks, D. N., & Lindsay, W. R. (1989). An evaluation of tailored psychological treatment of insomnia. *Journal of Behavior Therapy and Experimental Psychiatry, 20,* 143–154.

Espie, C. A., Lindsay, W. R., Brooks, D. N., Hood, E. M., & Turvey, T. (1989). A controlled comparative investigation of psychological treatments for chronic sleep-onset insomnia. *Behaviour Research and Therapy, 27,* 79–88.

Frances, A., Sweeney, J., & Clarkin, J. (1985). Do psychotherapies have specific effects? *American Journal of Psychotherapy, 39,* 159–174.

Frank, J. D. (1961). *Persuasion and healing.* Baltimore: Johns Hopkins University Press.

Frank, J. D. (1971). Therapeutic factors in psychotherapy. *American Journal of Psychotherapy, 25,* 350–361.

Frank, J. D. (1981). Therapeutic components shared by all psychotherapies. In J. H. Hawey & M. M. Parks (Eds.), *Psychotherapy research and behavior change* (pp. 9–37). Washington, DC: American Psychological Association.

Goldfried, M. R. (1980). Toward the delineation of therapeutic change principles. *American Psychologist, 35,* 991–999.

Goldfried, M. R., & Newman, C. (1986). Psychotherapy integration: An historical perspective. In J. C. Norcross (Ed.), *Handbook of eclectic psychotherapy* (pp. 25–61). New York: Brunner/Mazel.

Grencavage, L. M., & Norcross, J. C. (1990). Where are the commonalities among the therapeutic common factors? *Professional Psychology: Research and Practice, 21,* 372–378.

Gurman, A. S. (1980). Behavioral marital therapy in the 1980's: The challenge of integration. *American Journal of Family Therapy, 8,* 86–96.

Haaga, D. A. (1986). A review of the common principles approach to integration of psychotherapies. *Cognitive Therapy and Research, 10,* 527–538.

Hobbs, N. (1962). Sources of gain in psychotherapy. *American Psychologist, 17,* 741–747.

Imber, S. D., Pilkonis, P. A., Sotsky, S. M., Elkin, I., Watkins, J. T., Collins, J. F., Shea, M. T., Leber, W. R., & Glass, D. R. (1990). Mode-specific effects among three treatments for depression. *Journal of Clinical and Consulting Psychology, 58,* 352–359.

Jones, E. E., Cumming, J. D., & Horowitz, M. J. (1988). Another look at the nonspecific hypothesis of therapeutic effectiveness. *Journal of Consulting and Clinical Psychology, 56,* 48–55.

Karasu, T. B. (1986). The specificity versus nonspecificity dilemma: Toward identifying therapeutic change agents. *American Journal of Psychiatry, 143,* 687–695.

Kazdin, A. E. (1979). Nonspecific treatment factors in psychotherapy outcome research. *Journal of Consulting and Clinical Psychology, 47,* 846–851.

Kazdin, A. E. (1986). Comparative outcome studies of psychotherapy: Methodological issues and strategies. *Journal of Consulting and Clinical Psychology, 54,* 95–105.

Kazdin, A. E., & Wilson, G. T. (1978). *Evaluation of behavior therapy: Issues, evidence and research strategies.* Cambridge, MA: Ballinger.

Kempler, W. (1980). Some views on effective principles of psychotherapy. *Cognitive Therapy and Research, 4,* 269–306.

Lacks, P., Bertelson, A. D., Gans, L., & Kunkel, J. (1983). The effectiveness of three behavioural treatments for different degrees of sleep-onset insomnia. *Behavior Therapy, 14,* 593–605.

Lambert, M. J. (1986). Implications of psychotherapy outcome research for eclectic psychotherapy. In J. C. Norcross (Ed.), *Handbook of eclectic psychotherapy* (pp. 436–462). New York: Brunner/Mazel.

Lambert, M. J., Shapiro, D. A., & Bergin, A. E. (1986). The effectiveness of psychotherapy. In S. L. Garfield & A. E. Bergin (Eds.), *Handbook of psychotherapy and behavior change* (pp. 157–212). New York: Wiley.

Landman, J. T., & Dawes, R. M. (1982). Smith and Glass' conclusions stand up under scrutiny. *American Psychologist, 37,* 504–516.

Lewinsohn, P. M., Hoberman, H. M., Teri, L., & Hautzinger, M. (1985). In S. Reiss & R. R. Bootzin (Eds.), *Theoretical issues in behavior therapy* (pp. 331–361). New York: Academic Press.

Luborsky, L., Singer, B., & Luborsky, L. (1975). Comparative studies of psychotherapies. *Archives of General Psychiatry, 32,* 995–1008.

Mahrer, A. R. (1989). *The integration of the psychotherapies: A guide for practicing therapists.* New York: Human Sciences Press.

Messer, S. B. (1986). Eclecticism in psychotherapy: Underlying assumptions, problems, and trade-offs. In J. C. Norcross (Ed.), *Handbook of eclectic psychotherapy* (pp. 379–397). New York: Brunner/Mazel.

Messer, S. B., & Winokur, M. (1980). Some limits to the integration of psychoanalytic and behavior therapy. *American Psychologist, 35,* 818–827.

Messer, S. B., & Winokur, M. (1981). Therapeutic common principles: Are commonalities more apparent than real? *American Psychologist, 36,* 1547–1548.

Michelson, L. K., & Marchione, K. (1991). Behavioral, cognitive, and pharmacological treatments of panic disorder with agoraphobia: Critique and synthesis. *Journal of Consulting and Clinical Psychology, 59,* 100–114.

Norcross, J. C. (1981). All in the family? On therapeutic commonalities. *American Psychologist, 36,* 1544–1545.

Norcross, J. C. (Ed.). (1986). *Handbook of eclectic psychotherapy.* New York: Brunner/
    Mazel.
Norcross, J. C. (Ed.). (1987). Special section: Toward a common language for
    psychotherapy. *Journal of Integrative and Eclectic Psychotherapy, 4,* 165–205.
O'Connell, S. (1983). The placebo effect and psychotherapy. *Psychotherapy: The-
    ory, Research and Practice, 20,* 337–345.
Omer, H., & London, P. (1989). Signal and noise in psychotherapy: The role and
    control of non-specific factors. *British Journal of Psychiatry, 155,* 239–245.
Parsons, B. V., Jr., & Alexander, J. F. (1973). Short-term family interventions: A
    therapy outcome study. *Journal of Consulting and Clinical Psychology, 41,*
    195–201.
Patterson, C. H. (1989). Foundations for a systematic eclecticism in psychother-
    apy. *Psychotherapy, 26,* 427–435.
Paul, G. L. (1969). Outcome of systematic desensitization: II. Controlled inves-
    tigation of individual treatment technique variations and current status. In
    C. M. Franks (Ed.), *Behavior therapy: Appraisal and status.* New York:
    McGraw-Hill.
Pilkonis, P. A., Imber, S. D., Lewis, P., & Rubinsky, P. (1984). A comparative
    outcome study of individual, group, and conjoint psychotherapy. *Archives
    of General Psychiatry, 41,* 431–437.
Prioleau, L., Murdock, M., & Brody, N. (1983). An analysis of psychotherapy
    versus placebo studies. *Behavioral and Brain Sciences, 6,* 275–310.
Prochaska, J. O. (1984). *Systems of psychotherapy: A transtheoretical analysis* (2nd ed.).
    New York: Dorsey Press.
Rehm, L. P. (1977). A self-control model of depression. *Behavior Therapy, 8,*
    787–804.
Rehm, L. P. (1981). A self-control therapy program for treatment of depression.
    In J. F. Clarkin & H. Glazer (Eds.), *Depression: Behavioral and directive
    treatment strategies* (pp. 68–110). New York: Garland Press.
Rehm, L. P., Kaslow, N. J., & Rabin, A. S. (1987). Cognitive and behavioral
    targets in a self-control therapy program for depression. *Journal of Clinical
    and Consulting Psychology, 55,* 60–67.
Rosenthal, D., & Frank, J. D. (1956). Psychotherapy and the placebo effect.
    Psychological Bulletin, 53, 294–302.
Rosenzweig, S. (1936). Some implicit common factors in diverse methods of
    psychotherapy. *American Journal of Orthopsychiatry, 6,* 412–415.
Rush, A. J., Beck, A. T., Kovacs, M., Weissenberger, J., & Hollon, S. D. (1982).
    Comparison of the effects of cognitive therapy and pharmacotherapy on
    hopelessness and self-concept. *American Journal of Psychiatry, 139,* 862–866.
Shapiro, A. K., & Morris, L. A. (1978). The placebo effect in medical and
    psychological therapies. In S. L. Garfield & A. E. Bergin (Eds.), *Handbook
    of psychotherapy and behavior change: An empirical analysis* (2nd ed., pp.
    369–410). New York: Wiley.
Shapiro, D., & Shapiro, D. (1982). Meta-analysis of comparative therapy out-
    come studies. *Psychological Bulletin, 92,* 581–604.
Shoham-Salomon, V. (1990). Interrelating research processes of process research.
    Journal of Consulting and Clinical Psychology, 58, 295–303.
Shoham-Salomon, V., & Hannah, M. T. (1991). Client-treatment interaction in

the study of differential change processes. *Journal of Consulting and Clinical Psychology, 59,* 217–225.

Simons, A. D., Garfield, S. L., & Murphy, G. E. (1984). The process of change in cognitive therapy and pharmacotherapy for depression: Changes in mood and cognition. *Archives of General Psychiatry, 41,* 45–51.

Sloane, R. B., Staples, F. R., Cristol, A. H., Yorkston, N. J., & Whipple, K. (1975). *Psychotherapy versus behavior therapy.* Cambridge, MA: Harvard University Press.

Smith, M. L., & Glass, G. V. (1977). Meta-analysis of psychotherapy outcome studies. *American Psychologist, 32,* 752–760.

Smith, M. L., Glass, G. V., & Miller, T. J. (1980). *The benefits of psychotherapy.* Baltimore: Johns Hopkins University Press.

Steinmark, S. W., & Borkovec, T. D. (1974). Active and placebo treatment effects on moderate insomnia under counterdemand and positive demand instructions. *Journal of Abnormal Psychology, 83,* 157–163.

Stiles, W. B., Shapiro, D. A., & Elliott, R. (1986). Are all psychotherapies equivalent? *American Psychologist, 41,* 165–180.

Strupp, H. (1983, July). *The non-specific hypothesis of therapeutic effectiveness: My current view.* Paper presented at the meeting of the Society for Psychotherapy Research, Sheffield, England.

Thompson, J. R. (1987). *The process of psychotherapy: An integration of clinical experience and empirical research.* Frederick, MD: University Press of America.

Torrey, E. F. (1972). *The mind game.* New York: Bantam Books.

Turner, R. M., & Ascher, L. M. (1979). Controlled comparison of progressive relaxation, stimulus control, and paradoxical intention therapies for insomnia. *Journal of Consulting and Clinical Psychology, 47,* 500–508.

Turner, R. M., & Ascher, L. M. (1982). Therapist factor in the treatment of insomnia. *Behaviour Research and Therapy, 20,* 33–40.

Watson, G. (1940). Areas of agreement in psychotherapy. *American Journal of Orthopsychiatry, 10,* 698–709.

Weissman, M. M., Klerman, G. L., Prusoff, B. A., Sholomskas, D., & Padian, N. (1981). Depressed outpatients: Results one year after treatment with drugs and/or interpersonal psychotherapy. *Archives of General Psychiatry, 38,* 51–55.

Wilson, G. T. (1982). Psychotherapy process and procedure: The behavioral mandate. *Behavior Therapy, 13,* 291–312.

Zeiss, A. M., Lewinsohn, P. M., & Munoz, R. F. (1979). Nonspecific improvement effects in depression using interpersonal skills training, pleasant activity schedules, or cognitive training. *Journal of Consulting and Clinical Psychology, 47,* 427–439.

10

Relapse and Recurrence in Psychopathological Disorders

STEVEN D. HOLLON

RONALD COBB

Many psychopathological disorders show a variable course. In those disorders, a period of acute symptomatology may be followed by periods of relative freedom from symptoms, but the individual remains at elevated risk for symptom return. In such disorders, the return of symptoms following a symptom-free interval can have real implications for both theory and clinical practice.

In this chapter, we consider the nature and implications of symptom return following a well interval. Because our own expertise lies largely in the area of the affective disorders, we draw heavily on concepts and findings from that domain. Given that the affective disorders are largely episodic in nature, that is not an unhappy coincidence. Nonetheless, we try to extend the relevant concepts to other representative types of psychopathology.

The study of the temporal course of disorder dates at least to Kraepelin (1921). The central thesis of this chapter is that the study of the processes driving symptom return can both contribute to our understanding of the etiological mechanisms underlying the expression of the disorder and elucidate the mediators of therapeutic change.

AFFECTIVE DISORDERS

Relapse versus Recurrence

The affective disorders (i.e., depression and mania) have long been known to be episodic in nature (Beck, 1967). Although any given episode is typically self-limiting in that recovery tends to occur whether treatment is sought or not, the disorder tends to be recurrent in that most individuals who experience one episode will experience multiple episodes (Consensus Development Panel, 1985). A minority of such patients will experience only a single episode and another minority will exhibit a chronic course, but, for most such individuals, the course is one of recurrent symptomatic episodes separated by protracted symptom-free intervals (Keller, 1985).

In the affective disorders, there is a growing consensus regarding the need to distinguish between relapse versus recurrence. According to a recent MacArthur Foundation Task Force (Frank et al., 1991), *relapse* is best defined as the return of symptoms associated with the index episode, whereas *recurrence* represents the onset of a wholly new episode. Consistent with these conventions, *remission* is defined as the termination of symptoms associated with the index episode, whereas the term *recovery* is reserved for the end of the episode itself. Although these conventions are by no means universal (Prien, Carpenter, & Kupfer, 1991), they do represent an effort to establish a set of common definitions that are likely to be widely adopted in the field in the years to come.

Why distinguish between relapse and recurrence? An analogy can be drawn between the affective disorders and ear infections in young children. Typically, an infant with such an infection shows manifest signs and symptoms consistent with the disorder (e.g., fever, redness in the ear, and crying). Treating the child with an antibiotic usually results in a rapid amelioration of distress. However, withdrawing the medication prematurely (i.e., shortly after symptomatic relief has been achieved) often leads to a rapid return of the manifest symptoms. Presumably, the symptomatic expression of the disorder was merely being suppressed. The underlying infection is still in the infant's system, waiting to reassert itself if treatment is terminated prematurely. In most instances, several weeks of treatment are required to ensure that the underlying infection is eradicated. Only then can medication be safely withdrawn without undue risk of symptom return.

It is widely believed that a similar state of affairs may exist in the affective disorders. Most studies of the natural course of the affective disorders have observed that risk for symptom return is greatest during the first several months following remission (Keller, Shapiro, Lavori, & Wolfe, 1982; Lavori, Keller, & Klerman, 1984). This is particularly true when remission is induced pharmacologically (Hollon, Evans, & DeRubeis, 1990). It has become common clinical practice to continue antidepressant medications for several months following the cessation of symptoms in an effort to forestall relapse (Prien & Kupfer, 1986).

Nature of the Episode

What this suggests is that the underlying episode has a life of its own that runs its course regardless of whether symptoms are manifest (Hollon etal., 1990). Longitudinal studies predating the introduction of interventions known to be effective in the treatment of depression suggest that the typical untreated episode lasts about 6 to 12 months, with an interval of 3 to 4 symptom-free years before the next episode (Beck, 1967). Tricyclic antidepressants (TCAs), the current standard of treatment, typically produce clinical response within 4 to 6 weeks, well before the episode would remit spontaneously. Unless pharmacotherapy "turns off" the mechanisms responsible for the expression of the episode, such patients should be at elevated risk for relapse between the time of pharmacologically induced remission and the completion of true spontaneous recovery.

This period of risk is depicted in Figure 10.1. In this figure, the hatched portion represents a region of risk during which medication discontinuation is particularly likely to be followed by symptom return. During this interval, the mechanisms driving the episode are still in place; in essence, the individual is still "in episode," despite the fact that manifest symptoms are currently being suppressed by active medication. Following Frank and associates (1991) conventions, such individuals would be said to be symptomatically remitted, but not yet recovered from the underlying episode.

Two-Process Model of Risk

It may be that risk can best be described as the consequence of two independent risk processes, one involving the mechanisms that determine the course of the underlying episode (relapse), and the other involving the vulnerability factors that keep the individual at risk even after the episode has run its course (recurrence). According to this two-process risk model, relapse should be tied temporally to the treated episode such that risk declines as a function of time from most recent onset. The decline in risk for relapse should parallel the expected course of spontaneous recovery. Risk for recurrence, by constrast, is presumed to be relatively constant over time. Risk for relapse should be superimposed on risk for recurrence because there is no reason for the mechanisms controlling the latter to cease to exist just because an individual enters an active episode.

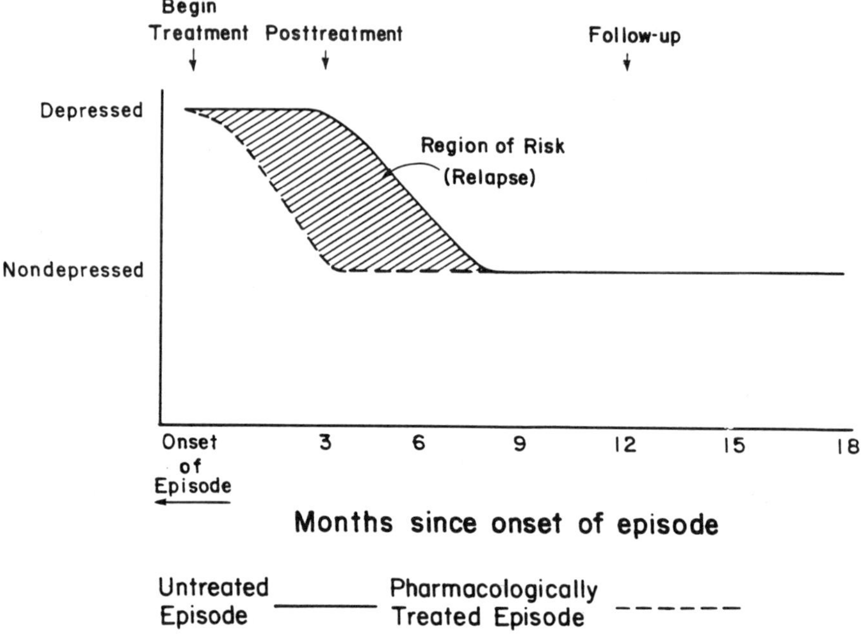

FIGURE 10.1. Course of untreated versus pharmacologically treated depressions. From "Cognitive Mediation of Relapse Prevention Following Treatment for Depression: Implications of Differential Risk" (p. 127) by S. D. Hollon, M. D. Evans, and R. J. DeRubeis, in R. E. Ingram (Ed.), *Contemporary Psychological Approaches to Depression,* 1990, New York: Plenum Press. Copyright 1990 by Plenum Publishing Corp. Reprinted by permission.

Figure 10.2 presents the cumulative risk that would be expected to result under such a two-process risk model. In this figure, risk is depicted as the number of months "survived" without a return of symptoms. (Survival is plotted semilogarithmically, in order to adjust for sampling without replacement. Failure to do so would result in a negatively accelerated curve, even when risk is constant. Such improperly plotted curves have sometimes been interpreted substantively to suggest that some process exists that reduces risk over time. As described by Sutton [1979], this has been particularly common in the substance abuse literature, a point we return to in a later section.) Under such a model, total risk should be greatest shortly following pharmacologically induced remission; it should then decline over the next several months in a manner that parallels the course of spontaneous recovery

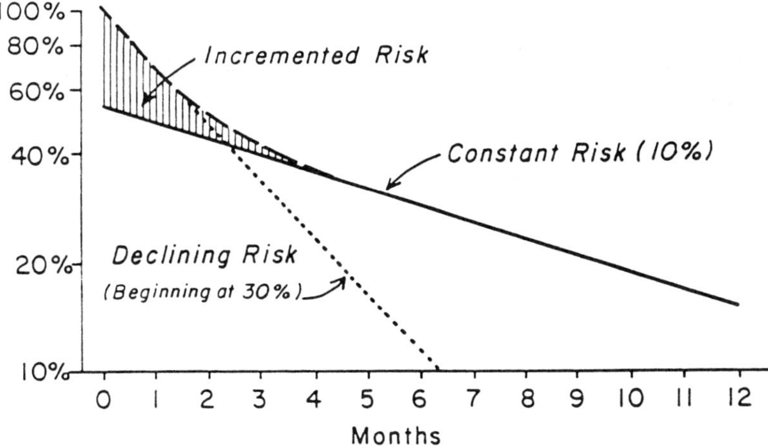

FIGURE 10.2. Two-process risk model plotted semilogarithmically. From "Cognitive Mediation of Relapse Prevention Following Treatment for Depression: Implications of Differential Risk" (p. 128) by S. D. Hollon, M. D. Evans, and R. J. DeRubeis, in R. E. Ingram (Ed.), *Contemporary Psychological Approaches to Depression*, 1990, New York: Plenum Press. Copyright 1990 by Plenum Publishing Corp. Reprinted by permission.

before finally "flattening" out to the lower rate associated with recurrence alone.

Figures 10.3 and 10.4 present data on placebo continuation patients from two of the largest and best known continuation medication trials (Glen, Johnson, & Shepherd, 1984; Prien et al., 1984). In each study, depressed outpatients were first treated to remission pharmacologically and then withdrawn from active medication. Consistent with a two-process model, risk following successful short-term pharmacotherapy was approximately three times as great during the first 6 to 12 months following medication withdrawal as it was during any subsequent period. It should be noted that the hypothetical curve depicted in Figure 10.2 was constructed on a priori theoretical grounds *before* inspecting the empirical literature.

Multiple Subtypes Model of Risk

Does this mean that relapse and recurrence are necessarily mediated by distinct processes? Not necessarily. As described by Lavori and colleagues

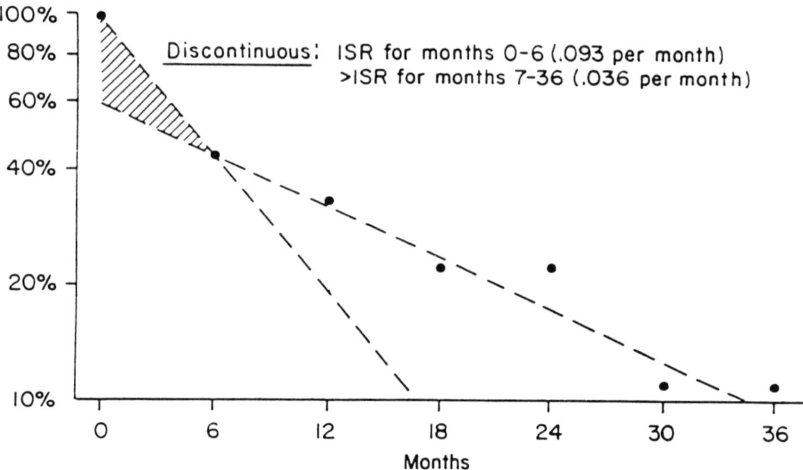

FIGURE 10.3. Semilogarithmic survivorship curve for placebo-continuation patients from Glen et al., 1984. From "Cognitive Mediation of Relapse Prevention Following Treatment for Depression: Implications of Differential Risk" (p. 129) by S. D. Hollon, M. D. Evans, and R. J. DeRubeis, in R. E. Ingram (Ed.), *Contemporary Psychological Approaches to Depression,* 1990, New York: Plenum Press. Copyright 1990 by Plenum Publishing Corp. Reprinted by permission.

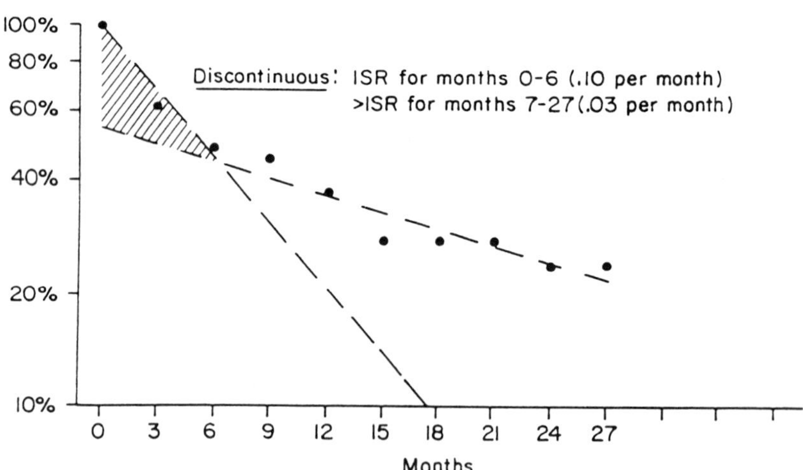

FIGURE 10.4. Semilogarithmic survivorship curve for placebo-continuation patients from Prien et al., 1984. From "Cognitive Mediation of Relapse Prevention Following Treatment for Depression: Implications of Differential Risk" (p. 130) by S. D. Hollon, M. D. Evans, and R. J. DeRubeis, in R. E. Ingram (Ed.), *Contemporary Psychological Approaches to Depression,* 1990, New York: Plenum Press. Copyright 1990 by Plenum Publishing Corp. Reprinted by permission.

(1984), there is at least one viable alternative model that would produce a comparable pattern of findings. If, instead of two distinct processes, there exist two or more subtypes of depression differing in risk for symptom return, the more rapid exit of the higher risk subtype(s) from the sample could produce a cumulative survival curve similar to that depicted in Figure 10.2. Such a model, labeled the *multiple subtypes* hypothesis, represents a viable alternative to the two-process hypothesis.

It is quite possible that distinct subtypes do exist that differ in risk. For example, patients with "double depression" (i.e., patients for whom the current episode of major depression is superimposed on a history of chronic dysthymia) have been found to be at higher risk than patients without a history of chronicity (Keller et al., 1982). In that same study, among patients without a history of chronicity, those patients with a history of multiple prior episodes were found to be at higher risk than those patients with no such history (Keller et al., 1982).

Nonetheless, we doubt that the observed findings can be accounted for solely by the presence of multiple subtypes. Such subtypes would have to be few in number and quite distinct in risk to account for the findings observed. We think it is more likely that two distinct sets of causal processes are shared universally by all depressed patients showing an episodic course, although subtypes also exist that vary in risk within each of those two processes. This issue could be tested empirically. For example, the multiple subtypes model would predict that discontinuity in risk is a consequence of sample heterogeneity; under such a model, no such discontinuity should be found in narrowly defined subsets of depressives (e.g., recurrent depressives with three or more prior episodes) regardless of when they are withdrawn from medication. Conversely, the two-process model would suggest that discontinuity in risk is a consequence of premature medication withdrawal; no such discontinuity should be found when medications are continued past the time required for the underlying episode to run its course.

The existing data are ambiguous. Keller and associates (1982) found little evidence of discontinuity among recurrent patients with three or more prior episodes withdrawn from medications while still within the period of risk for relapse, whereas Frank and colleagues (1990) found evidence of discontinuity among recurrent patients continued on medications well past the point of risk for relapse. Both sets of findings argue in favor of the multiple-subtypes model. By contrast, two other studies that continued medication past the point of risk for relapse found no evidence of any discontinuity in risk following medication withdrawal (Evans et al., 1992; Kane et al., 1982). These latter findings argue in favor of the two-process model. Clearly, additional research, designed with this question in mind, will be needed to resolve this issue.

Implications for Psychopathology Research

What would it mean for psychopathology research if risk for relapse were truly distinct from risk for recurrence in the affective disorders? Elsewhere, we have described how such a state of affairs might allow causal inferences to be drawn from purely correlational designs (Hollon et al., 1990). Such a design would capitalize on pharmacotherapy's symptom-suppressive status to deconfound the causes of the disorder from its consequences.

Consider first three different logical classes of phenomena relevant to depression. State-dependent symptoms represent the observable manifestations of the affective disorder. They are, in effect, the consequences of being depressed, but they are not themselves causal to the depression. Causal mechanisms represent the processes controlling the onset and offset of an episode. Most persons at risk for the affective disorders show a variable course; they are not invariably symptomatic. Thus, there must be some psychopathological or pathophysiological events that determine whether such people are in episode at any given time. External events, such as interpersonal loss or intrapersonal frustrations, may play a pre-cipitating role. We return to a discussion of this issue later in the chapter.) Finally, "stable" traits represent factors that may predispose an individual to become depressed, but do not themselves initiate the episode. As such, they contribute to risk, but they are not themselves sufficient to produce the symptomatic expression of the disorder. (We have put the term *stable* in quotes because these traits may change over time, but they must not wholly covary with the expression of either the underlying episode or the manifest symptoms.)

It is important to clarify the conceptual distinctions between these three logical classes of variables. Once again, an analogy may prove helpful. Consider the system used to light the typical room. Any such system consists of at least three components: the lights, the switch on the wall, and the wiring in the wall. The lights correspond to the state-dependent symptoms; when engaged, we have visible evidence that something is going on, but that "something" lies at the end of a causal chain that produces the phenomenon of illumination. Whether the lights shine has no effect on either the switch or the wiring; it is a purely state-dependent consequence of those other events. The switch on the wall corresponds to the mechanisms that control the onset and offset of the particular "episode." It must be thrown in the on position for the lights to shine. In that sense, it can be considered causal to the phenomenon of illumination (at the least, it can be said to play a mediational role). Finally, the wiring in the wall corresponds to the stable predisposing factors that contribute to, but are not sufficient to cause the episode to occur.

As shown in Table 10.1, the typical psychopathology design consists

TABLE 10.1. Design Logic for Deconfounding Symptoms, Mechanisms, and Traits

	Status with respect to depression						
	Symptomatic		Remitted		Recovered		Never
Symptoms:	Abnormal	>	Normal	=	Normal	=	Normal
Mechanisms:	Abnormal	=	Abnormal	>	Normal	=	Normal
Traits:	Abnormal	=	Abnormal	=	Abnormal	>	Normal

Note. From Hollon, Evans, and DeRubeis, 1990, p. 132. Copyright 1990 by Plenum Publishing Corp. Reprinted by permission.

of a minimal two cell comparison between a currently depressed sample (column 1) and a largely "never depressed" control sample (column 4). (We say "largely" never depressed because in many studies there is no attempt to control for prior history. Thus, some small portion of the control subjects can be expected to have a positive history for depression or exhibit risk factors for its subsequent occurrence.) The three rows represent three different classes of variables: state-dependent symptoms (the consequences of being depressed), causal mechanisms (the processes controlling the occurrence of an episode), and stable traits (factors that may predispose an individual to become depressed, but that do not themselves initiate the episode).

As shown in Table 10.1, the typical two-group psychopathology design does not permit separation of these three classes of variables; all three are abnormal in the currently depressed group, and all three are normal among the "never depressed" controls. The middle two cells, however, capitalize on the symptom suppressive status of pharmaco-therapy for the affective disorders to do just that.

As can be seen in Table 10.1 (reprinted from Hollon et al., 1990), the second column depicts the same group of depressed subjects shortly following successful treatment with tricyclic antidepressants, approximately 3 months after initiating treatment. By this time, treatment-responsive subjects should be in a state of clinical remission; that is, symptoms should have normalized, but not the underlying mechanisms or stable traits. The third column depicts this same group of patients at a still later point, approximately 12 months following the beginning of treatment. By this time, the patients should have moved through the period of risk for relapse; that is, the causal mechanisms driving the underlying episode should have resolved. In essence, patients should have recovered and no longer be at elevated risk for relapse.

Thus, each of the three classes of variables should show a different pattern of change over time relative to that exhibited by a "never depressed" control. Consequential symptoms should normalize with remission, mechanisms controlling the life of the particular episode should normalize with recovery, and predispositional traits should not normalize. As a final check, purported mechanisms should predict risk for relapse (but not necessarily recurrence), whereas stable traits should predict risk for recurrence (but not necessarily relapse). Although we are unaware of any study that has attempted to apply this logic, we think it has real promise for helping to disentangle causal status with respect to the affective disorders.

Implications for Treatment Research

Finally, we can ask what implications the distinction between relapse versus recurrence has for studies of treatment process. As shown in Table 10.2 (reprinted from Hollon et al., 1990), at least three kinds of intervention strategies can be defined, based on their locus of action with respect to the classes of relevant processes just described.

According to this scheme, *suppressive* interventions are those treatments that block the expression of the manifest symptoms. Such interventions do not directly affect the underlying mechanisms controlling the presence of the episode, and they do nothing to alter the predisposing traits that confer subsequent risk. Thus, such interventions provide symptomatic relief, but do nothing to alter subsequent risk, either for relapse or recurrence.

Curative interventions, by contrast, directly affect the mechanisms that control the life of the underlying episode. As such, they can be expected both to reduce symptomatic distress and to reduce risk for subsequent relapse. In effect, such interventions turn off the existing episode. What they do not do is reduce risk for subsequent episodes.

That is done by truly *prophylactic* interventions. Such interventions reduce risk for recurrence by directly affecting the stable traits (or subsequent pathophysiology) that give rise to the onset of new episodes. Such interventions might have little effect on an existing episode, either in terms of ameliorating existing symptoms or reducing risk for relapse, but should reduce subsequent risk following recovery.

TABLE 10.2. Three Modes of Treatment Efficacy

Suppressive	Blocks the expression of symptoms associated with an ongoing episode, but does not affect the course of that episode or reduce the probability of future episodes
Curative	Interrupts the course of the ongoing episode, both providing symptom relief and reducing risk for relapse, but does not reduce the probability of future episodes
Prophylactic	Reduces the probability of future episodes; need not necessarily reduce symptoms associated with an existing episode or reduce risk for relapse following remission

Note. From Hollon, Evans, and DeRubeis, 1990, p. 131. Copyright 1990 by Plenum Publishing Corp. Reprinted by permission.

It should be noted that this classification scheme is based upon the presumed locus of action. As such, it differs somewhat from definitions currently in conventional usage (see, for example, Quitkin, Rifkin, & Klein, 1976). For example, there is good evidence that providing ongoing pharmacotherapy for euthymic individuals with a history of multiple prior episodes of mania or depression prevents both relapse and recurrence (Frank et al., 1990; Glen et al., 1984; Prien et al., 1984). However, it remains unclear whether this preventive effect is mediated by the action of the medications on either underlying mechanisms or stable traits. It is quite possible that the preventive effect is obtained by the continued provision of a purely symptom–suppressive intervention. Careful attention to the differential impact of the various clinical interventions on response, relapse, and recurrence, along with the simultaneous study of the effects of those treatments on purported symptom, mechanism, and trait measures, should facilitate our understanding of the mechanisms of therapeutic action.

Predictors of Risk

Can any factors be said to predict differential risk for relapse versus recurrence following remission or recovery? Unfortunately, although a number of studies have followed the course of affectively disordered patients over time and attempted to identify factors that predicted risk, most have failed to distinguish between the two. Nonetheless, careful attention to the nature of the samples studied and the types and duration of treatment provided (if any) should allow some rough conclusions to be drawn.

In a recent comprehensive review, Belsher and Costello (1988) identified factors predictive of risk among depressed patients following successful treatment. Included among these factors were (1) time since remission, (2) nature of treatment, (3) recent environmental stress, (4) absence of social support, (5) history of prior episodes, (6) history of chronicity, and (7) persistent neuroendocrine dysregulation. To this list we would add (8) the presence of certain cognitive proclivities, particularly a negative attributional style, which we have found to be predictive of risk for relapse following successful treatment (Evans et al., 1992). We discuss each in turn.

Time Since Remission

In their review, Belsher and Costello (1988) report that although cumulative risk increases with time, the risk for symptom return in any given interval (interval specific risk, or ISR) tends to decline with the passage of time. Lavori and colleagues (1984) arrived at a similar conclusion in their quantitative review of a largely overlapping literature. What this means is that the probability that a given individual will experience a return of symptoms goes up the longer that individual is followed (e.g., symptoms are more likely to return within 12 months than within one month), but that the likelihood that they will return in a given month is greatest shortly after remission and declines thereafter (e.g., the likelihood that symptoms will return in the first month is greater than the likelihood that they will return in the twelfth month, given that they have not already done so).

Nonetheless, not all such studies show such a decline in interval specific risk. For example, an examination of the survival curves reported by Lavori and associates (1984) suggests that only those studies conducted after the introduction of the tricyclic antidepressants (Bratfos & Haug, 1968; Keller et al., 1982; Kolakowska, 1975; Murphy, Woodruff, Herjanic, & Fisher, 1974; Perris & D'Elia, 1966) show such a declining interval-specific rate of risk. Studies conducted prior to the introduction of those interventions (Brodwall, 1947; Huston & Locher, 1948; Lundquist, 1945; Seager, 1958) show little indication of any such decline. This suggests that relapse may be a largely treatment-dependent phenomenon. As has been previously suggested, it may be that what is needed to leave the patient in a state of elevated risk for symptom return shortly following remission is an intervention that suppresses symptom expression while leaving unaffected the underlying mechanisms driving the episode. In essence, a treatment must first be applied that suppresses manifest symptoms (but does not cure the underlying episode), and that treatment must then be taken away before that episode has had a chance to run its course, for the patient to be put at risk of relapse.

The ultimate implication, of course, is that relapse (as currently defined) is a largely treatment-dependent phenomenon; it exists only when a symptom-suppressive intervention is superimposed, temporarily, on a disorder with a natural course that is unaffected by that intervention. Recurrence, in contrast, represents the pure expression of the natural course of the disorder. Although it may be affected by truly prophylactic interventions (should any be found to exist), its existence as a natural phenomenon does not depend on the nature and timing of those interventions.

Nature of Treatment

Although there is ample evidence that antidepressant medications are effective in accelerating the course of symptomatic relief (Klein, Gittelman, Quitkin, & Rifkin, 1980), there is little indication that they are more than symptom-suppressive. Patients continued on medication for several months following short-term acute treatment are at far lower risk of symptom return than are patients discontinued from active treatment (Prien & Kupfer, 1986). Risk following medication discontinuation appears to be about three times as great following brief treatment (2–4 months) than following extended treatment (10–12 months) (Hollon et al., 1990). Although providing extended maintenance medication does appear to suppress subsequent recurrence (Frank et al., 1990), there is no evidence that prior medication does anything to reduce risk for subsequent symptom return following termination.

It has long been suggested that the various psychosocial interventions might produce change that survives the end of treatment, that is, that psychotherapy provides more than purely symptomatic change (Wolberg, 1967). With respect to depression, there is some reason to think that this might be the case, at least for some types of interventions. In recent years, there has been considerable interest in two relatively short-term interventions, interpersonal psychotherapy and cognitive therapy. Interpersonal psychotherapy, largely adapted from Sullivanian principles, focuses on dealing with problems and patterns in important interpersonal relationships (Klerman, Weissman, Rounsaville, & Chevron, 1984). Interpersonal psychotherapy has typically faired well in studies of acute response (Elkin et al., 1989; Weissman et al., 1979), and it appears to provide some protection against relapse (Klerman, DiMascio, Weissman, Prusoff, & Paykel, 1974) and recurrence (Frank et al., 1990), so long as it is continued or maintained. Nonetheless, there is, as yet, no direct evidence that it reduces risk following the termination of treatment (Weissman, Klerman, Prusoff, Sholomskas, & Padian, 1981), although there are some indications that it might indeed produce delayed improvements in interpersonal functioning (Weissman, Klerman, Paykel, Prusoff, & Hanson, 1974; Weissman et al., 1981).

Cognitive therapy is predicated on the notion that negative beliefs and maladaptive information processing contribute to the etiology and maintenance of depression (Beck, Rush, Shaw, & Emery, 1979). It has similarly fared well in controlled trials of acute response (see Hollon, Shelton, & Loosen, 1991, for a review; but see Elkin et al., 1989, for an exception). More critically for our current purposes, there are indications that it may reduce risk even following treatment termination (Hollon et al., 1991). Across four naturalistic follow-ups of controlled trials (Blackburn, Eunson, & Bishop, 1986; Evans et al., 1991; Kovacs, Rush, Beck, & Hollon, 1981; Simons, Murphy, Levine, & Wetzel, 1986), patients treated to remission with cognitive therapy (either alone or in combination with medications) have typically shown about half the risk following treatment termination as patients treated to remission pharmacologically.

Although not conclusive (the samples studied have been small and, as described in Hollon et al. [1991] the findings open to multiple interpretation), these studies do suggest that cognitive therapy may be more than simply symptom-suppressive. Even if the findings observed do reflect a "true" preventive effect, it remains to be seen whether this effect extends to recurrence. (In the existing trials, treatment was terminated well before the episode would have been expected to run its course, and the bulk of the instances of differential symptom return occurred during the period of risk for relapse.) In either event, the discovery of a preventive intervention holds great promise theoretically. If cognitive therapy proves to be prophylactic with respect to at least relapse, than those processes differentially affected by the intervention relative to pharmacotherapy are likely candidates as the mechanisms controlling episode onset and offset. If cognitive therapy proves to be preventive with respect to recurrence, then an examination of those processes differentially affected may facilitate the search for the risk factors contributing to vulnerability to the disorder (Hollon et al., 1990).

Recent Environmental Stress

Paykel and Tanner (1976) examined the relation of life events to symptom return in the context of a controlled trial of continuation pharmacotherapy. In this study, all patients were first treated to remission with 4 to 6 weeks of acute pharmacotherapy and then either continued on medication or withdrawn onto a pill-placebo or a no-pill condition. (These three levels of medication were crossed with two levels of psychotherapy, but that is of little concern for our present purposes.) Across the full sample, patients who relapsed during an ensuing 8-month continuation phase exhibited a significantly greater number of negative life events in the 3 months prior to relapse than did matched controls during that same period. No such relation was observed in two other studies (Faravelli, Ambonetti, Pallanti, & Pazzagli, 1986; Gonzales, Lewinsohn, & Clarke 1985), but may have been obscured by methodological limitations (see Belsher & Costello, 1988, for an extended discussion).

Conceptually, life events would be expected to be more closely related to recurrence than to relapse. Negative life events are generally seen as constituting the precipitating event in a diathesis–stress model. Nonetheless, there is no a priori reason why negative life events should not be related to symptomatic relapse.

Absence of Social Support

Two studies have found a relation between family interaction patterns and risk following treatment (Hooley, Orley, & Teasdale, 1986; Vaughn & Leff, 1976). In both studies, a high level of "expressed emotion," defined as a pattern of overinvolvement and verbalized hostility and criticism toward the patient, was found to be associated with greater risk for relapse. Positive family interaction patterns were found to be associated with lowered rates of risk following hospitalization in samples including, but not restricted to, previously hospitalized depressives (Breier & Strauss, 1984; Spiegel & Wissler, 1986).

History of Prior Episodes

Several studies have suggested that the number of prior episodes predicts subsequent risk. In their reanalysis of nine studies published between 1947 and 1982, Lavori and associates (1984) found that patients with more frequent prior episodes were at greater subsequent risk. Although it was not possible to determine whether risk pertained to relapse or recurrence, it is likely that it was the latter. In what was probably the most comprehensive study of relapse and recurrence following remission and recovery, Keller and colleagues (Keller & Shapiro, 1981; Keller, Lavori, Lewis, & Klerman, 1983; Keller et al., 1982) found the number of prior episodes to be a predictor of subsequent risk. Similarly, Gonzalez and colleagues (1985) found the of prior episodes to be predictive of subsequent relapse following successful treatment for depression.

Despite the robustness of the finding, it should be clear that an index like number of prior episodes is not a likely candidate as either a mechanism or a predispositional trait. It does appear to be a predictor, but it does not itself vary with the period of risk. Thus, it cannot be a mechanism. Similarly, although it can be thought of as a predispositional trait, it cannot itself enter into the causal process leading to the generation of risk (it cannot itself be the actual causal diathesis). It appears most reasonable to consider the number of prior episodes as a marker of risk, a correlate of the actual causal processes that are themselves predisposing factors in the underlying structure.

Such a recognition could have a salutary effect on research. Because of the number of prior episodes appears to covary with risk, it should prove possible to use number of prior episodes (controlling for age and age at first episode) to form groups for the purposes of subsequent hypothesis testing. Thus, those processes that differentiate patients with few versus many prior episodes are particularly likely to be *stable* traits that contribute to risk. Once again, we put the term "stable" in quotes, in this instance because it is quite possible that such factors can grow across time; that is, processes that predispose to subsequent risk may be acquired as a consequence of experience. This is a topic we return to in a subsequent section.

History of Chronicity

There are indications that a history of chronicity predicts greater risk, although these indications are not robust. In a particularly large and influential study, Keller and associates (1982) found that patients with "double depression," a current episode of major depression superimposed on a history of chronic dysthymia, are more likely to relapse following an 8-week period of minimal symptomatology than are patients without such a history. In a smaller study, Gonzales and colleagues (1985) reported a trend in the opposite direction. In their review, Belsher and Costello (1988) conclude that the Keller group's findings are likely to be the more reliable, but note that the methods used in the two trials were actually quite comparable. Clearly, additional research is needed to clarify this discrepancy.

Assuming that the relation between chronicity and risk does hold, one additional finding from Keller and associates (1982) becomes relevant. In that study, differential risk as a function of chronicity was most evident during the first several weeks after the period of minimal symptomatology; differences in interval specific rates of risk were not significant beyond the fourth week of follow-up. What this suggests is that patients with a history of chronicity never truly "recovered," even with treatment. It may well be the case that chronic depressives are chronic because they do not spontaneously recovery from any given episode. In terms of the earlier lighting system analogy, such patients may have a "switch on the wall" that never moves to the "off" position. If true, then one additional strategy for identifying the causal mechanisms that underly the course of a given episode may be to follow medicated patients across an extended continuation period and identify those processes that show differentially greater change in patients without a history of chronicity than in those with such a history.

Persistent Neuroendocrine Dysfunction

There are indications that persistent neuroendocrine dysregulation may contribute to subsequent risk. As described in greater detail elsewhere (Shelton, Hollon, Purdon, & Loosen, 1991), two types of dysregulation are of particular interest: dysfunction in the hypothalamic-pituitary-adrenal (HPA) axis and dysfunction in the hypothalamic-pituitary-thyroid (HPT) axis. The HPA axis plays an important role in the regulation of response to stress. Stressful life events trigger noradrenergic neurons in the brain stem to fire, which in turn stimulate the release of corticotropin releasing hormone (CRH) in the hypothalamus. The CRH stimulates the release of adrenocorticotropic hormone (ACTH) from the pituitary, which in turn stimulates the release of cortisol from the adrenals. The HPA dysfunction typically is indexed by the lack of cortisol suppression following the administration of the synthetic hormone dexamethasone (the dexamethasone suppression test, or DST), but can also be indexed by elevated basal cortisol or blunted ACTH release following CRH administration (Amsterdam, Maislin, Gold, & Winokur, 1989).

The HPT axis appears to be largely involved in the regulation of basal temperature. Changes in ambient temperature levels trigger firing of serotonergic neurons in the raphe nucleus, which stimulate the release of thyrotropin-releasing hormone (TRH) from the hypothalamus. The TRH in turn stimulates the release of thyrotropin stimulating hormone (TSH) from the pituitary, which in turn stimulates the release of the thyroid hormones T_3 and T_4 from the thyroid glands. The HPT dysregulation takes the form of blunted TSH release following administration of TRH (Loosen, 1986).

In a recent review, Arana, Baldessarini, and Orsten (1985) found that 77% of patients evidencing DST nonsuppression at recovery relapsed within the next several months, compared to only 19% of those patients showing DST suppression. Differences of a comparable magnitude have been noted as a function of persistent TSH-blunting following TRH administration, with patients showing blunting at greater risk (Loosen, 1986). Dysregulation in one axis is relatively independent of dysregulation in the other, with up to 60% of all patients evidencing dysregulation in one or both (Winokur, Amsterdam, Caroff, Snyder, & Brunswick, 1982). Although HPA-axis dysregulation is somewhat more common than HPT-axis dysregulation during the acute episode, dysregulation in the latter appears to be more stable following recovery. It is thus a better candidate as a vulnerability factor. It is now generally accepted that HPA-axis abnormalities are largely state-dependent. Further, HPA-axis dysregulation appears to be closely tied to the severity of the current episode. For example, in a review of 14 published trials, Khan and colleagues (1988) found an average rate of nonsuppression of only 20% among outpatients versus an average rate of 54% among inpatients. Thus, even though persistent HPA-axis dysregulation might predict relapse, the proportion of outpatients evidencing dysregulation at remission is so low as to limit its utility as a marker of risk.

Negative Cognitive Style

Cognitive theories of depression hold that negative beliefs and maladaptive information-processing styles represent cognitive diatheses that predispose to risk for depression. In the oldest and best known of these models, Beck (1967) has proposed that persons at risk for depression possess a depressotypic schema. According to this model, the propensity for depressotypic thinking lies dormant until triggered by negative life events; it then becomes activated and colors the way the individual interprets the self, the world, and the future (Kovacs & Beck, 1978).

In a closely related model, Seligman, Abramson, and colleagues

(Abramson, Metalsky, & Alloy, 1989; Abramson, Seligman, & Teasdale, 1978; Peterson & Seligman, 1984) have emphasized the role of negative attributional (or explanatory) style in the etiology of depression. According to this attributional reformulation of the learned helplessness model, individuals with a tendency to interpret negative life events in an internal, global, and stable fashion are seen as being at elevated risk for becoming depressed in the face of life stress. The two models are hardly incompatible, in that attributional styles could readily be seen as part of a larger schematic structure, but schema theory does posit the existence of a larger cognitive network, whereas the attributional reformulation places a particular emphasis on the role of a specific type of inferential process.

In general, the evidence for a causal role for either (or any) type of cognitive model is equivocal at best. Although persons who are currently depressed clearly are much more negative and process information in a different fashion than those who are not, it is not yet clear that differences can be detected between persons differing in risk when comparably euthymic (Barnett & Gotlib, 1988). In part, this may reflect a failure in research methodology; most such studies have treated depressotypic cognition as a stable trait rather than as the latent predisposition (Hollon, 1992) or have operationalized the attributional construct in a less than optimal fashion (Peterson & Seligman, 1984). In our own work, we have found that cognitive therapy produces greater change in attributional styles than does tricyclic pharmacotherapy, and that attributional style following successful treatment predicts (and may mediate) cognitive therapy's apparent relapse-preventive effect (Hollon et al., 1990). Whether this finding will replicate in subsequent studies and, if it does, whether it will extend to the prediction of recurrence remain to be seen, but, for the present, we consider such cognitive propensities to represent particularly interesting candidates as potential diatheses that deserve further exploration.

OTHER DISORDERS

Are there other disorders to which the relapse–recurrence distinction applies? There are other disorders for which some evidence exists for episodicity, or at least remission with subsequent recrudescence. We next consider several of these disorders.

Schizophrenia

The classic depiction of schizophrenia is of a chronic disorder with a deteriorating course (Kraepelin, 1921). Subsequent conceptualizations have deemphasized the notion of chronicity as a defining feature, but the implication remains that the disorder typically continues, with only a waxing and waning of symptoms, once it has begun (American Psychiatric Association, 1987). Although the more florid symptoms typically remit over time, a return to full premorbid levels of functioning is not common. The modal course is typically one of acute exacerbations superimposed on continued residual impairment.

It has become common to distinguish between positive symptoms (e.g., florid signs of acute disorder such as delusions, hallucinations, loosening of associations) versus negative symptoms (e.g., social withdrawal, flattening of affect, motivational decrements). The course of the disorder is typically divided into three stages: a *prodromal phase,* in which there is a clear deterioration from previous levels of functioning; an *active phase,* during which the psychotic symptoms become prominent; and a *residual phase,* which follows the active phase of disorder. Negative symptoms appear to be present during all three phases, but are typically overshadowed by the more florid positive symptoms during the active phase (American Psychiatric Association, 1987).

Two patterns predominate with respect to the course of the disorder (Ciompi, 1980). The first is marked by an acute onset, followed by an undulating course and a generally good recovery from the given episode. Subsequent episodes often occur, but are typically followed by a relatively rapid recovery. The second pattern involves a more gradual onset, followed by a chronic course and considerable residual impairment. Each pattern has been found to account for approximately one quarter of all cases, with various combinations of onset, course, and outcome accounting for smaller proportions of the remaining instances of the disorder.

It is not clear that recovery occurs in schizophrenia, at least not in the sense that the term is used with respect to the affective disorders. A complete cessation of symptoms, especially negative symptoms, appears to be unusual. Even among those patients showing the best long-term adjustment, subtle and not-so-subtle signs of residual deficit often remain (Lehmann & Cancro, 1985). Nonetheless, it is likely that at least some patients do show a relatively complete recovery, and many more show periods of at least partial or full remission. A number of factors appear to be predictive of better long-term prognosis, including acute onset, better premorbid adjustment, later age of onset, and presence of affective distress (Lehman & Cancro, 1985).

Antipsychotic medications remain the current standard of treatment in the schizophrenias, but there is a general consensus that a broad-based approach that combines medications with individual and family counseling is better still (Simpson & May, 1985). Although the antipsychotic medications are most clearly effective in suppressing the expression of the more florid positive symptoms, there are indications that they, perhaps in combination with changes in the nature of psychosocial treatment and milieu factors, may halt the progression to more distinctive manifestations of the disorder (Lehman & Cancro, 1985). Continuation medication strategies appear to reduce the rate of relapse, at least with respect to the reemergence of the acute phase and the associated expression of positive symptoms, but may not affect the course of negative symptoms as powerfully. In recent years, interventions targeted at modifying the behavior of family members toward the recovering patient have shown real promise in reducing the rate of relapse into acute psychotic states (Goldstein, 1991).

On the whole, although it is evident that the schizophrenias are less clearly episodic than the affective disorders, some indications of variability in course and outcome do exist. This is particularly true with respect to the positive symptoms of the disorder. Whether a distinction between relapse versus recurrence (or remission versus recovery) applies to the schizophrenias remains to be determined, but it does appear to have some promise

Panic and Anxiety Disorders

The panic disorders probably stand second only to the affective disorders with respect to their episodicity of course (Barlow, 1988). Although some individuals show a single episode and others display a chronic course, many such individuals exhibit a course in which episodes marked by frequent panic attacks are interspersed with periods of full remission or recovery. Precisely why this is the case remains unknown. Like the affective disorders, the panic disorders respond to a number of pharmacological agents (Klein, 1982), but show little evidence of reduction in subsequent risk once medication is terminated. Again like the affective disorders, there is evidence that relatively more enduring reductions in risk can be brought about by the application of psychosocial interventions, particularly cognitive–behavioral interventions targeted at catastrophic misinterpretations of relatively harmless proprioceptive physical sensations (Barlow & Cerny, 1988; Clark, 1986).

In contrast, most simple phobias are relatively situationally specific, but enduring in nature (Marks, 1969). Individuals with specific fears of objects or situations tend to retain those fears over time, unless steps are taken to deal with those fears in therapy. Although some recrudescence is likely to occur even in treated individuals with the passage of time, it is likely that this phenomenon reflects a deterioration of treatment effects rather than any truly temporal dimension of the pathophysiology of the underlying disorder.

General anxiety disorder is likely to be intermediate between these two extremes (Barlow, 1988). The basic propensity for the disorder appears to be largely chronic over time, but the actual experience of distress appears to wax and wane in a manner that may have some temporal component to it (Klein, 1981). The same appears to be true for obessive–compulsive disorder, with chronicity in the core disorder being the rule, but some variability in the expression of symptoms being the normal course (Rachman, 1985).

What this suggests is that the distinction between relapse and recurrence is more likely to be profitably extended to the panic disorders than to the simple phobias, with general anxiety disorder and obsessive–compulsive disorder intermediate. Whether such extensions prove to be of use remains to be determined.

Substance Abuse Disorders

Two models predominate in the substance abuse disorders (Marlatt, 1983). According to the disease model, addiction follows a progression in which the individual increasingly loses control over his or her capacity to restrict exposure to the substance (Jellinek, 1960). According to a social-learning theory model, dependency and excessive use are largely habit problems cued and conditioned by situational and psychological factors (Marlatt & Gordon, 1985).

Both models would predict high rates of relapse in the substance abuse disorders, but for different reasons. According to the disease model, addiction and dependency are largely physiologically determined; exposure to the substance inevitably leads to loss of control, and abstinence is the only legitimate goal of treatment. According to the social-learning model, it should be possible to learn to control patterns of exposure; insistence on abstinence is seen as only undermining the capacity to exercise voluntary control over subsequent use.

It is not clear that the distinction between relapse and recurrence is directly applicable to the substance abuse disorders. Clearly, individuals with a history of abuse are at elevated risk for resuming use after a period of abstinence, but it is not clear that there is any temporal component to this phenomenon. Early longitudinal studies suggested that risk stabilized after about 3 months of abstinence, but later work is not so sanguine (Brownell, Marlatt, Lichtenstein, & Wilson, 1986). As previously noted, some of the basis for hypothesized "safe" points with respect to subsequent relapse was derived from a simple failure to adjust plots of the data for sampling without replacement (Sutton, 1979). Precisely what role temporal factors play in the nature of risk following remission or recovery in the substance abuse disorders remains to be determined.

CONCLUSIONS

There are clear reasons for considering the role of temporal factors in the affective disorders. Relapse appears to be differentiable from recurrence, at least conceptually, and this differentiation may facilitate the search for the causal processes that control both the specific episode and underlying risk for the disorder. It is less clear that the exploration of temporality will prove as useful with respect to other major types of psychopathology, although that may still prove to be the case. Those disorders that show the clearest evidence of episodicity appear to be the most promising candidates. For those disorders, and most certainly for the affective disorders, a thorough exploration of the processes governing relapse and recurrence may provide a basis for understanding both the nature of the causal processes producing the disorders and the processes involved in their treatment.

REFERENCES

Abramson, L. Y., Metalsky, G. I., & Alloy, L. B. (1989). Hopelessness depression: A theory-based subtype of depression. A metatheoretical analysis with implications for psychopathology research. *Psychological Review, 96,* 358–372.

Abramson, L. Y., Seligman, M. E. P., & Teasdale, J. (1978). Learned helplessness in humans: Critique and reformulation. *Journal of Abnormal Psychology, 87,* 49–74.

American Psychiatric Association (1987). *Diagnostic and statistical manual of mental disorders* (3rd ed., rev.). Washington, DC: Author.

Amsterdam, J. D., Maislin, G., Gold, P., & Winokur, A. (1989). The assessment of abnormalities in hormonal responsiveness at multiple levels of the hypothalamic–pituitary–adrenocortical axis in depressive illness. *Psychoneuroendocrinology, 14,* 43–62.

Arana, G. W., Baldessarini, R. J., & Ornsteen, M. (1985). The dexamethasone suppression test for diagnosis and prognosis in psychiatry. *Archives of General Psychiatry, 42,* 1193–1204.

Barlow, D. H. (1988). *Anxiety and its disorders: The nature and treatment of anxiety and panic.* New York: Guilford Press.

Barlow, D. H., & Cerny, J. A. (1988). *Psychological treatment of panic.* New York: Guilford Press.

Barnett, P. A., & Gotlib, I. H. (1988). Psychosocial functioning and depression: Distinguishing among antecedents, concomitants, and consequences. *Psychological Bulletin, 104,* 97–126.

Beck, A. T. (1967). *Depression: Clinical, experimental, and theoretical aspects.* New York: Harper & Row.

Beck, A. T., Rush, A. J., Shaw, B. F., & Emery, G. (1979). *Cognitive therapy of depression.* New York: Guilford Press.

Belsher, G., & Costello, C. G. (1988). Relapse after recovery from unipolar depression: A critical review. *Psychological Bulletin, 104,* 84–96.

Blackburn, I. M., Eunson, K. M., & Bishop, S. (1986). A two-year naturalistic follow-up of depressed patients treated with cognitive therapy, pharmacotherapy and a combination of both. *Journal of Affective Disorders, 10,* 67–75.

Bratfos, O., & Haug, J. O. (1968). The course of manic–depressive psychosis: A follow-up investigation of 215 patients. *Acta Psychiatrica Scandinavia, 44,* 89–112.

Breier, A., & Strauss, J. S. (1984). The role of social relationships in the recovery from psychotic disorders. *American Journal of Psychiatry, 141,* 949–955.

Brodwall, O. (1947). The course of manic–depressive psychosis. *Acta Psychiatrica et Neurologica, 22,* 195–210.

Brownell, K. D., Marlatt, G. A., Lichtenstein, E., & Wilson, G. T. (1986). Understanding and preventing relapse. *American Psychologist, 41,* 765–782.

Ciompi, L. (1980). Catamnestic long-term study on the course of life and aging in schizophrenics. *Schizophrenia Bulletin, 6,* 607–618.

Clark, D. M. (1986). A cognitive approach to panic. *Behaviour Research and Therapy, 24,* 461–470.

Consensus Development Panel. (1985). NIMH/NIH consensus development conference statement on mood disorders: Pharmacological prevention of recurrences. *American Journal of Psychiatry, 142,* 469–476.

Elkin, I., Shea, M. T., Watkins, J. T., Imber, S. D., Sotsky, S. M., Collins, J. F., Glass, D. R., Pilkonis, P. A., Leber, W. R., Docherty, J. P., Fiester, S. J., & Parloff, M. B. (1989). NIMH Treatment of Depression Collaborative Research Program: I. General effectiveness of treatments. *Archives of General Psychiatry, 46,* 971–982.

Evans, M. D., Hollon, S. D., DeRubeis, R. J., Piasecki, J., Grove, W. M., Garvey, M. J., & Tuason, V. B. (1992). Differential relapse following cognitive therapy and pharmacotherapy for depression. *Archives of General Psychiatry, 49,* 802–808.

Faravelli, C., Ambonetti, A., Pallanti, S., & Pazzagli, A. (1986). Depressive relapses and incomplete recovery from index episode. *American Journal of Psychiatry, 143,* 888–891.

Frank, E., Kupfer, D. J., Perel, J. M., Cornes, C., Jarrett, D. B., Mallinger, A. G., Thase, M. E., McEachran, M. S., & Grochocinski, V. J. (1990). Three-year outcomes for maintenance therapies in recurrent depression. *Archives of General Psychiatry, 47,* 1093–1099.

Frank, E., Prien, R. F., Jarrett, R. B., Keller, M. B., Kupfer, D. J., Lavori, P. W., Rush, A. J., & Weissman, M. M. (1991). Conceptualization and rationale for consensus definitions of terms in major depressive disorder: Remission, recovery, relapse, and recurrence. *Archives of General Psychiatry, 48,* 851–855.

Glen, A. I. M., Johnson, A. L., & Shepherd, M. (1984). Continuation therapy with lithium and amitriptyline in unipolar depressive illness: A randomized, double-blind controlled trial. *Psychological Medicine, 14,* 37–50.

Goldstein, M. J. (1991). Schizophrenia and family therapy. In B. D. Beitman & G.

L. Klerman (Eds.), *Integrating pharmacotherapy and psychotherapy* (pp. 291–309). Washington, DC: American Psychiatric Press.

Gonzales, L. R., Lewinsohn, P. M., & Clarke, G. N. (1985). Longitudinal follow-up of unipolar depressives: An investigation of predictors of relapse. *Journal of Consulting and Clinical Psychology, 53,* 461–469.

Hollon, S. D. (1992). Cognitive theories of depression from a psychobiological perspective. *Psychological Inquiry, 3,* 250–253.

Hollon, S. D., Evans, M. D., & DeRubeis, R. J. (1990). Cognitive mediation of relapse prevention following treatment for depression: Implications of differential risk. In R. E. Ingram (Ed.), *Contemporary psychological approaches to depression* (pp. 117–136). New York: Guilford Press.

Hollon, S. D., Shelton, R. C., & Loosen, P. T. (1991). Cognitive therapy in relation to pharmacotherapy for depression. *Journal of Consulting and Clinical Psychology, 59,* 88–99.

Hooley, J. M., Orley, J., & Teasdale, J. D. (1986). Levels of expressed emotion and relapse in depressed patients. *British Journal of Psychiatry, 148,* 642–647.

Huston, P. E., & Locher, L. M. (1948). Manic–depressive psychosis: Course when treated and untreated with electric shock. *Archives of Neurology and Psychiatry, 60,* 37–48.

Jellinek, E. M. (1960). *The disease concept of alcoholism.* New Brunswick, NJ: Hill House Press.

Kane, J. M., Quitkin, F. M., Rifkin, A., Ramos-Lorenzi, J. R., Nayak, D. D., & Howard, A. (1982). Lithium carbonate and imipramine in the prophylaxis of unipolar and bipolar II illness. *Archives of General Psychiatry, 39,* 1065–1069.

Keller, M. B. (1985). Chronic and recurrent affective disorders: Incidence, course, and influencing factors. *Advances in Biochemical Psychopharmacology, 40,* 111–120.

Keller, M. B., Lavori, P. W., Lewis, C. E., & Klerman, G. L. (1983). Predictors of relapse in major depressive disorder. *Journal of the American Medical Association, 250,* 3299–3304.

Keller, M. B., & Shapiro, R. W. (1981). Major depressive disorder: Initial results from a one-year prospective naturalistic follow-up study. *Journal of Nervous and Mental Disease, 169,* 761–768.

Keller, M. B., Shapiro, R. W., Lavori, P. W., & Wolfe, N. (1982). Relapse in major depressive disorder. *Archives of General Psychiatry, 39,* 911–915.

Khan, A., Johnson, F., Avery, D. H., Cohen, S., Scherzo, B., & Dunner, D. L. (1988). DST results in nonpsychotic depressed outpatients. *American Journal of Psychiatry, 145,* 1153–1156.

Klein, D. F. (1981). Anxiety reconceptualized. In D. F. Klein & J. Rabkin (Eds.), *Anxiety: New research and changing concepts.* New York: Raven Press.

Klein, D. F. (1982). Medication in the treatment of panic attacks and phobic states. *Psychopharmacological Bulletin, 18,* 85–90.

Klein, D. F., Gittelman, R., Quitkin, F., & Rifkin, A. (1980). *Diagnosis and drug treatment of psychiatric disorders: Adults and children* (2nd ed.). Baltimore: Williams & Wilkins.

Klerman, G. L., DiMascio, A., Weissman, M., Prusoff, B., & Paykel, E. (1974).

Treatment of depression by drugs and psychotherapy. *American Journal of Psychiatry, 131,* 186–191.

Klerman, G. L., Weissman, M. M., Rounsaville, B., & Chevron, E. (1984). *Interpersonal psychotherapy of depression (IPT).* New York: Basic Books.

Kolakowska, T. (1975). The clinical course of primary recurrent depression in pharmacologically treated female patients. *British Journal of Psychiatry, 126,* 336–345.

Kovacs, M., & Beck, A. T. (1978). Maladaptive cognitive structures in depression. *American Journal of Psychiatry, 135,* 525–533.

Kovacs, M., Rush, A. J., Beck, A. T., & Hollon, S. D. (1981). Depressed outpatients treated with cognitive therapy or pharmacotherapy. *Archives of General Psychiatry, 38,* 33–39.

Kraepelin, E. (1921). *Manic–depressive insanity and paranoia.* Edinburgh: Livingstone Press.

Lavori, P. W., Keller, M. B., & Klerman, G. L. (1984). Relapse in affective disorders: A reanalysis of the literature using life table methods. *Journal of Psychiatric Research, 18,* 13–25.

Lehmann, H. E., & Cancro, R. (1985). Schizophrenia: Clinical features. In H. I. Kaplan & B. J. Sadock (Eds.), *Comprehensive textbook of psychiatry* (4th ed., pp. 680–713). Baltimore: Williams & Wilkins.

Loosen, P. T. (1986). Hormones of the hypothalamic–pituitary–thyroid axis: A psychoneuroendocrine perspective. *Pharmacopsychiatry, 19,* 401–415.

Lundquist, G. (1945). Prognosis and course in manic–depressive psychosis: A follow-up study of 319 first admissions. *Acta Psychiatrica et Neurologica, 35*(Suppl.), 1–93.

Marks, I. M. (1969). *Fears and phobias.* New York: Academic Press.

Marlatt, G. A. (1983). The controlled-drinking controversy: A commentary. *American Psychologist, 38,* 1097–1110.

Marlatt, G. A., & Gordon, J. R. (Eds.). (1985). *Relapse prevention: Maintenance strategies in the treatment of addictive behaviors.* New York: Guilford Press.

Murphy, G. E., Woodruff, R. A., Herjanic, M., & Fisher, J. R. (1974). Validity of the clinical course of primary affective disorder. *Archives of General Psychiatry, 30,* 757–761.

Paykel, E. S., & Tanner, J. (1976). Life events, depressive relapse and maintenance treatment. *Psychological Medicine, 6,* 481–485.

Perris, C., & D'Elia, G. (1966). A study of bipolar (manic–depressive) and unipolar recurrent depressive psychoses: Part IX. Therapy and prognosis. *Acta Psychiatrica Scandinavia, 194*(Suppl.), 153–171.

Peterson, C., & Seligman, M. E. P. (1984). Causal explanations as a risk factor for depression: Theory and evidence. *Psychological Review, 91,* 347–374.

Prien, R. F., Carpenter, L. L., & Kupfer, D. J. (1991). The definition and operational criteria for treatment outcome of major depressive disorder: A review of the current research literature. *Archives of General Psychiatry, 48,* 796–800.

Prien, R. F., & Kupfer, D. J. (1986). Continuation drug therapy for major depressive episodes: How long should it be maintained? *American Journal of Psychiatry, 143,* 18–23.

Prien, R. F., Kupfer, D. J., Mansky, P. A., Small, J. G., Tuason, V. B., Voss, C. B., & Johnson, W. E. (1984). Drug therapy in the prevention of recurrences in unipolar and bipolar affective disorders. *Archives of General Psychiatry, 41,* 1096–1104.

Quitkin, F., Rifkin, A., & Klein, D. F. (1976). Prophylaxis of affective disorders. *Archives of General Psychiatry, 33,* 337–346.

Rachman, S. J. (1985). An overview of clinical and research issues in obessional-compulsive disorders. In M. Mavissakalian, S. M. Turner, & L. Michelson (Eds.), *Obsessive–compulsive disorder* (pp. 1–47). New York: Plenum Press.

Seager, C. P. (1958). A comparison between results of unmodified and modified electroplexy. *Journal of Mental Science, 104,* 206–220.

Shelton, R. C., Hollon, S. D., Purdon, S. E., & Loosen, P. T. (1991). Biological and psychological aspects of depression. *Behavior Therapy, 22,* 201–228.

Simons, A. D., Murphy, G. E., Levine, J. E., & Wetzel, R. D. (1986). Cognitive therapy and pharmacotherapy for depression: Sustained improvement over one year. *Archives of General Psychiatry, 43,* 43–49.

Simpson, G. M., & May, P. R. A. (1985). Schizophrenia: Somatic treatment. In H. I. Kaplan & B. J. Sadock (Eds.), *Comprehensive textbook of psychiatry* (4th ed., pp. 680–713). Baltimore: Williams & Wilkins.

Spiegel, D., & Wissler, T. (1986). Family environment as a predictor of psychiatric rehospitalization. *American Journal of Psychiatry, 143,* 56–60.

Sutton, S. R. (1979). Interpreting relapse curves. *Journal of Consulting and Clinical Psychology, 47,* 96–98.

Vaughn, C. E., & Leff, J. P. (1976). The influence of family and social factors on the course of psychiatric illness. *British Journal of Psychiatry, 129,* 125–137.

Weissman, M. M., Klerman, G. L., Paykel, E. S., Prusoff, B., & Hanson, B. (1974). Treatment effects on the social adjustment of depressed patients. *Archives of General Psychiatry, 30,* 771–778.

Weissman, M. M., Klerman, G. L., Prusoff, B. A., Sholomskas, D., & Padian, N. (1981). Depressed outpatients one year after treatment with drugs and/or interpersonal psychotherapy (IPT). *Archives of General Psychiatry, 38,* 51–55.

Weissman, M. M., Prusoff, B. A., DiMascio, A., Neu, C., Goklaney, M., & Klerman, G. L. (1979). The efficacy of drugs and psychotherapy in the treatment of acute depressive disorders. *American Journal of Psychiatry, 136,* 555–558.

Winokur, A., Amsterdam, J., Caroff, S., Snyder, P. J., & Brunswick, D. (1982). Variability of hormonal responses to a series of neuroendocrine challenges in depressed patients. *American Journal of Psychiatry, 139,* 39–44.

Wolberg, L. R. (1967). *The techniques of psychotherapy.* New York: Grune & Stratton.

11

Community Care for Psychopathological Disorders

GRAHAM THORNICROFT

GERALDINE STRATHDEE

The further development of community-oriented psychiatric services in both the United Kingdom and the United States lies at a crossroads. In the United States the primary challenge is to generalize the best models of community care to areas so far neglected. In Britain, which is in many ways considerably behind the United States in establishing local services, the immediate issue is how to provide services successfully while most large psychiatric institutions are closing.

In this chapter our subject is community care for people with psychopathological disorders, and we shall begin by drawing out the main landmarks in the historical development of these ideas and practices. We also go to more contemporary issues: how to conceptualize a local psychiatric service that is being planned, developed, or modified; which principles should guide these decisions; and which logistical steps should be taken at each stage. We then add detail to this overall outline with two specific forms of care that have been empirically shown to enhance both the functional outcomes and the quality of life of people with disabling mental illnesses: psychosocial interventions and case management programs. In our final section we advocate that a rigorous form of discipline in both extending and evaluating community mental health is to set specific targets for our clinical and research activities. Throughout this chapter we indicate where the scientific evidence about each component of community psychiatric services is strong, weak, or missing and also indicate priorities for further research work.

In considering this transformation in psychiatric services it is important to keep a clear view of the scale of the problems addressed. The extent of psychiatric morbidity in the population is sobering (Bebbington, Hurry, Tennant, Sturt, & Wing, 1981; Mann, 1991). Primary care surveys have shown that at least 26% of the population consult their family doctor each year with a mental health problem (Goldberg, 1991). In addition, there is considerable indirect morbidity among patients' relatives and caregivers who often develop psychiatric symptoms from their burden of care (MacCarthy, Lesage, Brewin, Brugha, & Wing, 1989). The costs of mental ill health are also staggering: These problems in Britain account for 14% of days lost to work, 20% of total National Health Service (NHS) expenditure, 23% of inpatient costs, and 25% of pharmaceutical charges (Thornicroft & Strathdee, 1991). The total annual costs of mental illness are estimated at between £4.6 and £5.6 billion (Croft-Jeffreys & Wilkinson, 1985; Davies & Drummond, 1990), of which less than a third is for direct services. Therefore, mental illness, and especially persisting and seriously disabling mental illness, warrants forceful, coordinated, and sound service planning and implementation.

Although there are an estimated 2 million chronic mentally ill in the United States (Goldman, Morrisey, & Bachrach, 1983), there are fewer than 130,000 psychiatric inpatients (Scull, 1984). The vast majority of disabled patients now live outside hospitals. Although there has been considerable research interest in the quality of life (Lehman, 1983), problems of homelessness (Bachrach, 1984; Fischer & Breakey, 1986), organization of services (Stein & Test, 1980), use of case managers (Harris, Bergman, & Bachrach, 1986), financial resource allocation (Mechanic & Aiken, 1987), and governmental policy (Audit Commission, 1986; Griffiths, 1988) toward this patient group, there have been few attempts to evaluate the effectiveness of mobile services for the seriously mentally ill in deprived inner-city areas (Schulberg & Bromet, 1981; Tessler & Goldman, 1982; Avison & Speechley, 1987; Franklin, 1988). Within this overall context, therefore, the issues addressed in this chapter, community-based psychiatric services, focus on major public health challenges.

THE HISTORICAL DEVELOPMENT OF COMMUNITY MENTAL HEALTH CARE

The recent history of the treatment of those with severe and chronic mental illness must be one of the most significant social changes of our time. Although the processes of deinstitutionalization and of the development of alternative community services vary between countries (Mangen, 1988), there are common themes to both the British, and

American literatures. *Deinstitutionalization* has been well defined by Bachrach (1976) as the contraction of traditional institutional settings, with the concurrent expansion of community-based services. We will use this distinction to describe the components of these processes, which may be related more in hope than in practice. Brown (1975), then director of the National Institute of Mental Health, identified a further essential component of deinstitutionalization: the prevention of inappropriate mental hospital admissions. Another important distinction is that between asylums as institutions and asylum as a function: The provision of a place of safety or haven is not necessarily related to institutional size (Wasow, 1986; Rosenblatt, 1984; Wing & Furlong, 1986). Finally, the term *community care* requires careful specification. The concept ambiguously implies both care in and by the community, and so has united supporters of the former (libertarian radicals) and the latter (fiscal radicals). It may imply merely a change in the locus of care or, more thoroughly, in the methods and financing of care delivery (Goldman, Adams, & Taube, 1983).

In the United Kingdom the numbers of inpatients peaked at 148,100 in 1954 (Tooth & Brooke, 1961). On February 19, 1954, Kenneth Robinson addressed the House of Commons: "That this House . . . expresses its concern at the serious overcrowding of mental hospitals" (Jones, 1972, p. 289). A reduction in numbers was seen as the only humane option. In the following year Houston (1955) wrote in *Lancet:* "By incarceration we were aggravating the natural process of the disease. At last a new era is dawning and the doors of despair are being unlocked" (p. 1133). The decline in numbers of psychiatric inpatients has continued at an even rate since 1954 (Thornicroft, 1988). The average number of psychiatric beds occupied each day in 1985 in England and Wales was 64,800 (Audit Commission, 1986). This represents a return to the occupancy level last seen in 1895 (Scull, 1984).

The process of deinstitutionalization in Britain has been paralleled in the United States. From a maximum inpatient population of 558,900 in 1955, numbers had fallen to 132,164 by 1980 (Scull, 1984). At the peak of this process during the 1970s, the institutional population was diminishing by as much as 6% each year (Mechanic, 1986). The justifications for this transfer of long-stay patients from the larger psychiatric hospitals are many and varied, being associated with sociological, financial, pharmacological, administrative, and legal changes (Jones, 1972; Scull, 1984). Both within and without the psychiatric profession, a view criticizing the ill effects of prolonged stay within the large institutions emerged with increasing force during the 1950s (Miller, 1985). Barton (1959) described "institutional neurosis" as "a disease in its own right . . . characterised by apathy, lack of initiative, loss of interest."

Taking this view further, Goffman (1961) formulated the concept of the "total institution," central to which was "the handling of many human needs by the bureaucratic organisation of whole blocks of people," so that those admitted are "shaped and coded" into the roles of psychiatric patients (p. 18). Wing and Brown (1970) reinforced this view with their description of the "institutionalism" of chronic patients. From their study of long-stay patients in three British hospitals, they accepted the hypothesis that the social conditions under which a patient lives (particularly poverty of the social environment) are actually responsible for part of the symptomatology (particularly the negative symptoms), although they stressed that institutionalized practices were not confined to large facilities.

A series of inquiries into malpractice in British hospitals for the mentally ill provided further critical evaluation of psychiatric institutions. Martin (1984) has documented 14 investigations and inquiries in Britain from 1969 (Ely) to 1980 (Rampton). He sets out the recurring themes associated with established cases of ill treatment: isolation of the institutions, lack of staff support, poor reporting procedures, a failure of leadership, ineffective administration, inadequate financial resources, the divided loyalties of trade unions, poor staff training, and occasional negligent individuals. These influences combined to allow the substitution of secondary aims, such as the establishment of ward routines, for the primary aim of delivering care to patients. The effect of such inquiries was to reinforce the developing view that the large institutions were self-evidently harmful.

Treatment patterns have also shown widespread changes. Within 3 years of the formulation of chlorpromazine in 1952, its use as an antipsychotic agent was widespread (Jones, 1972). This was paralleled by innovations in patient management. Industrial therapy organizations were set up (Wing, 1960), therapeutic communities were developed (Clark, 1974), day hospitals appeared, hostels and half-way houses were established (Golomb & Kocsis, 1988), and in the United States community mental health centers were founded (Levine, 1981).

Government policy in Britain, as set out in the white paper *Better Services for the Mentally Ill* (Department of Health and Social Security [DHSS], 1975), was to establish a target of 47,900 inpatient psychiatric beds after the completion of the current program of closure of psychiatric hospitals. On these estimates, 84% of the planned reduction in long-stay psychiatric beds toward this goal from the high point in 1954 has already happened, and only the final sixth of long-stay patients remain to be relocated. Alongside this attrition, there has been a corresponding increase in the annual number of admissions: from 78,586 in 1955 to 185,514 in 1981 (Social Services Committee, 1985).

Of an estimated 1.7–2.4 million chronically mentally ill persons in the United States (Goldman, Adams, & Taube, 1983a), only 116,000 remained within state mental hospitals by 1983 (Bachrach, 1986). A government review of policy demonstrated that community-based facilities have been implemented "in the absence of a planned, well-managed and systematic approach." In response to this criticism, NIMH community support programs were established in 1977. Fifteen sites provided demonstration projects of services for chronic mentally ill patients (Scull, 1985). In reviewing the outcome of these initiatives, Tessler and Goldman (1982) see this program as "an incomplete reform." They found that the political trend toward shifting responsibility and costs for the chronic mentally ill from federal to state level threatened to undermine the benefit of these federal programs.

DEFINITIONS AND PRINCIPLES

Setting up community-based psychiatric services has been one of the foremost preoccupations of contemporary psychiatry. Reflecting the diversity of historical influences on their development, there is little agreement on what constitutes the "community." At its most basic, the term refers to the locality of services, commonly regarded as those outside the psychiatric hospital. Sabshin viewed (1966) the nature of the care to be more important than locality and proposed that

> community psychiatry involves the utilisation of the techniques, methods, theories of social psychiatry and other behavioural sciences to investigate and to meet the mental health needs of a functionally or geographically defined population over a significant period of time, and the feeding back of information to modify the central body of social psychiatric and other behavioural science knowledge.

Focusing on the organizational context, Hunter and Wistow (1987) consider that two themes have underpinned the development of community services: that they should be directed to meeting individual needs rather than producing services and that this objective is best met by replacing inherited service systems dominated by large institutions with a more balanced and flexible range of alternative services. As Wing (1977) has suggested, no system of care can be understood except in relation to the underlying social and political structures of the society it serves. The development of community services for the mentally ill is almost exclusively a product of the latter half of this century. Their evolution has been influenced by a complex interaction of factors including alterations and advances in mental health treatment practices, legislation, attitudes among the public and professions, the organization and extent of decentralization in health care systems, national political movements, the extent of state and private finance burdens in the provision of health, and local geography and health service history (Ramon, 1988; Mechanic, 1987; Klein, 1991).

The Principles of Community Psychiatric Services

Many organizations and groups have enunciated their views of the essential principles of community services and the summary here is based on the definitions of four disparate bodies: MIND, presented in *Common Concern* in 1983; Lord Glenarthur, speaking as government spokesman in 1985; the Royal College of Psychiatrists in *Caring for a Community* in 1990; and in the stimulating but practical *Towards a Model for a Comprehensive Community-based Mental Health System,* the National Institute of Mental Health's formulation (1987). They consider that:

> Services should be *local and accessible* and, to the greatest extent possible, delivered in the client's usual environment.
>
> Services should be *comprehensive* and address the diversity of needs of individuals with mental health disorders.
>
> Services should be *flexible* by being available whenever and for whatever duration. There should be a range of complementary models that provide individuals with choice and vary, depending on need, at any point in time.
>
> Services should be *consumer oriented,* that is, based on the needs of the client rather than those of providers. Achieving this balance is one of the major difficulties to be overcome in resource allocation. Central, highly resourced facilities, for example, hospital-based units, may appear more efficient and effective in terms of easy movement of staff between wards, training, information gathering, and reduction in staff isolation, but be inflexible in addressing patients' needs.
>
> Services should *empower clients* by using and adapting treatment techniques that enable clients to enhance their self-help skills and retain the fullest possible control over their own lives. This can take place at both the individual level and at all stages in the planning and development of a service. By integrating an educational component into treatment, patients can determine the strategies in terms of medications and manipulation of social environments that enable them to take part in secondary and tertiary prevention. At the services level, clients should be actively involved in planning and policy-making decisions and be represented on all relevant committees.
>
> Services should be *racially and culturally appropriate.* Mechanisms to ensure provision of appropriate and acceptable services include use of culturally appropriate needs-assessment tools, representation

on planning groups, cross-cultural training for staff, use of indigenous workers and bilingual staff, identification and provision of alternative basic facilities, and evaluation of the provision against accepted indicators.

Services should *focus on strengths.* They should be built on the skills and strengths of clients and help them maintain a sense of identity, dignity, and self-esteem. Patients should be discouraged from adopting the sick role and the service from developing an environment organized around permanent illness with lowered expectations.

Services should be *normalized and incorporate natural supports* by being in the least restrictive, most natural setting possible. The natural work, education, leisure and, support facilities in the community should be used in preference to specialized developments.

Services should *meet special needs,* with particular attention to those with physical disabilities, mental retardation, the homeless, or imprisoned.

Service should be *accountable* to the consumers and caregivers and evaluated to ensure their continuing appropriateness, acceptability, and effectiveness on agreed parameters.

STAGES IN SETTING UP COMMUNITY MENTAL HEALTH SERVICES

A series of steps is necessary to create a model plan for the development of community services. In such a plan we propose that there be four stages, starting with the creation of a consensus philosophy and vision, the gathering of appropriate information on which to base the developments, and an identification of some of the strategic, management, and organizational issues involved in the planning mechanisms. The preparation for implementation of any service is fundamental to its success, and throughout this section attention is focused on strategies likely to increase the success of innovative developments.

Step 1: The Philosophy and Vision of the Service

Fundamental to the development of any service is an agreement from the outset of whom the service should serve and what its objectives should be. The creation of a mission statement by the team of senior personnel and major stakeholders, including users, is a powerful process in developing team cohesion and in enabling each individual and organization to recognize the inherent strengths, skills, and biases of the others.

Step 2. Establishing Joint Planning Mechanisms

In planning a comprehensive service for individuals with mental health disorders, a wide range of needs must be considered and accommodated. At both the national and district level, there is therefore a need to create joint planning mechanisms and to involve and consult with a complex network of agencies, including the primary health care teams, social services and housing departments, the prison and probation services, advocacy groups, education, employment agencies, and the voluntary organizations and users. In an ideal model, a common and shared set of priorities would be evolved, based on clear policies produced by intensive, committed, forward-looking individuals, and having the prior benefit of substantive research demonstrating their primacy and efficacy.

Step 3. Models of Service Planning

A number of approaches have been adopted to planning community services, and we describe here three that are in common use. These we have termed the *needs model* (based on a bottom-up approach), the *components model* (a top-down approach), and the *functions model.*

A prime example of the needs model is the National Institute of Mental Health's formulation of a model plan (1987) for a comprehensive community-based mental health system. This attractive model first delineates the range of needs of individual patients and then formulates a series of steps to convert the cumulative needs of patients into the necessary elements of service.

The components model takes the approach of defining the necessary elements for the provision of a comprehensive service. A list of specific facilities are formulated, including inpatient beds, outpatient clinics, and day hospitals (MIND, 1983; DHSS, 1971, 1974; Hirsch, 1988).

The functions model focuses on the expected function of the service. For example, when an acute treatment facility is needed, the requirement may be for an environment in which removal from stress is the main attribute, whereas in others, the presence of highly skilled staff, provision of a temporary home, or containment of aggressive behaviors may be the predominant need.

Step 4. Information Systems Required

To set up and monitor locally based mental health services, a clear, systematic, continuing method of collecting clinical and social need and service usage data is required. The most comprehensive method to elicit, code, and store these data is the *case register,* which is defined as a local information system that records the contacts with designated social and medical services of patients or clients from a defined geographic area (Wing, 1989). Although such systems were formerly labor-intensive, the recent availability of on-site microcomputers and minicomputers has made their more widespread use a practical option in many districts. The routine collection of clinical contact data allows aggregate data to show patterns of service with respect to patterns of diagnoses (Der & Bebbington, 1987; Tansella & Williams, 1989), social class (Wiersma, Giel, de Jong, & Slooff, 1983), and geographical mobility (Lesage & Tansella, 1989). Further, the use of standardized coding and diagnostic systems allows comparisons of service use within local areas (Giel & ten Horn, 1982), within regions (Torre & Marinoni, 1985), and between countries (ten Horn, Giel, Gulbinat, & Henderson, 1986; Sytema, Balestrieri, Giel, ten Horn, & Tansella, 1989). Particular areas in which case registers have been shown to be invaluable include familial studies, the influence of ecological factors, the accumulation of new long-stay patients, the influences on readmissions, and the analysis of time trends. Such data can therefore indicate how variations in treated morbidity vary with local sociodemographic characteristics, with the nature and extent of local service provision, and with the service trends at the national level. Where one of the primary aims of developing local mental health services is to deliver services to identified priority groups of patients, then the detailed information produced by case registers will be required to ensure that the outcome of implementation is consistent with the declared aims of the service.

Step 5. Clarifying Strategic Issues

In planning community services, the organization of services is of paramount importance. As Tansella (1986) counsels, "What is important in community care is not only the number and characteristics of various services but the way in which they are arranged and integrated." Mechanisms must be found that enable effective service delivery and that are consistent with the three guidelines that have been enunciated by Paumelle, an early proponent of community care in France (Strathdee, 1991).

The first guideline is that *continuity of care* should be ensured. This, he believed, could best be achieved by ensuring that persons and families were dealt with at all stages and at all levels of illness by the same team. In turn, this meant assigning such teams and their associated structures such as beds and clinics to populations of manageable size. Given the range of needs of individuals with mental health problems, *coordination of care* was cited as the second fundamental guideline. Only by the introduction of multidisciplinary and interagency teams could the range of treatments necessary to overcome the impairment and disability of the mentally ill be delivered. *Integration of care* was regarded as the third essential based on the premise (WHO, 1983) that in any community first contact for individuals in distress is often not with the psychiatric specialist team, but rather persons in key positions of responsibility in the community such as teachers, police, public health nurses, community nurses, social workers, and general practitioners. The specialist team must therefore integrate its efforts with those of the nonspecialists, as well as taking the lead in educating and counseling nonspecialists.

In Great Britain these guidelines must be considered in the light of an important aspect of our health care system. There is a uniquely strong primary care tier of care. General practitioners play a major role in the care of those with both acute and chronic psychological disorders (Shepherd, Cooper, Brown, & Kalton, 1966; Goldberg & Blackwell, 1970; Sharp & Morrell, 1989; Paykel, 1990). For many patients with severe, long-term disorders, the general practitioner is indeed the only source of continuing care (Murray Parkes, Brown, & Monck, 1962; Lee & Murray, 1988; Johnstone, Owens, Gold, Crow, & Macmillan, 1984; Brown, Strathdee, Christie-Brown, & Robinson, 1988). As Jones (1972) concluded, "Unless attention is given to finding administrative solutions to the repeated official exhortations (DHSS, 1975, 1978, 1981; Griffiths, 1988) for collaboration and co-operation with GPs [general practitioners] we will fail to provide the mix of services needed."

Family doctors provide the overwhelming bulk of all care for psychiatric problems (Goldberg & Huxley, 1980), and about 8% of patients seen in primary care suffer from a chronic mental disorder (Wilkinson, Falloon, & Sen, 1985). The redeployment of psychiatric staff outside the psychiatric hospital has generated new forms of collaboration between the primary and secondary care services. More than one fifth of British psychiatrists now see patients in primary care centers (Strathdee & Williams, 1984). This may include a greater emphasis upon home visits, holding outpatient clinics in general practitioners' offices, seeing selected patients at the request of family doctors, acting as a consultant to the primary care team, or seeing patients jointly with their general practice colleagues (Mitchell, 1985; Monk-Jorgensen, 1986).

To achieve the principles of effective delivery of psychiatric care as delineated here, one approach has been hailed. Workers, both abroad (Lindholm, 1983; Hansson, 1989) and in Great Britain (Tyrer, Turner, & Johnson, 1989), consider that an essential prerequisite to the development of effective community psychiatric services is the delineation of small, geographically defined areas or sectors as the unit of service provision. The concept of the *psychiatrie de secteur* was first developed in France after 1947. By 1961, more than 300 sectors had been established in departments across half of the country. In 1963 the Kennedy Community Mental Health Centers (CMHC) Act in the United States was introduced, and with it the concept of a catchment area for each CMHC, which by 1975 provided for 40% of the U.S. population (Levine, 1981; Goldman, Adams, & Taube, 1983). In Europe, throughout the 1970s, the organizing principle of sectorization was widely applied to areas in West Germany (sector size 250,000), Netherlands (300,000), Denmark (60–120,000), Finland (100,000), Norway (40,000), and Sweden (25–50,000) (Lindholm, 1983), and the most comprehensive implementation of the concept is in Italy with sectors of in the range 50–200,000 population (Tansella, Salvia, & Williams, 1987). Evaluations have concentrated to a large extent on establishing whether sectorization would facilitate the development of community alternatives to inpatient hospital treatment. A number of advantages have been claimed for sectorized services. For example, in Nottingham, Tyrer and colleagues (1989) found the following reductions after sectorization: number of admissions (5%), duration of admissions (4%), use of inpatient beds (38%). One Swedish study (Hansson, 1989) found a decrease in the number of admissions (20%), bed days used (40%), and compulsory admissions (25%).

COMPONENTS OF A COMPREHENSIVE MENTAL HEALTH SERVICE

A comprehensive community care system must address the wide range of needs of individuals with mental health disorders. In the method of the components and functions model of planning described previously, this section focuses on some of the main components of community services and outlines some of the functions considered to be of importance. The categories delineated are not mutually exclusive, and as in any local settings, the organization and form of such services should ideally should be constructed on the basis of the local data available.

Crisis Response and Acute Care

One of the fundamental aims of mental health treatment must be the practice of secondary and tertiary prevention (Newton, 1987). There is a body of literature that indicates that adequate treatment, associated with client, family, and staff education and training, can prevent the onset of many crises (Birchwood et al., 1989). Falloon and Pederson (1985), for example, showed reductions in family disruptions, physical and mental disorders, and perceived burden after structured family interventions. Because of the episodic nature of the illness, however, there will be instances that require acute care and rapid-response crisis stabilization services. The aim of the services should be to enable the client, family members, and others to cope with the emergency while maintaining the client's status as a functioning community member to the greatest extent.

The services should be available on a 24-hour basis and be known to providers, families, clients, and the community. Immediate psychiatric consultation should be available for rapid evaluation, diagnosis, and chemotherapeutic interventions as indicated.

The traditional provision of crisis intervention has been through consultation at the local general practitioner's office (Murray Parkes et al., 1962), domiciliary consultation (Littlejohns, 1986; Fry & Sandler, 1988; Sutherby, Srinath, & Strathdee, 1991), and, in many districts, accident and emergency departments of general hospitals. With the development of community services, this has been extended by a range of options that include 24-hour telephone helpline, walk-in emergency clinics (Lim, 1983; Haw & Lanceley, 1987), community mental health center facilities and mobile outreach crisis intervention teams (Boardman, 1987), community crisis residential beds for temporary respite care outside the normal residential environment when needed, and inpatient beds in a variety of settings such as the psychiatric units of a district general hospital. In reviewing U.S. community care experience, Bachrach (1984) has cautioned that the decrease in beds has led to excessive use of emergency services by young psychotic patients who use no other facilities. The system of open access of British primary care services may result in primary care teams having an increasing role to play in this regard (Kendrick, Sibbald, Burns, & Freeling, 1991).

Acute treatment facilities should be available to provide assessment by a multidisciplinary team, investigation facilities to exclude an organic basis for a mental health disorder, supportive counseling and psychotherapeutic treatment, mechanisms for the provision and monitoring of medication to ensure education and maximal therapeutic effectiveness, and a range of residential facilities. The location of such services has been the subject of major debate. Particular attention has been paid to the question of the role of the hospital and the appropriateness of alternative facilities, including hospital hostels, home-based teams, and preadmission facilities. Tyrer (1985), in proposing his "hive" model, advocates that the hospital base should form the core of a system with closely coordinated subunits of care such as day hospitals, community clinics, or mental health centers located in areas of greatest morbidity.

Evaluation of Continuing Care and Outreach Services

Reviews of the community-oriented approach to continuing care (Braun, Kochansky, & Shapiro, 1981; Kiesler, 1982) have shown that outcome from assertive outreach programs is in no published case worse than for standard hospital-based treatment, and that it is often better. To date, however, these studies have not indicated which subgroups among the seriously mentally ill may be most and least likely to benefit from these forms of care (Mosher, 1983; Tantam, 1985). Further, they have often used service usage indices as the major outcome variables. With the exception of these few studies, however, most work describing community forms of psychiatric care has been methodologically very weak. Such evaluations should fulfill the following scientific criteria: random allocation to experimental and control programs, clear patient characterization, validated diagnoses, clearly described treatment programs, outcomes measured with properly validated instruments, follow-up of a high proportion of patients for an adequate period of time, and patient numbers sufficient to allow full statistical analysis.

Prompted by a growing body of evidence pointing to the pathological consequences of long-term institutionalization, the Program for Assertive Community Treatment (PACT) outreach model of service delivery to the seriously mentally ill was been pioneered by staff at the Mendota State Hospital in Madison, Wisconsin. Their approach assumes that such patients require the following elements to avoid frequent rehospitalization: material resources such as food, shelter, and clothing; coping skills; motivation; freedom from pathologically dependent relationships; community support and education; and a support system that assertively helps the patients *in vivo* (Stein & Test, 1980; Weisbrod, Test, & Stein, 1980).

Since the early 1960s, a number of studies have compared home-based care with hospital care (Test & Stein, 1980; Marks, Connolly, & Muijen, 1988). Despite differences in the models and evaluative methodologies used, these studies confirm a decrease in hospital admissions, improvement in clinical outcome and social functioning, and greater patient satisfaction from acute home-oriented care. Replication of this model in Sydney (Hoult, & Reynolds, 1984) and Montreal (Fenton, Tessier, Struening, Smith, & Benoit, 1982) has demonstrated that the approach can be successfully adapted, and an application of case management in inner-city Chicago has been shown to be cost-effective (Bond, 1984).

Consultation and Liaison Services

Until the past few decades, the majority of consultation services were conducted in hospital outpatient settings. Evaluation of the services indicates dissatisfaction with communication patterns (Pullen & Yellowlees, 1988) and clinical and referrer outcome (Kaeser & Cooper, 1971; Strathdee, 1990). The appropriateness of psychiatry's uncritical emulation of the model of general medicine, particularly for those with long-term disorders, has been questioned (Todd, 1984).

Two innovations in community provisions have begun to redress the deficiencies. First, there has been an evolution of outpatient clinics from hospital sites and the establishment of consultation clinics in primary care settings. In England and Wales 19% of all consultant general adult psychiatrists (Strathdee & Williams, 1984) and half the Scottish psychiatrists (Pullen & Yellowlees, 1988) work in this way. The evidence indicates that the clinics enhance continuity of care, particularly when the psychiatric team and their primary care colleagues work in an integrated manner. Additional advantages cited are that patients prefer the accessibility and nonstigmatizing setting of their local doctor's office, the general practitioners enhance their knowledge of psychiatric disorders and treatment techniques, and the psychiatric team has increased access to community resources and is better placed to intervene at an earlier stage in the development of illness and relapse (Mitchell, 1985; Creed & Marks, 1989; Tyrer, 1984; Joseph, Bridgewater, Ramsden, & El Kabir, 1990; Hansen, 1987). The involvement of psychiatrists with primary care practitioners is rapidly increasing, and by 1984, for example, Strathdee and Williams (1984) found that more than 20% of psychiatrists have such a liaison function.

Second, a growing number of community mental health centers have been established. Kingdon's survey (1989) indicates that they have been developed in 18% of districts, with plans afoot in another 40%. The American community mental health centers attempt to provide five services: inpatient, outpatient, partial hospitalization, emergency services, and consultation and education. In the United Kingdom those described have functioned more as a resource for crisis intervention, coordinators of multidisciplinary teams, and consultation services (Patmore & Weaver, 1991; Tufnell, Borras, Watson, & Brough, 1985).

Day Care and Respite Care

Day hospitals were begun in Britain in 1946 after their establishment in the Soviet Union a decade earlier. They provide a service that can compare favorably with standard inpatient treatment for those in acute relapse (Dick, Cameron, Cohen, & Barlow, 1985). Unless day hospitals are especially oriented to the needs of the chronic mentally ill (Aracharya & Ekdawi, 1982), however, such patients are more likely to attend Social Service day centers, which are less well staffed and oriented more toward support than treatment. Day-care facilities vary enormously. In a comprehensive review, Holloway (1988) defines five possible functions of the day hospital: an alternative to admission for the acutely ill; provision of support, supervision, and monitoring in the transition between hospital and home; source of long-term structure and support for those with chronic handicaps; site for brief intensive therapy for those with personality difficulties or severe neurotic disorders and those who require short-term focused rehabilitation; and an information, training, and communication resource.

The practices covered by the term *respite care* are of increasing importance in mental health service provision. Such respite care provides relatively brief planned periods of residential care, usually of between 1 week and 1 month, during which the patient may be fully reassessed, treatment can be modified, the family can benefit from relief of the burden of care, and the patient may be given temporary sanctuary from the demands of everyday life, which may include an emotionally charged atmosphere at home. To date, respite care has been most fully developed for people with learning difficulties (Gerard, 1990), with physical disabilities (Robinson, 1984), and for the elderly (Harper, 1988). Although there is evidence of substantial benefits for patients and their caregivers, within mental illness services, respite services are as yet poorly developed and await full evaluation.

Physical Health and Dental Care

Patients treated in the community are often the most severely ill and vulnerable, with significant requirements for physical as well as psychiatric care (Brugha, Wing, & Smith, 1989). In a study of 145 long-term users of hospital and social services' day psychiatric facilities, Brugha and associates (1989) found that 41% suffered medical problems potentially requiring care. Therefore, it is important to liaise with the providers of medical care, most often the primary care doctors. This aspect of need is advantaged when services are located in a general hospital.

Housing

The success of community-based services is crucially related to the nature and availability of accommodation. Within the British context, Wing and Furlong (1986) have described a tenfold typology of sheltered housing for people with severe psychiatric disorders. The level of least supervision is that of unsupervised housing, in which the individual lives alone or with family or friends. Contact with psychiatric services is through nonresidential staff. A variation of this arrangement is to afford a degree of administrative protection, for example, from eviction for arrears in rent. At the next level, supervised housing provides regular domiciliary supervision by a mental health practitioner to sustain standards of hygiene, nutrition, and household maintenance. In group homes, which may be arranged in clusters, several residents with psychiatric disorders share the same house, which may be supervised by a residential administrator, with support from visiting staff.

In supervised hostels, residents may each have a bedroom and share communal facilities, with residential staff offering close daily supervision (Goldberg, 1986). A higher level of supervision is required for residents more disabled by psychiatric or physical conditions: the hostel model can be supplemented with a night nursing staff, the provision of meals, and the supervision of budgeting. For those with severe behavioral disturbance, an intensive supervision hostel (or hostel–ward) may be needed, characterized by high staffing levels, a structured regimen, a perimeter area, and the rapid availability of extra staff (Garety & Morris, 1984). Finally, a form of basic nursing unit is necessary for people who are incontinent, immobile, or disoriented.

In the United States, these gradations of care have been provided in a range of different settings. A level of support similar to supervised housing is provided in sheltered lodging, or board-and-care homes (Linn, Caffey, Klett, & Hogarty, 1977). These are often privately owned homes or hotels that provide lodgings, meals, and medication management for an unlimited period (Blaustein & Viek, 1987). In 1977 approximately 20% of the 2 million chronic mentally ill people in the United States were living in such homes (Goldman, 1981). A further variation of this form of hostel is required for residents with severe physical disabilities, and in the United States nursing homes are the most frequently used provision for the elderly chronically mentally ill (Linn et al., 1985). It is argued, both by professionals (Lamb, 1982) and by the users of these forms of accommodation (Castenada & Sommer, 1986), that a comprehensive psychiatric service must include a flexible range of accommodation, with many levels of professional support varying with the changing needs of each resident.

Where do long-term patients live? Leavitt (1984) made estimates for the 55,000 patients who would have been in state hospital beds, had deinstitutionalization not occurred in California. He proposed that 45% were in board-and-care residential homes, 22% were independent or with their families, 7% were in locked facilities, 7% were in halfway houses, and 9% were inpatients. The remaining 9% were untreated and mostly homeless. In Britain, Jones (1985) followed 34 long-stay patients in York for 1 to 2 years after discharge. They had been inpatients continuously for more than 12 months before discharge, and 68% had a diagnosis of functional psychosis. She showed that 44% lived largely independently in their own homes or in lodgings, and as many lived in sheltered homes or hostels.

Evaluations of differing residential settings have been largely unsatisfactory, either because they were uncontrolled or inappropriately matched, or because residential provisions were only one among many variables in an alternative package of care delivered to discharged patients. The quality of life of patients discharged to new residential facilities has been reviewed by Lehman (1983). In an uncontrolled study, Lehman, Reed, & Possidente (1982) administered the Quality of Life Interview to

278 randomly selected residents of board-and-care homes in Los Angeles. The respondents were most consistently dissatisfied with unemployment, poverty, housing, and their relationships with friends and family. In an extension of this project, Lehman, Possidente, and Hawker (1986) compared quality of life between long-term hospital patients and residents in board-and-care homes. Regardless of their length of stay, the community residents perceived their living conditions more favorably, had more financial resources, and were less likely to have been assaulted in the last year.

These findings are supported by the 5- to 9-year follow-up of 120 Feighner-criteria chronic schizophrenic patients discharged from Shenley hospital in North London (Johnstone, Owens, Gold, Crown, & MacMillan, 1981). In the 66 cases for whom social information was available, 35% lived with a spouse; 39% lived with other family members, usually parents; 11% lived alone; and 15% lived in residential accommodations. Although severe emotional, social, and financial problems were commonplace, not one patient in this study sought readmission to the hospital, and few relatives favored this course. These studies plainly demonstrate the great variation in location at follow-up, with the majority needing continuing supported accommodation. This work also emphasizes the need for effective monitoring and tracing systems for relocated patients.

That institutionalism may be independent of the size of the facility has been shown in a West German study of 961 chronic patients in nursing homes, group homes, and a state hospital. Kunze (1985) demonstrated that the nursing homes manifested the most impoverished social environment, housed the most chronic and severely disabled schizophrenic patients, and were at least as likely to foster the features of institutionalism as the state hospital (Wing & Brown, 1970).

A considerable concern is that discharged patients will rapidly lose contact with services, although remaining symptomatic or socially disabled. An uncontrolled interview study in Los Angeles of 101 residents of board-and-care homes who had been recently discharged from a hospital found that initially more than half had contact with community occupational rehabilitation services, but in only a quarter of cases was this maintained (Lamb, 1979).

Garety (1988), in a comprehensive review, examines the range of provisions evolving and indicates the principles that should guide their future development. They include sheltered accommodation, hostels, and foster-family care schemes. To the greatest extent possible, individuals should exercise choice and control over their living environment. The skills training, supports, and services needed to enable clients to reside successfully in their own homes in normal community settings should be available and accessible, regardless of where the individuals are living. There should also be a small number of supervised, structured settings for extremely dysfunctional individuals. Similarly, Carling and Ridgway (1985) have asserted that individuals have a basic right to affordable, acceptable housing available in the normal housing arrangements typically used in the community. In terms of the research data available, the issue of residential mobility in the North American context was studied by Caton and Goldstein (1984) in Manhattan. One year after discharge, half of the study group of 119 chronic schizophrenics had changed their living arrangements at least once. Typically, different housing placements were arranged after each readmission.

To ensure the success of community housing provisions, liaison with community members and caring agencies is essential. Practical guidelines for the functioning of community hostels can be defined as follows: They should be within easy access of shops, sports facilities, cinemas, day centers, workshops, and pubs; a clear plan for medical cover should be formulated before the admission of residents; and there should be detailed discussion with all staff members, especially general practitioners if they are to be involved, and agreement about spheres of responsibility, emergency work, prescribing, and communication. Aside from permanent housing, homeless individuals who are mentally ill require additional living situations with varying degrees of supervision and structure, including emergency shelters (Fischer & Breakey, 1986).

Studies suggest mental illness rates among the homeless in 41–93%, alcohol dependency in more than 60%, and chronic medical and dental problems in more than 40% of this group (Morrisey & Levine, 1987, Bassuk, 1984; Kroll, Carey, Hagedorn, Dog, & Benavides, 1986). These individuals characteristically have restricted social support networks, little contact with psychiatric services, lower readmission rates than their domiciled counterparts, and little likelihood of referral to long-term care facilities (Appleby & Desai, 1985). Local psychiatric facilities clearly do not serve these homeless mentally ill at all adequately (Lamb, 1984). Even so, it is important to avoid overgeneralizations about the homeless mentally ill, who have been shown to demonstrate considerable variations between the sites of detailed studies (Bachrach, 1992), for example, in the proportion of such people who originated in the local area.

Advocacy

The importance of advocacy and user involvement at all levels within services has been increasingly acknowledged (Brandon & Brandon, 1987; World Psychiatric Association, 1991). Bassett, Braisby, Edwards, and Newbiggin (1991) define four categories of involvement. At the individual clinical level, active participation can include having access to documentation and involvement in goal setting and reviews. Involvement of users at all stages of the planning process may facilitate alliances between professionals and their clients and ensure more effective implementation of the services. User participation in the monitoring and management of the service and in training and education is also important. Users' charters emphasize the rights of patients to privacy, consultation, information, and choice. Mechanisms to inform individuals and their families of their legal rights are the responsibility of the services.

Family and Community Education and Support

Many persons with severe, disabling mental illness reside with their families, with consequences that must be addressed. The process of daily care for relatives who have severe social and behavioral disturbances takes place at the cost of disruption to family routine, resulting physical and psychological morbidity to the health of the other family members, and the diminished economic viability of the family unit. There should be assistance to families that provides education on the nature of the illness, consultation and supportive counseling on handling daily problems and intermittent crisis situations, appropriate involvement in the treatment-planning process, respite care, and referrals to family support groups and advocacy organizations such as the national or local mental health associations. In addition, to facilitate community integration and acceptance, practical support and education should be available to landlords, employers, educationors, community agencies, and others.

The paramount need for consistent, carefully organized support is a recurrent theme in the literature on deinstitutionalization (Brown, 1985; Mechanic & Aiken, 1987). For the public, such support means education to address disproportionate fears. For patients' relatives, support translates into psychoeducational intervention and counseling about the range of financial, vocational, domestic, and mutual-help services available (Falloon & Pederson, 1985; Grunebaum, 1986; Creer & Wing, 1974). The employees and proprietors of public and private residential facilities in turn face the risk of isolation unless they receive professional consultation and statutory monitoring of their quality of care (Blaustein & Viek, 1987; Scull, 1985). The needs and views of staff during the transition from the hospital must be addressed directly (Bachrach, 1976; Towell & McAusland, 1984) if misunderstanding and resistance are to be avoided. Finally, administrative support must be rendered to institutions in decline to maintain morale, adequate staffing levels, and treatment standards and to avoid staff burnout (Lamb, 1982).

The Influence of Patients' and Public Attitudes

Do long-stay inpatients wish to leave the hospital? There is a notable lack of information about this topic. Abrahamson and Brenner's survey (1982) showed that patients with more than 10 years of hospitalization are more likely to wish to remain in the hospital and usually give realistic reasons. Conversely, patients' attitudes toward hospitalization may strongly predict their length of hospital stay and their likelihood of readmission (Drake & Wallach, 1988; Kalman, 1983).

Ambivalent or adverse public attitudes toward the discharged mentally ill may further attenuate the security of former patients (Appelbaum, 1987). The seminal work of Nunnally (1961) on public attitudes toward the mentally ill demonstrated that they were regarded with fear, distrust, and dislike by the general public. Their behavior was seen to be characteristically unpredictable (Cumming & Cumming, 1957). Psychotics were held in lower esteem than neurotics. There was a much narrower range of attitudes than of knowledge. More recent work has suggested that public attitudes may be favorably influenced by educational programs or by direct personal contact with former patients (Trute & Loewen, 1978). The reprovision of services may have developed in advance of the public education necessary for these services to function effectively. Peterson (1986), for example, has described a community counseling center where a series of open meetings forged alliances between service users and members of the local community.

Rehabilitation and Resettlement Services

Rehabilitation services are critical for most individuals living in the community. The functions of rehabilitation can be enabling the individual to acquire or regain the practical skills needed to live and socialize in the community; teaching clients how to cope with their disabilities; assistance in developing social skills, interests, and leisure activities that provide a sense of participation and personal worth and that include opportunities for age-appropriate, culturally appropriate daytime and evening activities; and providing activities to the extent possible in the natural setting, where the client lives, works, learns, and socializes, that teach daily and community living skills such as diet, personal hygiene, cooking, shopping, budgeting, housekeeping, and use of transportation and other community resources, in other words, social network building. There should be a range of vocational services and employment opportunities available to assist clients to prepare for, obtain, and maintain employment. They could include vocational assessment and counseling, prevocational job readiness, career development, on-the-job-training, job sharing, transitional employment, job development with local employers, and innovative approaches to using those who are recovering as mental health workers.

The significance of daily occupation is illustrated by the finding of Wing & Brown (1970) in the Three Hospital Study that the amount of time patients spent doing nothing was directly related to their levels of primary symptoms. Occupation may usefully be seen as either work, a purposeful activity requiring effort and discrimination that has social significance, or employment, an economic exchange relationship in which effort is rendered for payment (Hartley, 1980). Occupation may confer a sense of mastery through the performance of social roles. It may also bring social status and social contacts. Finally, it can be a criterion of recovery (Shepherd, 1984). Many long-term psychiatric inpatients are involved with occupational therapy, but very few indeed maintain competitive employment (Ford, Goddard, & Lansdall-Welfare, 1987).

To respond to this need for occupational rehabilitation, a clubhouse model of day care has been developed, based upon Fountain House in New York (Beard, 1978). The chronic mentally ill become members of a club that offers a center where they can drop in for social activities or refreshment. There are also concurrent programs of vocational training, explicitly emphasizing empowerment and participation by members. As an extension of the clubhouse approach, transitional employment programs, also originating at Fountain House (Beard, 1978), are gaining popularity in the United States. Each program is an agency that negotiates positions for unskilled labor with local employers and guarantees that there will be no employee absences. If a program employee does not attend work, the vacancy is filled immediately from the pool of other workers or by one of the program staff (Beard, 1978).

Anthony (1972; Anthony, Cohen, & Vitalo, 1978) has reviewed literature on the specific effects of occupational rehabilitation programs on performance outside the hospital. Overall, the proportion of patients who are readmitted increases as the period of follow-up lengthens (Pryor & Distefano, 1986). Five to 10 years after discharge, only 25–30% of the patients had avoided readmission. Several treatment variables were indicators of outcome. Day center attendance was associated with lower readmission rates (Kruzich & Borg, 1985; Dickey, Cannon, McGuire, & Gudeman, 1986), as were medication compliance and contact with psychiatric supervision. Contact with occupational centers is also highly associated with their geographic accessibility (Lamb, 1979).

Inpatient Facilities

The NIMH guidelines advocate for each locality consumer self-help groups and consumer-operated services that are self-defined and consumer-controlled. These services are voluntary and based on choice and the patients' basic needs for survival, friendship, and a sense of community. The services generally supplement the formal mental health system and meet a variety of social and support needs through, for example, peer-support groups that meet regularly to share ideas and information and provide mutual support, or drop-in centers that can offer welfare benefits or housing advice.

PSYCHOSOCIAL APPROACHES

A wealth of research over the last 20 years has demonstrated that the quality of life of people disabled by chronic schizophrenia can be substantially improved by an approach combining social, psychological, and pharmacological interventions (Barrowclough & Tarrier, 1984). Patients receiving such integrated treatment have been shown to have fewer relapses, to spend less time in the hospital, to make fewer demands on their relatives, and to show less clinical and social impairment. Balanced and effective care must blend four types of intervention: skills training interventions, pharmacological methods, community support interventions, and family treatments (Fuhrer, 1987). The stress in current research is on the importance of combining these approaches to maximize the therapeutic benefit.

Expressed Emotion

Research conducted on discharged long-term psychiatric patients 30 years ago suggested that patients who went to live in lodgings or with siblings did best, whereas outcome was worst for those discharged to hostels or to live with their parents (Brown, 1959). In addition, the patients who lived with their parents and who had more daily contact with them fared worst of all. Pursuing this, a subsequent prospective study with more than 100 schizophrenic discharged patients revealed that it was the parents' and not the patient's behavior that best predicted outcome, and in particular that high levels of "emotional involvement" were associated with more frequent relapse. More recent studies have refined both the measures of family involvement with the Camberwell Family Interview and the concepts used to describe the components of family interactions (Brown & Rutter, 1966; Vaughn & Leff, 1976), which became known as *expressed emotion* (EE). The five components of a rating of high EE are a high level of critical comments, a high rating on overinvolvement, the demonstration of hostility toward the patient, low warmth, and few positive remarks. The method used most frequently is to tape-record an interview with the relative and rate for the three constituents later. Relatives with a score of 6 or more critical comments, any degree of hostility, or a rating of 3 or more for overinvolvement are assigned to a high-EE group (Leff, Kuipers, Berkowitz, Eberlein-Fries, & Sturgeon, 1982).

Evidence is now accumulating that the concept of expressed emotion may be meaningful and important across cultures. A study among low-income Mexican–Americans in Los Angeles, for example, found that a high level of EE on the part of key relatives significantly increases the risk of relapse among schizophrenic patients recently discharged from the hospital. Compared with the London and Anglo–American studies (Vaughan et al., 1982), the Mexican–American families less often demonstrated high EE levels, and the authors proposed that this difference may in part explain the better prognosis for schizophrenia in developing countries (Karno et al., 1987). A further part of the WHO Determinants of Outcome study (Sartorius, 1986) showed that critical comments could be rated reliably in Hindi and that relatives in rural Chandigarh in India expressed fewer critical comments, fewer positive remarks, and less overinvolvement than both their local urban counterparts and families studied in Denmark. At 1-year follow-up, the patients from high-EE families again showed poorer outcome in rural Chandigarh, and the authors suggest that the improved prognosis as compared with London is largely attributable to the lower proportion of high-EE relatives in the Indian sample.

From the observations that high levels of expressed emotion were associated with poor outcome for schizophrenic patients, several intervention trials during the last decade have specifically sought to improve patterns of communication within the families (Falloon, 1988). The aim of this technique is to enable family members to express their feelings and needs in a direct and specific way that can facilitate efficient conflict resolution and reduce the harmful effects of critical comments toward the patient. The results showed considerable clinical and social gains by the family therapy group. At 9 months follow-up they had fewer positive symptoms of schizophrenia, a lower relapse rate, and improve social adjustment and social role performance; were more effective on problem solving; showed a higher compliance rate with medication; and required lower doses. At 2-year follow-up, five sixths of the experimental group remained improved, compared with only one sixth of the control group (Falloon & Pederson, 1985).

Social Skills Training

Social skills training may be defined as those methods that use the specific principles of learning theory to promote the acquisition, generalization, and durability of skills needed in interpersonal situations (Liberman, Wallace, Falloon, & Vaughn, 1981). Social skills training is therefore a systematic psychological treatment that aims to develop patients' social competence and needs to be distinguished from nonspecific socialization group activities. In one such intervention trial, Hogarty and colleagues

(1986) showed no relapses for patients receiving both family intervention and social skills training, compared with 41% in the first year for patients receiving neither. The training seeks to enhance both verbal and non-verbal social behavior and to develop more accurate social perception and judgment. One widely used model (Liberman, Cardin, McGill, Falloon, & Evans, 1987) categorizes the social behaviors necessary to communicate as acknowledging positive behavior, active listening skills, making positive requests, expressing negative feelings, and requesting a temporary break in the communication.

Different approaches have been taken to evaluating the outcome of social skills training. A study in Los Angeles that also used family education methods found improvement in household functioning, work, studying, decision making, and establishing friendships outside the home (Falloon, Boyd, & McGill, 1985). In addition this study showed clear advantages for family interventions for days of admission to hospital (mean 0.83 versus 8.39 for control group) and for relapse rates (6% versus 44%). Earlier work in Los Angeles had compared intensive social skills training and family therapy with a combined regimen of holistic therapies and insight-oriented psychotherapy. Outcome was rated primarily on mental state according to the Present State Examination and the Psychiatric Assessment Scale, and no significant differences were reported in the relapse rates at 9 months follow-up between the experimental group (29%) and the control group (50%) (Liberman et al., 1981). Similar results have emerged from social skills programs in Italy (De Isabella & Meneghelli, 1983) and Switzerland (Brenner et al., 1980).

A wide range of outcomes have been used to rate improvement after social rehabilitation programs, including readmission, employment, social behavior, social role performance, and quality of life. It is apparent, however, that the majority of intervention trials have incorporated social skills training within a wider psychosocial package of interventions, and there is only modest evidence on the enduring effectiveness of social skills training conducted in isolation.

Relatives of People Disabled by Serious Mental Disorders

For many long-term inpatients who are discharged to community-based facilities, there is no remaining contact with any family member. Younger schizophrenic patients often either live with or have frequent contact with their relatives (Goldman, 1981). These relatives experience major disruption in their patterns of life and financial resources, and one follow-up study found that nearly two thirds complained of the patients' hostility, poor personal hygiene, and bizarre behavior (Hoenig & Hamilton, 1966). There are often disabling social consequences for the relatives themselves.

The Scottish Schizophrenia Research Group (1987) found that after the first admission of the schizophrenic patients, most relatives experienced transient disturbance of their social and leisure activities and persisting disruption of their marital relationships. As expected, this distress was usually proportional to the severity of the patient's symptoms and behavioral disturbance.

There is strong evidence that the burden of care sustained by relatives of schizophrenic patients can be experienced as psychological distress. One study of first admissions for schizophrenia found significant mood disorder among three quarters of relatives, compared with 20% of the normal population (Scottish Schizophrenia Research Group, 1987). Much of this distress persists. At 1 year follow-up, although the relatives' degree of anxiety had reduced, there were continuing high levels of somatic symptoms.

A wide-ranging survey of the experiences and needs of 80 families of schizophrenic patients mainly living in south eastern England found that relatives most often complained of the loss of meaningful social contact with their schizophrenic relatives (Creer & Wing, 1974). Three quarters also mentioned difficulties in that the patients showed slowness, a lack of conversation, and few leisure interests. Many had tried different forms of social contact and had concluded that interaction was painful or exhausting for the patient, and that a degree of withdrawal was protective. Two thirds of the relatives also reported concerns that the patients had very limited social performance. The majority of patients did not live with a marital partner and contributed little to household finances or maintenance. They offered little companionship to their family and played no part in social life outside the home. Almost half of the relatives said that the effects on their health of living with the schizophrenic relative had been severe. The majority felt dissatisfied with the support offered by psychiatric services, and they described difficulties at every stage of referral, treatment, and follow-up, with a particular shortage of day care and staffed residential facilities. Despite the wide range of difficulties suffered by the families, they nevertheless strongly preferred to keep the affected relative at home (Grad & Sainsbury, 1968). Indeed, in one large follow-up study in North London, not one family preferred the patient to be readmitted to the hospital, even though many had little or no contact with psychiatric services (Johnstone et al., 1984).

The concept of the burden of care has become prominent in the recent literature examining the family effects of living with a schizophrenic relative (Kuipers & Bebbington, 1985). *Burden* can be defined as the presence of problems, difficulties, or adverse events that affect the lives of psychiatric patients' significant others (Platt, 1985). Burden exists for relatives where the usual reciprocal balance that exists in social exchanges within the family breaks down and one member is experienced as a drain on social, psychological, and financial resources. A number of rating schedules have been developed to measure the burden experienced by family members. The Social Behaviour Assessment Scale provides standardized measures of the degree of interference with family life that can be attributed to the patient, as well as the individual distress caused by the burden of care to family members. Similarly, the Burden on Family Interview Schedule produces subscores of burden in the areas of financial loss, disruption of routine family activities, family leisure, family interaction, and the effects on physical and mental health. A similar approach was used in the study of experimental community-based treatment of patients with chronic mental disorder in Madison, Wisconsin (Test & Stein, 1980). In comparison with traditional inpatient-oriented treatment, the experimental program produced no greater family burden when measured with a modified Grad & Sainsbury scale, which included six objective and one subjective measures of family burden. The authors concluded that community-based care was no more burden on the family in this study because of the large amount of support that staff gave to patients and their caregivers.

To summarize the research on family burden, several points are clear. First, the process of daily care for relatives who have severe social and behavioral disturbance takes place with the costs of disruption to family routine, costs to the physical and psychological health of other family members, and costs to the economic viability of the family unit. Professional support rendered to such families, experimental and model projects aside, is often extremely inadequate. Where such supportive services are provided, the burden of care is no greater than for orthodox hospital care. Finally, almost without exception, where meaningful contact exists with the family, relatives are unwilling to see the patient admitted to the hospital for the long term. In the next section, active and structured programs of family involvement, with the aim of reducing the risk of relapse of schizophrenic episodes, are described.

Psychosocial Treatment Interventions

The methods described under the general heading of psychosocial interventions have the following aims in common: to reduce the risk of relapse for patients suffering from schizophrenia, to improve the quality of life of both patients and families, and to teach skills to manage and minimize the primary symptoms, the secondary distress, and the tertiary consequent social disability (Falloon & Pederson, 1985). From early 1970s, work conducted in Pittsburgh suggested that social interventions could enhance the effects of maintenance antipsychotic medications in reducing the risk of relapse for schizophrenia (Hogarty, Goldberg, & Collaborative Study Group, 1973). The social interventions used were termed *sociother-*

apy; later modifications of this program, which were described as "major role therapy" (MRT), included individual casework and vocational rehabilitation counseling. The authors concluded that such interventions led to fewer relapses and improved social adjustment for the less symptomatic patients.

The methods used in psychoeducational treatment include family workshops in which families are given straightforward information about schizophrenia and a series of meetings of the therapist, the patient, and the family (Anderson, Hogarty, & Reiss, 1986). The family meetings are held every 2 or 3 weeks for up to 1 year. The psychoeducational approach has more recently emphasized the improvement of communication patterns within the family by using techniques derived from family therapy (Anderson, Hogarty, & Reiss, 1986). There are four stages in this process: connection with the family, teaching family survival skills, the application of these skills to everyday life, and disengagement (Hogarty et al., 1973, 1979).

In the initial phase, the cooperation of the family is invited through reviewing the case history, open discussion about the problems and feelings of the family members, decreasing the guilt they experience, and establishing a written treatment contract. The survival skills are usually taught in small groups including several families; they begin with specific information about schizophrenia. They go on to provide concrete recommendations about clear and emotionally restrained methods of communication, setting limits on behavior that disturbs any member of the family, and modifying excessive expectations by parents and siblings. The subsequent phases of treatment invite the family to practice these techniques at home, report back on difficulties, and then withdraw gradually from supervised treatment.

Giving information to relatives is an integral part of such combined family programs, and the methods used have included lectures, video presentations, and written summaries. The experience of these researchers suggests that any educational programs should attend to the following issues: First, before giving information, there is a need to understand the patient's and the family's perceptions of the disorder. Second, information should focus on the particular patient's problems and symptoms rather than on general information about schizophrenia. Third, the information conveyed must be selective, in that few items of information can be retained. Fourth, clinicians need to assess the amount of information that the families have understood and be ready to repeat the information-giving sessions. Finally, teaching the family to use a model in which family interactions are understood to influence the patient's condition is easiest soon after the onset of the disorder (Tarrier & Barrowclough, 1986) by using, for example, an approach such as the Knowledge about Schizophrenia Interview (Barrowclough et al., 1987).

What is the functional value of teaching information about schizophrenia to families? A research team in Manchester (Barrowclough et al., 1987) used the Knowledge about Schizophrenia Interview to assess the useful knowledge conveyed by two educational sessions for 17 families during the first 2 weeks after discharge. Relatives showed improved factual knowledge after the sessions, and also there was significant change from functionally negative or neutral responses toward positive responses to the patient after the program. Although from a small trial with brief follow-up, these results do suggest that the educational component of psychoeducational programs can have important therapeutic benefits in improving communication within the family of schizophrenic patients.

Structured problem solving can be taught as a series of six steps (Falloon, 1988). First, a specific problem or desired goal is identified. This is often a clear, circumscribed, and achievable goal that the family members agree is an example of a larger area of difficulty. For example, a family may set as a goal that the patient should clean his or her room once a week for at least half an hour, rather than aim to change more globally the patient's reluctance to be involved in housework. The second step is to list alternative solutions to the specific problem identified. This can be achieved during a brief session in which a wide range of ideas are written down without, at this stage, any evaluation.

The third stage is to list the positive and negative features of each alternative and to use this list to choose the preferred practical course of action. The next step is to draw up a detailed action plan to implement the option chosen. This will include specific, small-scale tasks for each family member and a clear and agreed timetable for their completion. Finally, subsequent meetings review the outcome of these actions and amend the methods used in the light of the progress made. Each stage of the process is written down in negotiation with the family. At present this work is being extended to include more behaviorally oriented strategies such as social skills training, operant conditioning methods to deal with positive and negative symptoms of schizophrenia, and specific identified deficits in communication skills (Falloon, 1988).

The accumulating evidence from this body of research, especially from the controlled trials, is that interventions using combined packages of social and psychological methods can reduce symptomatic and social suffering for the schizophrenic patient and reduce the burden falling upon the family. These methods appear to be most effective where the aims of treatment are clearly established at the outset and are agreed among the whole family. The lessons of the earlier trials are that treatment groups must be diagnosed with standardized methods and their sociodemographic features fully described.

CASE MANAGEMENT

Defining *Case Management*

Case management is a strategy for coordinating service delivery on behalf of patients (Modrcin, Rapp, & Chamberlain, 1985). It is a generic term that encompasses the following functions: the coordination, integration, and allocation of individualized care within limited resources. Many more precise definitions have been put forward that emphasize aspects of this range of activities and reflect the various levels at which case management is intended to operate. At the individual level, for example, case management has been defined as the coordination of care for patients who require a multiplicity of services (Clifford, Craig, & Sayce, 1988). At the project level, case management has been used to describe a method of organizing the delivery of care for a defined patient group, which clarifies and allocates the responsibilities of the staff team. At the program level, case management has been characterized as an approach that provides services on the basis of need, avoids duplication of effort between agencies, and seeks to offer an adequate range of services to target groups of patients, such as those with diagnoses both of psychosis and substance abuse (Fariello & Scheidt, 1989). This third level may be more accurately called *care* (or *system*) *management.*

Three issues deserve closer attention. First, the definitions of *case management* more often refer to treatment principles (see next section) than to treatment practices (Modrcin et al., 1985). Second, most accounts of case management are generalized elaborations of such principles and are not precisely defined (Bachrach, 1989). Third, descriptions of case management programs for long-term mental illness refer to a very wide range of practices (Robinson & Bergman, 1989). It is clear, therefore, that descriptions of case management programs should specifically set out their structure and working methods to allow useful comparison with similar projects.

The Development of the Case Manager Concept

The origins of case management lie in social casework (Robinson & Bergman, 1989), which has long stressed the value of interventions with distressed individuals that encourage the development of self-reliance and adaptation (Lee & Kenworthy, 1929). Within the mental health services the coordination function was first formally recognized in the United States in 1963 by the Community Mental Health Centers Act, and its 1975 amendments explicitly required the centers to link with other agencies providing care for long-term patients. There has, however, been an increasing recognition in the United States over the last 25 years that community-based services for long-term mental illness were still too often fragmented (Braun et al., 1981; Kiesler, 1982; Mechanic & Aiken, 1987). Methods of drawing together the health and social service care components were developed, especially in federally funded initiatives such as the Community Support Program (Tessler & Goldman, 1982). These models were rapidly disseminated. In 1981, for example, no Medicaid-supported case management programs were operating in the United States. By 1986, 19 states had more than 651,000 patients enrolled in such programs (Spitz, 1987). A parallel development in Britain has been the rapid expansion of community mental health centers (many of which include case-managed care for long-term patients), of which 87 had opened by 1987 (Sayce, Craig, & Boardman, 1991).

The Core Tasks of Case Management

There is considerable consensus about the range of tasks that case management can offer (Modrcin et al., 1985; Renshaw, 1987; Charnley & Davies, 1987; Knapp et al., 1990). Patient identification requires first the definition of the target group for the case management service. This may be clearly established from current contact with services or may include, for example, forms of outreach to identify patients with no previous or current contact who nevertheless require psychiatric care (Charnley & Davies, 1987). The next stage is to assess the social, clinical, vocational, physical health, and residential needs of each patient (Brewin, Wing, Mangen, Brugha, & MacCarthy, 1987; Worley, Drago, & Hadley, 1990). This may require interviews with several members of the care team to establish the extent of disability in each domain. On the basis of this thorough assessment of need, the case manager decides, within the resources available, which services should be offered, how often, where, and by whom. Where interventions are distributed across agencies, the details of each agreed service may be set out in joint care plans or may be itemized in formal contract specifications (House of Commons, 1990). Whether the case manager acts as service broker or direct caregiver, the effectiveness of care next needs to be evaluated, formally or informally. Where quality standards have been included in the service contract, the process of care may be set against agreed expectations. Patient satisfaction with care is increasingly used as an important indicator of the adequacy of interventions. It is often preferable, in addition, to use outcome measures of clinical and social function to establish the effectiveness of care (Hall, 1979).

Twelve Axes to Define Case Management in Practice

There are as many ways to implement the principles of case management as there are case management programs. Several authors have attempted to bring order to this disarray by developing contrasting models of case management (Lamb, 1980; Bachrach, 1980; Dill, 1987; Renshaw, 1987; Schwab, Drake, & Burghardt, 1988). For example, they commonly distinguish between direct care and service broker applications of case management. It may be more useful, however, to consider each program in terms of 12 axes that, together, precisely define the characteristics of its practice.

Axis 1. *Individual–team case management.* Most case management programs give clear responsibility for a given patient group either to an individual (Breakey, 1989) or to a team of staff (Intagliata, 1982). Test (1979) has described four advantages to team case management: continuous coverage, continuity in the absence of individuals, better-quality planning, and better support between caregivers. Individual case loads may intensify the staff–patient relationship and provide better continuity of care (Renshaw et al., 1988), but can act at the expense of effective delegation to the most appropriate worker.

Axis 2. *Direct care–service brokerage.* At one extreme of this axis lie brokerage models in which the case manager may have little or no direct continuing contact with the patient, but whose primary role is to ensure that a range of other care staff provide the necessary level of care (Lamb, 1980; Schwab et al., 1988). In contrast, direct care staff gain a personal understanding of the patient and family, but may undertake tasks that conflict with or fall outside their competence or expertise, and that can produce boundary disputes about the proper therapeutic tasks for each specialty.

Axis 3. *Intensity of interventions.* The frequency of case management contacts may vary from at least daily to less than monthly (Robinson & Bergman, 1989). The intensity of the therapeutic, material, and social support that can be offered to the patient is importantly constrained by the frequency of contact, and this in turn is closely associated with the target group served and the caseload.

Axis 4. *Degree of budgetary control.* The effectiveness of case managers for long-term mental illness is often closely associated with the degree of control they exercise over the budget for patient services. Where such decentralized control exists, case managers may have flexibility for care substitution, the better to match resources to patients' needs. Financial autonomy may ensure accountability and encourage creativity (Davies, 1987). Conversely, budgetary control at the level of the case manager can introduce inequitable resource allocation, may produce inconsistent expenditure decisions between practitioners, and, unless closely supervised, may encourage overspending. It can operate best where patients have detailed individual treatment plans and budgets (Knapp et al., 1990). In the United States, for example, considerable advantages have been described from a capitation system of payments to the case manager, who has wide discretion about which services to purchase (Goldman & Taube, 1988), and conversely case managers with clinical responsibility but little financial discretion may be unable to act fully in the patients' interests.

Axis 5. *Health or social service staff.* Case management teams may be established within health or social service settings and may contain staff from either or both of these agencies (Clifford et al., 1988). Alternatively, staff with a range of professional training may be employed by an independent agency such as locally based mental health consortium or housing partnership. There is some evidence that a predominantly social work orientation is associated with more and more frequent contacts with patients with neurotic rather than psychotic disorders (Levine, 1981), and clinical practice in British community mental health centers also suggests that this tendency is reinforced by poor managerial direction and by individual discretion by case managers about which referrals to accept (Sayce et al., 1991). The clear implication here is that clear lines of managerial accountability are required, preferably with agreed guidelines about the mix of diagnoses within individual case loads.

Axis 6. *Status of case manager.* Case managers with professional qualifications may offer long-term psychiatric patients greater expertise in assessment and psychological intervention, and are themselves more costly to employ, but may be unwilling to do more mundane tasks, such as negotiate social welfare benefit entitlements. For these reasons, and especially within the context of psychiatric hospital closure, new community caregivers or care assistants (Griffiths, 1988), with relatively little formal training and professional status, are increasingly being used to provide direct care to the long-term mentally ill.

Axis 7. *Specialization of the case manager.* Case management teams show considerable variation in whether staff members work as generic case managers or as specialists. As nonspecialists, case managers may be allocated irrespective of their formal training and offer a common core service. In contrast, patients who need help with regular medication, for example, may be allocated to psychiatric nurses in the team, whereas patients on no medication but with substantial debts may be allocated to a social work colleague. The issue of specialization is likely to become increasingly important because of the distinction drawn between health care and social care in the National Health Service and Community Care Act of 1990.

Axis 8. *Staff-to-patient ratio.* Sustained quality in case management services to the long-term mentally ill depends on a relatively restricted caseload. Direct care models usually operate within a range of 10 to 25 patients per staff member, but ratios of more than 1:15 run the risk of rapidly diminishing benefits (Harris & Bergman, 1988). The broker model of indirect care may allow the ratio to extend to 1:40 (Robinson & Bergman, 1989).

Axis 9. *Degree of patient participation.* Case management teams show great variation in the emphasis given to patient participation. One pole of the axis includes programs that aim to establish treatment and care targets jointly with the patient; at the other extreme lie approaches in which patients' needs are defined by third parties and in which outcome includes no reference to patients' satisfaction with services.

Axis 10. *The point of contact.* Case management programs may make contact with patients in a wide range of settings, including their family homes (Breakey, 1989), in hotel rooms (Bond, 1984), in the team offices (Stein & Diamond, 1985), or in primary care facilities. Contact can be established at the point of first referral (Marks et al., 1988) or after discharge from the hospital (Wasylenki, Goeing, Lancee, Balantyne, & Farkas, 1985).

Axis 11. *Level of intervention.* Case management interventions may take place at the individual, network, or systems level (Ross, 1979). Individual care includes those activities previously referred to as core tasks, including, for example, advocacy services for individual patients. At the network level, services can be offered to other formal caregivers, to family and other natural supports, or to specialized groups such as those fostering self-help. In systems terms, the case manager may offer public education on mental disorders or advocate for resource allocation to the long-term mentally ill.

Axis 12. *The target population.* Whereas case management is conceptually well suited to the continuing service needs of the long-term mentally ill, case managers may in fact spend much of their time with people suffering from briefer or more intermittent forms of mental disorder. More specifically, where community mental health centers aiming to offer a comprehensive service to the catchment population have no formal priority for defined patient groups, then patients with more severe conditions are selectively undertreated (Levine, 1981). Indeed, Stein and Diamond (1985) have described the characteristics most likely to benefit from "assertive" case management: those who are unwilling to attend hospital-based services, who show poor medication compliance and poor ability to monitor themselves, and who have frequent crises.

Evaluations of Case Management

The use of case management for long-term mental illness has increased rapidly in the United States over the last 25 years, and most published accounts that describe process and outcome evaluations are American, although few are methodologically rigorous. The federally funded Community Support Program (CSP), for example, established and evaluated case management programs at 18 demonstration sites for 1,471 patients (Tessler & Goldman, 1982). The patient group was in many ways typical of the long-term mentally ill usually targeted by case management programs. The mean age of patients was 42, with an average 18 years of psychiatric contact, including three previous admissions. Their most frequent problems were with transport, money management, taking prescribed medications, getting meals, and finding companionship.

The size of the staff:patient ratio has crucial implications for the range and quality of services that can be provided. A study in New York State that evaluated changes as this ratio increased from 1:15 to 1:50 found that staff progressively became more reactive than proactive, spent less time assessing needs, acted for patients rather than assisting patients to act on their own behalf, and focused on documentation rather than direct patient contact (Baker & Intagliata, 1984).

Case management programs may therefore have important roles to play. First, they may ensure that patients with long-term mental illness do maintain contact with services, especially for rehabilitation. Indeed, evidence is emerging that case managers may be a necessary but not sufficient component of adequate continuing care, and that vocational training is particularly important in influencing the long-term outcome of younger severely disabled psychiatric patients (Solomon, Davis, & Gordon, 1984). Second, they may offer an array of interventions that the patient may value and benefit from, and that the patient collaborates in choosing. Third, they may avoid both gaps and redundancy in service provision. Finally, they may determine, through continuing regular review, when services should be varied or discontinued. Case management is a unifying concept that promises to represent a patient group that has been neglected, to integrate services that have been fragmented, and to offer care shaped by the needs of the patients rather than of service providers. Careful evaluation will allow us to judge how far these opportunities can be realized.

CONCLUSIONS

In this final section we develop the view that clinicians, planners, managers, and researchers should set specific targets for performance, outcome, and quality for the mental health services they develop. There are already some illustrations of this approach (WHO, 1981, 1991). There has been, for example, considerable debate about the numbers of psychiatric beds that are necessary (Wing, 1971). The 1975 British White Paper (DHSS, 1975) suggests targets of 50 district general hospital beds per 100,000 of the population, together with 35 for the elderly severely mentally infirm and 17 for "new" long-stay patients. More recently, the House of Commons Social Services Committee report on community care (1985) noted that "a smaller number of in-patients beds is now thought necessary for general psychiatric services," and a Royal College of Psychiatrists working party has specified this number as 44 acute beds for a population of 100,000 (Hirsch, 1988).

Within the British context, for example, we propose that mental health targets be set at five levels of intervention that define responsibilities at national, regional, service purchaser district, provider (local service unit), and patient levels. In advancing these targets and their associated indicators, our intention is to stimulate widespread debate among health and social agencies, service users, and the voluntary sector that will generate ambitious and detailed mental health targets to be incorporated in the planned Act of Parliament.

The targets we propose are of three kinds: structure, process, and outcome. In terms of service structure, a wide consensus has emerged over the last decade on the characteristics that locally based services should assume (Murphy, 1991), and we propose that regions and districts should first make an inventory of the range, character, and size of local facilities and then draw up a time scale during which services should be reoriented against specific targets. Evidence to date suggests that the worst of service provision is very poor. The majority of health districts, for example, have no mental health respite care facilities (Thornicroft, 1990). At the district level, one of the most fundamental barriers to rational planning and evaluation has been the lack of even basic information infrastructures (Wing, 1989; WHO, 1991). Strategic guidance from both regional and national levels has been minimal, and although local ownership of such systems is crucial to their success, the provision of acknowledged expert consultants could expedite the development of systems relevant to planning (Strathdee, 1990).

Over the course of the last 30 years, the pernicious effects of the institutionalized handling of psychiatric patients have become recognized, and a few model programs have demonstrated that under favorable conditions community-based services can provide a quality of care that the recipients value highly. The challenge for the remainder of this century is to continue to build on this firm foundation, so that the best of services are generalized, the worst of services are brought up to a level that is at least acceptable, and we continue to evaluate our service innovations and interventions so that we may more precisely understand how they can function most effectively.

REFERENCES

Abrahamson, D., & Brenner, D. (1982). Do long-stay patients want to leave hospital? *Health Trends, 14,* 95–97.

Anderson, C., Hogarty, G., & Reiss, D. (1986). Family treatment of adult schizophrenic patients: A psycho-educational approach. *Schizophrenia Bulletin, 6,* 490–505.

Anthony, W. (1972). Efficacy of psychiatric rehabilitation. *Psychological Bulletin, 78*, 447–456.

Anthony, W., Cohen, A., & Vitalo, R. (1978). The measurement of rehabilitation outcome. *Schizophrenia Bulletin, 4*, 365–381.

Appelbaum, P. (1987). Crazy on the streets. *Commentary, 83*, 34–39.

Appleby, L., & Desai, P. (1985). Documenting the relationship between homelessness and psychiatric hospitalisation. *Hospital and Community Psychiatry, 36*, 732–735.

Aracharya, S., & Ekdawi, M. (1982). Day hospital rehabilitation, a six year study. *Social Psychiatry, 17*, 1–5.

Audit Commission. (1986). *Making a reality of community care.* London: Her Majesty's Stationery Office.

Avison, W., & Speechley, K. (1987). The discharged psychiatric patients: A review of social, social–psychological, and psychiatric correlates of outcome. *American Journal of Psychiatry, 144*, 10–18.

Bachrach, L. (1976). Deinstitutionalisation: An analytical review and sociological perspective. Rockville, MD: U.S. Department of Health, Education and Welfare, National Institute of Mental Health.

Bachrach, L. (1980). Overview: Model programs for chronic patients. *American Journal of Psychiatry, 137*, 1023–1031.

Bachrach, L. (1984). *The homeless mentally ill and mental health services: An analytical review of the literature.* Washington, DC: U.S. Department of Health and Human Services.

Bachrach, L. (1986). Deinstitutionalisation: What do the numbers mean? *Hospital and Community Psychiatry, 37*, 118–121.

Bachrach, L. (1989). Case management: Towards a shared definition. *Hospital and Community Psychiatry, 40*, 883–884.

Bachrach, L. (1992). What we know about homelessness among mentally ill persons? *Hospital and Community Psychiatry, 43*, 453–464.

Baker, F., & Intagliata, L. (1984). The New York State community support system, *Hospital and Community Psychiatry, 35*, 39–44.

Barrowclough, C., & Tarrier, N. (1984). "Psychosocial" interventions with families and their effects on the course of schizophrenia: A review. *Psychological Medicine, 14*, 629–642.

Barrowclough, C., Tarrier, N., Watts, S., Vaughn, C., Bamrah, J., & Freeman, H. (1987). Assessing the functional value of relatives' knowledge about schizophrenia: A preliminary report. *British Journal of Psychiatry, 151*, 1–8.

Barton, R. (1959). *Institutional neurosis.* Bristol, England: John Wright.

Bassett, T., Braisby, D., Edwards, S., & Newbiggin, K. (1991). Involving service users in community mental health services. In E. Echlin (Ed.), *Community mental health centres/teams* (pp. 31–42). London: Good Practices in Mental Health.

Bassuk, E. (1984). The homelessness problem. *Scientific American, 251*, 40–46.

Beard, J. (1978). The rehabilitation services of Fountain House. In L. Stein & M. Test (Eds.), *Alternatives to mental hospital treatment* (pp. 97–118). New York: Plenum Press.

Bebbington, P., Hurry, J., Tennant, C., Sturt, E., & Wing, J. (1981). Epidemiology of mental disorders in Camberwell. *Psychological Medicine, 11*, 561–579.

Birchwood, M., Smith, J., Macmillan, F., Hogg, B., Prasad, R., Harvey, C., & Bering, S. (1989). Predicting relapse in schizophrenia: The development and implementation of an early signs monitoring system using patients and families as observers, a preliminary investigation. *Psychological Medicine, 19,* 649–656.

Blaustein, M., & Viek, C. (1987). Problems and needs of operators of board-and-care homes: A survey. *Hospital and Community Psychiatry, 38,* 750–753.

Boardman, J. (1987). *The mental health advice centre in Lewisham. Service usage: Trends from 1978–1984* (Research Report No. 3). Lewisham, England: The National Unit for Psychiatric Research and Development.

Bond, G. (1984). An economic analysis of psychosocial rehabilitation, *Hospital and Community Psychiatry, 35,* 356–362.

Brandon, D., & Brandon, A. (1987). Consumers as colleagues. In *Power in strange places: User involvement in mental health services.* London: Good Practices in Mental Health.

Braun, P., Kochansky, G., & Shapiro, R. (1981). Overview: Deinstitutionalisation of psychiatric patients, a critical review of outcome studies. *American Journal of Psychiatry, 138,* 736–749.

Breakey, W. (1989). Integrating training and research with clinical services in a community setting. *Hospital and Community Psychiatry, 40,* 1175–1179.

Brenner, H., Stramke, W., & Mewes, J. (1980). Erfahrungen mit einem spezifishcen Therapieprogramm zun Training kognitiver kommunikativer Faehigkeiten in der Rehabilitation chronisch schizophrener 20 Patienten [Experiences with a specific program of cognitive and communication skills training in the rehabilitation of chronic schizophrenic patients]. *Nervenartz, 51,* 106–112.

Brewin, C., Wing, J., Mangen, S., Brugha, T., & MacCarthy, B. (1987). Principles and practice of measuring needs in the long-term mentally ill, the Medical Research Council Needs for Care assessment. *Psychological Medicine, 17,* 971–981.

Brown, B. (1975). *Deinstitutionalisation and Community Support Systems.* Statement by Director, National Institute of Mental Health, 4 November. Bethesda, Maryland: NIMH.

Brown, G. (1959). Experiences of discharged schizophrenic mental hospital patients in various types of living group. *Millbank Memorial Fund Quarterly, 37,* 105–131.

Brown, G., & Rutter, M. (1966). The measurement of family activities and relationships. *Human Relations, 19,* 241–263.

Brown, P. (1985). *The transfer of care: Psychiatric deinstitutionalisation and its aftermath.* London: Routledge & Kegan Paul.

Brown, R., Strathdee, G., Christie-Brown, J., & Robinson, P. (1988). A comparison of referrals to primary care and hospital outpatient clinics. *British Journal of Psychiatrists, 153,* 168–173.

Brugha, T. S., Wing, J. K., & Smith, B. L. (1989). Physical ill-health of the long-term mentally ill in the community. Is there an unmet need? *British Journal of Psychiatry, 155,* 777–782.

Carling, P., & Ridgway, P. (1985). Community residential rehabilitation: An emerging approach to meeting housing needs. In P. Carling & P. Ridgway

(Eds.), *Providing housing and supports for people with psychiatric disabilities* (pp.121–148). Rockville, MD: National Institute of Mental Health.

Castenada, D., & Sommer, R. (1986). Patients' housing options as viewed by parents of the mentally ill. *Hospital and Community Psychiatry, 37,* 1238–1242.

Caton, C., & Goldstein, J. (1984). Housing change of chronic schizophrenic patients: A consequence of the revolving door. *Social Science and Medicine, 1,* 758–764.

Challis, D., & Davies, B. (1986). *Case management in community care.* Aldershot, England: Gower.

Charnley, H., & Davies, B. (1987). *Blockages and the performance of the core tasks of case management* (Personal Social Services Research Unit Discussion Paper No. 473). Canterbury: University of Kent.

Clark, D. (1974). *Social therapy in psychiatry.* Harmondsworth, England: Pelican.

Clifford, P., Craig, T., & Sayce, L. (1988). *Towards co-ordinated care for people with long-term, severe mental illness.* London: National Unit for Psychiatric Research and Development.

Creed, F., & Marks, B. (1989). Liaison psychiatry in general practice: A comparison of the liaison-attachment scheme and the shifted outpatient clinic models. *Journal of the Royal College of General Practitioners, 39,* 514–517.

Creer, C., & Wing, J. (1974). *Schizophrenia at home.* Surbiton, Surrey, England: National Schizophrenia Fellowship.

Croft-Jeffreys, C., & Wilkinson, G. (1985). Estimated costs of neurotic disorder in UK general practice. *Psychological Medicine, 19,* 549–558.

Cumming, E., & Cumming, J. (1957). *Closed ranks: An experiment in mental health.* Cambridge, MA: Harvard University Press.

Davies, B. (1987). Review article: Making a reality of community care. *British Journal of Social Work, 18,* 173–186.

Davies, L., & Drummond, M. (1990). The economic burden of schizophrenia. *British Journal of Psychiatry, 154,* 522–525.

De Isabella, G., & Meneghelli, A. (1983). Training di abilita sociali per la rehabilitatzione di pazient psicotici [Training in social skills in the rehabilitation of chronic psychotic patients]. *Riv Speriment di Freniatria, 5,* 1194–1204.

Department of Health and Social Security. (1971). *Hospital services for the mentally ill.* London: Her Majesty's Stationery Office.

Department of Health and Social Security. (1974). *Providing a comprehensive district psychiatric service for the adult mentally ill.* London: Her Majesty's Stationery Office.

Department of Health and Social Security. (1975). *Better services for the mentally ill* (Cmnd. 6233). London: Her Majesty's Stationery Office.

Department of Health and Social Security. (1978). *Collaboration in community care. Central Health Services Council.* London: Her Majesty's Stationery Office.

Department of Health and Social Security. (1981). *Care in action.* London: Her Majesty's Stationery Office.

Der, G., & Bebbington, P. (1987). Depression in inner London. A register study. *Social Psychiatry, 22,* 73–84.

Dick, P., Cameron, L., Cohen, D., & Barlow, N. (1985). Day and full-time psychiatric treatment: A controlled comparison. *British Journal of Psychiatry, 147,* 246–250.

Dickey, B., Cannon, N., McGuire, T., & Gudeman, J. (1986). The Quarterway House: A two year cost study of an experimental residential program. *Hospital and Community Psychiatry, 37,* 1136–1143.

Dill, A. (1987). Issues in case management for the mentally ill. In D. Mechanic (Ed.), *Improving mental health services: What the social sciences can tell us.* San Francisco: Jossey Bass.

Drake, R., & Wallach, M. (1988). Mental patients' attitudes toward hospitalisation: A neglected aspect of hospital tenure. *American Journal of Psychiatry, 145,* 29–34.

Falloon, I. (1988). The prevention of morbidity in schizophrenia. In I. Falloon (Ed.), *Handbook of behavioural family therapy* (pp. 316–349). London: Hutchinson.

Falloon, I., Boyd, J. L., & McGill, C. W. (1984). *Family care of schizophrenia.* New York: Guilford Press.

Falloon, I., & Pederson, J. (1985). Family management in the prevention of morbidity of schizophrenia. The adjustment of the family unit. *British Journal of Psychiatry, 147,* 156–163.

Fariello, D., & Scheidt, S. (1989). Clinical case management of the dually diagnosed patient. *Hospital and Community Psychiatry, 40,* 1065–1067.

Fenton, F., Tessier, L., Struening, E., Smith, F., & Benoit, C. (1982). *Home and hospital psychiatric treatment.* London: Croon Helm.

Fischer, P., & Breakey, W. (1986). Homelessness and mental health: An overview. *International Journal of Mental Health, 14,* 6–41.

Ford, M., Goddard, C., & Lansdall-Welfare, R. (1987). The dismantling of the mental hospital? Glenside Hospital surveys 1960–1985. *British Journal of Psychiatry, 150,* 479–485.

Franklin, L. (1988). Case management: A dissenting view. *Hospital and Community Psychiatry, 39,* 921.

Fry, J., & Sandler, G. (1988). Domiciliary consultations: Some facts and questions. *British Medical Journal, 297,* 337–338.

Fuhrer, M. (1987). Overview of outcome analysis in rehabilitation. In M. Fuhrer (Ed.), *Rehabilitation outcomes* (pp. 1–15). Baltimore: Brookes.

Garety, P. (1988). Housing. In A. Lavender & F. Holloway (Eds.), *Community care in practice.* Chichester, England: Wiley.

Garety, P., & Morris, I. (1984). A new unit for long-stay psychiatric patients: Organisation, attitudes and quality of care. *Psychological Medicine, 14,* 183–192.

Gerard, K. (1990). Determining the contribution of residential care to the quality of life of children with severe learning difficulties. *Child Care Health and Development, 16,* 177–188.

Giel, R., & ten Horn, G. (1982). Patterns of mental health care in a Dutch register area. *Social Psychiatry, 17,* 117–123.

Goffman, E. (1961). *Asylums.* Harmondsworth, England: Pelican.

Goldberg, D. (1986). Implementation of mental health policies in the North West of England. In G. Wilkinson & H. Freeman (Eds.), *The provision of mental health services in Britain: The way ahead* (pp. 61–69). London: Gaskell (Royal College of Psychiatrists).

Goldberg, D. (1991). Filter to care: A model. In R. Jenkins & S. Griffiths (Eds.), *Indicators for mental health in the population* (pp. 31–37). London: Her Majesty's Stationery Office.

Goldberg, D. P., & Blackwell, B. (1970). Psychiatric illness in general practice: a detailed study using a new method of case identification. *British Medical Journal, 2,* 439–443.

Goldberg, D. & Huxley, P. (1980). *Mental illness in the community—The pathway to psychiatric care.* London: Tavistock.

Goldman, H. (1981). Defining and counting the chronically mentally ill. *Hospital and Community Psychiatry, 32,* 21–27.

Goldman, H., Adams, N., & Taube, C. (1983). Deinstitutionalisation; The data demythologised. *Hospital and Community Psychiatry, 34,* 129–134.

Goldman, H., Morrissey, J., & Bachrach, L. (1983). Deinstitutionalisation in international perspective: Variations on a theme. *International Journal of Mental Health, 11,* 153–165.

Goldman, H., & Taube, C. (1988). High users of outpatients mental health services: II. Implications for practice and policy. *American Journal of Psychiatry, 145,* 24–28.

Golomb, S., & Kocsis, A. (1988). *The halfway house.* New York: Brunner/ Mazel.

Grad, J., & Sainsbury, P. (1968). The effects that patients have on families in a community care and a control psychiatric service: A two year follow-up. *British Journal of Psychiatry, 114,* 265–278.

Griffiths, R. (1988). *Community care: An agenda for action.* London: Her Majesty's Stationery Office.

Grunebaum, H. (1986). Families, patients and mental health professionals. *American Journal of Psychiatry, 143,* 1420–1421.

Hall, J. (1979). Assessment procedures used in studies on long-stay patients. *British Journal of Psychiatry, 135,* 330–335.

Hansen, V. (1987). Psychiatric service within primary care. Mode of organisation and influence on admission rates to a mental hospital. *Acta Psychiatrica Scandinavica, 76,* 121–128.

Hansson, L. (1989). Utilisation of psychiatric in-patient care. *Acta Psychiatrica Scandinavica, 79,* 571–578.

Harper, N. (1988). Planned short-stay admission to a geriatric unit: One aspect of respite care. *Age and Aging, 17,* 199–204.

Harris, M., & Bergman, H. (1988). Misconceptions about use of case management services by the chronic mentally ill: A utilisation analysis. *Hospital and Community Psychiatry, 39,* 1276–1280.

Harris, M., Bergman, H., & Bachrach, L. (1986). Individualised network planning for chronic psychiatric patients. *Psychiatric Quarterly, 58,* 51–56.

Hartley, J. (1980). Psychological approaches to unemployment. *Bulletin of the British Psychological Society, 32,* 309–314.

Haw, C., & Lanceley, C. (1987). Patients at a psychiatric walk-in clinic: Who, how, why and when. *Bulletin of the Royal College of Psychiatrists, 11,* 329–332.

Hirsch, S. (1988). *Psychiatric beds and resources: Factors influencing bed use and service planning.* London: Gaskell (Royal College of Psychiatrists).

Hoenig, J., & Hamilton, M. (1966). The schizophrenic patient in the community and his effect on the household. *International Journal of Social Psychiatry, 12,* 165–176.

Hogarty, G., Anderson, C., Reiss, D., Kounblith, S., Greenwald, D., Javnac, & Madonia, M. (1986). Family psycho-education, social skills training, and maintenance chemotherapy in the aftercare treatment of schizophrenia. *Archives of General Psychiatry, 43,* 633–642.

Hogarty, G., Goldberg, S., & Collaborative Study Group. (1973). Drug and sociotherapy in the aftercare of schizophrenic patients. *Archives of General Psychiatry, 28,* 54–64.

Hogarty, G., Schooler, N., Ulrich, R., Miussare, F., Ferro, P., & Herron, P. (1979). Fluphenazine and social therapy in the aftercare of schizophrenic patients. *Archives of General Psychiatry, 36,* 1283–1294.

Holloway, F. (1988). Day care and community support. In A. Lavenders & F. Holloway, (Eds.), *Community care in practice* (pp. 161–186). Chichester, England: Wiley.

Hoult, J., & Reynolds, I. (1984). Schizophrenia: A comparative trial of community oriented and hospital oriented psychiatric care. *Acta Psychiatrica Scandanavica, 69,* 359–372.

House of Commons. (1985). *Second report from the Social Services Committee, Session 1984–85, community care.* London: Her Majesty's Stationery Office.

House of Commons. (1990). *The national health service and community care act.* London: Her Majesty's Stationery Office.

Houston, F. (1955). A project for a mental-health village settlement. *Lancet, i,* 1133–1134.

Hunter, D., & Wistow, G. (1987). Mapping the organisation context. I. Central departments, boundaries and responsibilities. In *Community care in Britain: Variations on a theme.* London: King Edward's Hospital Fund for London.

Intagliata, J. (1982). Improving the quality of care for the chronic mentally disabled: The role of case management. *Schizophrenic Bulletin, 8,* 655–674.

Johnstone, E., Owens, D., Gold, A., Crow, T., & MacMillan, J. (1981). Institutionalisation and the defects of schizophrenia. *British Journal of Psychiatry, 139,* 195–203.

Johnstone, E., Owens, D., Gold, A., Crow, T., & Macmillan, F. (1984). Schizophrenic patients discharged from hospital: A follow-up study. *British Journal of Psychiatry, 145,* 586–590.

Jones, K. (1972). *A history of the mental health services.* London: Routledge and Kegan Paul.

Jones, M. (1985). *After hospital: A study of long-term psychiatric patients in York, 1985.* York, England: Department of Social Policy and Social Work, University of York.

Joseph, P., Bridgewater, J. A., Ramsden, S. S., & El Kabir, D. J. (1990). A psychiatric clinic for the single homeless in a primary care setting in inner London. *Psychiatric Bulletin, 14,* 270–271.

Kaeser, A. C., & Cooper, B. (1971). The psychiatric out-patient, the general practitioner and the out-patient clinic; an operational study: A review. *Psychological Medicine, 1,* 312–325.

Kalman, T. (1983). An overview of patients' satisfaction with psychiatric treatment. *Hospital and Community Psychiatry, 34,* 48–54.

Karno, M., Jenkins, J., de al Selva, A., Santana, F., Telles, C., Lopez, S., & Mintz,

J. (1987). Expressed emotion and schizophrenic outcome among Mexican–American families. *Journal of Nervous and Mental Diseases, 175,* 143–151.

Kendrick, A., Sibbald, B., Burns, T., & Freeling, P. (1991). Role of general practitioners in care of long term mentally ill patients. *British Medical Journal, 302,* 508–511.

Kiesler, C. (1982). Mental hospitals and alternative care. *American Psychologist, 37,* 349–360.

Kingdon, D. (1989). Mental health services: Results of a survey of English district plans. *Psychiatric Bulletin, 13,* 77–78.

Klein, R. (1991). The politics of change. *British Medical Journal, 320,* 1102–1103.

Knapp, M., Cambridge, P., Thomsaon, C., Beecham, J., Allen, C., & Darton, R. (1990). *Care in the community* (Newsletter No. 9). Canterbury: University of Kent, Personal Social Services Research Unit.

Kroll, J., Carey, K., Hagedorn, D., Dog, P., & Benavides, E. (1986). A survey of homeless adults in urban shelters. *Hospital and Community Psychiatry, 37,* 283–286.

Kruzich, J., & Berg, W. (1985). Predictors of self-sufficiency for the mentally ill in long-term care. *Community Mental Health Journal, 21,* 198–207.

Kuipers, L., & Bebbington, P. (1985). Relatives as a resource in the management of functional psychosis. *British Journal of Psychiatry, 147,* 465–470.

Kunze, H. (1985). Rehabilitation and institutionalisation in community care in West Germany. *British Journal of Psychiatry, 147,* 261–264.

Lamb, H. (1979). The new asylums in the community. *Archives of General Psychiatry, 36,* 129–134.

Lamb, H. (1980). Board-and-care home wanderers. *Archives of General Psychiatry, 37,* 135–137.

Lamb, H. (1982). *Treating the long-term mentally ill.* San Francisco: Jossey-Bass.

Lamb, H. (1984). Deinstitutionalisation and the homeless mentally ill. *Hospital and Community Psychiatry, 35,* 899–907.

Leavitt, A. (1984). *The impact of deinstitionalisation on ten San Francisco Bay area counties.* San Francisco: Department of Public Health, City and County of San Francisco.

Lee, A. S., & Murray, R. M. (1988). The long-term of outcome Maudsley depressives. *British Journal of Psychiatry, 153,* 741–751.

Lee, P., & Kenworthy, M. (1929). *Mental hygiene and social work.* New York: Commonwealth Fund.

Leff, J., Kuipers, L., Berkowitz, R., Eberlein-Fries, R., & Sturgeon, D. (1982). A controlled trial of social intervention in schizophrenic families. *British Journal of Psychiatry, 141,* 121–134.

Lehman, A. (1983). The well-being of chronic mental patients. *Archives of General Psychiatry, 40,* 369–374.

Lehman, A., Possidente, S., & Hawker, F. (1986). The quality of life of chronic patients in a state hospital and in community residences. *Hospital and Community Psychiatry, 37,* 901–907.

Lehman, A., Reed, S., & Possidente, S. (1982). Priorities for long-term care: Comments from board and care residents. *Psychiatric Quarterly, 54,* 181–189.

Lesage, A., & Tansella, M. (1989). Mobility of schizophrenic patients, nonpsychotic patients and the general population in a case register area. *Social Psychiatry and Psychiatric Epidemiology, 24,* 271–274.

Levine, M. (1981). *The history and politics of community mental health.* London: Oxford University Press.

Liberman, R., Cardin, V., McGill, C., Falloon, I., & Evans, C. (1987). Behavioural family management of schizophrenia: Clinical outcome and costs. *Psychiatric Annals, 17,* 610–619.

Liberman, R., King, L., DeRisi, W. & McCann, M. (1975). *Personal effectiveness: Guiding people to express their feelings and improve their social skills.* Champaign, IL: Research Press.

Liberman, R., Wallace, C., Falloon, I., & Vaughn, C. (1981). Interpersonal problem-solving therapy for schizophrenic patients and their families. *Comprehensive Psychiatry, 22,* 627–630.

Lim, M. H. (1983). A psychiatric emergency clinic: A study of attendances over six months. *British Journal of Psychiatry, 143,* 480–486.

Lindholm, H. (1983). Sectorised psychiatry. *Acta Psychiatrica Scandinavica, 67*(Suppl. 304), 1–127.

Linn, M., Caffey, E., Klett, J., & Hogarty, G. (1977). Hospital vs community (foster) care for psychiatric patients. *Archives of General Psychiatry, 34,* 78–83.

Linn, M., Gurel, L., Williford, O., Overall, J., Gurland, B., Laughlin, P., & Barchiesi, A. (1985). Nursing home care as an alternative to psychiatric hospitalisation. *Archives of General Psychiatry, 42,* 544–551.

Littlejohns, P. (1986). Domiciliary consultations—who benefits? *Journal of Royal College of GP's, 36,* 313–315.

MacCarthy, B., Lesage, A., Brewin, C., Brugha, T., & Wing, J. (1989). Needs for care among the relatives of long term users of day care. *Psychological Medicine, 19,* 725–736.

Mangen, S. (1988). Implementing community care: An international perspective. In A. Lavender & F. Holloway (Eds.), *Community care in practice* (pp. 27–50). Chichester, England: Wiley.

Mann, A. (1991). Public health and psychiatric morbidity. In R. Jenkins & S. Griffiths (Eds.), *Indicators for mental health in the population* (pp. 6–17). London: Her Majesty's Stationery Office.

Marks, I., Connolly, J., & Muijen, M. (1988). The Maudsley daily living programme. *Bulletin of the Royal College of Psychiatrists, 12,* 22–24.

Martin, L. (1984). *Hospitals in trouble.* Oxford: Blackwell.

Mechanic, D. (1986). The challenge of chronic mental illness: A retrospective and prospective view. *Hospital and Community Psychiatry, 37,* 891–896.

Mechanic, D. (1987). Correcting misconceptions in mental health policy: Strategies for improved care of the seriously mentally ill. *Millbank Quarterly, 65,* 203–230.

Mechanic, D., & Aiken, L. (1987). Improving the care of patients with chronic mental illness. *New England Journal of Medicine, 317,* 1634–1638.

Miller, A. (1985). Deinstitutionalisation in retrospect. *Psychiatric Quarterly, 57,* 160–171.

MIND. (1983). *Common concern.* London: MIND Publications.

Mitchell, A. (1985). Psychiatrists in primary health care settings. *British Journal of Psychiatry, 147,* 371–379.

Modrcin, M., Rapp, C., & Chamberlain, R. (1985). Case management with psychiatrically disabled individuals: Curriculum and training programme. Lawrence: University of Kansas School of Social Work.

Monk-Jorgenson, P. (1986). General practitioners' selection of patients for treatment in community psychiatric services. *Psychological Medicine, 16,* 611–619.

Morrisey, J., & Levine, I. (1987). Researchers discuss latest findings, examine needs of homeless mentally ill persons. *Hospital and Community Psychiatry, 38,* 811–812.

Mosher, L. (1983). Radical deinstitutionalisation: The Italian experience. *International Journal of Mental Health, 11,* 129–136.

Murphy, E. (1991). Community mental health services: A vision for the future. *British Medical Journal, 302,* 1064–1065.

Murray Parkes, C., Brown, G. W., & Monck, E. M. (1962). The general practitioner and the schizophrenic patient. *British Medical Journal, 1,* 972–976.

National Institute of Mental Health. (1987). *Towards a model for a comprehensive community-based mental health system.* Washington, DC: Author.

Newton, J. (1987). *The prevention of mental illness.* London: Routledge Kegan Paul.

Nunnally, J. (1961). *Popular conceptions of mental health.* New York: Holt, Rhinehard & Winston.

Patmore, C., & Weaver, T. (1991). *Good practices in mental health. Community mental health teams: Lessons for planners and managers.* London: Good Practices in Mental Health.

Paykel, E. (1990). Innovations in mental health in the primary care system. In I. Marks & R. Scott (Eds.), *Mental health service evaluation.* Cambridge, England: Cambridge University Press.

Peterson, C. (1986). Changing community attitudes toward the chronic mentally ill through a psychosocial program. *Hospital and Community Psychiatry, 37,* 180–182.

Platt, S. (1985). Measuring the burden of psychiatric illness on the family: An evaluation of some rating scales. *Psychological Medicine, 15,* 383–393.

Pryor, M., & Distefano, M. (1986). Follow-up of participants in vocational rehabilitation program at a state hospital. *Hospital and Community Psychiatry, 37,* 1261–1262.

Pullen, I., & Yellowlees, A. (1988). Scottish psychiatrists in primary health care settings: A silent majority. *British Journal of Psychiatry, 153,* 633–636.

Ramon, S. (1988). Community care in Britain. In A. Lavender & F. Holloway (Eds.), *Community care in practice.* Chichester, England: Wiley

Renshaw, J. (1987). Care planning and case management. *British Journal of Social Work, 18,* 79–105.

Renshaw, J., Hampson, R., Thomsaon, C., et al. (1988). *Care in the community: The first steps.* Aldershot, England: Gower.

Robinson, A. (1984). *Respite care services for families with a handicapped child.* London: National Children's Bureau.

Robinson, G., & Bergman, G. (1989). *Choices in case management.* Washington, DC: Policy Resources.

Rosenblatt, A. (1984). Concepts of the asylum in the care of the mentally ill. *Hospital and Community Psychiatry, 35,* 244–250.

Ross, H. (1979). *Proceedings of the conference on the evaluation of case management programs.* Los Angeles: Volunteers for Services to Older Persons.

Rothman, D. (1971). *The discovery of the asylum.* Boston: Little Brown.

Royal College of Psychiatrists. (1988). A carer's perspective. *Bulletin of the Royal College of Psychiatrists, 11,* 237–239.

Royal College of Psychiatrists (1990). *Caring for a community: 1. The model mental health service.* London: Royal College of Psychiatrists.

Sabshin, M. (1966). Theoretical models in community and social psychiatry. In L. Roberts, S. Halbeck, & M. Loeb (Eds.), *Community psychiatry.* Madison: University of Wisconsin Press.

Sartorius, N. (1986). Early manifestations and first-contact incidence of schizophrenia in different cultures. *Psychological Medicine, 16,* 909–928.

Sayce, L., Craig, T., & Boardman, A. (1991). The development of community mental health centres in the UK. *Social Psychiatry and Psychiatric Epidemiology, 26,* 14–20.

Schulberg, H., & Bromet, E. (1981). Strategies for evaluating the outcome of community services. *American Journal of Psychiatry, 138,* 930–935.

Schwab, D., Drake, R., & Burghardt, E. (1988). Health care of the chronically mentally ill: The culture broker model. *Community Mental Health Journal, 24,* 174–184.

Scottish Schizophrenia Research Group. (1987). The Nithsdale schizophrenia survey. VI: Relatives' expressed emotion: Prevalence, patterns and clinical assessment. *British Journal of Psychiatry, 150,* 640–644.

Scull, A. (1984). *Decarceration* (2nd ed.). Cambridge: Polity.

Scull, A. (1985). Deinstitutionalisation and public policy. *Social Science and Medicine, 5,* 545–552.

Sharp, D., & Morrell, D. (1989). The psychiatry of general practice. In P. Williams, G. Wilkinson & K. Rawnsley (Eds.), *Scientific approaches on epidemiological and social psychiatry: Essays in honour of Michael Shepherd.* London: Routledge.

Shepherd G. (1984). *Institutional care and rehabilitation.* London: Longman.

Shepherd M., Cooper B., Brown A. & Kalton G. (1966). Psychiatric Illness in General Practice. Oxford University Press, Oxford.

Social Services Committee 1984/85 session, second report. (1985). *Community care with special reference to adult mentally ill and mentally handicapped people.* London: Her Majesty's Stationery Office.

Solomon, P., Davis, J., & Gordon, B. (1984). Discharged state hospital patients' characteristics and use of aftercare: Effects on community tenure. *American Journal of Psychiatry, 141,* 1566–1570.

Spitz, B. (1987, Spring). A national survey of Medicaid case management programs. *Health Affairs,* 61–86.

Stein, L., & Diamond, R. (1985). A programme for difficult to treat patients. *New Directions in Mental Health Services, 26,* 29–39.

Stein, L., & Test, M. (1980). Alternative to mental hospital treatment. *Archives of General Psychiatry, 37,* 392–397.

Strathdee, G. (1990). The delivery of psychiatric care. *Journal of the Royal Society of Medicine, 83,* 222–225.

Strathdee, G. (1991). The interface between psychiatry and primary care in the management of schizophrenic patients in the community. In R. Jenkins, V. Field, & R. Young (Eds.), *The primary care of schizophrenia.* London: Her Majesty's Stationery Office.

Strathdee, G., & Williams, G. (1984). A survey of psychiatrists in primary care: The silent growth of a new service. *Journal of the Royal College of General Practitioners, 34,* 615–618.

Sutherby, K., Srinath, S., & Strathdee, G. (1991). *The domiciliary consultation service: Outdated anachronism or essential part of community psychiatric outreach?* Unpublished research report.

Sytema, S., Balestrieri, M., Giel, R., ten Horn, G. & Tansella, M. (1989). Use of mental health services in South-Verona and Groningen. *Acta Psychiatrica Scandinavica, 79,* 153–162.

Tansella, M. (1986). Community psychiatry without mental hospitals—the Italian experience: A review. *Journal of the Royal Society of Medicine, 79,* 664–669.

Tansella, M., de Salvia, D., & Williams, P. (1987). The Italian psychiatric reform: Some quantitative evidence. *Social Psychiatry, 22,* 37–48.

Tansella, M., & Williams, P. (1989). The spectrum of psychiatric morbidity in a defined geographical area. *Psychological Medicine, 19,* 765–770.

Tantam, D. (1985). Alternatives to psychiatric hospitalisation. *British Journal of Psychiatry, 146,* 1–4.

ten Horn, G., Giel, R., Gulbinat, W., & Henderson, J. (Eds.). (1986). *Psychiatric case registers in public health: A worldwide inventory, 1960–1985.* Amsterdam: Elsevier.

Tessler, R., & Goldman, H. (1982). *The chronic mentally ill, assessing the community support program.* Cambridge, England: Ballinger.

Test, M. (1979). Continuity of care in community treatment. *New Directions for Mental Health Services, 1,* 15–23.

Test, M., & Stein, L. (1980). Alternative to mental hospital treatment: III social cost. *Archives of General Psychiatry, 37,* 409–412.

Thornicroft, G. (1988). Progress towards D.H.S.S. targets for community care. *British Journal of Psychiatry, 153,* 257–258.

Thornicroft, G. (1990). Are England's psychiatric services for schizophrenia improving? *Hospital and Community Psychiatry, 41,* 1073–1075.

Thornicroft, G., & Breakey, W. (1991). The COSTAR programme (1). Improving the social networks of the long-term mentally ill. *British Journal of Psychiatry, 159,* 245–249.

Thornicroft, G., & Strathdee, G. (1991). The health of the nation: Mental health. *British Medical Journal, 303,* 410–412.

Todd, J. W. (1984). Wasted resources. Referral to hospital. *Lancet, ii,* 1089.

Tooth, G., & Brooke, E. (1961). Trends in mental hospital population and their effect on future planning. *Lancet, 1,* 710–713.

Torrey, E. (1986). Continuous treatment teams in the care of the chronic mentally ill. *Hospital and Community Psychiatry, 37,* 1243–1247.

Torre, E., & Marinoni, A. (1985). Register studies: Data from four areas in Northern Italy. *Acta Psychiatrica Scandinavica,* (Suppl) *316,* 87–94.

Towell, D., & McAusland, T. (1984). Managing psychiatric services in transition. *Health and Social Services Journal, 25,* 1–8.

Trute, B., & Loewen, A. (1978). Public attitude toward the mentally ill as a function of prior personal experience. *Social Psychiatry, 13,* 79–84.

Tufnell, G., Borras, N., Watson, J. P., & Brough, D. I. (1985). Home assessment and treatment in a community psychiatric service. *Acta Psychiatrica Scandinavica, 72,* 20–28.

Tyrer, P. (1984). Psychiatric clinics in general practice: An extension of community care. *British Journal of Psychiatry, 145,* 9–14.

Tyrer P. (1985). The "hive" system: A model for a psychiatric service. *British Journal of Psychiatry, 146,* 571–575.

Tyrer, P., Turner, R., & Johnson, A. (1989). Integrated hospital and community psychiatric services and use of inpatient beds. *British Medical Journal, 299,* 298–300.

Vaughn, C., & Leff, J. (1976). The influence of family and social factors on the course of psychiatric illness: A comparison of schizophrenic and depressed neurotic patients. *British Journal of Psychiatry, 129,* 125–137.

Vaughn, C., Snyder, K., Freeman, W., Janes, F., Falloon, I., & Liberman, R. et al. (1982). Family factors in schizophrenic relapse: A replication. *Schizophrenia Bulletin, 8,* 425–427.

Wasow, M. (1986). The need for asylum for the chronically mentally ill. *Schizophrenia Bulletin, 12,* 162–167.

Wasylenki, D., Goeing, P., Lancee, W., Balantyne, R., & Farkas, M. (1985). Impact of a case manager program on psychiatric aftercare. *Journal of Nervous and Mental Disease, 173,* 303–308.

Weisbrod, B., Test, M., & Stein, L. (1980). Alternative to mental hospital treatment. *Archives of General Psychiatry, 37,* 400–405.

Weisman, G. (1985). Crisis-oriented residential treatment as an alternative to hospitalisation. *Hospital and Community Psychiatry, 36,* 1302–1305.

Wiersma, D., Giel, R., de Jong, A. & Slooff, C. (1983). Social class and schizophrenia in a Dutch cohort. *Psychological Medicine, 13,* 141–150.

Wilkinson, G., Falloon, I., & Sen, B. (1985). Chronic mental disorders in general practice. *British Medical Journal, 291,* 1302–1304.

Wing, J. (1960). Pilot experiment in the rehabilitation of long-term hospitalised male schizophrenic patients. *British Journal of Preventative and Social Medicine, 14,* 173–180.

Wing, J. (1971). How many psychiatric beds? *Psychological Medicine, 1,* 189–190.

Wing, J. (1989). *Health services planning and research.* London: Gaskell (Royal College of Psychiatrists).

Wing, J., & Brown, G. (1970). *Institutionalism and schizophrenia.* Cambridge: Cambridge University Press.

Wing, J., & Furlong, R. (1986). A haven for the severely disabled within the context of a comprehensive psychiatric community service. *British Journal of Psychiatry, 149,* 449–457.

World Health Organization. (1981). *Global strategy for health for all by the year 2000.* Geneva: Author.

World Health Organization. (1983). *First contact mental health care.* Copenhagen: WHO Regional Office for Europe.

World Health Organization. (1991). *Implications for the field of mental health of the European targets for attaining health for all.* Copenhagen: Author.
World Psychiatric Association. (1991). WPA statement and viewpoints on the rights and legal safeguards of the mentally ill. *WPA Bulletin, 1,* 32–33.
Worley, N., Drago, L., & Hadley, T. (1990). Improving the physical health–mental health interface for the chronically mentally ill: Could nurse case managers make a difference? *Archives of Psychiatric Nursing, 2,* 108–113.

INDEX